Neuromuscular Disease

NEUROMUSCULAR DISEASE

Evidence and Analysis in Clinical Neurology

By

MICHAEL BENATAR, MBChB, MS, DPhil

Department of Neurology,
Emory University School of Medicine,
Atlanta, GA

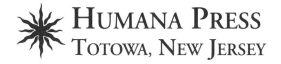

HUMANA PRESS
TOTOWA, NEW JERSEY

© 2006 Humana Press Inc.
999 Riverview Drive, Suite 208
Totowa, New Jersey 07512

www.humanapress.com

Cover design by Patricia F. Cleary

For additional copies, pricing for bulk purchases, and/or information about other Humana titles, contact Humana at the above address or at any of the following numbers: Tel.: 973-256-1699; Fax: 973-256-8341, E-mail: orders@humanapr.com; or visit our Website: www.humanapress.com

This publication is printed on acid-free paper. ∞
ANSI Z39.48-1984 (American National Standards Institute) Permanence of Paper for Printed Library Materials.

Printed in the United States of America. 10 9 8 7 6 5 4 3 2 1

e-ISBN 159745-106-1

Library of Congress Cataloging-in-Publication Data
Benatar, Michael.
  Neuromuscular disease : evidence and analysis in clinical neurology / by Michael Benatar.
    p. ; cm.
  Includes bibliographical references and index.
  ISBN 1-58829-627-X (alk. paper)
  1. Neuromuscular diseases. 2. Neurology.
  [DNLM: 1. Neuromuscular Diseases--diagnosis. 2. Neuromuscular
Diseases--therapy. 3. Review Literature. WE 550 B456n 2006] I. Title.
  RC925.B43 2006
  616.7'44--dc22
                                                                        2005029391

To my brothers

PREFACE

A Certain Kind of Wisdom

In Plato's *Apology*, the Greek philosopher Socrates is on trial to defend himself against the allegation of corrupting the youth of Athens. Socrates denies this charge and offers an alternate reason for why he is on trial. He explains, "[w]hat has caused my reputation is none other than a certain kind of wisdom. What kind of wisdom? Human wisdom, perhaps *(1)*." He proceeds to tell the story of his friend Chaerophon, who once asked the Oracle at Delphi whether there was anyone wiser than Socrates. The Oracle answered that there was not. Socrates did not agree and thought that he would try to prove the Oracle wrong. And so he set about seeking out Athenians with a reputation for wisdom in various regards in order to test their claims to knowledge through questioning. He discovered many with false claims to knowledge and none with genuine wisdom and ultimately concluded that he was the wisest. He reached this conclusion not because of any special knowledge he possessed that others did not, but rather because he recognized his own lack of knowledge and strived to learn more, while others thought that they were knowledgeable but were not.

Socrates' conclusion that there is wisdom in recognizing the limitations of accepted knowledge represents the motivation for this book. In the process of asking questions and delving into the neuromuscular literature in an effort to find answers, one is left with the impression that we know less about the diagnosis, treatment, and prognosis of a range of neuromuscular disorders than we perhaps realize. It is not expected that everyone will accept this premise, but *Neuromuscular Disease: Evidence and Analysis in Clinical Neurology* has been written as much for those who doubt this claim as for those who already accept it.

Although Socrates did not claim to be knowledgeable, he believed that knowledge could be acquired by engaging in a series of questions to test someone else's claim to knowledge. This method of enquiry, known as "Socratic dialogue," entails a series of questions traded back and forth between the questioner and his interlocutor. Although this approach is not easily reproduced in written form, the present book employs a question–answer format in an effort to emulate the style (and, it is hoped, the effectiveness) of the Socratic dialogue.

Obstacles to Knowledge

If the first step to wisdom is the recognition that our knowledge is limited, then the second step requires discerning the reasons for this limitation. The answer seems to be that there are numerous obstacles to the acquisition of knowledge, including a relative paucity of high-quality evidence and difficulties that arise in the understanding and interpretation of the available evidence, as well as inadvertent misrepresentation of the published data.

Lack of High-Quality Evidence

In many instances, our collective lack of knowledge results from to a simple lack of good-quality data. For example, the lack of high-quality data is responsible for our uncertainty as to which patients, if any, will benefit from surgery for the management of cervical spondylotic myelopathy, whether steroids or other immunosuppressive therapy should be used to treat patients with ocular myasthenia gravis, what sort of immunosuppression is most appropriate for patients with vasculitic peripheral neuropathy, or what the indications are for surgical treatment of ulnar neuropathy at the elbow.

There are numerous reasons, many of them complex, for the paucity of high-quality evidence. In some instances, a particular treatment modality has become sufficiently well established that clinical equipoise no longer exists and so a randomized placebo-controlled trial cannot be justified. The use of steroids in the management of generalized myasthenia gravis is one such example. A second problem is that many individual neuromuscular disorders are quite rare, the consequence of which is that it is difficult for one (or even a selection) of neurologists to recruit sufficient number of patients with the disorder in question within a reasonable period of time to participate in a controlled trial. A third problem arises from the difficulty of marrying clinical practice and clinical research. The pressures of the daily practice of medicine frequently do not permit clinicians the luxury to gather the sort of detailed information in a scientifically rigorous fashion that will be required to reach unbiased conclusions.

Yet another reason relates to the limitations of clinical investigators' knowledge of study design. This is less of a problem for studies of therapeutic interventions because most investigators and clinicians are aware of the methodological advantages of the randomized controlled trial and recognize the limitations of other study designs such as case series, case–control, and cohort studies. But even within the realm of the randomized controlled trial, there are many aspects of study design, such as allocation concealment, patient and observer blinding, the proportion of patients who are lost to follow-up, and other sources of bias that often receive less attention. Limited knowledge of study design is an even greater problem for studies of diagnostic tests and prognosis. The STAndards for Reporting Diagnostic tests (STARD) initiative has recently drawn attention to the serious shortcomings in much of the literature on diagnostic studies, pointing out the importance of issues such as the use of a clearly identified and well established reference standard and the need for investigator blinding in the interpretation of the diagnostic test under investigation *(2)*.

Inadequate Understanding and Interpretation of the Evidence

The basic tools of clinical research are founded on the principles of epidemiology and biostatistics and yet relatively few clinical researchers and even fewer clinicians have any formal training in the methodology of clinical research. This state of affairs has two unfortunate consequences. The first is that those who are engaged in clinical research often do not have the necessary skills to design and perform clinical studies that conform to the rigorous standards required in order to reduce random error and bias (systematic error). This issue is discussed in the previous section. The second consequence is that those who read the literature have limited ability to critically appraise publications and to discern the strengths and limitations of the studies being read.

Moreover, it is commonplace for people to skip over the methodology section of a paper (and perhaps even the results section as well) and to read only the introduction and discussion. Frequently, the abstract of a paper is all that will be read. If the methods section of a paper is not read carefully, there is no chance that the reader will be able to discern the strengths and shortcomings of the study. The natural tendency to skip over the methodology section of a paper is fostered by the recent trend among journals (even prominent journals such as *Neurology*) to decrease the size of the font in which the methodology section is printed. These trends place a greater burden on journal editors and reviewers to carefully scrutinize manuscripts for methodological shortcomings and to insist that authors adequately address these issues. Unfortunately, this burden is not easily shouldered by reviewers because they too frequently lack any formal training in clinical research methodology. And there is covert pressure on authors to emphasize the strengths and to minimize the weaknesses of their studies in order to maximize the chances of publication in a reputable journal.

The result of all of this is that the published literature is often interpreted as providing evidence for some conclusion, when in fact this is not the case. Investigations of diagnostic studies are especially prone to this particular problem. Investigators frequently choose to study the utility of a diagnostic test in a population of subjects that is not representative of the patient population in which the test will be used. For example, many studies of the accuracy of single-fiber electromyography for the diagnosis of myasthenia gravis have examined patients who are already known to have myasthenia and have compared them with subjects who are known to be healthy or to have some other disease *(3–6)*. Similarly, studies of the utility of nerve conduction studies for the diagnosis of chronic inflammatory demyelinating polyradiculoneuropathy (CIDP) have compared patients known to have CIDP with those known to have other diseases such as diabetic polyneuropathy or amyotrophic lateral sclerosis *(7–10)*. Studies such as these provide estimates of the sensitivity and specificity of the test in question, but do not provide information about how useful the test will be in clinical practice because the positive and negative predictive values of the test will be determined by the pretest probability of disease, which is strongly influenced by the prevalence of the disease in the population in which the test is being used. A better approach is to evaluate the performance of a diagnostic test in the broader patient population in which the test will be used. Studies that only include subjects with already established disease as well as either healthy subjects or those with other diagnoses are susceptible to a form of selection bias known as "spectrum bias," in which only a select component of the full spectrum of patients with the disease is studied. Such issues have historically been neglected and the result is that our knowledge of the accuracy of tests used in the diagnosis of neuromuscular disease is quite limited, even if not widely recognized.

Such problems are not restricted to studies of the accuracy of diagnostic tests. The literature is filled with case series (often mistakenly described as cohort studies) in which the clinical manifestations or clinical outcome of a group of patients with a particular disorder are described. These case series are most frequently based on patient populations seen in tertiary referral centers and so are less likely to be representative of the spectrum of manifestations of the disease that would be encountered in the general population. Very often, such case series do not include consecutive patients, further increasing the potential for selection bias. The result is that such studies do not provide meaningful information about the sensitivity of a particular clinical finding or the sensitivity of the results of a diagnostic study. Because these case series almost invariably include only patients who have the condition of interest (rather than all patients who were initially thought to possibly have the condition of interest), it is not possible to determine the specificity of the clinical findings or results of diagnostic studies. The consequence of such methodological shortcomings is that much of the literature turns out to be not very informative and certainly not very scientific. To make matters worse, such studies are often mistakenly regarded as definitive.

Misrepresentation of the Evidence

There are a number of practices that have, albeit unintentionally, the consequence of providing misleading information about the available evidence. It is commonplace, for example, for authors to cite review articles rather than original data in referencing a particular claim. In researching the literature to write this book, I have frequently tried to track down the primary data that supports a particular claim, but have been frustrated to find that the reference cited to support the claim is a review article, which in turn references a review article or provides no reference at all. A related problem is that although an article with primary data is referenced, the primary data does not adequately support the claim that has been made.

The second practice, which is perhaps even more worrying than the first, is the publication of evidence-based guidelines that make statements or recommendations under the guise of being based on evidence but that, in reality, are based on very little (if any) real evidence. For example, the practice parameter published by the American Academy of Neurology recommends that percutaneous endoscopic gastrostomy (PEG) feeding tube placement should be performed before the forced vital capacity (FVC) falls to less than 50% of predicted *(11)*. As discussed in much more detail in Chapter 5, the evidence does not really support this claim, and it is certainly the case that the quality of data cited by this practice parameter is sufficiently poor that some qualification of the recommendation to place a PEG before FVC falls to less than 50% would be in order. The evidence-based guidelines published by the American College of Cardiology regarding indications for pacemaker placement in patients with myotonic dystrophy are subject to the same criticism *(12,13)*. These guidelines were revised and updated between 1998 and 2002, with the revised guidelines indicating that pacemaker placement should be considered in patients with myotonic dystrophy in the presence of even first or second degree heart block *(13)*. Interestingly, the revised guidelines do not cite any new literature to support this new "evidence-based" recommendation.

The Goals and Scope of This Book

The goal of *Neuromuscular Disease: Evidence and Analysis in Clinical Neurology* is to review the literature with respect to the diagnosis, treatment, and prognosis of a range of neuromuscular disorders and to present a description, analysis, and discussion of the quality of this literature. The intention is not simply to provide the reader with an easy reference to the publications that are most clinically relevant to neurologists who evaluate and treat patients with neuromuscular disease. The intention is also to offer an analysis of the evidence in the form of a critique of study methodology such that the reader will be aware not just of the content of the literature but also of its quality. The hope is that the analyses presented will also help the reader to think more critically about the design of clinical research studies in general and to be more inquisitive about study methodology when reading and evaluating publications in the future.

The scope of *Neuromuscular Disease: Evidence and Analysis in Clinical Neurology* is fairly broad within the field of neuromuscular disease, but is by no means exhaustive.

It could not possibly be as extensive as many readers might like, given the space constraints of a book such as this. But an effort has been made to cover those neuromuscular disorders that the adult neurologist is likely to encounter in routine clinical practice. Almost without exception, individual chapters are devoted to particular disorders with relatively well defined etiologies whereas such syndromic diagnoses as brachial and lumbosacral plexopathy that are not unitary disorders have been excluded. Although it would be possible to review the literature pertinent to the diagnosis of these disorders, the specific treatment and prognosis will very much depend upon etiology. Similarly, disorders that manifest primarily in childhood, even if there is survival into adulthood (such as with the dystrophinopathies), have not been included.

Within each chapter, there are sections devoted to the diagnosis, treatment, and prognosis of the relevant neuromuscular disease. In order to mirror this individual chapter structure, introductory chapters describing the epidemiological and biostatistical principles relevant to diagnosis, treatment, and prognosis have been included.

There are several important differences between *Neuromuscular Disease: Evidence and Analysis in Clinical Neurology* and the systematic reviews published by the Cochrane Collaboration. First, although the chapters in this book are not as comprehensive as the Cochrane reviews, they do provide much broader coverage of individual diseases insofar as they focus not only on treatment, but also on issues related to diagnosis and prognosis. Second, because the methodology for meta-analysis of observational studies has not yet been adequately refined, the Cochrane reviews have focused almost exclusively on the content of randomized controlled trials (although data from observational studies are often included in the discussions that accompany the systematic reviews). This book considers evidence not only from randomized controlled trials, but also from observational studies. Some might be critical of the present work for this reason, but it is not possible to explore issues related to the diagnosis and prognosis of neurological disease without considering these other types of studies. *Neuromuscular Disease: Evidence and Analysis in Clinical Neurology*, therefore, should be seen as complementary to the systematic reviews that are published in the Cochrane Database of Systematic Reviews.

Conclusion

It is not only in the realm of neuromuscular disease that our knowledge is limited. The impediments to understanding that I have described are also relevant to a range of other disciplines within neurology. The hope is that this book will be the first in a series of books dedicated to an analysis of the evidence within a range of subspecialties within neurology. Already in preparation is a text devoted to the field of neuro-ophthalmology. The intention is that this book, and others that follow, will help to encourage the Socratic approach, and that this will lead to greater awareness of the limitations of our current knowledge. It is hoped that insight into the shortcomings of the available literature will provide a stimulus for further research to address the clinical questions that, until now, have remained unanswered.

Michael Benatar, MBChB, MS, DPhil

References

1. Plato. Apology, 360 BCE.
2. Bossuyt PM, Reitsma JB, Bruns DE, et al. Towards complete and accurate reporting of studies of diagnostic accuracy: the STARD initiative. Br Med J 2003;326:41–4.

3. Kelly JJ, Daube JR, Lennon VA, Howard FM, Younge BR. The laboratory diagnosis of mild myasthenia gravis. Ann Neurol 1982;12:238–242.

4. Sanders DB, Howard JF. AAEE Minimonograph #25: Single fiber electromyography in myasthenia gravis. Muscle & Nerve 1986;9:809–819.

5. Oh SJ, Kim DE, Kuruoglu R, Bradley RJ, Dwyer D. Diagnostic sensitivity of the laboratory tests in myasthenia gravis. Muscle & Nerve 1992;15:720–724.

6. Milone M, Monaco M, Evoli A, Servidei S, Tonali P. Ocular myasthenia: diagnostic value of single fiber EMG in the orbicularis oculi muscle. J Neurol Neurosurg Psychiatry 1993;56:720–721.

7. van den Bergh PY, Pieret F. Electrodiagnostic criteria for acute and chronic inflammatory demyelinating polyradiculoneuropathy. Muscle & Nerve 2004;29:565–574.

8. Nicolas G, Maisonobe T, Le Forestier N, Leger J-M, Bouche P. Proposed revised electrophysiological criteria for chronic inflammatory demyelinating polyradiculoneuropathy. Muscle & Nerve 2002;25:26–30.

9. Haq RU, Fries TJ, Pendlebury WW, Kenny MJ, Badger GJ, Tandan R. Chronic inflammatory demyelinating polyradiculoneuropathy. A study of proposed electrodiagnostic and histologic criteria. Arch Neurol 2000;57:1745–1750.

10. Bromberg MB, Feldman EL, Albers JW. Chronic inflammatory demyelinating polyradiculoneuropathy: comparison of patients with and without an associated monoclonal gammopathy. Neurology 1992;42:1157–1163.

11. Miller R, Rosenberg J, Gelinas D, et al. Practice parameters: the care of the patient with amyotrophic lateral sclerosis (an evidence-based review). Neurology 1999;52:1311–1323.

12. Gregoratos G, Cheitlin M, Conill A, et al. ACC/AHA Guidelines for Implantation of Cardiac Pacemakers and Antiarrhythmia Devices: Executive Summary — a report of the American College of Cardiology/American Heart Association Task Force on Practice Guidelines (Committee on Pacemaker Implantation). Circulation 1998;97:1325–1335.

13. Gregoratos G, Abrams J, Epstein AE, et al. ACC/AHA/NASPE 2002 Guidelines Update for Implantation of Cardiac Pacemakers and Antiarrhythmia Devices — Summary Article. A report of the American College of Cardiology/American Heart Association Task Force on Practice Guidelines (ACC/AHA/NASPE Committee to Update the 1998 Pacemaker Guidelines). J Am Coll Cardiol 2002;40:1703–1719.

CONTENTS

I Methodology

1

Basic Principles of Epidemiology and Biostatistics

1. INTRODUCTION

Epidemiology is a discipline that studies the distribution and determinants of disease. The applications of epidemiology are diverse and include identifying causal mechanisms of disease, diagnostic testing, determining prognosis, and testing new treatments. The goal of an epidemiological study is valid measurement. To understand this goal, it is necessary to understand what it is that is being measured and what is meant by the term validity. The epidemiologist is usually interested in measuring the relationship or association between some exposure and some outcome. The first step is to measure the frequency of the exposure and/or the frequency of the outcome (e.g., disease) of interest. It is then possible to compare these measures of frequency between two populations. The demonstration that disease occurs more frequently within a population exposed to some risk factor than within a population without such exposure provides insight into the association between the exposure and the disease. "Validity" describes the extent to which a measurement is correct (i.e., reflects the truth). A major difficulty is that we typically do not know the truth. Ensuring validity, therefore, requires that we take precautions to minimize error. Broadly speaking, epidemiological studies are susceptible to two types or error—systematic error (also known as bias) and random error. Error is reduced by an awareness of its origins and by the use of appropriate study design.

This introductory chapter will focus on some of the basic principles of epidemiology, including basic study design, measures of frequency and of association, and sources of error in epidemiological studies, as well as fundamental ideas in statistics such as test statistics, p values, and confidence intervals.

2. MEASURES OF FREQUENCY AND MEASURES OF ASSOCIATION

Measures of frequency and measures of association are the basic tools in epidemiology and it is important to understand the difference between these two sorts of measures. Measures of frequency provide information about the distribution of disease within

From: *Neuromuscular Disease: Evidence and Analysis in Clinical Neurology*
By: M. Benatar © Humana Press Inc., Totowa, NJ

populations. The primary measures of frequency include risk, rate, prevalence, and odds. Measures of association, on the other hand, provide a means of comparing the frequency of disease in two populations and, as such, inform on the determinants of disease. Broadly speaking, measures of association can be classified as "difference" measures or as "ratio" measures. Risk difference is an example of the former, whereas the risk ratio and the odds ratio are examples of the latter.

2.1. Measures of Frequency

The term *risk* is used synonymously with *cumulative incidence*. It is a proportion that can be calculated by dividing the number of people who develop the disease during the time period of interest by the number of people who were followed during the time period of interest. This proportion describes the probability of developing disease within a specified time interval and may assume any value between 0 and 1.

To illustrate how risk is calculated, consider the following 2×2 table.

	Disease	No disease
Exposed	a	b
Not exposed	c	d

The risk of disease among those with exposure $= \dfrac{a}{a+b}$

One distinct advantage of using risk as a measure of disease frequency is that it is extremely intuitive. We can easily understand that the risk of developing a particular disease over a 1-year period translates as the probability of developing the disease within this time frame.

One distinct disadvantage of risk as a measure of disease frequency is that it requires knowledge of the number of people in the population who were followed over a specified period of time. The problem is that this number may not be constant because subjects may die from some other cause (competing risk) or be lost to follow-up.

Use of *rate*, also known as *incidence density*, as a measure of disease frequency overcomes this problem in that it is calculated as the number of people who develop the disease divided by a measure of time. The measure of time is calculated as the summation of the follow-up time (e.g., years) experienced by all subjects in the study. Those who were followed for 5 years contribute 5 years of "person time" and those who were followed for 10 years contribute 10 years of "person time." As an example, consider the following hypothetical data.

	Exposed	Not exposed
Cases	100	20
Person years	100,000	100,000

The rate of disease among the exposed group $= \dfrac{100}{100,000} = 1$ per 1000 person years.

The rate of disease among the nonexposed = $\dfrac{20}{100,000}$ = 0.2 per 1000 person years.

Therefore, in contrast with risk, which provides a measure of the probability of developing disease within a particular period of time, rate is an expression of the rapidity with which disease develops. Both risk and rate are measures of disease incidence in that they provide a time-dependent estimate of the occurrence of new instances of the disease within a population. Risk requires specification of the relevant time period whereas the expression of rate incorporates a measure of time.

Prevalence differs from risk and rate (both measures of new cases) in that it provides a measure of the proportion of the population with the disease. Prevalence is more accurately termed *point prevalence* in that it estimates the proportion of people with disease at a given point in time.

With the possible exception of those who spend their days at the race track, odds is a concept that is less well understood. The unintuitive nature of odds probably derives from the fact that it is a ratio measure rather than a proportion. For example, the odds of exposure among those with disease is calculated as the ratio of the proportion of those with disease who are exposed divided by the proportion of those without the disease who are exposed. This is illustrated with the following table.

	Disease	*No disease*
Exposed	a	b
Not exposed	c	d

The proportion of those with disease who were exposed = $\dfrac{a}{a+c}$

The proportion of those with disease who were not exposed = $\dfrac{c}{a+c}$

The odds of exposure among those with disease is calculated as the ratio of these two

proportions: $= \dfrac{\dfrac{a}{a+c}}{\dfrac{c}{a+c}} = \dfrac{a}{c}$

The odds ratio is an even more confusing ratio of two ratios (but we shall return to this later).

2.2. Measures of Association

Measures of association provide the tools for comparing disease frequency between two populations and thus provide a mechanism for discerning the determinants of disease. Disease frequency in different populations may be compared on either an additive or a multiplicative scale. Difference measures (risk difference, rate difference) permit comparison on an additive (absolute) scale whereas ratio measures (risk ratio, rate ratio, odds ratio) facilitate comparison on a multiplicative (relative) scale.

The following hypothetical 2×2 table can be used to illustrate these concepts.

	Disease	No disease
Exposed	a	b
Not exposed	c	d

We have already established that the risk of disease among

those with exposure $= \dfrac{a}{a+b}$

The risk of disease among those without exposure $= \dfrac{c}{c+d}$

The risk difference is calculated as $\dfrac{a}{a+b} - \dfrac{c}{c+d}$

The risk ratio is calculated as $\dfrac{a}{a+b} \div \dfrac{c}{c+d}$

The rate difference and rate ratios are calculated in a similar fashion.

The odds ratio deserves special mention. Although it is the least intuitive measure of association (given that it is a ratio of two ratios), it is the most versatile. In contrast with risk and rate ratios, which can only be determined from studies that provide incident data (i.e., follow-up studies), the odds ratio can be estimated not only from follow-up studies but also from case–control data. It turns out that the odds ratio is also extremely useful as a measure of association for logistic regression (but we shall deal with this idea in more detail in the chapter on prognosis).

To understand the derivation of the odds ratio, we return to the following 2×2 table.

	Disease	No disease
Exposed	a	b
Not exposed	c	d

We have already established that the odds of exposure among

those with disease $= \dfrac{a}{c}$.

Using the identical approach, the proportion of those without disease who

were exposed is calculated as $\dfrac{b}{b+d}$.

And the proportion of those without disease who were not exposed $= \dfrac{d}{b+d}$.

The odds of exposure among those without disease is calculated as the ratio of these

two proportions: $\dfrac{\frac{b}{b+d}}{\frac{d}{b+d}} = \dfrac{b}{d}$.

The (exposure) odds ratio is calculated as the ratio

$$\text{of these two ratios} = \left.\frac{a}{c}\middle/\frac{b}{d}\right. = \frac{ad}{bc}.$$

The odds ratio is also known as the "cross-products ratio."

Because risk is an intuitive concept and odds is not, it is tempting to think of the odds ratio as equivalent to the risk ratio. Although these two ratios are not the same, it turns out that the odds ratio is a reasonably good surrogate for the risk ratio when the frequency of the disease is low. The odds ratio, therefore, is said to estimate the risk ratio when the rare disease assumption is met.

3. TYPES OF EPIDEMIOLOGICAL STUDIES

Broadly speaking, there are only three types of study designs: (1) follow-up studies, which include cohort studies and clinical trials, (2) case–control studies, and (3) cross-sectional studies. The term "case" is used to describe individuals who are affected or who have the disease of interest. The term "control" is used to describe those who are unaffected. A "cohort" refers to any group of subjects who are followed over time.

The characteristic feature of a follow-up study (either a cohort or a clinical trial) is that subjects are followed from exposure (or lack thereof) until outcome (disease). In a clinical trial, for example, subjects may be randomized to receive an active treatment (exposure) or a placebo (nonexposure), and these subjects are then followed over time to determine the frequency with which disease occurs in each group. A cohort study has similar characteristics, the difference being that subjects are assigned to the exposure or nonexposure groups via some method other than randomization. A case–control study, by contrast, is characterized by the identification of subjects who have the outcome or disease (i.e., cases) and subjects who do not (i.e., controls). The investigator then looks back in time to ascertain whether the subjects were exposed or not. In the cohort study and clinical trial, the investigator compares the frequency of disease among those who were exposed with that of those who were not exposed. In the case–control study the investigator compares the frequency of exposure among those with the disease to the frequency of exposure among those without the disease. A common misconception is that the case–control study, but not the cohort study, includes both cases and controls. This is not so. Any good epidemiological study includes both cases and controls.

The terms "prospective" and "retrospective" may sometimes cause confusion. Both case–control and cohort studies can be performed either prospectively or retrospectively. For example, it is possible to review medical records to identify subjects with and without exposure and to then ascertain (from the chart) whether they developed the outcome of interest. This would be an example of a retrospective cohort study.

A unifying feature of follow-up and case–control studies is that they have a longitudinal design. What this means is that information about exposure and disease are collected at different points in time. A cross-sectional study, by contrast, represents a snap-shot in time in that the characteristics of a study population (both potential risk factors and disease status) are ascertained at a single time point. Cross-sectional studies provide estimates of the prevalence of disease and the prevalence of certain risk factors among those with and those without particular diseases. But cross-sectional studies do not assess disease incidence and so provide no information about the risk or rate of developing disease.

4. SOURCES OF ERROR

Broadly speaking, epidemiological studies are susceptible to two types or error– random error and systematic error (also known as bias). Random errors are statistical fluctuations in the measured data that reflect the limited precision of measurement, either on the part of the person making the measurement or the instrument being used to make the measurement. Random errors may lead to over or under-estimation and the direction of the error is variable. If the sample size is large enough, then this random error will, on average, approximate zero. Systematic error, on the other hand, reflects reproducible inaccuracy that is consistently in the same direction (i.e., there is consistently either over or underestimation). One way to conceptualize the difference between systematic and random error is to ask whether the magnitude of the error would be reduced by increasing the sample size. Error that is reduced by increasing sample size is random error. Error that is unaffected by sample size is systematic.

4.1. Systematic Error (Bias)

In order to detect systematic error in published studies and to avoid such bias in the design and conduct of a study, it is useful to classify systematic error into three categories—selection bias, information (misclassification) bias, and confounding. There is overlap between these categories, but this classification nevertheless provides a useful conceptual framework within which systematic error can be evaluated. We shall consider each of these in turn.

4.1.2. SELECTION BIAS

Selection bias describes the error that results from differences in the association between exposure and disease between those who participate in the study and those who do not. A common and important example of selection bias is that which results from the inclusion in a study of patients evaluated at a tertiary referral center rather than a population-based sample. It might be expected that those patients who are referred to a tertiary center are more likely to have more severe or more complicated disease. A prognostic study, therefore, might report a less favorable outcome than would be observed had the study population been more representative of the full spectrum of patients with the disease in question. Another common and important example of selection bias results from loss to follow-up in a clinical trial. If follow-up information is not available for a substantial proportion of subjects who entered the study because they dropped out, it is possible that those who remain in the study differ in some systematic way from those who do not. It is for this reason that studies with high drop-out rates have the potential for significant bias.

4.1.3. INFORMATION BIAS

Information bias describes the error that results from the misclassification of exposure or disease status. If the goal of an epidemiological study is to measure the frequency of disease or to measure the association between exposure and disease, the validity of these measures will critically depend on correctly classifying subjects with exposure as being exposed and classifying those with the disease as having the disease. The term misclassification bias is also used to describe this type of bias. In evaluating information bias, a distinction should be made between *differential* and *nondifferential* misclassification. If the misclassification of one variable depends on the level or status of another variable, then the misclassification is said to be differential. Classification of exposure in case-control studies is one important potential source of differential misclassification bias. Subjects who have acquired the disease of interest may be more likely to recall exposure to a potential variable than those without the disease of interest. Similarly, the investigator may subconsciously probe affected subjects more intensely than unaffected subjects in order to elicit a history of exposure to the variable of interest. These two forms of differential misclassification bias are often referred to as recall bias and observer bias respectively. The error that results from such differential misclassification is often described as bias away from the null, meaning that there is a bias towards a stronger exposure-disease association.

Nondifferential misclassification bias has the opposite effect in that it tends to produce bias toward the null. This means that it is more difficult to demonstrate an association between exposure and disease. To understand why, consider the extreme example of a case–control study in which neither those with the disease nor those without the disease can recall their true exposure status and so randomly guess. On average, one-half of those with the disease will report having been exposed and half of those without the disease will report the same. Such a scenario will clearly make it impossible to detect any real association between exposure and disease.

Incorporation bias is another example of misclassification bias that frequently arises in diagnostic studies. In this form of bias, the result of the diagnostic test that is being evaluated is used to determine whether subjects are classified as having the disease or not. Use of a positive test result (even in part) to designate disease as present will have the effect of inflating the estimate of the sensitivity of the test in question.

4.1.4. CONFOUNDING

Confounding is best conceptualized as a "mixing up" of effects. What this means is that the effect of the exposure on disease is mixed up or confused with the effect of some extraneous variable. Two criteria must be met for a variable to cause confounding—the extraneous (confounding) variable must be associated with the exposure variable (but not as a consequence of exposure) and it must also be associated with the outcome variable. Confounding differs from other forms of systematic bias in that its presence can be demonstrated by a change in the strength of the exposure–disease relationship when the effect of the extraneous variable are taken into account. A number of approaches may be used to control for confounding, either in the design or analysis phase of a study. One of the primary reasons for randomization in clinical trials is to ensure the even distribution of both known and unknown risk factors between the two treatment groups. The equal distribution of risk factors (potential confounders) between groups ensures, by definition, that there is no association between the potential confounder and the exposure variable. Restriction and stratification are other methods that may be used to control for confounding, in the design and analysis phases of a study, respectively. Each involves evaluating the exposure–disease relationship within a single level of the potential confounder, and this uniformity or homogeneity of the extraneous variable ensures that there cannot be imbalance in the distribution of the extraneous variable between the treatment groups. A modeling approach may also be used to control for confounding, but the details are beyond the scope of this chapter.

4.2. Random Error

Random error is the error that remains once systematic error has been removed. It reflects the variability in the data that cannot be explained on the basis of systematic error. The study of the distribution and determinants of disease in a population typically involves the evaluation of a sample derived from the population of interest. By analyzing this sample it is possible to obtain an *estimate* of the true disease frequency in the entire population. Once systematic error has been removed, random error describes the precision with which the estimate reflects the true population parameter of interest. One way to quantify the precision of the estimate is to report both a point estimate of the parameter as well as the confidence interval around the point estimate. A narrow confidence interval indicates a high degree of precision whereas a broad confidence interval reflects poor precision. The width of the confidence interval thus provides a measure of random error inherent in the estimate. Increasing the sample size leads to improved precision, which is reflected in a narrower confidence interval. We typically describe 90% or 95% confidence intervals (although any confidence interval could be calculated). A 95% confidence is defined as follows. If the identical study were repeated many times over, the confidence interval would include within it the correct value of the parameter of interest 95% of the time. This is often loosely translated into the statement that we can be 95% confident that this interval includes the true value. Although not quite accurate statistically, this description is somewhat more intuitive and will probably suffice.

The p value, which is described in more detail later in this chapter, similarly provides a measure of the magnitude of the random error. The confidence interval and the p value, therefore, are closely related concepts in that both provide a quantification of random error.

5. INTERACTION AND CONFOUNDING

These are two important concepts that are often confused. Confounding, as has already been discussed, describes a mixing up of effects in which there is an apparent association between one variable and the outcome of interest. The mixing up occurs because of some other association that exists between the variable of interest and the confounding variable as well as the association between the confounding variable and the outcome of interest.

Confounding represents a threat to the internal validity of a study. It is a nuisance that distorts the true association between the exposure and disease of interest.

Interaction, also known as effect modification, on the other hand, describes the scenario in which the effect of a variable on the outcome of interest differs depending on the level of some other extraneous factor (the effect modifier). When present, interaction should be identified and reported upon. There are a variety of available methods for detecting interaction. One simple method is to stratify data on the basis of the potential effect modifier and to compare the stratum-specific measures of association between the strata. Differences in the stratum-specific measures of association indicate the presence of interaction (effect modification) and under such circumstances, the stratum-specific measures of association should be reported. If there is no interaction (i.e., the stratum-specific measures of association are essentially the same), then an adjusted measure of association (e.g., Mantel Haenszel odds ratio) should be calculated and this adjusted measure compared with the crude measure of association (i.e., that obtained prior to stratification). Meaningful differences between the crude and adjusted measures of association indicate the presence of confounding.

6. THE NULL HYPOTHESIS AND STATISTICAL TESTING

The null hypothesis, for most study designs, assumes that there is no difference between two groups. It usually takes the form of the expression that the frequency of disease is no different between two groups, that the mean of some outcome measure is no different between two groups, or that the frequency of exposure is no different between two groups. The alternate hypothesis expresses that the two populations differ with respect to the outcome measure of interest. The idea of a statistical test is to provide some summary measure of the data such that it is possible to determine the probability of obtaining the observed results or of observing more extreme results (assuming that the null hypothesis is true). By "more extreme" we mean results that are less consistent with the null hypothesis. The p value is simply an expression of this probability. A common misconception is to think that the p value provides a measure of the probability that the null hypothesis is correct. Instead, the p value provides an estimate of the probability of obtaining the observed results (or more extreme results), given the assumption that the null hypothesis is correct. That is to say, the statistical test is based on the assumption that there is no meaningful difference between the two groups in the outcome measure of interest. The p value then provides an estimate of how consistent the data are with the null hypothesis. A high p value indicates that chances are great that the observed differences between the two groups are due to chance and that the null hypothesis should be accepted. A low p value, on the other hand, indicates that there is a small probability that the observed differences are due to chance and hence, that the null hypothesis should be rejected.

It is customary to regard a p value that is less than 0.05 as "statistically significant." A p value of 0.05 simply means that there is only a 5% chance of obtaining the observed results, or more extreme results, assuming that the null hypothesis is true. If we select a p value of 0.05 as the cut-off for determining "statistical significance," what we are saying is that we are willing to accept that we will be wrong 5% of the time. That is to say, in 5% of cases, we will reject the null hypothesis and conclude that there is in fact a meaningful difference between the two treatment groups when in fact there is not.

7. CONCLUSION

In reading and critically reviewing the medical literature, it is helpful to know something about the basic principles of epidemiology and biostatistics. The aim of this and the following three chapters is to provide the reader with some insight into these basic principles. One should not assume that the authors of a peer-reviewed and published paper necessarily know enough about these principles. It is commonplace, for example, for case series to be described as cohort studies. Often, it is clear that the authors of a paper have themselves not fully appreciated the difference between a case–control study and a cohort study. Authors frequently overinterpret p values, concluding that p values of 0.049 indicate statistical significance whereas p values of 0.052 do not. The reader should not assume that the authors' description of the study or the conclusions that are drawn are correct. Instead, the reader should try to ascertain the authors' hypothesis and study design based on the data presented. The reader should consider potential sources of error—both systematic and random—and try to draw independent conclusions about the validity of the study.

2 Diagnosis

1. INTRODUCTION

The clinical decision-making process is based on probability. Based on certain clinical information such as risk factors, family history, and findings on physical examination, the clinician obtains some estimate of the probability of disease (the pretest probability). Diagnostic tests are performed in order to improve the estimate of this probability. If the test is negative, the probability of disease should fall and if the test is positive, then the probability of the disease should rise. Useful diagnostic tests will produce marked shifts in the probability of disease based on whether the results of the test are positive or negative.

In this chapter, we will explore the science of diagnostic testing from two perspectives. We shall first consider the methodological principles that underpin the design and conduct of studies of diagnostic tests. We shall then explore the epidemiological principles that guide the use and interpretation of diagnostic test results.

2. BASIC PRINCIPLES

Studies of the accuracy of diagnostic tests are generally of poor quality (1) and the ability to read and critically appraise the literature on diagnostic testing therefore requires some understanding of how to assess the quality of these studies. In evaluating the quality of a study of a diagnostic test, it is necessary to consider the process whereby participants were selected, the nature of the gold or reference standard that was used to determine the presence or absence of disease, whether the test under investigation (the index test) formed part of the reference standard, and whether the investigators who performed the index test were blind to the results of the reference standard. These issues have to do with the external validity of the study. That is to say, how easily can the results of this study be generalized to populations of patients encountered in clinical practice?

A diagnostic test is useful only insofar as it distinguishes between conditions that might otherwise be confused. A study that evaluates the ability of a test to distinguish two unrelated disorders or to distinguish individuals severely affected by a disease from healthy controls does not mimic the conditions encountered in clinical practice and so provides relatively little information about the real diagnostic value of the test. It is

From: *Neuromuscular Disease: Evidence and Analysis in Clinical Neurology*
By: M. Benatar © Humana Press Inc., Totowa, NJ

remarkable how often this basic principle is ignored in studies of diagnostic tests. This is a theme that will recur throughout this book. Furthermore, in reporting the results of a study of a diagnostic test, the authors should specify the setting in which subjects were recruited and whether study subjects represent a consecutive series or whether subjects were selected for inclusion on the basis of having received the index test or reference standard. Each of these factors are relevant to the external validity of the study.

In order to evaluate the performance of a diagnostic test it is also necessary to know something about the standard against which the results of the test were compared. In other words, it is necessary to know the criteria that were used as the gold or reference standard to determine whether the outcome of interest (e.g., disease) is present or absent. Reliable and robust gold standards do exist, but frequently they are not available in routine clinical practice. Pathological evidence for the presence of a disease might be considered the gold standard for certain diseases, but biopsy or autopsy material may not always be available, which makes it difficult to rely on pathology as the gold standard for a diagnostic test. As a compromise, investigators frequently rely on some set of clinical criteria in order to evaluate the accuracy of a diagnostic test. In doing so, it is crucial to avoid incorporating the results of the test of interest into the criteria that will be used as the surrogate gold standard (an error referred to as "incorporation bias"). Although this recommendation is intuitive based on common sense, it is ignored with surprising frequency (as shall be illustrated repeatedly throughout the course of this book).

Blinding of the investigator to the results of the reference standard is also of fundamental importance to the validity of a study of a diagnostic test. Knowledge of the results of the reference standard may influence (consciously or subconsciously) the interpretation of the index test and thus introduce significant bias.

Various methods for evaluating the quality of diagnostic studies have been reported (2,3). Most prominent among these is the Standards for Reporting of Diagnostic Accuracy (STARD) initiative, which represents an attempt to improve the quality of studies that are designed to investigate the accuracy of diagnostic studies. Among the methodological issues highlighted by the STARD document are the need for a clear definition of the population under study with explicit inclusion and exclusion criteria, the need for clear articulation of the gold (reference) standard against which the diagnostic test is being compared, the necessity of blinding of the examiner to the results of the gold standard, and the need for a clear discussion of how indeterminate results were handled. The STARD recommendations have received broad acceptance and will likely play an important role in the definition of a new standard by which studies of diagnostic tests will be judged.

3. SENSITIVITY AND SPECIFICITY

It is extremely unlikely that a positive test will always imply the presence of disease and that a negative test will always indicate the absence of disease. Because every test is likely to be fallible, there are four possible outcomes for any test in which the result is reported only as either positive or negative (i.e., no indeterminate results). These possible results are illustrated in the following table.

	"Truth"	
Test result	Disease	No disease
Positive	a True positive (TP)	b False positive (FP)
Negative	c False negative (FN)	d True negative (TN)

Those with the disease for whom the test is positive are labeled as true positive (a).

Those without the disease for whom the test is positive are labeled as false positive (b).

Those with the disease for whom the test is negative are labeled as false negative (c).

Those without the disease for whom the test is negative are labeled as true negative (d).

The sensitivity of a diagnostic test is defined as the proportion of people with the disease who test positive. That is say, sensitivity $= \dfrac{a}{a+c} = \dfrac{TP}{TP+FN}$.

For a test with high sensitivity, most individuals with the disease will test positive. Because there are few false negatives, a negative test result provides good evidence that the disease is not present. Tests with high sensitivity are typically most useful for ruling out a particular disease. This is the sort of test that would be most useful as a screening test, in that a negative result reliably excludes disease. Subjects with positive results, however, will require more detailed testing to determine whether the disease is truly present.

The specificity of a diagnostic test is defined as the proportion of people without the disease who test negative. That is say, specificity $= \dfrac{d}{b+d} = \dfrac{TN}{TN+FP}$.

For a test with high specificity, most individuals without the disease will test negative. Because there are few false positives, a positive test result provides good evidence that the disease is present. Tests with high specificity are most useful for ruling in a particular disease.

Diagnostic accuracy is the term used to describe the combination of sensitivity and specificity. Accuracy can be estimated from the area under the receiver operating characteristic (ROC) curve (explained in "Cut-Points and ROC Curves").

Although sensitivity and specificity are properties of the diagnostic test, the performance of the test may vary among different populations *(4)*; hence the importance of evaluating the performance of the diagnostic test in the population of patients in which it will ultimately be used clinically. To illustrate how the performance of a test may vary from population to population, consider the example of the use of single-fiber electromyography (SFEMG) for the diagnosis of myasthenia gravis. Evaluation of the accuracy of SFEMG by comparing healthy subjects with those who have seropositive generalized myasthenia gravis may show that the test is both sensitive and specific. If the accuracy of SFEMG is instead evaluated using patients with mitochondrial disease or oculopharyngeal muscular dystrophy as controls and myasthenics with purely ocular disease as cases, both the sensitivity and specificity of the test might be expected to be reduced.

4. CUT-POINTS AND ROC CURVES

Sensitivity and specificity, therefore, are terms used to describe the performance of a test relative to some external gold standard. The sensitivity and specificity of a test depend, to a large extent, on the threshold or cut-point that is used to discriminate between a positive test result and a negative test result. In general, if the threshold for a positive (abnormal) test result is raised (i.e., making the test less likely to produce a positive result), then the sensitivity will fall and the specificity will rise. If, on the other hand, a low threshold for a positive test is used, then the test will be more likely to detect a greater proportion of subjects who have the disease (i.e., increased sensitivity), but this may come at the price of more frequent positive test results even among those without the disease (i.e., lower specificity). In general, good (i.e., useful) diagnostic tests combine high sensitivity with high specificity. The utility of a diagnostic test using different cut-points can be explored by plotting a ROC curve as shown in Graph 2.1., in which sensitivity on the y-axis is plotted against 1-specificity on the x-axis.

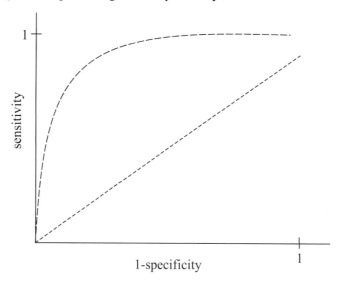

Graph 2.1

Tests in which improved sensitivity are accompanied by a fall in specificity of similar magnitude have no discriminative value. The ROC curve for such a test is illustrated by the straight 45° line. The diagnostic accuracy of such a test, which may be calculated from the area under the curve, is 50%. Such a test performs as well as the flip of a coin in determining whether disease is present or not.

Graph 2.1 shown above also illustrates the ROC curve for a test with almost perfect diagnostic accuracy. Specificity remains close to 100% at every test threshold until sensitivity also reaches almost 100%. This ROC curve ascends almost vertically along the y-axis from 0 to 1 and then extends almost horizontally along the x-axis from 0 to 1. The area under this curve is close to 100%, indicating that the test has an almost perfect discriminative value between disease and no disease. In reality, no test conforms to such specifications, but these hypothetical examples serve to illustrate the characteristics of a useful diagnostic test. The more toward the upper left-hand corner of the graph the ROC curve is located, the better the diagnostic accuracy of the test. The point of inflection of the ROC curve indicates the cut-point at which the combination of sensitivity and specificity is maximized.

5. PREDICTIVE VALUE

In contrast with sensitivity and specificity, which characterize the diagnostic accuracy of a test, the positive and negative predictive values are two estimates that directly address the probability of disease.

	"Truth"	
Test result	Disease	No disease
Positive	a	b
	True positive	False positive
Negative	c	d
	False negative	True negative

The positive predictive value represents the probability of disease being present if the test is positive. Using the hypothetical 2×2 table above, it is calculated as

$$\frac{a}{a+b} = \frac{TP}{TF+FP}.$$

The negative predictive value similarly represents the probability of disease being absent if the test is negative. It is calculated as $\frac{d}{c+d} = \frac{TN}{TN+FN}.$

Use of the predictive values illustrates the point that the utility of a test depends on the population in which the test is being applied. The pretest probability of disease depends on the prevalence of disease within the specified population. The positive predictive value will be greater and the negative predictive value will be reduced in populations with high disease prevalence (i.e., high pretest probability).

6. LIKELIHOOD RATIOS

The likehood ratio (LR) is the ratio of the probability of a particular test result for a person with the disease divided by the probability of that same result for a person without the disease. The LR indicates by how much a given diagnostic test result will raise or lower the pretest probability of the disease in question.

The LR for a positive test (LR+) is defined as the probability of a positive test result for a person with the disease divided by the probability of a positive test result for a person without the disease. LR+ may be calculated as $\dfrac{sensitivity}{1-specificity}$. Similarly, the LR for a negative test (LR–) is defined as the probability of a negative test result for a person with the disease divided by the probability of a negative test result for a person without the disease. LR– may be calculated as $\dfrac{1-sensitivity}{specificity}$.

Test results may, for example, be categorized as indicating high probability of disease, moderate probability, low probability, or no probability of disease. Within each level of the test result it is possible to calculate the LR and to use this ratio to estimate the posttest probability of disease.

LRs ratios greater than 10 and less than 0.1 generate large and often definitive changes from pretest to posttest probability, LRs between 5 and 10 and between 0.1 and 0.2 lead to moderate changes in pretest to posttest probability, and LRs between 2 and 5 and between 0.2 and 0.5 result in small changes in probability. LRs between 1 and 2 and between 0.5-1 rarely alter pretest probability *(5)*.

The utility of the LR is that it can be used to estimate the posttest probability of disease. The strategy for doing so is illustrated as follows:

1. Determine the pretest probability of disease (this is typically based on an assessment of risk factors, family history, personal history, and physical examination).
2. Convert pretest probability to pretest odds (divide by 1 – pretest probability).
3. Multiple pretest odds by the LR to yield the posttest odds.
4. Convert the posttest odds to the posttest probability (divide by 1 + posttest odds).

7. CONCLUSION

The principles that should guide the conduct of a study of a diagnostic test should be born in mind when reading and evaluating the relevant literature. A study's failure to include an appropriate population, its susceptibility to incorporation bias, or the inadequacy of blinding should lead to caution in the interpretation of the results. Studies of diagnostic tests do not always frame their findings using the appropriate terminology (sensitivity, specificity, LR), but where possible, every effort should be made to tabulate data in such a way as to permit estimation of these parameters. So doing will permit the reader to think in terms of probability and to evaluate the utility of diagnostic tests in terms of a test's ability to move the posttest probability toward either very low or very high likelihood of disease.

REFERENCES

1. Reid M, Lachs M, Feinstein A. Use of methodological standards in diagnostic test research: getting better but still not good. JAMA 1995;274:645–651.
2. England J, Gronseth G, Franklin G, et al. Distal symmetric polyneuropathy: A definition for clinical research: Report of the American Academy of Neurology, the American Association of Electrodiagnostic Medicine, and the American Academy of Physical Medicine and Rehabilitation. Neurology 2005; 64:199–207.

3. Bossuyt PM, Reitsma JB, Bruns DE, et al. Towards complete and accurate reporting of studies of diagnostic accuracy: the STARD initiative. Br Med J 2003;326:41–44.
4. Jaeschke R, Guyatt G, Lijmer J. Diagnostic tests. In: (Guyatt G, Rennie D, eds.) User's Guide to the Medical Literature. A Manual for Evidence-Based Clinical Practice. American Medical Association Press, Chicago: 2002:121–140.
5. Jaeschke R, Guyatt G, Sackett D. Users' guides to the medical literature. III. How to use an article about a diagnostic test. B. What are the results and will they help me in caring for my patients? The Evidence-Based Medicine Working Group. JAMA 1994;271:703–707.

3 Treatment

1. INTRODUCTION

The randomized controlled trial (RCT) is a powerful experimental technique for demonstrating the efficacy of a therapeutic strategy. The goal of the RCT is to obtain a valid measure of the efficacy of a particular intervention. Validity is maximized by strict adherence to the design elements of the RCT that aim to minimize bias, confounding, and random error.

Clinical trials are characterized by a number of important features. They are always prospective, always involve an intervention of some sort, and always include a control group against which the intervention is compared. The crucial feature that distinguishes an RCT from any other sort of clinical trial is the fact that study subjects are randomly assigned to the intervention group or the control group. The goal of randomization is to ensure that the control and intervention groups are comparable at baseline with respect to all important prognostic factors such that any difference in outcome may reasonably be attributed to the intervention.

A clinical trial should be motivated by a primary research question or hypothesis. Every clinical trial should have a primary outcome measure that has been specified in advance. The anticipated effect of the intervention on this primary outcome measure forms the basis for determining the required sample size.

A study may be powered to show that one intervention is better than another (superiority trial) or to show that two interventions have similar efficacy (equivalence study). The finding that two interventions are equivalent is not the same as failing to demonstrate the superiority of one intervention over another.

In this chapter, we consider a number of important aspects of the design and analysis of an RCT. We shall first explore the theoretical basis for sample size estimation, because the failure to adequately power a study may lead to unacceptably high random error and result in the study's failure to demonstrate the efficacy of a treatment that does in fact work. We then turn our attention to the randomization process and the need for blinding of both the examiner and the study subjects as well as a number of issues relevant to the analysis of data from an RCT.

From: *Neuromuscular Disease: Evidence and Analysis in Clinical Neurology*
By: M. Benatar © Humana Press Inc., Totowa, NJ

2. SAMPLE SIZE ESTIMATION

Every clinical trial should include a sufficient number of participants in order to provide adequate power to detect differences between treatment groups that are regarded as clinically meaningful. The essential, but often misunderstood, concept is that sample size determination critically depends on estimation of the magnitude of the clinical effect that the investigator proposes to demonstrate (i.e., the effect size that is regarded as clinically meaningful).

The first step in estimating sample size is to determine the response or outcome variable that will be used to measure the effectiveness of the treatment or intervention that is being studied. Broadly speaking, there are three types of response variables, and the method used to estimate sample size will depend on the nature of the response variable. The three types of response variables are dichotomous, continuous, and time-to-an-event. Stroke and death are examples of dichotomous outcome variables in which the event either occurs or does not occur. Sample size estimation for dichotomous variables is based on a comparison of the event rates—i.e., a comparison of the proportion of subjects who experience the event in the active treatment group (P_1) with the proportion of who experience the event in the control group (P_0). Examples of continuous variables are blood pressure, weight, or the score of a particular clinical scale such as the National Institutes of Health stroke scale (NIHSS; this is actually an ordinal scale, but such data are often analyzed as though continuous). Sample size estimation is based on a comparison of the mean score in the active treatment group (μ_1) with the mean score in the control group (μ_0). Time-to-event outcome variables describe the time period that elapses between entry into the study and the occurrence of some predefined event such as stroke, death, or relapse from cancer remission. Sample size estimates rely on a comparison of the hazard rates in the active treatment (λ_1) with control groups (λ_0). The example of a dichotomous outcome variable is used here for the purposes of illustrating the process of sample size estimation.

In order to determine the required sample size, the investigator must estimate the event rate in the control population (P_0). This estimate may be obtained either from the literature or from a preliminary study performed by the investigator. The investigator will then need to estimate the anticipated event rate in the intervention group (P_1). This is typically done by estimating the smallest difference in event rates (i.e., $P_0 - P_1$) that would be regarded as clinically meaningful. If, for example, stroke is expected to occur in 20% (0.2) of the control population, the investigator might decide that an absolute risk reduction of 5% would be clinically meaningful, in which case P_1 is estimated at 15% (0.15). Any difference less than 5% would be taken to imply no difference in event rates between the intervention and control groups.

Having estimated these two event rates, the investigator must decide the false-positive and false-negative rates that she is willing to accept for the clinical trial. To understand what is meant by false-positive and false-negative rates, it is helpful to turn to the concepts of the null and alternate hypotheses. The null hypothesis for this clinical trial could be stated as $P_0 - P_1 = 0$ (i.e., there is no difference in the event rates between the control and intervention groups, where "no different" implies that the difference is less than 5%). The alternative hypothesis would state that $P_0 \ P_1$ (i.e., the event rates are different between the control and intervention groups, where "different" implies at least a 5%

difference). Incorrectly rejecting the null hypothesis in favor of the alternative hypothesis (i.e., deciding that there is a difference between P_0 and P_1 when in truth no difference exists) is a false-positive result. Accepting the null hypothesis when the truth is that there is a real difference between P_0 and P_1 is a false-negative result (also know as β). The power of a study describes the ability of the study to correctly reject the null hypothesis and is calculated as $1 - \beta$ (i.e.,1 minus the false-negative rate).

It is customary to accept a false-positive rate of 5% (i.e., α set at 0.05). An adequately powered study should have at least an 80% chance of demonstrating a true difference between the event rates in the intervention and control groups (i.e., β of at most 0.2). But the investigator must decide whether to endow the study with even greater power (e.g., 90%). Clearly, greater power implies a stronger study design, but increasing power comes at the expense of increasing the sample size that will be required.

Sufficient concepts have been introduced that it is now possible to consider the formula for sample size estimation for a study comparing event rates between the two treatment groups.

$$n = \frac{\left(Z_\alpha + Z_\beta\right)^2 \times 2\overline{p}\left(1 - \overline{p}\right)}{\left(P_1 - P_0\right)^2}$$

where Z_α = z-value for α

Z_β = z-value for β

$\overline{p} = \dfrac{P_1 + P_0}{2}$

P_1 = event rate in the intervention group

P_0 = event rate in the control group

From this equation, it should be clear that sample size is inversely proportional to the difference in the event rates in the intervention and control groups. That is to say, the smaller the difference in event rates, the larger the sample size that will be required. Furthermore, the sample size is proportional to the power of the study, implying that increasing the power of the study will require an increase in the necessary sample size.

3. RANDOMIZATION

Randomization describes the process whereby study subjects are assigned to the different treatment groups in such a way that each subject has an equal chance of being assigned to any particular treatment group. This method of randomization is sometimes referred to as *simple randomization* in order to distinguish it from *stratified* and *blocked* randomization (which are discussed later). The goal of randomization is to control for confounding.

It will be recalled that confounding describes a mixing up of effects and the potential for confounding exists when a feature or variable is unequally distributed between two treatment groups. Randomization ensures that the control and intervention groups are comparable at baseline with respect to all important prognostic factors such that any difference in outcome may reasonably be attributed to the intervention. A strategy of stratification could similarly produce equal distribution of known prognostic factors between two treatment groups, but the strength of randomization lies in the fact that it will result in the equal distribution of both known and unknown prognostic factors between the two treatment groups.

An essential, but sometimes underrecognized aspect of the randomization process is concealment of allocation. Allocation of the study subject to one treatment group or another should be unknown (i.e., concealed) to the investigator. It is possible for treatment assignment to be randomized but not concealed. To understand how this may occur, consider the example of the study in which a random number generator is used to assign study subjects to one treatment group or another, but these treatment assignments are listed on paper for the investigator to see. The investigator, therefore, knows that the next patient who is enrolled in the study will receive a particular treatment. This knowledge may influence the investigator's decision to include a particular patient in the clinical trial. If, for example, the investigator holds a bias in favor of the active treatment arm but suspects that the next potential study subject has a poor prognosis, he might decide not to recruit this subject to participate in the trial if the next assignment is to the active treatment group. Allocation concealment can be achieved either by sealing each treatment group assignment inside an opaque envelope to be opened only after the subject has been entered into the study, or by using a central randomization center. Once an investigator has entered a subject into the study, she may call the central randomization center to determine the treatment group to which this study subject will be assigned. Allocation concealment, therefore, is central to preserving the validity of the randomization process. Without it, both selection bias and confounding may result.

A description of the randomization process would not be complete without reference to the concepts of blocking and stratification. Blocked randomization aims to avoid any serious imbalance in the number of subjects assigned to each treatment group. A simple randomization process might result in more subjects being assigned to one treatment group than the other by chance alone, especially if the sample size is relatively small. In blocked randomization, an equal number of study subjects are randomized to each treatment group within blocks of a predetermined size. For example, for a block size of four, two subjects are assigned to one treatment and two subjects are assigned to the alternate treatment, with the order of treatment assignment within each block being randomly determined. Such a strategy ensures that at any point in time the difference in the number of subjects assigned to each treatment group cannot differ by more than two. One potential problem with blocking is that the investigator may have been able to discern the treatments received by the first three patients in the block of four and hence be able to predict the treatment group to which the next patient will be assigned. This problem can be avoided by varying the size of the blocks in some random fashion.

Stratified randomization helps to ensure the balance of a particular prognostic factor across treatment groups. Because it is possible, by chance alone, for simple randomization to produce an imbalance of a particular prognostic factor between treatment groups, stratification is sometimes used prior to randomization in order to ensure even distribution of the most important prognostic factor. Stratified randomization involves measurement or determination of the prognostic factor prior to randomization, assignment to a particular stratum, and then randomization to one treatment group or another within that stratum. If more than one variable is used for stratification, then the number of strata represents the product of the number of subgroups and the number of strata. For example, stratification according to age (e.g., three age groups) and gender (two groups) will yield six strata.

4. BLINDING

Blinding describes the process whereby the investigators and study subjects are masked to the treatment group to which subjects are assigned. Blinding is important because it helps to minimize the bias that may otherwise result if either the investigator or the study subject is aware of the treatment received.

The ideal study is double-blind in that neither the investigator nor the study subject are aware of the treatment received. Bias may result if either the investigator or the study subject is aware of the treatment received. If the investigator is aware that a subject has been assigned to the placebo group, he may be tempted (consciously or subconsciously) to prescribe some other concomitant therapy. Similarly, knowledge of the treatment received may influence the investigators' reporting of outcome. The investigator who favors the active treatment may be inclined to overestimate the benefit of the active treatment and underestimate the benefit of the placebo treatment. The bias may also work in the opposite direction if, for example, the investigator believes that the active treatment is unlikely to be effective. Bias may also arise if the study subject is aware of the treatment group to which he has been assigned. If he knows that he is receiving placebo he may be more inclined to drop out of the study or to report little improvement in the outcome measure.

Double-blinding, however, may not always be possible. In studies that compare a medical intervention with a surgical treatment, for example, it is impossible to mask treatment assignment among the study subjects. Investigator blinding, however, may be partially preserved by hiding the surgical scar, instructing the study subject not to inform the investigator of the treatment received, and using someone who is not directly involved in providing care to measure outcome. Under these circumstances, the person who evaluates outcome is typically not the same person who is providing routine medical care to the subject.

Subject blinding may be difficult even in drug trials in that it may not be possible to produce placebo tablets that are identical in size, weight, appearance, and taste. Such differences are particularly important in cross-over studies in which subjects will receive both forms of treatment at some stage.

At the end of a study, it may be worthwhile to evaluate the success of blinding. This can be accomplished by asking the investigators and study subjects to guess the treatment arm to which they were assigned. In a trial in which one-half of the study participants received active drug and half received placebo, 50% would be expected to correctly guess their treatment assignment. The extent to which the proportion of subjects who correctly guess the treatment received deviates from 50% provides a measure of the extent to which blinding was unsuccessful.

5. ANALYSIS OF RESULTS

Ideally, all subjects who were randomized to one of the study treatments groups should be included in the final analysis, because the exclusion of some study subjects may lead to bias either in favor of or against the intervention under investigation. The temptation to exclude some study subjects may arise from various sources. It may be that a subject is randomized to one treatment group, but for some reason or another ends up receiving the other treatment, or a subject is poorly compliant with the treatment that he was randomized to receive. Alternatively, a subject may be entered into the study and randomized but subsequently found not to meet all of the study inclusion criteria. The problem with excluding any of the subjects who fall into these various categories is that it may introduce a form of selection bias and defeat the purpose of the randomization. The term "intention-to-treat" is used to describe the sort of analysis in which the outcomes of all study participants are analyzed according to the treatment that they were randomized to receive. This is widely regarded as the most appropriate (albeit, the most stringent) method of data analysis.

At times, it may be impossible to include all randomized subjects in the analysis because study subjects withdrew or were lost to follow-up, and so data regarding the final outcome measure may be missing. High rates of withdrawal or loss to follow-up may also introduce significant selection bias, because the subjects included in the final analysis may differ in some important respect from those study subjects who were not included in the final analysis. Sometimes withdrawal and loss to follow-up are unavoidable and various analytic techniques must be employed to compensate for these losses. One approach for those who withdraw from the study (i.e., stop taking the study medication) is to continue to follow these study subjects and to measure the outcome variable in this group at the end of the study. When this is not possible (i.e., when subjects are lost to follow-up), it may be necessary to use some technique to impute the missing data. There are various methods available for imputing missing data, but all have their limitations and none adequately avoids the bias that may result from loss to follow-up of study subjects. One of the commonly used data imputation techniques is to use what is known as the "last observation carried forward" (LOCF). The technique involves using the most recent measure of the outcome variable in the final analysis. It may be that the study called for measurement of the outcome variable at various time points prior to the study end-point. For this technique, data from an earlier evaluation are assumed to remain constant until the end of the study. In this way, the last available data on the study subject are carried forward to the final analysis. LOCF makes substantial assumptions, which may not always hold true. An alternative technique that may be used to deal with missing data is to perform a sensitivity analysis. This requires assuming two different extreme values for the missing data. For example, one assumption might be that all subjects lost to follow-up experienced the outcome event of interest, whereas a second assumption is that none of the subjects experienced the outcome of interest. By analyzing the data separately using each of these assumptions, it is possible to set "confidence limits" around an estimate of the outcome measured from the study subjects for whom final outcome data are actually available. Whichever technique is used, it should be recalled that loss to follow-up may introduce bias and no analytic technique entirely compensates for the lost data.

6. SUMMARY

The focus of this chapter has been on the design and analysis of data from randomized controlled trials. We have explained why randomization is so important as well as some of the considerations that are relevant to maintaining the benefits of randomization, including adequate concealment of allocation, blinding of both the investigator and the study subjects, and the intention-to-treat analysis. We have also touched on issues related to sample size estimation and have emphasized the need to determine the smallest effect that would be considered clinically meaningful in order to be able to adequately estimate the sample size that will be required.

4 Prognosis

1. INTRODUCTION

Determining the prognosis of a disease involves a prediction of the probable outcome. The term natural history is sometimes used synonymously with prognosis, but it is probably better used to describe a particular sort of prognosis—that which ensues in the absence of any therapeutic intervention. The most reliable information about the outcome of a disease is usually derived from the experience of other patients with the same disorder. To estimate prognosis, therefore, we typically examine the outcome of a group of patients who all have the same disorder. To refine our estimate of the prognosis, we compare outcome among subgroups of patients based, for example, on age, gender, comorbidity, or some other variable. Variables or factors that really do predict outcome are known as *prognostic factors*. Prognostic factors are really just examples of risk factors. In the same way that risk factors predict the occurrence of disease, prognostic factors predict the outcome of disease.

The study of prognosis and prognostic factors is very similar to the study of risk and risk factors and similarly involves the use of cohort and case–control study designs. Clinical trials also provide information about prognosis in that the outcome of patients within each treatment group can be determined and the extent to which the different treatments under investigation affect outcome can be studied. In effect, treatment received represents a prognostic variable. In addition, there are a number of analytic techniques, such as regression and survival analysis, that lend themselves particularly well to the study of prognosis. The focus of this chapter is on these analytic techniques as well as on the basic epidemiological principles that should govern studies of prognosis.

2. STRATIFICATION

One of the simplest ways to evaluate prognosis is compare the outcome in two groups of subjects. Examples include comparing outcome among those who receive a placebo with that of those who receive an active drug, or comparing outcome between men and women, both of whom received the same treatment. This process of dividing subjects into groups is known as stratification. This is a useful strategy when sample size is large and there is no need to carve up the study population into too many strata. The problem with

From: *Neuromuscular Disease: Evidence and Analysis in Clinical Neurology*
By: M. Benatar © Humana Press Inc., Totowa, NJ

too many strata is that the sample size within each stratum may become quite small and the reduced sample size impairs the precision with which estimates of outcome can be made. For example, to determine the prognostic significance of gender, smoking history, and asbestos exposure with regard to the risk of lung cancer, it would be necessary to stratify on each of these variables, i.e., to divide the data into 8 (2^3) strata. Another shortcoming of stratification is that the investigator ends up relying on only a subset of the data (rather than the entire data set) to determine outcome. To return to the example cited above, a comparison of outcome among male smokers with asbestos exposure with that among male smokers without asbestos exposure would involve using only a fraction of the entire data set. The limitations of stratification, however, may be overcome by using modeling (*see* "Regression Analysis" and "Survival Analysis").

3. REGRESSION ANALYSIS

Regression is an analytic technique that entails the fitting of a simple equation to observed (measured) data points. There are a number of different forms of regression analysis, with linear and logistic regression being the two that are most commonly used. For any regression analysis we have a response variable (sometimes known as the dependent variable) as well as at least one predictor variable (also known as the independent variable). Because one of the goals of regression analysis is to determine the extent to which the response variable is predicted by the independent variables, it should be clear why this analytic technique is so relevant to the study of prognosis.

The term "modeling" is sometimes used to describe regression analysis. The reason for this is that regression involves the development of a model that best summarizes and explains the observed (measured) data. The model building process requires that the investigator determine the optimal combination of independent variables that best fit or describe the data. For linear regression, the least squares method is used to determine the best fit and for logistic regression, the maximum likelihood method is used. The details of these methods will be explained elsewhere in this chapter, but for now it will suffice to understand that these forms of regression each employ a different mathematical formula to determine the best fit of the data. Of course, linear and logistic regression differ in other respects as well. In linear regression, the outcome variable is a normally distributed continuous variable. In logistic regression, the outcome variable is a binomially distributed dichotomous variable.

To develop a better understand these analytic techniques, we shall now consider examples of both linear and logistic regression. The examples provided are theoretical because the necessary data to develop these models are not available.

3.1. Linear Regression

Suppose we are faced with a patient who has amyotrophic lateral sclerosis (ALS) with some impairment of respiratory function that we have quantified by measuring the forced vital capacity (FVC). The patient would like to know the rate at which his respiratory muscle function is likely to decline and how long it will be before he is faced with the need for a ventilator. The outcome or response variable that we would like to predict, therefore, is the FVC. FVC is a continuous variable and, based on the assumption that values for FVC are normally distributed, we can use linear regression to predict the rate with which we expect FVC to decline. In order to develop a linear regression model to predict FVC, we need to study FVC in a large cohort of patients with ALS and to gather information about the variables which we think might be useful in determining FVC. These variables might include age, gender, duration of disease, and site of onset of disease (bulbar vs limb).

For the purpose of illustrating the method of linear regression, we shall consider only a single variable (e.g., duration of disease). Consider the following scatter plot of a hypothetical data set (Graph 4.1)

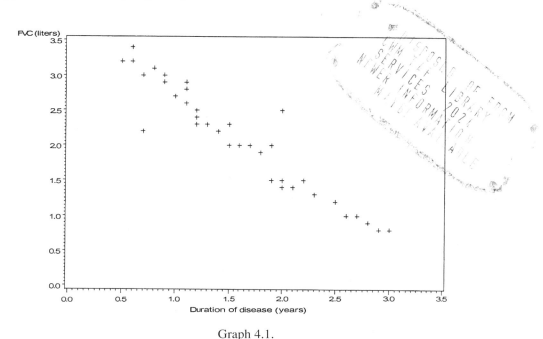

Graph 4.1.

Linear regression involves determining the equation for a straight line that best fits this data. The equation will take the form $y = \beta_0 + \beta_1 X$

where y = predicted FVC
       X = duration of disease (years)
       β_0 = intercept (value of y when $X = 0$)
       β_1 = slope of the straight line

As noted before, the least squares method is used to determine the best fit straight line. "Best fit" is defined as the line that produces the smallest square distance from the mean (i.e., the line that produces the "least square" distance from the mean).

As illustrated in Graph 4.2, the determination of the least square involves computing the sum of square distance of each data point from the extrapolated line. One can imagine extrapolating a number of different lines, calculating the sum of the square distance of each data point from the line and then comparing the sum values obtained for each line. The line that produces the smallest sum of these square values represents the linear regression line with the least squares (i.e., best fit).

Linear regression analysis of the data set used to derive this scatter plot yields the following best-fit equation for a straight line: FVC = 3.77 – (1.03 × disease duration).

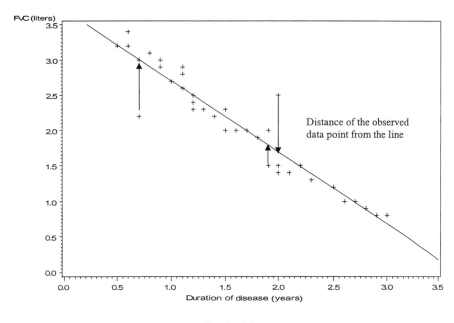

Graph 4.2

The value 1.03 represents the slope of the regression line. The interpretation of this value is that the FVC declines by 1.03 L per each 1-year increase in disease duration.

Before accepting this model, however, we need ask two further questions. The first is, "how well does the model describe the data?" Put another way, we need to ask how much of the variability in the data is explained by the model. We can obtain a partial answer to this question by inspecting the scatter plot with the superimposed liner regression line and ask how close the observed data points lie to the regression line. The closer the data points are to the line, the better the fit. Linear regression provides a numerical estimation of the extent to which the model explains the variability in the data. This is known as the R-square value. In the hypothetical data presented here, the R-square value is 0.88, indicating that the regression line explains 88% of the variability in the data.

The second question we must answer is, "how strong a relationship is there between the predictor variable and the outcome variable?" The slope estimate provides an answer to this question. The larger the absolute value of the slope estimate, the better the independent variable predicts the response variable. To understand why, remember that the slope value represents the magnitude of the change in the y-variable (FVC) per unit change in the x-variable (yearly increment in disease duration).

Armed with these data, we can now return to our patient with newly diagnosed ALS whose FVC is measured as 3.5 L. We have established that the model is a good one in that duration of disease explains most of the variation in the values of FVC and that disease duration is a good predictor of FVC. We can use the data from this model to estimate that it will take approximately 3 years for our patient's FVC to fall below the 1-L mark.

Multivariate linear regression is really just an extension of the univariate method described above. For multivariate linear regression, the model contains more than one variable. Thus $y = \beta_0 + \beta_1 X_1 + \beta_2 X_2 + \beta_3 X_3$, where X_1, X_2 and X_3 may represent duration of disease, age, and site of disease onset. β_1, β_2, and β_3 represent the slope estimates for each of these variables. The slope estimate for each individual variable is calculated while the other variables remain constant, which is to say that the other variables have been controlled. Multivariate analysis allows the investigator to determine the relative predictive value of different variables and to include in the final model only those variables that have meaningful predictive value.

3.2. Logistic Regression

Consider the example of the patient with newly diagnosed ALS who asks about her risk of death over the ensuing few years. We would like, therefore, to know the risk of death and whether this risk is modified by any particular variables such as age, gender, or the site of disease onset (limb vs bulbar). The outcome death is dichotomous and so linear regression is not suitable. Instead we turn to logistic regression.

For the purposes of illustrating the method of logistic regression, we shall consider only a single variable (e.g., age at onset of disease). In logistic regression, we directly model the log of the odds of an event, in this case death, but we can always use this information to determine the risk (probability) of the event. The logistic equation takes the following form.

Log odds = Exp $(\beta_0 + \beta_1 X_1)$

Instead of using the least squares method to determine the best fit for the data as we did for linear regression, we use the maximum likelihood function to determine the best fit for the data when doing logistic regression. Likelihood may be defined as the probability of observing the data that was observed and the goal is to find the model that maximizes this likelihood. The description of the maximum likelihood function that follows is not essential to understanding logistic regression, but is presented here for those who are more mathematically minded. Others may simply skip this section.

To illustrate the maximum likelihood function, consider the following small hypothetical dataset in which the variable death is coded as 1 for those who died during the 3-year study period and as 0 for those who did not die during the 3-year study period.

Age at onset	Death
63	1
35	0
56	1
58	1
39	0

In order to calculate the likelihood function, it should be recalled that the probability of death is represented by the expression

$$\frac{Exp(\beta_0 + \beta_1)}{1 + Exp(\beta_0 + \beta_1)}$$

and the probability of survival is represented

by the expression $\dfrac{1}{1 + Exp(\beta_0 + \beta_1)}$.

Likelihood =

$$\left[\frac{e^{(\beta_0 + 63\beta_1)}}{1 + e^{(\beta_0 + 63\beta_1)}}\right]\left[\frac{1}{1 + e^{(\beta_0 + 35\beta_1)}}\right]\left[\frac{e^{(\beta_0 + 56\beta_1)}}{1 + e^{(\beta_0 + 56\beta_1)}}\right]\left[\frac{e^{(\beta_0 + \beta 58_1)}}{1 + e^{(\beta_0 + 58\beta_1)}}\right]\left[\frac{1}{1 + e^{(\beta_0 + 39\beta_1)}}\right]$$

The computer will try multiple iterations of β_0 and β_1 and will present final values for the logistic model by selecting the combination of β_0 and β_1 that maximize this likelihood function.

Consider now a slightly larger data set constructed similarly to the small data set illustrated above, for which the maximum likelihood function returns the following results.

Parameter	DF	Estimate	Std. Error	Wald Chi-Square	Pr > ChiSq
Intercept	1	4.9774	2.3435	4.5111	0.0337
Age at onset	1	−0.0917	0.0423	4.6949	0.0303

To apply these results, we return to the logistic equation : Log odds = Exp $(\beta_0 + \beta_1 X_1)$ β_0 is the estimate of the intercept and β_1 is the estimate of the coefficient for X_1. Substituting these values, we obtain the formula:

Log odds = Exp [4.9774 −(0.0917 × age at onset)]

We can now use this formula to estimate the log odds of death for a person diagnosed with ALS at, for example, the age of 40.

$$\text{Log odds} = Exp\left[4.9774 - (0.0917 \times 40)\right]$$
$$\text{Log odds} = Exp(1.3094)$$
$$\text{Odds} = 3.7$$
$$\text{Risk} = \frac{\text{odds}}{1 + \text{odds}} = \frac{3.7}{1 + 3.7} = 0.66$$

There is, therefore, a 66% risk of death. For this estimate to have meaning, we have to know the time period over which this risk applies. To know this, we must return to the study in which the data was gathered for the logistic model. We see that death was determined over a 3-year study period. The 3-year risk of death, therefore, for a person diagnosed with ALS at the age of 40 is 66%.

Multivariate logistic regression is no more complicated. If additional variables are included in the model, then the logistic equation expands to accommodate them as follows:

Log odds = Exp ($\beta_0 + \beta_1X_1 + \beta_2X_2 + \beta_3X_3$, etc.)

The algorithm to maximize the likelihood function will now return estimates for each of the β's (coefficients). If X_1, X_2 and X_3 represent age at onset, gender, and site of disease onset, respectively, with gender coded 1 for males and 0 for females, and site of disease onset coded 0 for limb and 1 for bulbar onset, we can use the estimates of the coefficients to determine the 3-year probability of death for a 40-yr old man with bulbar onset, a 56-yr-old woman with limb onset disease, or any other combination of these predictor variables.

3.3. Conclusion

From the examples provided here, it should be clear that linear and logistic regression are very powerful analytic tools that can be used to determine prognosis, provided, of course, that adequate studies of the outcome of interest using a wide range of predictor variables have been performed. As will become evident through the material presented in this book, relatively few studies of the prognosis of neuromuscular disorders have been done using these analytic techniques.

4. SURVIVAL ANALYSIS

Survival analysis describes the analytic techniques that are applicable to data in which the outcome variable is "time until an event occurs." The event may represent death, diagnosis of disease, relapse from remission, or any other dichotomous event. The term "survival time" is used in a generic sense to describe the duration of follow-up from study entry even though it does not always really describe survival time.

The concepts of the "survival" and the "hazard" are central to an understanding of survival analysis. Survival is the complement of risk and can be calculated using the formula:

survival = 1 – risk.

Whereas risk describes the probability of an event up until a specified time point *(t)*, survival describes the probability of survival beyond *t*.

The "hazard function" is quite a bit more difficult to understand. In many respects, hazard can be thought of as a "rate" in that it describes the probability of the outcome event over a very short time period. The probability described by the hazard function is conditional in so far as it reflects the probability of the outcome event given survival until time *t*. The hazard function may be calculated using the formula:

$$h(t) = \lim \Delta t \to 0 \frac{P(t \leq T < t + \Delta t \,|\, T \geq t)}{\Delta t}$$

What this formula specifies is that the hazard function is calculated using a very short time interval (i.e., Δt approaches zero) and that it reflects the probability of an event during this short time interval (between t and $t + \Delta t$). The term "$|T \geq t$" describes the conditional probability "given that the subject has already survived beyond time t." We shall return to the concept of hazard under "Cox Proportional Hazards Regression."

To understand the utility of survival analysis, consider the hypothetical data set presented in the previous section, which examined the risk of death from ALS. It may not always be the case that all subjects are enrolled in a study at the same time, and so a study that lasts for 3 years may include 3-year follow-up for only those patients who were enrolled very early on. Shorter periods of follow-up (e.g., 1–2 years) will likely be available for the other subjects who were enrolled over the course of the 3-year study. Similarly, some subjects who were enrolled may have been lost to follow-up, with there being no knowledge of whether they have died or remain alive. The elegance of survival analysis is that it allows the investigator to utilize all of the available follow-up data. To understand why this is the case, consider the hypothetical data set in Graph 4.3.

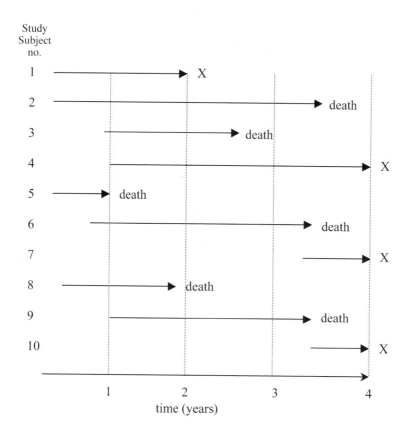

Graph 4.3

In Graph 4.3, X indicates that the subject was censored. A subject is censored when the event of interest (in this case, death) does not occur. A subject may be censored either because of loss to follow-up or because the subject survives to the end of the study period without the event of interest occurring. In this example, death occurred in subjects 2, 3, 5,

6, 8, and 9. Subject 1 was lost to follow-up after 2 years, and subjects 4, 7, and 10 survived until the end of the study. The data from this study may be summarized as follows:

Subject number	Survival time (yr)	Event (1)/censored (0)
1	2	0
2	3.5	1
3	1.5	1
4	3	0
5	1	1
6	2.5	1
7	0.8	0
8	1.5	1
9	2.5	1
10	0.5	0

Each subject, therefore, is able to contribute some "survival time" to the study, even athough subjects entered and left the study at varying time points. Survival analysis, therefore, provides a very powerful tool that enables the investigator to make full use of the data. Having acquired data of the sort outlined in the table above, the investigator may construct a survival curve and/or perform Cox modeling to estimate the survival and hazard functions (do not worry if you do not know what these are—they are described under "Survival Curves" and "Cox Proportional Hazards Regression").

4.1. Survival Curves

Two commonly used techniques for constructing survival curves are the Kaplan-Meier and the Life Tables methods. Kaplan-Meier survival analysis requires individual event-time data such as that provided in the table above. The goal is to construct a series of follow-up periods that are demarcated by the occurrence of an event and to estimate the proportion of subjects at risk for each time period and the proportion of subjects who survive each time period. The basic method is illustrated below.

1. Arrange subjects in order of increasing survival times:

Subject no.	Survival time	Event/censored
10	0.5	0
7	0.5	0
5	1.0	1
3	1.5	1
8	1.5	1
1	2.0	0
6	2.5	0
9	2.5	1
4	3.0	0
2	3.5	1

2. Construct a table indicating the time periods, number at risk, and number of events:

Time	No. at risk	Events	Censored	No. surviving	Probability survival	Cumulative survival
$0 < t \leq 1$	10	0	2	10	1.0	1.0
$1 < t \leq 1.5$	8	1	0	7	0.88	$1 \times 0.88 = 0.88$
$1.5 < t \leq 2.5$	7	2	1	5	0.7	$0.88 \times 0.7 = 0.6$
$2.5 < t \leq 3.5$	4	1	2	3	0.75	$0.75 \times 0.6 = 0.45$
$t \geq 3.5$	1	1	0	0	0	0

3. Construct a Survival Curve (*see* Graph 4.4).

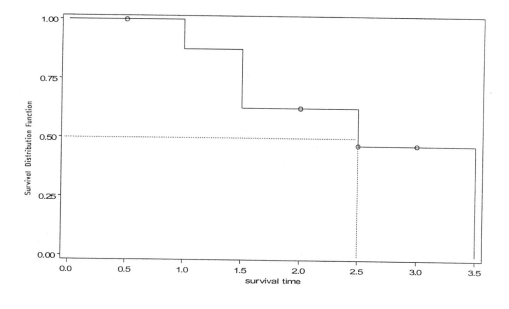

Graph 4.4

In Graph 4.4, each vertical step represents an event (death). The circles (○) represent censored subjects. It is important to note that the estimates of survival at later time periods are based on fewer subjects, the implication of which is reduced precision with which these estimates are made.

The Life Tables method for estimating survival (and generating survival curves) has many similarities to the Kaplan-Meier method. The primary difference is the use of larger time intervals that are not determined by every event as in the Kaplan-Meier method. For this reason, it is computationally simpler, but this consideration is of little significance in the computer era.

The median survival is one estimate of prognosis. As shown by the dotted line, 50% of patients with ALS are still alive at 2.5 years. The Kaplan-Meier and Life Tables methods can be used to evaluate the prognostic value of particular variables. For example, to investigate the prognostic value of gender would simply require the construction of two survival curves (using the same approach as outlined previously), one for each gender.

There are a number of methods for determining whether two survival curves are different. One approach is to simply "eyeball" the curves and use intuition to decide whether they are meaningfully different. Another approach is to compare the median survival for each group. The third technique involves the use of the Log-Rank statistic. The details of this statistical test will not be reviewed here, but suffice it to say that this statistic provides an overall measure of whether the two survival curves differ. Meaningful differences between the survival curves would indicate that gender is of prognostic significance.

4.2. Cox Proportional Hazards Regression

The strategy outlined in the previous section for comparing the prognostic value of a particular variable (e.g., gender) represents a form of a stratified analysis—the data are separated into two strata based on gender and the survival function of men and women are examined separately. One problem with stratification is that it becomes increasingly difficult as the investigator wishes to examine the effects of an increasing number of covariates. Whereas examination of the effect of gender requires only two strata, an investigation into the effect of gender and site of disease onset (limb vs bulbar) will require four strata. Increasing the number of strata has the effect of reducing the effective sample size within each stratum, and this reduces the precision with which the effect of each variable can be estimated. Modeling offers a solution to this problem, and the Cox Proportional Hazards model is a regression technique that is commonly used for the analysis of survival data. The utility of Cox modeling is that it permits estimation of hazard and survival as a function of multiple covariates

To understand this modeling technique it is necessary to understand what is meant by the terms "hazard" and "proportional hazard." We have already discussed "hazard." Briefly, "hazard" describes the instantaneous rate of the event of interest given survival until a particular time. It is calculated as the conditional probability of the event during a very short period of time (between time t and time $t + \Delta t$) given that the subject has already survived to time t.

One of the advantages of Cox modeling is that it is not necessary to know the hazard of the outcome. However, this analytic technique does require that the hazard of the outcome in the two groups of interest remain proportional over time. To understand what is meant by this, we return to the example of the analysis of survival of ALS patients. Imagine that we wish to compare the hazard of death between men and women with ALS. To use the Cox modeling technique, the ratio of the hazard of death in men to the hazard of death in women must be constant over time. This is not to say that the hazard must be constant over time, but rather that the ratio of the hazards in the two groups is constant. There are a variety of methods that may be used to determine whether this proportionality assumption is met and, hence, whether Cox modeling can legitimately be used, but the details of these methods are beyond the scope of this chapter. For now, it will suffice to understand what is meant by the term proportional hazards.

The Cox model takes the following form: $h(t) = h_0(t)e^{\beta_1 X_1 + \beta_2 X_2}$

where $h(t)$ is the hazard at time t

$h_0(t)$ is the baseline hazard

X_1 and X_2 are the prognostic variables of interest (e.g., age, gender, race)

β_1 and β_2 are the estimates of the regression coefficients

The best fit for the Cox model is determined using a maximum likelihood function that is analogous (although different) to that used in logistic regression.

The results of Cox modeling are typically presented in the form of a hazards ratio (HR). The HR is simply the ratio of two hazards and is derived from the formula:

$$HR = \frac{h_0(t)\,e^{\beta_1 X_1 + \beta_2 X_2}}{h_0(t)\,e^{\beta_1 X_1 + \beta_2 X_2}}$$

It can be seen that the baseline hazard, $h_0(t)$, that is present in both the numerator and denominator will cancel (which is why it is not necessary to know the baseline hazard in order to calculate the HR).

To understand the final step involved in determining the HR, it is necessary to know how the data was coded. X_1, for example might represent gender (coded 0 for females and 1 for males), and X_2 might represent age (coded continuously). To calculate the HR comparing the hazard for a 30-year-old man to that of a 20-year-old woman, we simply substitute as follows:

$$HR = \frac{h_0(t)\,e^{\beta_1(1)X_1 + \beta_2 X_2(30)}}{h_0(t)\,e^{\beta_1(0)X_1 + \beta_2 X_2(20)}} = e^{\beta_1 + 10\beta_2}$$

In running the Cox model, the computer will have generated estimates for β_1 and β_2. These values are simply substituted into this equation and the HR is estimated.

5. CONCLUSION

In this chapter, we have examined the analytic techniques that are suitable for determining prognosis and for estimating the prognostic significance of potential predictor variables. Prognosis and prognostic variables are analogous to risk and risk factors and can be determined using the same sorts of study designs (case–control and follow-up) that are used to estimate risk. The choice of analytic technique for determining prognosis largely depends on the nature of the outcome variable. Linear regression is appropriate for continuous variables and logistic regression for dichotomous variables. Survival analysis and Cox proportional hazards modeling are well suited to studies in which the outcome variable is an estimate of time to an event.

II Spinal Cord, Anterior Horn Cell, and Nerve Roots

5 Amyotrophic Lateral Sclerosis

1. INTRODUCTION

Amyotrophic lateral sclerosis (ALS) is a degenerative disorder characterized by loss of motor neurons in the spinal cord, brainstem, and cerebral cortex. It is an uncommon disease with an incidence in the range of 1–2.5 cases per 100,000 population. Incidence increases with age and there is a slight male preponderance. The etiology is unknown, and the progression of the disease is almost uniformly relentless, resulting in death.

The term ALS is sometimes used interchangeably with motor neuron disease (MND) but, strictly speaking, MND is a broader term that encompasses a range of neurodegenerative disorders characterized by loss of motor neurons. When the dominant symptoms are related to speech and swallowing, the term "progressive bulbar atrophy" is used. "Progressive muscular atrophy" refers to an isolated lower motor neuron syndrome, and the designation "primary lateral sclerosis" is used when signs of upper motor neuron dysfunction predominate.

The diagnosis of ALS is not difficult when advanced, but may be challenging initially when the differential diagnosis is broad. As there are no biomarkers for the disease, the diagnosis remains a clinical one. It is important, therefore, to know something about the accuracy of the proposed diagnostic (El Escorial) criteria for ALS as well as the utility of paraclinical investigations, such as electromyography (EMG) in evaluating patients with suspected ALS. This is one major focus on this chapter, but attention is also paid to a number of important therapeutic issues, including the indications for and timing of placement of a percutaneous endoscopic gastrostomy (PEG) feeding tube. The chapter concludes with a discussion of the natural history of the disease with an emphasis on those factors that predict prognosis.

2. DIAGNOSIS

2.1. What Are the El Escorial Criteria for the Diagnosis of ALS?

The World Federation of Neurology convened a workshop at El Escorial in Spain in 1990 that led to the publication of the El Escorial criteria for the diagnosis of ALS *(1)*. According to these criteria, the diagnosis of ALS requires:

From: *Neuromuscular Disease: Evidence and Analysis in Clinical Neurology*
By: M. Benatar © Humana Press Inc., Totowa, NJ

A. The presence of:
- Evidence of lower motor neuron (LMN) degeneration (by clinical, electrophysiological or neuropathological examination);
- Evidence of upper motor neuron (UMN) degeneration (by clinical examination);
- Progressive spread of symptoms or signs within a region or to other regions (as determined by history or examination).

B. The absence of:
- Electrophysiological and pathological evidence of other disease processes that might explain the signs of LMN and/or UMN degeneration;
- Neuroimaging evidence of other disease processes that might explain the observed clinical and electrophysiological signs.

These criteria recognize four regions of the central nervous system (CNS)—bulbar, cervical, thoracic and lumbosacral. Progression of signs within a region and, even more importantly, progression of signs to involve other regions is a crucial feature for the clinical diagnosis of ALS. The clinical diagnosis may be made with varying degrees of certainty. Recognized categories include (a) clinically definite ALS, (b) clinically probable ALS, (c) clinically possible ALS and (d) clinically suspected ALS. Clinically definite ALS requires the presence of UMN and LMN dysfunction in three of the four regions of the CNS. Involvement of only two regions satisfies criteria for clinically probable ALS.

The role of electrophysiological studies in the diagnosis of ALS is to confirm LMN dysfunction in clinically affected regions, to detect electrophysiological evidence of LMN dysfunction in clinically uninvolved regions and to exclude other pathophysiological processes. No neuroimaging tests are required to positively support the diagnosis of ALS, but should be used to exclude other conditions that might cause UMN and/or LMN signs.

2.2. How Accurate Are These Criteria for the Diagnosis of ALS?

There are limited data available to answer this question. In one study, 32 patients were followed from the time of diagnosis to death, and the proportions of patients meeting the El Escorial criteria at diagnosis and shortly before death were compared (2). The El Escorial criteria shortly before death were used as the gold standard for the diagnosis of ALS. Eight of 32 patients (25%) in this study died without meeting the El Escorial criteria for definite or probable ALS (Table 5.1A). A larger prospective population-based study of the natural history of ALS in Ireland showed similar results (Table 5.1B) (3).

In each of these studies, the "gold standard" for the diagnosis of ALS was the clinical diagnosis shortly before death. This seems reasonable, given that the diagnosis is typically not in doubt at this advanced stage of the disease. The data from these two studies differ somewhat, but they both show that the sensitivity of these criteria for the diagnosis of ALS at the time of initial presentation is quite low, ranging from 31–57%. It is not possible to calculate the specificity, however, because neither study included any sort of control group.

2.3. How Useful Is EMG for the Diagnosis of ALS?

Nerve conduction studies and electromyography play an important role in the diagnostic work up of patients with suspected ALS. In general terms, these neurophysiological tests may be used to exclude other disease processes that may mimic ALS and may also be useful for demonstrating evidence for LMN pathology when the clinical findings are insufficient for the diagnosis.

Table 5.1A
Diagnostic Accuracy of the El Escorial Criteria

El Escorial category	Proportion of subjects with specified degree of diagnostic confidence	
	Time of diagnosis	Shortly before death
Definite	1 (3%)	8 (25%)
Probable	9 (28%)	16 (50%)
Possible	12 (38%)	5 (16%)
Suspected	10 (31%)	3 (9%)

Data from ref. 2.

Table 5.1B
Diagnostic Accuracy of the El Escorial Criteria

El Escorial category	Proportion of subjects with specified degree of diagnostic confidence	
	Time of diagnosis	Shortly before death
Definite	131 (34%)	179 (71%)
Probable	87 (23%)	49 (19%)
Possible	136 (36%)	32 (9%)
Suspected	29 (8%)	3 (1%)

Data from ref. 3.

Lambert proposed a series of criteria for the diagnosis of ALS in 1957 (revised in 1969), which required (1) normal sensory and motor nerve conduction studies (apart from slowing of conduction velocity that might accompany a markedly reduced motor response amplitude) and (2) the presence of ongoing denervation changes (fibrillations and positive sharp waves) as well as fasciculations in two of three (cranial, cervical, and lumbosacral) segments of the nervous system, and (3) the finding of chronic reinnervation changes. Lambert did not, however, specify the number of muscles in a given segment that should show ongoing denervation or chronic reinnervation changes in order for these criteria to be met. Nor did he specify whether chronic reinnervation changes should be required in more than one segment.

The El Escorial criteria for the diagnosis of ALS (initially proposed in 1991 and revised in 1997) are more specific (1). As with Lambert's criteria, El Escorial endorsed the idea that EMG may be used to demonstrate the presence of LMN pathology that is not clinically apparent. The requirements for demonstrating LMN pathology electromyographically, however, are more precisely defined and include the presence of both ongoing denervation and chronic reinnervation changes. For the cranial and thoracic segments, it is sufficient to show these abnormalities in a single muscle. For the cervical and lumbosacral segments, these changes should both be present in at least two muscles innervated by different roots and peripheral nerves.

There has been limited investigation of the diagnostic accuracy (sensitivity and specificity) of these criteria. The study by Behnia and Kelly (4) provides some insight into the sensitivity (true-positive rate) of Lambert's criteria, but does not inform on the specificity (true-negative rate) because there was no control group. This study included 133 patients

Table 5.2
Diagnostic Accuracy of Thoracic Paraspinal Electromyograph (EMG)

	ALS	OND	Totals
Abnormal TPSP EMG	43	2	45
Normal TPSP EMG	12	13	25
Totals	55	15	70

Data from ref. 5.

ALS, amyotrophic lateral sclerosis; OND, other neurological disease; TPSP, thoracic paraspinal muscles.

with ALS based on clinical presentation and results of electrodiagnostic testing. EMG was entirely normal in 5 patients and ongoing denervation changes were present in only a single segment in a further 30 patients (10 of whom had widespread chronic reinnervation changes and 13 of whom had denervation changes in the contralateral limb of the same segment). The sensitivity of Lambert's criteria, therefore was approximately 74%.

Although there have been no studies of the diagnostic accuracy of the El Escorial electrodiagnostic criteria, a number of studies have addressed the utility of specific findings such as the presence of ongoing denervation changes in thoracic paraspinal muscles (5) and the utility of needle examination of the sternocleidomastoid (6,7) and cranial muscles other than the tongue (8) for demonstrating involvement of the cranial segment.

The study by Kuncl and colleagues that examined the diagnostic utility of thoracic paraspinal EMG warrants some discussion (5). The authors indicate that they prospectively studied 76 patients referred for EMG with a suspected diagnosis of ALS. ALS was eventually diagnosed in 55 of these patients based on accepted clinical criteria and Lambert's EMG criteria without consideration given to paraspinal muscle findings (thus avoiding the problem of incorporation bias). They compared the EMG findings in the 55 patients with ALS to those in 54 patients with other neurological diseases (15 of these control patients seem to have been derived from the original cohort of patients referred for evaluation for possible ALS, but the authors do not report what happened to the remaining 6 patients). Thoracic paraspinal muscles were considered abnormal only if fibrillation potentials and/or positive sharp waves were clearly identified. With an average of 3.3 vertebral segments between T7-T10 examined, abnormalities were identified in 43 of 55 ALS patients (78%) and in 10 of 54 (19%) patients with other neurological disorders (cervical and lumbar spondylosis, peripheral neuropathy, myeloradiculopathy, and polymyositis). The sensitivity of abnormalities of thoracic paraspinal muscles was reduced to 67% if only 1–2 segments were examined. An attempt to estimate the specificity of the findings of abnormal thoracic paraspinal EMG abnormalities is limited by the incomplete presentation of data from the original 76 patients that were evaluated for suspected ALS. Based on these data (with the results from 6 patients with other neurological diseases omitted), the sensitivity of thoracic paraspinal muscle EMG for the diagnosis of ALS is 78% and the specificity is 87% (Table 5.2) (5).

Two studies have addressed the diagnostic utility of EMG examination of the sternocleidomastoid muscle (6,7). One study included 36 patients with ALS, 32 patients with cervical spondylotic myelopathy (CSM), and 33 patients in whom the diagnosis was originally unclear (29 of whom were subsequently diagnosed with ALS and 4 of whom were found to have CSM). In total, therefore, this study included 65 ALS patients and 36 CSM patients. Electromyographic abnormalities included the presence of fibrillations and/or positive sharp waves as well as neurogenic motor unit potentials; from the data reported, it is not possible to determine how many patients showed abnormal spontaneous activity and how many displayed neurogenic motor unit potentials. This study showed EMG of sternocleidomastoid had a sensitivity of 97% and a specificity of 100%. The inclusion of a large number of patients with already established ALS (spectrum bias) artificially elevated the estimate of sensitivity (6). In a second study that examined the diagnostic utility of EMG of sternocleidomastoid, Li and colleagues prospectively evaluated 21 newly diagnosed ALS patients with high ALS functional rating scores (ALFRS) indicating that the disease was mild in most patients (7). The control group in this study included healthy individuals and those known to have cervical spondylosis. For all patients (limb and bulbar onset) combined, they found a sensitivity of 57% and a specificity of 100% (7).

These two studies also provided data about the comparable utility of EMG examination of the sternocleidomastoid and the tongue (6,7). In the study by Kang and Fen, sensitivity of EMG of the tongue for the diagnosis of ALS was 63% (compared with 97% for the sternocleidomastoid), although again, this estimate may be inflated by the inclusion of patients with more advanced disease (6). In the study by Li and colleagues, the sensitivity of EMG of the tongue was 29% (compared with 57% for sternocleido-mastoid) (7). Among those patients with no bulbar symptoms at the time of EMG, the sensitivity of examination of sternocleidomastoid was 71% compared with 14% for examination of the tongue. Sensitivity of examination of these two muscles was comparable among patients with bulbar symptoms (7).

Finally, Preston and colleagues examined the relative sensitivities of facial, glossal, and masticatory muscles for the diagnosis of ALS (8). They studied 21 patients with ALS who had symptoms for an average of 18 months. The authors do not specify how far advanced the disease was in these patients, thus limiting application of these results to the diagnosis of ALS. Furthermore, this study did not include a control group, and so it is not possible to estimate specificities. The results of this study show that chronic reinnervation changes alone were quite common, ranging from 33% in the temporalis muscle to 67% in the tongue and 71% in the masseter (Table 5.3). Both ongoing denervation and chronic reinnervation changes in the same muscle, however, were relatively infrequent, being found in the tongue in only 29% of patients (and even less frequently in other muscles) (8).

3. TREATMENT

3.1. What Is the Role of Noninvasvive Positive Pressure Ventilation in Patients With ALS?

The current recommendation, based on the report of the Quality Standards Subcommittee of the American Academy of Neurology (AAN), is to consider noninvasive positive pressure ventilation (NPPV) when the forced vital capacity (FVC) falls to less than 50% of predicted (9). This recommendation, however, seems to be based on relatively little data.

Theoretically, the utility of NPPV might be evaluated from a number of perspectives. What effect does NPPV have on spirometric measures of respiratory muscle function? Does it alleviate the symptoms of respiratory insufficiency? How well is it tolerated and

Table 5.3
Sensitivity of Cranial Muscle Electromyography

Muscle examined	Denervation changes (fibrillations)	Reinnervation changes	Denervation and reinnervation
Tongue	38%	67%	29%
Masseter	19%	71%	19%
Temporalis	0%	33%	0%
Frontalis	25%	45%	14%
Mentalis	27%	64%	18%

Data from ref. 8.

does it improve the quality of life for patients with ALS? And finally, does NPPV improve survival in patients with ALS?

There are a limited number of studies that have attempted to address these questions, and each of the relevant studies is significantly limited by methodological quality (Table 5.4). Three studies were retrospective (10–12) and four were prospective (13–16). The choice of control groups varied substantially–usually, groups were chosen by default rather than in a prospectively planned fashion. One study was randomized, but did not report any results comparing outcome in the two groups (15). In three studies, the control group comprised those patients who could not tolerate (11,12) or who declined (16) NPPV. Recognizing these various limitations, most studies reported outcome in terms of the impact of NPPV on survival or quality of life. Only two studies reported outcome using spirometric measures, with one showing a slower rate of decline of FVC following initiation of NPPV compared with that prior to initiation of NPPV (16) and another showing slower rates of decline in FVC among those patients with greater tolerance for NPPV (11).

In answer to the questions posed in the introduction to this section, there really are no data to indicate that NPPV alleviates the symptoms of respiratory insufficiency; it is tolerated by a sizable proportion of patients with declining respiratory function, it does appear to improve the quality of life, particularly with regard to the vitality and cognitive scores of the SF-36, and probably does improve survival. All of these conclusions, however, should be tempered by the very limited quality of the available data.*

3.2. What Are the Risks and Benefits of PEG Placement in Patients With ALS?

A significant proportion of patients with ALS and bulbar dysfunction develop dysphagia manifesting as coughing and choking with attempted eating and drinking. The potential consequences include dehydration, malnutrition, and aspiration pneumonia. The options for enteral nutritional support include placement of a nasogastric (NG) feeding tube and placement of a PEG feeding tube. Important questions that arise relate to the timing and safety of placement of a PEG feeding tube as well as the utility of a PEG feeding tube in terms of preventing malnutrition and prolonging survival.

---

*The results of a randomized controlled trial of NPPV have been published while this book has been in press. See Burke et al. Lancet Neurology 2006; 5:140–147 for details.

Table 5.4
The Role of Noninvasive Positive Pressure Ventilation in Patients With Amyotrophic Lateral Sclerosis (ALS)

Study design	Symptoms	Quality of life	Spirometry	Tolerance	Survival	Ref.
Prospective n = 20 Study subjects—those with abnormal blood gas 1st 10 assigned palliative Rx and 2nd 10 NPPV	Not reported	Improvement, but not significant (but small sample size)	No significant differences	Not reported	Improved % alive at 3 yr –74% (NPPV) vs 0% (controls)	Pinto (13)
Retrospective Tracheostomy-IPPV vs nasal-IPPV	Not reported	All patients were glad they chose nasal-IPPV	Not reported	Poorly tolerated in bulbar patients	Nasal IPPV patients survived 6–64 mo	Cazzolli (10)
Retrospective n = 22 Patients offered BiPAP if FVC<50% or symptoms of respiratory failure. Three groups: (1) BiPAP >4 h/d (2) BiPAP <4 h/d (3) no BiPAP	Not reported	Not reported	Slower rate of FVC decline in group 1 (–3.5%/mo) vs group 2 (–5.9%/mo) & group 3 (–8.3%/mo)	31% group 1 26% group 2 43% group 3	Improved Average survival was 14 mo (group) 1, 7 mo (group 2) and 6 mo (group 3)	Kleopa (11)
Retrospective n = 47 Two groups (1) tolerant of NPPV (2) intolerant of NPPV	Not reported	Improved	No effect	Tolerated in 48.9% of patients	Improved median survival 20 mo (tolerant) 5 mo (intolerant)	Aboussouan (12)

(continued)

Table 5.4
The Role of Noninvasive Positive Pressure Ventilation in Patients With Amyotrophic Lateral Sclerosis (ALS)

Study design	Symptoms	Quality of life	Spirometry	Tolerance	Survival	Ref.
Prospective Randomized—early BiPAP vs BiPAP when FVC < 50% Blinded	Improved in 5 of 6 patients	Improved SF-36 vitality score in 5 of 6 patients	Not reported	Not Reported	Not Reported	Jackson (15)
Prospective n = 27 BiPAP for symptoms of sleep disordered breathing with evidence of respiratory muscle weakness, hypoventilation and sleep disordered breathing (n = 16) Controls—ALS patients with normal diaphragm function (n = 11)	Not reported	Improved vitality score of SF-36	Not reported	Not reported	Not reported	Lyall (14)
Prospective n = 22 NPPV offered to 17 patients for symptoms, ↑pCO$_2$,↓ nocturnal O$_2$ sat.—15 accepted vs 2 declined (controls)	Improved (Epworth Sleepiness Scale)	Improved cognitive function on SF-36	Slowed rate of decline of FVC: −2.5%/mo (pre-NPPV) −1.1%/mo (post-NPPV)	Poor compliance/ tolerance in those in bulbar dysfunction	Longer survival in NPPV group, but very small	Bourke (16)

NPPV, noninvasive positive pressure ventilation; IPPV, intermittent positive pressure ventilation; BiPAP, bilevel positive airway pressure; FVC, forced vital capacity.

The ALS practice parameter published by the Quality Standards Subcommittee of the AAN recommends placement of a PEG feeding tube when the initial, more conservative management of dysphagia fails, with the advice to place the PEG tube before the FVC falls to less than 50% of the predicted normal value in order to minimize peri-procedural complications (9). The evidence supporting this recommendation, however, is somewhat limited.

The superiority of a PEG feeding tube rather than a nasogastric tube in patients with ALS was shown in a controlled trial of 40 patients with neurogenic dysphagia (of which 16 patients had ALS). These subjects were randomized to receive nutritional enteral support either via an NG tube or via a PEG tube (17). The primary outcome was the frequency of treatment failure (defined as failure to place the tube, excessively frequent blockages of the tube, or patient refusal to continue with efforts at tube placement). The volume of food delivered was a secondary outcome measure. The failure rate among those randomized to receive an NG tube was 95%, compared with zero failures in the PEG tube group (17). Those with a PEG tube successfully received 93% of the target feed volume, compared with 55% in the NG tube group. The complication rate was low, with two patients developing an aspiration pneumonia and one patient developing an infection at the PEG tube site. These results indicate that a PEG feeding tube can be placed safely in patients with ALS, and that it offers more effective delivery of enteral nutritional support as evidenced by feed volume administered and weight gain.

The remaining literature evaluating the safety of PEG feeding tubes, the potential benefits regarding improved nutrition, and improved quality of life and survival as well as the appropriate timing of PEG tube placement with regard to measurements of FVC is made up entirely of retrospective and uncontrolled studies.

In the one study of 68 ALS patients who were referred for enteral nutritional support, subjects were divided into two groups—those eligible and those ineligible for PEG tube placement. Eligibility was determined by a combination of patient preference, the results of spirometry (FVC > 1 L), and blood gas analysis (pCO_2 > 45 mmHg). Among the 55 patients eligible, a PEG tube was successfully placed in 49. There were no differences in survival between the PEG-eligible and-ineligible patients, and the mean FVC at the time of referral for PEG tube placement was 46% of predicted (Table 5.5) (18).

Conflicting results were reported in another study in which a PEG feeding tube was offered to 69 ALS patients with dysphagia and weight loss of greater than 5% body weight (19). Thirty-four patients accepted PEG tube placement (it was successful in 31), and 35 declined (controls). Body mass index and survival were significantly better among patients who elected to have a PEG tube placed than among controls. The mean survival time (onset of symptoms to death) was 38 months among those with a PEG compared with 30 months among controls (19). Among the PEG tube patients, survival was better among those with an FVC > 50% predicted (19).

Kasarskis and colleagues reported the experience with PEG tube placement in ALS patients who participated in the BDNF and CNTF trials (20). It is important to note that these studies were not designed to address the indications for and timing of PEG tube placement. The results are simply descriptive of the characteristics of the patients in these trials who had a PEG tube placed (Table 5.5). They noted that in the BDNF trial, post-PEG mortality was related to the degree of FVC reduction, arguing that PEG tubes should be placed sooner rather than later. On the other hand, post-PEG mortality was higher in

Table 5.5

Ventilatory Status and Outcome of Amyotrophic Lateral Sclerosis Patients Undergoing Percutaneous Endoscopic Gastrostomy (PEG) Placement

	Mathus-Vliegen (18)	Mazzini (19)	BDNF trial (20)	CNTF trial (20)	Chio (30)	Gregory (21)
Sample size	55	31	136	36	50	33
Mean age	58.8	60.9	59.2	56.3	61.7	–
FVC at time of PEG placement	45.8%	30.6%	53%	41.6%	68.9%	35.7%
24-h mortality	3.6%	0	0.7%	0	0	0
30-d mortality	11.5%	9.7%	9.6%	6.3%	2%	6%
Survival (days)	122	393	260	151	185	204

FVC, forced vital capacity.

the BDNF trial (9.6%) compared with that in the CNTF trial (6.3%), and mean FVC was higher in the latter study (53% compared with 41.6% in the CNTF study).

In a more recent publication, Gregory et al. described their experience with PEG tube placement in 33 patients with FVC less than 50% predicted (21). Each patient received respiratory support with NPPV and oxygen through a nasal mask while continuous pulse oximetry was recorded. A PEG tube was successfully placed endoscopically in 29 patients and the remaining 4 required surgical placement. The mean FVC at the time of PEG tube placement in these patients was 35.7% (Table 5.5). Although not directly comparable with the results from other studies that required higher FVC values, the peri-procedural mortality rates and median survival times do not seem to differ significantly (Table 5.5).

In summary, PEG tube placement in patients with ALS seems to offer the advantage of improved enteral nutritional support (17), which may result in improved body mass index (19). Whether survival is also improved is more controversial, because the published data are contradictory (18,19). The optimal timing (with regard to FVC) of PEG tube placement remains unclear. Although the AAN has recommended PEG tube placement before the FVC falls below 50% predicted, the published (retrospective and uncontrolled data) is somewhat contradictory with some studies suggesting increased mortality among those with lower FVC (20) whereas others have suggested that a PEG tube may be safely placed in ALS patients with FVC closer to 35% predicted, as long as noninvastive ventilatory support is provided (21). A definitive answer to these questions will likely require a prospective randomized controlled study.

3.3. What Are the Benefits of Riluzole for Patients With ALS?

The efficacy of riluzole in the treatment of patients with ALS has been examined in three prospective placebo-controlled trials (22–24). In the first study, by Bensimon et al., 155 patients with probable or definite ALS were randomized to receive either placebo (n = 78) or 100 mg riluzole per day (n = 77). Randomization was stratified according to whether disease was of limb (n = 123) or bulbar onset (n = 32). The primary outcome measures were tracheostomy-free survival and functional status after 12 months of treatment. No patients were lost to follow-up.

Table 5.6
Effects of Riluzole on 12-Month Survival in Patients
With Amyotrophic Lateral Sclerosis

Relative risk of death at 12 mo[a]	95% Confidence interval	Reference
0.61	0.39 – 0.97	Bensimon (22)
0.71	0.54 – 0.92	Lacomblez (23)
0.99	0.79 – 1.25	Bensimon (24)
0.78	0.65 – 0.92	Miller (25)

[a]Comparing risk of death in riluzole-treated patients with risk in placebo-treated patients.

The second trial of riluzole was similar in design to the first, but incorporated a dose-ranging design as well as a longer period of follow-up and a larger number of patients (23). Patients were stratified according to limb or bulbar onset, and the design was double-blind and placebo-controlled. A total of 959 patients were enrolled (295 with bulbar onset and 664 with limb onset) and randomized to receive placebo or 50 mg, 100 mg or 200 mg of riluzole. Tracheostomy-free survival (at 18 months) was again chosen as the primary outcome measure.

The third randomized controlled trial (24), which was also similar to the first in design, was carried out in parallel with the second (23) in order to accommodate those patients who were ineligible for participation in the second study (i.e., patients older than 75 years and those with more advanced disease, as evidenced by FVC less than 60% predicted or progression of disease over longer than 5 years). The dose of riluzole in this study was again 100 mg per day. One hundred sixty-eight patients were enrolled, a smaller number than required for the study to be adequately powered to detect an effect of riluzole. Randomization appeared inadequate because there were a variety of differences between the riluzole and placebo groups at study entry.

Tracheostomy-free survival was the primary outcome measure in all three studies. The results of the three individual studies as well as the combined results from a Cochrane collaboration meta-analysis are summarized in the Table 5.6. A survival advantage at 12 months was observed in the first two studies, but not in the third study, which included older patients and those with more advanced disease.

In the first study, by Bensimon and colleagues, separate analysis of the bulbar-and limb-onset groups showed that the 12-month survival advantage conferred by riluzole was entirely due to the improved survival in the bulbar-onset group. There was no significant difference in the endpoint of tracheostomy-free survival at 1 year in the subgroup of patients with limb-onset disease (22). This discrepancy was not observed in the larger study, by Lacomblez and colleagues (23).

In the Cochrane meta-analysis, the authors calculated the difference in survival between those treated with placebo and those who received 100 mg riluzole. Data were pooled for all patients at all time periods. The increase in median survival for the riluzole group was only 2 months (25). The absolute reduction in risk of death was 9%, with a number-needed-to-treat of 11 in order to delay death until after 12 months.

Other outcome measures included muscle strength and modified Norris scale scores. A beneficial effect on muscle strength was observed in the first trial but not in the subsequent two, and meta-analysis failed to show any overall benefit *(25)*. No individual study showed a beneficial effect on bulbar function using the Norris scale, but a small benefit was observed in the meta-analysis. A small positive benefit in limb function was observed in the second study *(23)* and also in the meta-analysis *(25)*. Any effect on quality of life is more difficult to discern based on the published data, with the authors of the Cochrane review concluding that patients treated with riluzole remained longer in a more moderately affected health state than did placebo-treated patients.

The overall conclusion seems to be that Riluzole 100 mg per day prolongs life by about 2 months in younger patients in the early stages of ALS. Benefit has not been show for older patients, those with more advanced disease, and those with disease duration of more than 5 years, although further study is needed.

3.4. Is Vitamin E of Any Benefit to Patients With ALS?

This question was addressed in a large multicenter study conducted in France *(26)*. Two hundred eighty-nine patients with probable or definite ALS (according to El Escorial criteria) were randomized to receive either the combination of α-tocopherol (500 mg twice daily) and riluzole (50 mg twice daily) or the combination of placebo and riluzole. Changes in the functional status as determined by modified Norris limb scale scores were used as the primary outcome measure of efficacy. Secondary outcome measures included tracheostomy-free survival, muscle strength (measured with manual muscle testing), and the ALS Health State Scale (AHSS) score. The study was powered to detect a seven-point difference in Norris limb scale scores between the two treatment groups. Analysis was performed on the intention-to-treat principle. One hundred forty-six patients did not complete 12 months of follow-up and the "last observation carried forward" method was used to impute the missing data *(26)*. Norris limb scale scores were no different between the two treatment groups at the end of the 12-month period of follow-up and the Kaplan-Meier curves (compared with the log rank test) showed no difference in survival between the two treatment groups. A statistically significant difference (favoring the α-tocopherol group) was found ($p = 0.045$) between the proportions of patients with mild and severe AHSS scores, suggesting the possibility of some effect of α-tocopherol in slowing progression of the disease *(26)*.

This study was reported as being double-blind, but there is no discussion of the methods used to ensure patient and observer blinding. It is also not clear whether treatment allocation was concealed. Finally, a significant proportion of subjects (51%) did not complete the 12-month period of treatment and follow-up, which necessitated data imputation. The publication describing the results of this study does not include an analysis or discussion of the impact of these losses to follow-up on outcome *(26)*. The conclusion from this study is that vitamin E is not beneficial in the treatment of ALS. The finding that fewer patients in the α-tocopherol group progressed from AHSS stage A (mild disease) to stage B (more severe disease) should be interpreted with caution, given that it was a secondary outcome measure, that these results only barely reached statistical significance, and that the authors do not report confidence intervals for the precision with which the study estimated the benefit of α-tocopherol for this outcome measure.

Table 5.7
Natural History of Amyotrophic Lateral Sclerosis

Median survival (onset)	Median survival (diagnosis)	3-yr survival (onset)	3-yr survival (diagnosis)	5yr survival (onset)	5yr survival (diagnosis)	Ref.
32 mo	19 mo				7%	31
	16 mo				25%	32
36 mo						33
30 mo	14 mo					34
	16.5 mo					35
	21 mo		29%		4%	36
24 mo						37
30.5 mo	19 mo	40.5%	29%	24.7%	20%	38

3.5. Is There Evidence for Benefit of Any Other Antioxidants for Patients With ALS?

This question has been addressed by a number of randomized controlled trials and was the subject of a recent Cochrane systematic review in which 12-month survival was used as the primary outcome measure (27). This meta-analysis included the results of three studies—one examining the efficacy of α-tocopherol (26) (see previous section), one examining the efficacy of acetylcysteine (28), and another the combination of L-methionine, vitamin E, and selenium (29)—and found no beneficial effect on the primary outcome measure. The authors of this review did note, however, that the literature on the use antioxidants is generally of poor quality and underpowered to show a clinically meaningful effect (27).

4. PROGNOSIS

4.1. What Is the Natural History of ALS?

The natural history of ALS is one of almost inexorable progression culminating in death. In studies of the natural history of ALS, it may be important to make a distinction between population-based studies and those that have examined patients at referral centers, because the reasons for referral might create a bias in the latter population. Table 5.7 summarizes the median survival as well as the 3- and 5-year survival rates in a series of published population-based studies. Note that studies have differed in terms of whether survival time was calculated from the time of symptom onset or from the time of diagnosis.

Median survival from symptom onset, therefore, is approximately 30 months and median survival from the time of diagnosis is approximately 14.5 months. Three-year survival from diagnosis is consistent at around 29%, but 5-year survival following diagnosis is more variable, ranging from 4% to 25%.

Table 5.8
Prognostic Factors for Survival in Amyotrophic Lateral Sclerosis (ALS)

Study design	Prognostic factors	Reference
Prospective, Kaplan-Meier, Cox regression	Older age Female gender Bulbar onset Shorter latency to diagnosis Greater severity of disease at time of diagnosis	del Aguila (31)
Retrospective, Kaplan-Meier, Stratified analysis	Older age ALS vs progressive muscular atrophy	Mortara (32)
Retrospective, Kaplan-Meier, Stratified analysis	Bulbar onset	Gubbay (33)
Prospective, Kaplan-Meier, Multivariate regression	Older age Bulbar onset	Norris (39)
Prospective, Kaplan-Meier, Multivariate regression	Old age (univariate) Female gender (multivariate) Bulbar onset (univariate)	Chancellor (34)
Retrospective, Kaplan-Meier, multivariate	Older age Bulbar onset Shorter latency to diagnosis LMN > UMN involvement	Tsynes (35)
Retrospective, Kaplan-Meier, univariate	Bulbar onset	Bettoni (40)
Retrospective, Kaplan-Meier, Cox regression	Older age Female gender Bulbar onset	Lee (36)
Retrospective, Kaplan-Meier, Cox regression	Older age Bulbar onset Combined UMN and LMN involvement	Forbes (37)
Prospective, Kaplan-Meier, Cox regression	Older age Bulbar onset More rapid decline of FVC Requirement for PEG Lower limb weakness	Chio (38)

LMN, lower motor neuron; UMN, upper motor neuron; FVC, forced vital capacity; PEG, percutaneous endoscopic gastrostomy.

4.2. Which Factors Predict Survival in ALS?

Many of the population-based studies that examined survival in patients with ALS have also tried to determine which clinical factors have prognostic value in predicting outcome. The statistical approaches used in these studies, however, have varied, with some using univariate and some multivariate analysis. Although the latter method is preferable, the results of studies that employed either type of analysis are summarized in Table 5.8.

Poor prognostic factors that are consistent across these studies include older age and bulbar-onset as opposed to limb-onset disease. Female gender was found to indicate a poor prognosis in some but not all studies. The effect of some of these other variables are more difficult to determine because they have not consistently been examined in all studies, but there is limited data suggesting (perhaps not surprisingly) that more severe disease at the time of diagnosis and more rapid progression of disease during the initial follow-up period also indicate a worse prognosis.

5. SUMMARY

- The El Escorial criteria require the presence of both upper and lower motor neuron findings in three of four regions (cranial, cervical, thoracic, and lumbosacral) for the diagnosis of definite ALS.
- The sensitivity of the El Escorial criteria for the diagnosis of ALS at the time of initial presentation ranges from 31% to 57%; published data do not permit estimation of the specificity of these criteria for ALS.
- The primary role for EMG in the diagnosis of ALS is to exclude other disorders and to demonstrate the presence of LMN abnormalities in multiple segments. For the cranial and thoracic segments, it is sufficient to show both ongoing denervation and chronic reinnervation changes in a single muscle. For the cervical and lumbosacral segments, these electromyographical changes should be present in at least two muscles innervated by different roots and peripheral nerves.
- There have been no studies of the diagnostic accuracy of the El Escorial electrodiagnostic criteria.
- The results of single study suggest that the sensitivity of finding ongoing denervation changes (fibrillations and/or positive sharp waves) in the thoracic paraspinal muscles for the diagnosis of ALS is 78% and that the specificity is 87%.
- Estimates of the sensitivity of finding fibrillations and positive sharp waves as well as neurogenic motor unit potentials in the sternocleidomastoid muscle vary from 57% to 97%; this variability may reflect differences in the study populations from whom these estimates were derived (early vs late-stage ALS). The specificity of sternomastoid EMG is approximately 96–100%.
- Estimates of the sensitivity of tongue EMG for the diagnosis of ALS have ranged from 29% to 63%.
- The diagnostic yield of EMG of other cranial muscles is poor (Table 5.3).
- The available data regarding the benefits of NPPV are mostly of poor quality, but suggests that it is reasonably well tolerated by a sizable proportion of patients with declining respiratory function, that it does improve the quality of life, particularly with regard to the vitality and cognitive scores of the SF-36, and that it probably does improve survival (these conclusions are supported by a recently published RCT).
- PEG tube placement in patients with ALS seems to offer the advantages of improved enteral nutritional support, which may result in improved body mass index, but the evidence regarding beneficial effects on survival is controversial.
- The optimal timing (with regard to FVC) of PEG tube placement remains unclear. Although the AAN has recommended PEG tube placement before the FVC falls below 50% predicted, there is some data which suggest that a PEG tube may be safely placed

in ALS patients with FVC as low as 35% predicted, as long as noninvasive ventilatory support is provided during the procedure.

- Riluzole 100 mg per day probably prolongs life by approximately 2 months in younger patients in the early stages of ALS; benefit has not been show for older patients, those with more advanced disease and those with disease duration of more than 5 years.
- Data from a single randomized controlled trial do not support the use of vitamin E in the treatment of patients with ALS.
- Median survival from symptom onset is approximately 30 months and median survival from the time of diagnosis is approximately 14.5 months; 3-year survival from diagnosis is approximately 29%.
- Older age of onset and bulbar-onset disease portend a poorer prognosis.

REFERENCES

1. Brooks BR. El Escorial World Federation of Neurology Criteria for the diagnosis of amyotrophic lateral sclerosis. J Neurol Sci 1994;124(Suppl.):96–107.
2. Chaudhuri KR, Crump S, Al-Sarraj S, Anderson V, Cavanagh J, Leigh PN. The validation of El Escorial criteria for the diagnosis of amyotrophic lateral sclerosis: a clinicopathological study. J Neurol Sci 1995;129(Suppl.):11–12.
3. Traynor BJ, Codd MB, Corr B, Forde C, Frost E, Hardiman OM. Clinical features of amyotrophic lateral sclerosis according to the El Escorial and Airlie House diagnostic criteria. A population-based study. Arch Neurol 2000;57:1171–1176.
4. Behnia M, Kelly JJ. Role of electromyography in amyotrophic lateral sclerosis. Muscle Nerve 1991;14:1236–1241.
5. Kuncl RW, Cornblath DR, Griffin JW. Assessment of thoracic paraspinal muscles in the diagnosis of ALS. Muscle Nerve 1988;11:484–492.
6. Kang DX, Fan DS. The electrophysiological study of differential diagnosis between amyotrophic lateral sclerosis and cervical spondylotic myelopathy. Electromyogra. Clin. Neurophysiol. 1995;35:231–238.
7. Li J, Petajan J, Smith G, Bromberg M. Electromyography of sternocleidomastoid muscle in ALS: a prospective study. Muscle Nerve 2002;25:725–728.
8. Preston D, Shapiro B, Raynor E, Kothari M. The relative value of facial, glossal, and masticatory muscles in the electrodiagnosis of amyotrophic lateral sclerosis. Muscle Nerve 1997;20:370–372.
9. Miller RG, Rosenberg JA, Gelinas DF, et al. Practice parameter: the care of the patient with amyotrophic lateral sclerosis (an evidence-based review). Neurology 1999;52:1311–1323.
10. Cazzolli PA, Oppenheimer EA. Home mechanical venilation for amyotrophic lateral sclerosis: nasal compared to tracheostomy-intermittent positive pressure ventilation. J Neurol Sci 1996;139(Suppl.):123–128.
11. Kleopa KA, Sherman M, Neal B, Romano GJ, Heiman-Patterson T. Bipap improves survival and rate of pulmonary function decline in patients with ALS. J Neurol Sci 1999;164:82–88.
12. Aboussouan LS, Khan SU, Banerjee M, Arroliga AC, Mitsumoto H. Objective measures of the efficacy of noninvasive positive-pressure ventilation in amyotrophic lateral sclerosis. Muscle Nerve 2001;24:403–409.
13. Pinto A, Evangelista T, Carvalho M, Alves M, Sales Luis ML. Respiratory assistance with a non-invasive ventilator (Bipap) in MND/ALS patients: survival rates in a controlled trial. J Neurol Sci 1995;129(Suppl.):19–26.
14. Lyall RA, Donaldosn N, Fleming T, et al. A prospecitve study of quality of life in ALS patients treated wtih noninvasive ventilation. Neurology 2001;57:153–156.
15. Jackson CE, Rosenfeld J, Moore DH, et al. A preliminary evaluation of a prospective study of pulmonary function studies and symptoms of hypoventilation in ALS/MND patients. J Neurol Sci 2001; 191:75–78.
16. Bourke SC, Bullock RE, Williams TL, Shaw PJ, Gibson GJ. Noninvasive ventilation in ALS. Indications and effect on quality of life. Neurology 2003;61:171–177.

17. Park R, Allison M, Lang J, et al. Randomized comparison of percutaneous endoscopic gastrostomy and nasogastric feeding in patients with persisting neurological dysphagia. Br Med J 1992;304:1406–1409.
18. Mathus-Vliegen LM, Louwerse LS, Merkus MP, Tytgat GN, Vianney de Jong JM. Percutaneous endoscopic gastrostomy in patients with amyotrophic lateral sclerosis and impaired pulmonary function. Gastrointest Endosc 1994;40:463–469.
19. Mazzini L, Corra T, Zaccala M, Mora G, Del Piano M, Galante M. Percutaneous endoscopic gastrostomy and enteral nutrition in amyotrophic lateral sclerosis. J. Neurol. 1995;242:695–698.
20. Kasarskis EJ, Scarlata D, Hill R, Fuller C, Stambler N, Cedarbaum JM. A retrospective study of percutaneous endoscopic gastrostomy in ALS patients during the BDNF and CNTF trials. J Neurol Sci 1999;169:118–125.
21. Gregory S, Siderowf A, Golaszewski AL, McCluskey L. Gastrostomy insertion in ALS patients with low vital capacity: respiratory support and survival. Neurology 2002;58:485–487.
22. Bensimon G, Lacomblez L, Meininger V. A controlled trial of riluzole in amyotrophic lateral sclerosis. N Engl J Med 1994;330:585–591.
23. Lacomblez L, Bensimon G, Leigh PN, Guillet P, Meininger V, and the Amyotrophic lateral sclerosis/ Riluzole study group II. Dose-ranging study of riluzole in amyotrophic lateral sclerosis. Lancet 1996; 347:1425–1431.
24. Bensimon G, Lacomblez L, Delumeau JC, et al. A study of riluzole in the treatment of advanced stage or elderly patients with amyotrophic lateral sclerosis. J Neurol 2002;249:609–615.
25. Miller RG, Mitchell JD, Lyon M, Moore DH. Riluzole for amyotrophic lateral sclerosis (ALS)/motor neuron disease (MND). Cochrane Database Systematic Reviews 2002;2:CD001447.
26. Desnuelle C, Dib M, Garrel C, Favier A. A double-blind, placebo-controlled randomized clinical trial of α-tocopherol (vitamin E) in the treatment of amyotrophic lateral sclerosis. Amyotroph Lateral Scler Other Motor Neuron Disord 2001;2:9–18.
27. Orrell RW, Lane JM, Ross MA. Antioxidant treatment for amyotrophic lateral sclerosis/motor neuron disease. Cochrane Database Syst Rev 2004;CD002829.
28. Louwerse ES, Weverling GJ, Bosuyt PM, Meyjes FE, de Jong JM. Randomized, double-blind, controlled trial of acetylcysteine in amyotrophic lateral sclerosis. Arch Neurol 1995;52:559–564.
29. Stevic Z, Nicolic A, Blagjevic D, et al. A controlled trial of combination of methionine and antioxidants in ALS patients. Jugoslavenska Medicinska Biokemija 2001;20:223–228.
30. Chio A, Finocchiaro E, Meineri P, Bottacchi E, Schiffer D, and the ALS Percutaneous Endoscopic Gastrostomy Study Group. Safety and factors related to survival after percutaneous endoscopic gastrostomy in ALS. Neurology 1999;53:1123–1125.
31. del Aguila MA, Longstreth WT, McGuire V, Koepsell TD, van Belle G. Prognosis in amyotrophic lateral sclerosis. A population-based study. Neurology 2003;60:813–819.
32. Mortara P, Chio A, Rosso MG, Leone M, Schiffer D. Motor neuron disease in the province of Turin, Italy, 1966–1980. Survival analysis in an unselected population. J Neurol Sci 1984;66:165–173.
33. Gubbay SS, Kahana E, Zilber N, Cooper G, Pintov S, Leibowitz Y. Amyotrophic lateral sclerosis. A study of its presentation and prognosis. J Neurol 1985;232:295–300.
34. Chancellor AM, Slattery JM, Fraser H, Swingler RJ, Holloway SM, Warlow CP. The prognosis of adult-onset motor neuron disease: a prospective study based on the Scottish Motor Neuron Disease Register. J Neurol 1993;240:339–346.
35. Tysnes OB, Vollset SE, Larsen JP, Aarli JA. Prognostic factors and survival in amyotrophic lateral sclerosis. Neuroepidemiology 1994;13:226–235.
36. Lee JR, Annegers JF, Appel SH. Prognosis of amyotrphic lateral sclerosis and the effect of referral selection. J Neurol Sci 1995;132:207–215.
37. Forbes R, Colville S, Parratt J, Chancellor A, Davenport R, Swingler R. Ten year survival data from the Scottish MND Register. J Neurol Neurosurg Psychiatry 2002;73:217. Abstract.
38. Chio A, Mora G, Leone M, et al. Early symptom progression rate is related to ALS outcome. A prospective population-based study. Neurology 2002;59:99–103.
39. Norris F, Shepherd R, Denys E, et al. Onset, natural history and outcome in idiopathic adult motor neuron disease. J Neurol Sci 1993;118:48–55.
40. Bettoni L, Bazzani M, Bortone E, Dascola I, Pisani E, Mancia D. Steadiness of amyotrophic lateral sclerosis in the province of Parma, Italy, 1960–1990. Acta Neurol Scand 1994;90:276–280.

6
Cervical Spondylosis

1. INTRODUCTION

Cervical spondylosis is a disorder characterized by degenerative disc disease, the formation of spondylotic ridges and osteophytes, facet and uncovertebral joint arthritis, ossification of the posterior longitudinal ligament, redundancy of the ligamentum flavum, and vertebral body listhesis. Injury to nerve roots or the spinal cord may occur either directly via mechanical trauma or compression, or indirectly via arterial insufficiency or venous stasis.

The clinical manifestations of cervical radiculopathy include neck and shoulder pain; pain, paresthesia, and sensory loss in the arms in a radicular distribution; muscle weakness and/or atrophy, as well as reflex loss. The manifestations of cervical spondylotic myelopathy (CSM), on the other hand, include weakness and spasticity due to motor long-tract dysfunction, sensory impairment due primarily to dorsal column involvement, and bladder dysfunction. The syndrome of CSM should be distinguished from isolated neck pain and isolated radicular symptoms.

How useful are electromyography (EMG) and magnetic resonance imaging (MRI) for the diagnosis of cervical radiculopathy? What is the role of MRI in the diagnosis of CSM? How should patients with radiculopathy or myelopathy from cervical spondylosis be treated? Are conservative measures sufficient to treat these disorders? When, if ever, is surgery indicated? What is the prognosis for patients with cervical spondylosis, and are there any clinical or radiological features that predict response to a particular form of therapy? These and other questions are the subject of this chapter.

2. DIAGNOSIS

2.1. How Accurate Is Electromyography for the Diagnosis of Cervical Radiculopathy?

Determining the sensitivity and specificity of EMG for the diagnosis of cervical radiculopathy requires that it be compared with some gold standard. In the absence of a true gold standard, it seems most appropriate to rely on the clinical features (symptoms and signs) for the diagnosis. From a clinical perspective, cervical radiculopathy typically manifests with pain in the neck that radiates into the arm in a radicular distribution and may or may not be accompanied by segmental neurological deficits (weakness, atrophy, sensory loss, and/or reflex loss). In a recent review, the American Academy of Electrodiagnostic Medicine suggested the use of the following six criteria to evaluate the

From: *Neuromuscular Disease: Evidence and Analysis in Clinical Neurology*
By: M. Benatar © Humana Press Inc., Totowa, NJ

quality of studies reporting the accuracy of EMG for the diagnosis of cervical radiculopathy *(3)*: (1) prospective study design, (2) diagnosis of cervical radiculopathy independently of electrodiagnostic findings, (3) exclusion of other upper extremity pathology that could confound the EMG results, (4) sufficient description of the electrodiagnostic procedure, (5) clearly stated criteria for the electrodiagnosis of cervical radiculopathy, and (6) results presented in sufficient detail to permit determination of the sensitivity and/or specificity of EMG. There are seven studies that meet at least four of these criteria, indicating adequate methodological quality (Table 6.1) *(4–10)*. The sensitivity of EMG for the diagnosis of cervical radiculopathy has ranged between 47% *(5)* and 95% *(4)*, with most studies suggesting sensitivity of approximately 50–70%. In the studies that separately reported the sensitivty of EMG for patients with segmental neurological deficits and for those patients with purely pain and sensory symptoms, the sensitivity was generally higher among patients with segmental deficits, with values ranging from 61% *(5)* to 100% *(10)*. One study indicated higher sensitivity among patients with symptoms of shorter duration *(7)*. There have been no studies examining the specificity of EMG for the diagnosis of cervical radiculopathy.

The overall impression is that the sensitivity of EMG for the diagnosis of cervical radiculopathy, using the presence of either fibrillations/positive sharp waves or chronic neurogenic changes in motor unit potential morphology, is around 50–70%, with sensitivity being higher in the presence of segmental neurological deficits.

2.2. What Is the Value of CT/MRI for the Diagnosis of Cervical Radiculopathy?

In order to answer this question, it would be helpful to know something about the frequency with which abnormalities of the cervical spine are detected on MRI in individuals who are entirely asymptomatic. There is a single study that sheds light on this question *(11)*. In this study, investigators reviewed the cervical cord MRI scans of 100 patients in whom MRI was performed for the evaluation of laryngeal disease. The MRI scans of 35 patients were reviewed retrospectively and 65 patients were recruited prospectively. In the retrospective cohort, medical records were reviewed for evidence of symptoms referable to the cervical spine. In the prospective cohort, patients completed a questionnaire enquiring whether they had ever experienced symptoms referable to the cervical spine. The frequencies with which various degenerative changes were observed on MRI were similar in the two cohorts (Table 6.2). The salient features are that MRI of the cervical spine was normal in only 29% of patients and that, although degenerative changes were present in the majority of subjects, obliteration of the intra-foraminal epidural fat, which indicates nerve root compression, was not seen in any patient *(11)*. In general, the frequency of degenerative disease in the cervical spine increased with advancing age. This study indicates that although degenerative disc disease in the cervical spine is common in asymptomatic individuals, it is extremely unusual to find asymptomatic narrowing of the neural foramen with compression of a cervical nerve root.

It is against this background that we now turn to consider those studies that have tried to determine the sensitivity of neuroimaging for the diagnosis of cervical radiculopathy *(12–16)* (Table 6.3). All of these studies were retrospective in design, and blinding of the neuroradiologist to the clinical details was maintained at least partially in all but one study *(16)*. The results from these studies are not easily compared because there is substantial

Table 6.1
Sensitivity of Electromyography for the Diagnosis of Cervical Radiculopathy

Reference	n	Study population	EMG criteria	Sensitivity	Comments
Tackmann (4)	20	Patients with radicular sensory symptoms (n = 4) and segmental neurological deficit (n = 16)	Fibrillations/PSWs or chronic reinnervation changes	95%	There was a frequent lack of correlation between the clinical root level and the EMG level, suggesting low specificity
Berger (5)	34	Patients with neck pain (n = 16) and segmental neurological deficits (n = 18)	Fibrillations/PSWs or chronic reinnervation changes	47%	Sensitivity of 61% for those with segmental deficits vs 31% for those with only neck pain
So (6)	14	All patients had segmental neurological deficits	Fibrillations/PSWs or chronic reinnervation changes	71%	High sensitivity may reflect the homogeneity of study population—all with segmental neuro. deficits
Partanen (7)	77	Patients with neck/shoulder pain ± segmental neurological deficits	Fibrillations/PSWs or chronic reinnervation changes	57%	Sensitivity of 67% for those with symptoms of < 3 mo duration vs 54% for symptoms > 3 mo. Sensitivity no better among those with weakness and/or atrophy
Leblhuber (8)	24	"Clinical unequivocal cervical radiculopathy" (disc herniation confirmed by myelography/CT)	Fibrillations/PSWs or chronic reinnervation changes	67%	—
Tsai (9)	32	Patients with neck pain ± segmental neurological deficits	Fibrillations/PSWs or chronic reinnervation changes	56%	—
Yiannikas (10)	30	Patients with sensory symptoms in the arms (n = 10) & segmental neurological deficits (n = 10)	Fibrillations/PSWs	50%	Sensitivity of 100% in those with segmental deficits and 0 in those with purely sensory symptoms

PSW, positive sharp waves; EMG, electromyography; CT, computed tomography

Table 6.2
Cervical Spine Magnetic Resonance Imaging (MRI) Abnormalities in Asymptomatic Subjects

MRI abnormality	Retrospective cohort	Prospective cohort
None	29%	29%
Disk space narrowing	60%	48%
Disk protrusion	49%	42%
Osteophytes	20%	26%
Spinal cord impingement	23%	19%
Spinal cord compression	6%	8%

Numbers do not total 100% within each cohort because many subjects displayed more than one abnormality. Data from ref. *11*.

heterogeneity between them with respect to the patient population studied, the imaging technique used to evaluate the cervical spine, and the criteria used to define the presence of radiological abnormalities.

One study included all patients with neck pain that radiated into the arm to below the elbow irrespective of the presence of neurological deficits or the results of EMG *(15)*; another study included only those patients with suspected cervical radiculopathy in whom there were EMG abnormalities in at least three limb muscles *(13)*; and the remaining studies included only those patients with radiculopathies of sufficient severity to warrant surgery *(12,14,16)*. Two studies evaluated the sensitivity of computed tomography (CT) *(12,13)*, whereas the other three examined the diagnostic accuracy of MRI *(14–16)*. In most studies the radiologic criteria that were used to define the presence of an abnormality of the nerve root were explicitly declared (Table 6.3).

Estimates of the sensitivity of CT for the diagnosis of cervical radiculopathy varied from 73% *(12)* to 92% *(13)* and estimates of the sensitivity of MRI ranged from 48% *(15)* to 93% *(16)*. This variability is likely attributable to the substantial heterogeneity between these studies (discussed above). Clearly, the sensitivity of neuroimaging will depend on the patient population being evaluated. The study population evaluated by Nardin et al. most closely resembles the patient population in whom MRI is likely to be used in clinical practice *(15)*. This study suggests that the sensitivity of MRI for the diagnosis of cervical radiculopathy is relatively low (48%). Although nonspecific degenerative changes will frequently be seen on MRI, the specificity of finding neural foraminal narrowing and impingement of the cervical nerve root is extremely high *(11)*.

2.3. What Is the Value of MRI for the Diagnosis of Cervical Spondylotic Myelopathy?

There appear to be very few published data that shed light on this question. The study by Teresi and colleagues of patients who underwent MRI of the neck to evaluate for diseases of the larynx is perhaps the most useful *(11)*. It will be recalled that the subjects included in this study were recruited both retrospectively (*n* = 35) and prospectively (*n* = 65) and that review of the medical records (retrospective cohort) and completion of a

Table 6.3
Sensitivity of Neuroimaging for the Diagnosis of Cervical Radiculopathy

Reference	n	Study population	Sensitivity	Comments
Daniels (12)	24	Analysis of cervical roots (rather than patients) in those undergoing surgery. The root was declared "symptomatic" if pain, EMG findings and surgery all implicated the same root as that identified by CT	73%	Neuroradiologists were blinded to clinical details and were asked to determine whether there was obliteration of neural foraminal epidural fat and hence compression of the nerve root based on **CT scan** Selection bias may have resulted from inclusion only of patients who underwent surgery (i.e., tendency to include more severe cases)
Katirji (13)	20	Patients were selected for inclusion based on very strict EMG criteria (fibs/PSWs in at least 3 muscles innervated by 2 different peripheral nerves)	65%	**CT/myelographic** criteria included the presence of root sleeve cut and/or lateral recess obliteration Selection bias may have resulted from inclusion only of patients with very strictly defined EMG abnormalities (i.e., tendency to include more severe cases)
Wilson (14)	40	Included patients with cervical radiculopathy who were treated surgically.	92%	Effacement of the subarachnoid space in the vicinity of the nerve root on **MRI** was used to define abnormality Selection bias is likely given the inclusion only of patients who were treated surgically (perhaps implying more severe disease).
Nardin (15)	27	Included patients with neck pain that radiated into the arm to below the level of the elbow	48%	Authors report simply the presence of "clinically relevant **MRI** abnormality" without indicating whether this indicates neural-foraminal narrowing or merely the presence of degenerative changes at the appropriate root level.
Ashkan (16)	45	Included patients with cervical radiculopathy who were treated surgically.	93%	Foraminal stenosis on **MRI** appears to have been the criterion used for documenting an abnormality Selection bias is likely given the inclusion only of patients who were treated surgically.

PSW, positive sharp waves; EMG, electromyography; CT, computed tomography; MRI, magnetic resonance imaging.

questionnaire (prospective cohort) were used to determine that the study participants were free of symptoms referable to the cervical cord. Spinal cord impingement, defined as the presence of a concave defect in the spinal cord adjacent to the site of a disc bulge/herniation or posterior osteophyte but without obliteration of the subarachnoid space, was present in 19% (prospective cohort) to 23% (retrospective cohort) of patients. Spinal cord compression, defined as the presence of a concave defect in the spinal cord associated with obliteration of the subarachnoid space, was present in 6% (retrospective cohort) to 8% (prospective cohort) of patients *(11)*. It seems that the designation "cord impingement" really describes the presence of a concave defect in the thecal sac without obliteration of the subarachnoid space (in which case, it does not really constitute spinal cord involvement), but this distinction is not entirely clear from the paper. On the assumption that spinal cord impingement is taken to imply pressure on the thecal sac rather than on the cord itself, these data show that 6–8% of asymptomatic subjects may show cord compression on MRI. One caveat is that these patients were not examined, and so one cannot be sure that mild dorsal column dysfunction, brisk reflexes, or extensor plantar responses were not present.

Therefore, the specificity of finding MRI evidence of cord compression for the diagnosis of CSM is relatively high, but does not appear to be 100%. There are no published data on the sensitivity of MRI for the diagnosis of CSM.

3. TREATMENT

3.1. Is Surgery More Effective Than Conservative Measures for the Treatment of Cervical Radiculopathy?

There is a single randomized study that has addressed this question *(17)*. In this study, 81 patients with "clinical and radiological findings indicating root compression" were randomized to one of three treatment groups—immobilization of the neck with a cervical collar, physical therapy or surgery. Outcome was measured using a visual analog scale to determine pain intensity, as well as with two measures of health quality—the Sickness Impact Profile (SIP) and the Mood Attenuation Check List. Outcome was measured 14–16 weeks after randomization and again 12 months later. The treatment groups were well balanced at baseline. Visual analog pain scores were improved in the surgical group at the first evaluation (14–16 weeks postrandomization) whereas scores in the other two groups were unchanged. SIP scores were improved at the time of the first evaluation in the surgery and physical therapy groups, but not in those treated with a collar. At the second evaluation (after 12 months), there were no significant differences between the treatment groups on any of the outcome measures. The authors conclude that surgery, physical therapy, and a collar are equally effective treatments in the long-term.

There are many methodological problems with this study. The method of randomization is not described, and no mention is made of whether the evaluating physician was blinded to the treatment that each patient received. The authors did not specify a primary outcome measure, and there is no discussion of whether the study was adequately powered to detect a difference between the three treatment modalities. Therefore, the conclusion that surgery, physical therapy, and immobilization of the neck with a cervical collar are equally effective should be tempered by the recognition that the relative efficacies of these treatments have not been adequately studied.

Table 6.4
Medical Management of Cervical Spondylotic Myelopathy

Study	No. of patients	Percentage of patients		
		Improved	Unchanged	Worse
Lees & Turner *(25)*	28	61	25	14
Roberts *(2)*	24	29	37	33
Nurick *(1)*	36	22	44	33
Clark & Robinson *(24)*	22	64	36	0
Arnasson *(21)*	4	0	100	0
Campbell *(22)*	13	77	23	0
TOTAL (weighted averages)	117	42%	44%	13%

3.2. How Effective Are Conservative Measures for the Treatment of CSM?

The options for nonsurgical management of CSM include avoidance of activities that might aggravate the disease process, immobilization of the neck with a collar, and traction. Measures such as physical therapy, muscle relaxants, and analgesics might be used to relieve associated symptoms of cervical spondylosis such as neck pain, but these are not symptoms of the myelopathy *per se*. One problem encountered in evaluating the literature dealing with the conservative management of CSM is that it is presented in a very heterogeneous fashion. That is to say, different investigators have used different methods for assessing outcome and some have used measures (such as pain) that, although due to the spondylotic process, are not necessarily related to the severity of the myelopathy. Some investigators have simply categorized subjects as improved, unchanged, or worse without specifying how these determinations were made. The outcome of patients treated conservatively is reported in this way in a number of studies (Table 6.4). Overall, approximately 42% of patients improve, 44% remain unchanged, and the remaining 13% deteriorate. These results, however, are difficult to interpret without knowing the initial disability of these subjects. For example, the outcome "no change" might indicate a favorable response if the initial disability was mild, but might indicate a poor outcome if the initial disability was severe. Although summary estimates are presented here, these are not robust, given the heterogeneity of the individual studies. The least-biased conclusion would be that the effects of conservative treatment for CSM are unknown.

3.3. What Are the Surgical Options for the Treatment of Cervical Spondylosis?

Surgery may be performed either by the anterior of the posterior approach and may involve either a single or multiple cervical segments. Anterior cervical discectomy and fusion (ACDF) implies removal of the offending disc and osteophytes with fusion via either a bony graft or instrumentation (e.g., cage or plate). The alternative is a vertebrectomy (also known as corpectomy), in which the relevant vertebral body is removed. The posterior approach involves either a laminectomy or some form of a laminoplasty. Whereas the former involves removal of the lamina, the latter technique aims to enlarge the spinal canal by preserving and elevating the lamina roof over the dura and, typically, has less potential than laminectomy to cause spinal instability.

3.4. How Effective Is Surgery for the Treatment of CSM?

The literature reporting the efficacy of laminectomy is comprised entirely of retrospective case series. For the most part, the criteria used for evaluating outcome are not clearly stated and it is difficult to combine the results of these various studies into a single analysis given the differences between the patient populations studied, the varying inclusion and exclusion criteria, the variable degree of disability prior to surgery, and the differences in surgical technique between the various surgeons. Notwithstanding these sources of heterogeneity, the results of those studies, for which outcome can be classified as improved, unchanged, or worse, are summarized in Table 6.5. These crude estimates suggest that 61% of patients improve with surgery, 31% remain unchanged, and around 8% deteriorate.

Concerns have been raised about the complications of laminectomy related to nonfusion, including spinal deformity, spinal instability, and late neurological deterioration. These concerns led to the development of laminoplasty as an alternative technique to laminectomy for the treatment of CSM. A variety of laminoplasty techniques have been developed, all of which represent variations on the theme of expansion of the spinal canal by posterior displacement of the preserved laminae. Ratliff and Cooper recently reviewed the English-language literature, focusing on the putative benefits of laminoplasty over laminectomy (18). Their review encompassed 71 clinical series with 2580 patients and outcome was evaluated using the Japanese Orthopedic Association (JOA) scale. The results were reported separately for the different types of laminoplasty. Most studies used the JOA scale to record mean pre- and postoperative scores and to calculate what has been termed a "recovery rate" based on the formula:

$$\text{Recovery rate } (\%) = \left[\frac{Postoperative\ score\ -\ preoperative\ score}{17 - preoperative\ score} \right] \times 100$$

In truth, the term "recovery rate" is misleading because this formula really estimates the extent to which the postoperative score (recovery) approximates the maximum score (return to normal). Many studies did not report data in terms of the proportion of subjects, treated surgically, who showed signs of improvement. Notwithstanding the limitations of the JOA scale and the recovery rate for evaluating outcome, the only available data have been presented using this scoring system. The results, which are summarized in Table 6.6, show that the mean recovery rate was approximately 55%, with no clear benefit of one technique over another. They concluded that there was no clear evidence that laminoplasty produces a better outcome that laminectomy (18).

3.5. What Are the Relative Efficacies of Surgery and Conservative Measures for the Treatment of Cervical Spondylotic Myelopathy?

There are limited data upon which to base an answer to this question. There have been two prospective cohort studies in which outcome in patients treated surgically and nonsurgically were compared (19,20), as well as a single randomized study that has addressed this question (17). In addition, there have been three retrospective cohort studies of patients treated either conservatively or surgically (1,21,22).

The three retrospective cohort studies included 142 patients, 89 of whom were treated surgically and 53 of whom were managed medically. Campbell and Philips did not specify the nature of the operative procedure used, whereas some combination of a

Table 6.5
Laminectomy for Cervical Spondylotic Myelopathy (Case Series Data)

Study	No. of patients	Percentage of patients		
		Improved	Unchanged	Worse
Gonzales-Feria (34)	20	85	5	10
Fager (35)	66	59	32	9
Scoville (36)	36	65	35	0
Bishari (37)	59	61	25	13
Pipegras (38)	36	44	53	3
Ebersold (39)	51	35	25	35
Hamanishi (40)	69	84	15	1
Inoue (41)	50	88	8	4
Laterre (42)	17	59	41	0
Yuhl (43)	26	37	52	11
Peserico (44)	47	38	55	7
Haft (45)	16	44	44	12
Guidetti (46)	150	77	11	12
Stoops (47)	42	83	17	0
Total (Weighted averages)	685	61%	30%	8%

posterior approach (typically laminectomy) and an anterior approach (anterior discectomy and fusion) were used in the other two studies. The duration of follow-up was not specified in any of these studies, and Nurick's was the only one to employ a clinical grading system with a clear definition of what constituted an improvement or deterioration (1). The results, summarized in Table 6.7, show great variability, with improvement ranging from 8 to 62% in the surgical group and from 0 to 77% among those treated medically. Similarly, the rate of deterioration ranged from 9 to 28% among those undergoing surgery, compared with approximately 12% in the medically treated group. The heterogeneity of these studies and the disparate results make it extremely difficult to draw any firm conclusions.

The one prospective cohort study included 62 patients, 31 of whom underwent surgical treatment (20). Medical management comprised pharmacological therapy, bed rest, cervical traction, neck bracing, and epidural injections. Surgical treatment took the form of a posterior approach (with foraminotomy and/or laminotomy and laminectomy), an anterior approach (anterior cervical discectomy), or a combination of the two. A variety of different outcome measures were used, including a subjective rating of neurological symptoms, ratings of functional status and the degree of independence with activities of daily living (ADL), the severity of pain, and overall patient satisfaction. Small but significant improvements in pain and overall functional status were found in the surgical group (comparing baseline with follow-up after approximately 1 year) (20). A limitation of this study, apart from those inherent to a cohort study (compared with a randomized controlled trial), is the use of outcome measures that are entirely subjective and which do not necessarily reflect changes in the severity of the underlying myelopathy. Pain, for

Table 6.6
Laminoplasty for Patients With Cervical Spondylotic Myelopathy

Technique	Mean recovery rate (range)	Percent improved cases (range)
Hattori	84%	Not reported
Hirabayashi	60% (41–81%)	77 (55–100)
Kurokawa	52% (20–76%)	81 (70–92)
Laminoplasty with fusion	51%	Not reported
Hardware augmentation	56%	82 (66.7–100)

Data from Ratliff and Cooper *(18)*.

example, is not a symptom of myelopathy, and so improvements in pain scores do not inform on the outcome of the spinal cord syndrome caused by the spondylotic changes.

In the other prospective cohort study, by King and colleagues, consecutive patients with CSM were recruited from a Veterans Affairs neurosurgery clinic *(19)*. Patients were evaluated at baseline and again at least 6 months later. The details of how patients were managed nonsurgically were not reported. The surgical approach (anterior vs posterior and the extent of decompression, fusion, and instrumentation) was left to the discretion of the operating surgeon. Outcome was evaluated using a broad range of measures including a series of disease specific scales (Nurick, Harsh, Cooper, and modified Japanese Orthopedic Assocation [mJOA] scales), general measures of quality of life (SF-36), and general measures of health values (standard gamble, time trade-off, visual analog scale, and willingness to pay) as well as overall patient satisfaction (using a seven-point Likert scale) *(19)*. The study included 28 patients treated surgically and 34 patients treated nonsurgically. Baseline characteristics were similar in the operative and nonoperative groups. Median follow-up in the surgical and nonsurgical groups were 244 and 216 days, respectively. In the surgical group, there were no significant changes between baseline and follow-up in most of the outcome measures. Two scales did show changes, but in opposite directions. VAS scores showed improvement, whereas mJOA scores showed decline from preoperative state. There were no changes from baseline in the nonsurgical group on any of the outcome measures used. Multivariate regression analysis was used to compare outcome in the operative and nonoperative groups while adjusting for baseline characteristics. There was a trend toward better outcome in the surgical group when using the Nurick scale, but a trend towards better outcome in the nonoperative group using the Cooper leg scale. With no differences in outcome between the two groups using this wide range of outcome measures, the authors concluded that there was no difference in outcome between the two groups *(19)*. The limitations of this study are the relatively small sample size, the lack of randomization, and the relatively short duration of follow-up. Nevertheless, the quality of the data presented in this study exceeds by far the quality of most of the literature that describes outcome in patients with CSM.

There has been only one randomized controlled trial of surgery for the treatment of CSM *(23)*. That study's investigators recruited 48 consecutive subjects with clinical signs and symptoms of mild to moderate CSM (mJOA score > 12). Patients were random-ized by coin toss into two groups—medical or surgical treatment—and were followed for

Table 6.7
Retrospective Cohort Studies of Surgery vs Conservative Therapy for Cervical Spondylotic Myelopathy

| | Improved | | Unchanged | | Worse | |
	Surgical	Medical	Surgical	Medical	Surgical	Medical
Nurick (1)	8% (n = 3)	7 % (n = 3)	64% (n = 29)	81% (n = 29)	28% (n = 12)	12% (n = 4)
Campbell (22)	58% (n = 7)	77% (n = 10)	25% (n = 3)	23% (n = 3)	17% (n = 2)	0%
Arnasson (21)	62% (n = 21)	0%	29% (n = 10)	100% (n = 4)	9% (n = 3)	0%

Roberts *(2)*

Follow-up disability	Initial Disability			
	Mild	Moderate	Severe	Very severe
Mild	5	4	-	-
Moderate	-	8		-
Severe	-	4	1	1
Very severe	-	1	-	-

Nurick *(1)*

Follow-up disability	Initial Disability			
	Mild	Moderate	Severe	Very severe
Mild	18	1	1	1
Moderate	8	3	-	-
Severe	-	-	-	-
Very severe	1	1	-	2

Follow-up disability	Initial Disability			
	Mild	**Moderate**	**Severe**	**Very severe**
Mild	23	5	1	1
Moderate	8	11	-	-
Severe	-	4	1	1
Very severe	1	2	-	2

☐ Improved
▨ Unchanged
▨ Deteriorated

Present classification	Nurick	Roberts
Mild	1. Signs of spinal cord disease, but no difficulty walking 2. Slight difficulty walking that does not prevent full-time employment	1. Moderate inconvenience in normal daily acitivity
Moderate	3. Difficulty walking, preventing full-time employment or ability to do all housework, but not requiring assistance to walk	2. Activities severely limited but able to get around alone
Severe	4. Able to walk only with assistance	3. Inability to get about without help
Very Severe	5. Chair-bound or bedridden	4. Bed or chair-bound

Fig. 6.1. Prognosis for patients with cervical spondylotic myelopathy, after Roberts *(2)* and Nurick *(1)*.

2 years. Outcome measures included the mJOA score, a timed 10-m walk, and an evaluation of activities of daily living (ADLs) by blinded observers as well as a subjective patient self-evaluation. Three types of surgical procedure were employed—anterior decompression in 13 (9 of which included an osseous graft), corpectomy in 5, and laminoplasty in 3. Conservative treatment comprised use of soft collar, anti-inflammatory drugs, intermittent bed rest, and active discouragement of high-risk physical activities. Patients in the surgical group underwent conservative treatment similar to that of the patients in the conservative group. Outcome was assessed using an intention-to-treat analysis.

The medical and surgical groups included 27 and 21 patients, respectively. There were no differences in mJOA scores or recovery rates at 6, 12, and 24 months. There were no significant differences in ADL scores within the conservatively managed group at the 6-, 12- or 24-month follow-ups, but a significant decline was observed in surgically treated patients. There were no differences between the two groups in the timed 10-m walk. Finally, there was no change in the subjective evaluation in the conservatively treated group, but surgically treated patients reported deterioration between the 6- and 12-month, and between the 6- and 24-month, follow-ups.

In conclusion, therefore, there were no significant differences in the objective outcome measures of patients with mild to moderate forms of CSM and long duration of symptoms, irrespective of whether the patients were treated conservatively or surgically. Caution should be exercised in the interpretation of these results, given the relatively small sample size and the lack of discussion about the power of the study. Finally, this study did not address the role of surgery in patients with more severe or rapidly progressive forms of CSM.

4. PROGNOSIS

4.1. What Is the Natural History of Untreated Cervical Spondylotic Myelopathy

The importance of knowing something about the natural history of CSM was expressed simply and eloquently by Nurick in 1972 when he wrote that "[i]n order to define the place of surgery in the treatment of CSM, it is necessary to ... know the natural history of the disorder" (1). This statement remains true even today, particularly given the lack of prospective controlled data. Regrettably, however, we are little closer to understanding the natural history of the disease as well as the role for surgery in its management than we were 30 years ago.

The natural history of CSM is difficult to determine from the available literature in part because of the paucity of reports, but in also part because the term "natural history" has been used in the CSM literature to describe the outcome of the disease among patients who were either treated conservatively (i.e., nonsurgically) or among those who were not treated at all, with the results for these two groups of patients often not reported separately. Here, we shall consider only those studies that reported results for subjects who were genuinely untreated.

In their 1956 series of 120 patients with CSM, Clark and Robinson included 26 patients who remained untreated (24). Although they did not provide numerical data to quantify outcome, they reported their results descriptively and indicated that in the majority (75%) of patients, the disease was characterized by episodes, during which new signs and symptoms developed, and in between these episodes the disease either progressed gradually (two-thirds of patients) or remained stable (one-third). Therefore, overall their impression was that progression was usually slow and that spontaneous improvement was rare.

The 1963 study by Lees and Turner is often cited as providing data on the natural history of CSM (25). In reality, the data are somewhat fuzzy. This study included 44 patients with CSM, 28 of whom were managed conservatively and 11 of whom were not treated at all. Surgery was undertaken in eight patients (including three patients from the first group who failed conservative therapy). The authors provide baseline and follow-up data regarding disability, but do not provide sufficient information for us to know how the disability status related to the treatment received. All they reported about the 11 untreated patients was the final disability status—no disability (1), mild disability (2), moderate disability (7), and severe disability (1). Without knowing the initial disability status, it is impossible to ascertain whether these patients improved, remained unchanged, or worsened.

Based on these data, it seems reasonable to conclude that significant uncertainty persists regarding the natural history of CSM.

4.2. What Is the Prognosis in Terms of Disability for Patients With CSM?

The studies by Roberts (2) and Nurick (1) reported data in terms of disability status before and following medical management. Although they used slightly different grading schemes to describe the degree of disability (a four-point scale in the study by Roberts and a five-point scale in Nurick's study), the descriptions of the different grades can be used to create categories of mild, moderate, severe, and very severe disability to facilitate a

Table 6.8
Prognostic Factors for Outcome Following Surgery

Reference	Study design	Factors examined	Results
Takahashi (26)	Retrospective review of 31 patients with CSM treated surgically, for whom clinical evaluation & MRI were available. A 4-point scale used to grade the severity of the myelopathy. Univariate analysis only.	T2 signal changes	Favorable outcome in 44% of patients with T2 lesions compared with 85% of patients without T2 lesions.
Mehalic (27)	Retrospective review of 16 patients with CSM treated surgically. No formal grading system for myelopathy severity. Univariate analysis only.	T2 signal changes Age Duration of symptoms	"The intensity of the preoperative T2 signal abnormality seemed to correlate with the postoperative clinical outcome" (no numerical analysis).
Matsuda (28)	Retrospective review of 29 patients with CSM treated surgically. JOA used to grade myelopathy. Univariate analysis only.	T2 signal changes	Worse outcome (JOA score) in those with T2 signal changes, but baseline JOA scores were worse in this group. With analysis of covariance to control for baseline differences, outcome still worse in the group with T2 changes.
Okada (29)	Retrospective review of 74 CSM patients. JOA used to grade myelopathy. Recovery rate used as the outcome variable. Multivariate linear regression analysis.	Duration of disease T2 signal changes Preop transverse area of the cord	Positive correlation between transverse area of cord and recovery rate ($r = 0.586$). Positive correlation between T2 signal intensity and recovery rate ($r = 0.426$). Negative correlation between duration of disease and recovery rate ($r = -0.401$).
Wada (30)	Retrospective review of 50 CSM patients treated with open-door laminoplasty. JOA used to grade myelopathy. Recovery rate used as the outcome measure. Multivariate linear regression analysis.	Age Duration of symptoms Myelopathy severity No. blocks (myelogram) AP-canal diameter Transverse area of cord T2 signal changes	The combination of disease duration, AP-canal diameter and transverse area of the spinal of the spinal cord provided the best prediction of surgical outcome (i.e., better outcome with shorter disease duration, larger AP diameter and larger transverse area of the cord).

Morio (31)	Retrospective review of 72 CSM patients treated with expansive laminoplasty. JOA used to grade myelopathy. Recovery rate used as the outcome measure. Multivariate linear regression analysis.	Age Duration of symptoms Myelopathy severity Preop T2 changes on MRI	Recovery rate correlated negatively with age (slope = − 1.28), negatively with duration (slope = − 0.33), and negatively with the presence of T2 signal changes (slope = −31.9)
Suri (32)	Prospective study of 146 patients with CSM undergoing surgery. Nurick scale used to grade myelopathy. Multiple outcome measures assessed (results for disability summarized here). Multivariate regression analysis.	Age Duration of symptoms No. prolapsed discs Surgical approach (anterior vs posterior) Signal intensity changes in cord	OR = 2.17 (95% CI: 0.61–9.1) Inconsistent effect. NS in multivariate model. One vs 3 levels: OR=2.9 (95% CI 0.7–10.4) Two vs 3 levels: OR = 2.6 (95% CI 0.4–8.9) OR = 7.15 (95% CI 1.8–17) T2 vs T1 + T2: OR = 3.23 (95% CI 1.2–1.6)
Papadopoulos (33)	Retrospective review of 42 consecutive CSM patients treated with decompression surgery. JOA used to grade myelopathy. Recovery rate used as the outcome measure. Univariate analysis.	T2 signal changes Spinal cord deformity	Recovery rates were better among those with no T2 signal changes (66%) and with single level T2 changes (71.5%) compared with patients with multilevel T2 changes in the cord (34.6%)

Recovery rate (%) = [(postop. score − preop. score) / (17 − preop.score)] × 100. CSM, cervical spondylotic myelopathy; MRI, magnetic resonance imaging; JOA, Japanese Orthopedic Association; AP, anterior/posterior; NS, not significant; OR, odds ratio; CI, confidence interval.

combined analysis of the data from the two studies (Fig. 6.1). These data suggest that the majority of patients have either mild or moderate disability and remain stable over time.

4.3. Are There Any Factors That Predict Clinical Outcome Following Surgery?

It would be useful to know whether there are any preoperative clinical or radiological features that predict a better outcome following surgery. Many studies have addressed this question, but each and every one has significant methodological flaws (26–33). Perhaps as a result of their varying and often poor quality, the results of these studies have not always been consistent (Table 6.8).

All of these were retrospective studies except for one (32) and only about one-half employed multivariate analytic techniques (29–32). There appears to be a serious problem with the analyses reported in the one prospective study (32). In a multivariate regression analysis, these authors found that younger age, use of an anterior (rather than a posterior) surgical approach, the presence of disease confined to 1–2 cervical segments, and the presence of T2 signal-intensity changes in the spinal cord (compared with the combination of both T1 and T2 signal-intensity changes) each predicted a better outcome in terms of less disability (32). Although the authors report these variables as being significantly associated with improved outcome with p values all less than 0.05, the 95% confidence intervals for each point estimate span unity (except T2 signal-intensity changes in the cord), indicating that the observed results are consistent with both an improved and a worse outcome.

Advancing age was found to correlate with worse outcome in one other study (31), but not in another (30). Most studies that examined the effect of disease duration reported improved outcome with shorter disease duration (29–31), but one study found disease duration to have no effect (32). The prognostic value of increased T2 signal intensity changes in the cervical spinal cord has been evaluated in most studies, but the results are inconsistent. Most studies have found that the presence of T2 signal-intensity changes in the cord are associated with worse outcome (26,28,31–33), but some have reported an association with improved outcome (27,29) whereas others have found no correlation (30).

In view of the variable quality of the available studies as well as their inconsistent results, it can only be concluded that it remains unclear which, if any, factors predict a response to surgical treatment for patients with CSM.

5. SUMMARY

- Estimates of the sensitivity of EMG for the diagnosis of cervical radiculopathy range from 50 to 70%, with higher diagnostic yield among patients with segmental neurological deficits.
- The sensitivity of MRI among patients with suspected cervical radiculopathy based on the presence of radicular pain (with or without segmental neurological deficits) is approximately 50%; the specificity, however, of finding neural foraminal stenosis is in excess of 90%.
- The sensitivity of MRI for the diagnosis of CSM is not known, but the specificity is in excess of 90%.
- The available retrospective data, albeit of limited quality, suggest that surgery, physical therapy and immobilization of the neck with a collar are equally effective in the long-term management of cervical radiculopathy.

- The available data, from a single randomized controlled trial, suggest that surgery and immobilization of the neck with a cervical collar are equally effective in the management of CSM.
- The available data are limited, but suggest that disability remains mild-to-moderate in most patients with CSM.
- There are no clinical or radiological factors that reliably predict outcome following surgery for CSM.

REFERENCES

1. Nurick S. The natural history and the results of surgical treatment of the spinal cord disorder associated with cervical spondylosis. Brain 1972;95:101–108.
2. Roberts A. Myelopathy due to cervical spondylosis treated by collar immobilization. Neurology 1966; 16:951–954.
3. American Association of Electrodiagnostic Medicine, and American Academy of Physical Medicine and Rehabilitation. The electrodiagnostic evaluation of patients with suspected cervical radiculopathies: literature review on the usefulness of needle electromyography. Muscle Nerve 1999;22:S213–S221.
4. Tackmann W, Radu EW. Observations on the application of electrophysiological methods in the diagnosis of cervical root compressions. Eur Neurol 1983;22:397–404.
5. Berger AR, Busis NA, Logigian EL, Wierzbicka M, Shahani BT. Cervical root stimulation in the diagnosis of radiculopathy. Neurology 1987;37:329–332.
6. So Y, T, Olney RK, Aminoff MJ. A comparison of thermography and electromyography in the diagnosis of cervical radiculopathy. Muscle Nerve 1990;13:1032–1036.
7. Partanen J, Partanen K, Oikarinen J, Niemitukia L, Hernesniemi J. Preoperative electroneuromyography and myelography in cervical root compression. Electromyogr Clin Neurophysiol 1991;31:21–26.
8. Leblhuber F, Reisecker F, Boehm-Jurkovic H, Witzmann A, Deisenhammer E. Diagnostic value of different electrophysiologic tests in cervical disk prolapse. Neurology 1988;38:1879–1881.
9. Tsai CP, Huang CI, Wang V, et al. Evaluation of cervical radiculopathy by cervical root stimulation. Electromyogr Clin Neurophysiol 1994;34:363–366.
10. Yiannikas C, Shahani BT, Young RR. Short-latency somatosensory-evoked potentials from radial, median, ulnar, and peroneal nerve stimulation in the assessment of cervical spondylosis. Comparison with conventional electromyography. Arch Neurol 1986;43:1264–1271.
11. Teresi LM, Lufkin RB, Reicher MA, et al. Asymptomatic degenerative disk disease and spondylosis of the cervical spine: MR imaging. Radiology 1987;164:83–88.
12. Daniels DL, Grogan JP, Johansen JG, Meyer GA, Williams AL, Haughton VM. Cervical radiculopathy: computed tomography and myelography compared. Radiology 1984;151:109–113.
13. Katirji MB, Agrawal R, Kantra TA. The human cervical myotomes: an anatomical correlation between electromyography and CT/myelography. Muscle Nerve 1988;11:1070–1073.
14. Wilson DW, Pezzuti RT, Place JN. Magnetic resonance imaging in the preoperative evaluation of cervical radiculopathy. Neurosurgery 1991;28:175–179.
15. Nardin RA, Patel MR, Gudas TF, Rutkove SB, Raynor EM. Electromyography and magnetic resonance imaging in the evaluation of radiculopathy. Muscle Nerve 1999;22:151–155.
16. Ashkan K, Johnston P, Moore AJ. A comparison of magnetic resonance imaging and neurophysiological studies in the assessment of cervical radiculopathy. Br J Neurosurg 2002;16:146–148.
17. Persson LC, Carlsson CA, Carlsson JY. Long-lasting cervical radicular pain managed with surgery, physiotherapy, or a cervical collar. A prospective, randomized study. Spine 1997;22:751–758.
18. Ratliff JK, Cooper PR. Cervical laminoplasty: a critical review. J Neurosurg (Suppl.) 2003; 98:230–238.
19. King JT, Moossy JJ, Tsevat J, Roberts MS. Multimodal assessment after surgery for cervical spondylotic myelopathy. J Neurosurg Spine 2005;2:526–534.
20. Sampath P, Bendebba M, Davis JD, Ducker TB. Outcome of patients treated for cervical myelopathy. Spine 2000;25:670–676.
21. Arnasson O, Carlsson CA, Pellettieri L. Surgical and conservative treatment of cervical spondylotic radiculopathy and myelopathy. Acta Neurochirurgica (Wien) 1987;84:48–53.

22. Campbell AB, Phillips DG. Cervical disk lesions with neurological disorder. Differential diagnosis, treatment and prognosis. Br Med J 1960:481–485.
23. Kadanka Z, Bednarik J, Vohanka S, et al. Conservative treatment versus surgery in spondylotic cervical myelopathy: a prospective randomised study. Eur Spine J 2000;9:538–544.
24. Clarke E, Robinson PK. Cervical myelopathy: a complication of cervical spondylosis. Brain 1956; 79:483–510.
25. Lees F, Turner JW. Natural history and prognosis of cervical spondylosis. Br Med J 1963;2:1607–1610.
26. Takahashi M, Yamashita Y, Sakamoto Y, Kojima R. Chronic cervical cord compression: clinical significance of increased signal intensity on MR images. Radiology 1989;173:219–224.
27. Mehalic TF, Pezzuti RT, Appelbaum BI. Magnetic resonance imaging and cervical spondylotic myelopathy. Neurosurgery 1990;26:217–226.
28. Matsuda Y, Miyazaki K, Tada K, et al. Increased MR signal intensity due to cervical myelopathy. Analysis of 29 surgical cases. J Neurosurg 1991;74:887–892.
29. Okada Y, Ikata T, Yamada H, Sakamoto R, Katoh S. Magnetic resonance imaging study on the results of surgery for cervical compression myelopathy. Spine 1993;18:2024–2029.
30. Wada E, Yonenobu K, Suzuki S, Kanazawa A, Ochi T. Can intramedullary signal change on magnetic resonance imaging predict surgical outcome in cervical spondylotic myelopathy? Spine 1999;24:455–461.
31. Morio Y, Teshima R, Nagashima H, Nawata K, Yamasaki D, Nanjo Y. Correlation between operative outcomes of cervical compression myelopathy and MRI of the spinal cord. Spine 2001;26:1238–1245.
32. Suri A, Chabbra RP, Mehta VS, Gaikwad S, Pandey RM. Effect of intramedullary signal changes on the surgical outcome of patients with cervical spondylotic myelopathy. Spine J 2003;3:33–45.
33. Papadopoulos CA, Katonis P, Papagelopoulos PJ, Karampekios S, Hadjipavlou AG. Surgical decompression for cervical spondylotic myelopathy: correlation between operative outcomes and MRI of the spinal cord. Orthopedics 2004;27:1087–1091.
34. Gonazlez-Feria L. The effect of surgical immobilization after laminectomy in the treatment of advanced cases of cervical spondylotic myelopathy. Acta Neurochirurgica (Wien) 1975;31:185–193.
35. Fager CA. Posterior surgical tactics for the neurological syndromes of cervical disc and spondylotic lesions. Clin Neurosurg 1978;25:218–244.
36. Scoville WB, Dohrmann GJ, Corkill G. Late results of cervical disc surgery. J Neurosurg 1976;45:203–210.
37. Bishara SN. The posterior operation in treatment of cervical spondylosis with myelopathy: a long-term follow-up study. J Neurol Neurosurg Psychiatry 1971;34:393–398.
38. Piepgras DG. Posterior decompression for myelopathy due to cervical spondylosis: laminectomy alone versus laminectomy with dentate ligament section. Clin Neurosurg 1976;24:508–515.
39. Ebersold MJ, Pare MC, Quast LM. Surgical treatment for cervical spondylitic myelopathy. J Neurosurg 1995;82:745–751.
40. Hamanishi C, Tanaka S. Bilateral multilevel laminectomy with or without posterolateral fusion for cervical spondylotic myelopathy: relationship to type of onset and time until operation. J Neurosurg 1996;85:447–451.
41. Inoue H, Ohmori J, Ishida Y, Suzuki K, Takatsu T. Long-term follow-up review of suspension laminotomy for cervical compression myelopathy. J Neurosurg 1996;85:817–823.
42. Laterre C, Stroobandt G. Changes in clinical signs after decompressive laminectomy in cervical spondylosis with myelopathy. Acta Neurol Belg 1976;76:286–290.
43. Yuhl ET, Hanna D, Rasmussen T, Richter RB. Diagnosis and surgical therapy of chronic midline cervial disk protrusions. Neurology 1955;5:494–509.
44. Peserico L, Uihlein A, Baker GS. Surgical treatment of cervical myelopathy associated with cervical spondylosis. Acta Neurchirurgica (Wien) 1962;10:365–375.
45. Haft H, Shenkin HA. Surgical end results of cervical ridge and disk problems. JAMA 1963;186:312–315.
46. Guidetti B, Fortuna A. Long-term results of surgical treatment of myelopathy due to cervical spondylosis. J Neurosurg 1969;30:714–721.
47. Stoops WL, King RB. Chronic myelopathy associated with cervical spondylosis. Its response to laminectomy and faramenectomy. JAMA 1965;192:281–284.

7 Lumbar Spondylosis

1. INTRODUCTION

In considering an approach toward the diagnosis, management, and prognosis of lumbar spine disease, a distinction can be made between acute lumbar disc herniation ("soft" disease) and degenerative lumbar spondylosis ("hard" or "bony" disease). The spectrum of the clinical manifestations of lumbar spine disease is broad, and includes back pain, with radiation into the leg (sciatica), lumbar radiculopathy (signs and symptoms of nerve irritation and/or radicular neurological deficit), and neurogenic intermittent claudication (pain and/or weakness that increases with walking and subsides with rest). The term spinal stenosis refers to any narrowing of the spinal canal, the nerve root canals, or the intervertebral foramina. Central (or canal) stenosis leads to impingement on the dura and cauda equina, whereas lateral (foraminal or lateral recess) stenosis results in compression of the nerve roots. Although there is no clear correlation between the nature of the underlying disease (i.e., soft vs hard disease) and the clinical symptomatology, it is useful to recognize these distinctions for the purposes of understanding the pathophysiology of lumbar spine disease because, at least in theory, different therapeutic approaches may be appropriate.

The literature on lumbar spine disease is large and often difficult to interpret. In part, this is because many important studies have included patients on the basis of symptomatology (e.g., sciatica) rather than underlying disease. Sciatica, for example, may result from acute herniation of a lumbar intervertebral disc as well as from encroachment on the nerve root pathway as it courses through the lateral recess *en route* to the intervertebral foramen (lateral recess stenosis). The variable use of terminology also contributes to the complexity of the literature. For example, the term *spinal stenosis* is often used to imply bony degenerative changes or spondylosis. Such usage of the term is not entirely accurate because acute herniation of a single disc may cause foraminal stenosis. Nevertheless, such usage of the term has been preserved in this chapter and should be taken to imply degenerative bony disease unless otherwise specified.

Although it is likely that degeneration of the intervertebral disc plays an important role in the pathophysiology of both acute disc herniation and lumbar spondylosis, it is not intuitive that these conditions (or stages of the disease process) are both likely to respond to the same treatments. Therefore, failure to take into account the underlying stage of the disease as well as the proximate cause of a particular symptom, like sciatica, is likely to confound treatment trials that recruited patients based on symptoms alone.

From: *Neuromuscular Disease: Evidence and Analysis in Clinical Neurology*
By: M. Benatar © Humana Press Inc., Totowa, NJ

In this chapter, an effort has been made to consider the evidence from the perspective of these different clinical and pathological entities, but this is not always possible. For example, a number of studies have lumped together patients with lower back pain and those with sciatica, or those with sciatica due to either a herniated disc or lumbar stenosis. Furthermore, sciatica has been variably defined by different authors, with some simply implying radiation of pain into the leg and others implying root injury with evidence of nerve root irritation and radicular neurological deficit. Finally, the data from prospective controlled trials in patients with lumbar spine disease are limited. It is useful, therefore, to know something about the natural history of acute disc herniation and spinal stenosis in order to place in the proper perspective those studies that have examined (either retrospectively or prospectively) the outcome of a particular form of treatment.

With these caveats in mind, the focus of this chapter is on the use of electrophysiological and neuroimaging modalities that may be useful for the diagnosis of lumbar spine disease as well as questions regarding the optimal treatment of patients with symptomatic lumbar spine disease.

2. DIAGNOSIS

2.1. What Is the Accuracy of Abnormal F-Wave Responses for the Diagnosis of Lumbosacral Radiculopathy?

F-waves are late responses that can be recorded from a muscle following supramaximal stimulation of the nerve innervating the muscle. The electrical stimulus travels along the motor nerve antidromically and excites a variable number of anterior horn cells, which in turn generates an impulse that travels orthodromically along the motor nerve to generate the F-wave. In eliciting F-waves, a series of stimuli are typically delivered, yielding 10–20 responses. A number of F-wave parameters can be measured, including the shortest and longest latencies with which an F-wave is recorded (F-min and F-max), the difference between the F-min and F-max (F-diff), which is a measure of the temporal spread (chronodispersion) of the F-responses, the average latency of the F-responses (F-mean), and the duration of the F-response from initial deflection to final return to baseline (F-duration).

Because F-waves depend on conduction velocity along proximal nerve segments (including nerve roots), it is theoretically possible that they might prove useful in the electrodiagnosis of radiculopathy. The actual utility of F-response in the electrodiagnosis of lumbosacral radiculopathy has been the subject of a number of studies (Table 7.1).

In examining the diagnostic accuracy of these various F-wave parameters, it is necessary to consider the criteria used to distinguish normal from abnormal responses. Broadly speaking, there are two approaches to this problem. The first is to define absolute values beyond which recordings are considered abnormal. The second, which is applicable only when considering unilateral pathology, is to compare recordings from the affected side with those from the unaffected side. As shown in Table 7.1, both of these approaches have been used.

The utility of the minimal F-latency (F-min), the F-wave parameter most commonly recorded in routine clinical practice, has been the subject of most of these studies, although a few have considered other F-wave parameters. The sensitivity of finding an abnormal minimal F-wave latency has varied from 13% (1) to 31% (2). When other F-wave param-

Table 7.1

Accuracy of F-Wave Responses in the Diagnosis of Lumbosacral Radiculopathy

Reference	N	Patient population	Parameter	Criteria for abnormality	Sensitivity	Comments
Aminoff (5)	28	Radicular pain and/or segmental neurological deficit	F-min	>52 ms (women) >55 ms (men)	18%	
Kalyon (6)	80	"Clinical evidence of L5 or S1 root compression"	F-mean	>2.5 ms prolongation compared to unaffected side	61%	Myelography & EMG abnormal in all patients
Toyokura (4)	100	Lumbosacral disc herniation confirmed operatively or with myelogram	F-min F-max F-diff[a] F-duration Rt-Lt-diff	Peroneal[b] Tibial[b] >29.4 ms >29.5 ms >33.0 ms >31.7 ms >8.0 ms >7.0 ms >11.7 ms >16.8 ms >3.5 ms >3.5 ms	70%	Abnormality was defined on the basis of an abnormality in at least one of the F-wave parameters studied
Mebrahtu (2)	91	Back pain with radiation to the leg AND segmental weakness, numbness or reflex loss AND paraspinal denervation at L5 or S1	F-min F-diff[a]	Criteria for abnormal F-min not defined. Abnormal F-diff defined as >95% percentile of that in healthy subjects—13 ms (peroneal) & 9.2 ms (tibial)	31% (F-min) 6–11% (F-diff)	
Toyokura (36)	27	Unilateral sciatica and/or weakness of toe flexion and/or calf muscles	F-duration	Duration exceeding upper limit of control population (i.e., >16.7 ms)	30%	Sensitivity improved to 60% by comparing F-duration on the affected and unaffected sides
Aiello (3)	24	"Clinically unequivocal L5 radiculopathy" with disc protrustion confirmed operatively or radiologically	F-min F-mean F-max	Study refers to normal values, but no mention of how these data were obtained	37.5%	
Fisher (8)	60	Back pain with or without radiculopathy	F-mean	Values exceeding the 95% confidence intervals of a linear regression line estimated from healthy controls	47%	
Kuruoglu (1)	100	Back pain with radiation to the leg and/or segmental neurological deficit	F-min	Not specified	13%	

[a]F-diff refers to the difference between F-min and F-max (i.e., chronodispersion).

[b]These values seem remarkably short, but are what were used in this study.

Study by Tonzola et al. (47) excluded because results for H-reflexes and F-waves not reported separately. EMG, electromyography.

eters are considered, the sensitivity may increase to 37.5% *(3)* or even 70% *(4)*. Although there are limited studies addressing this question, no single F-wave parameter appears to offer greater sensitivity than any other.

What accounts for the great variability in estimates of diagnostic sensitivity between the various studies? In part, this likely reflects the criteria used to select patients for inclusion in a particular study. Studies reporting low sensitivity included patients with radicular symptoms but did not require the presence of segmental neurological deficit *(1,5)* whereas those reporting higher sensitivity included only patients in whom lumbosacral disc herniation was confirmed operatively or myelographically *(4)*. It is not possible, however, to determine whether the greater sensitivity reported in the latter study reflects the inclusion of patients with more severe disease or the use a wider range of F-wave parameters. The fact that a similar diagnostic sensitivity has been found in other studies employing a single F-wave parameter suggests that much of the variability may reflect the patient population studied *(6)*.

Notwithstanding the heterogeneity of these studies, the overall impression is that abnormalities of F-responses are relatively insensitive for the diagnosis of lumbosacral radiculopathy. Moreover, none of the available studies offer any insight into the specificity of F-wave recordings for the diagnosis of radiculopathy.

2.2. What Is the Accuracy the H-Reflex for the Diagnosis of Lumbosacral Radiculopathy?

The H-response is a monosynaptic reflex that can be obtained reliably in the adult by stimulating the tibial nerve in the popliteal fossa and recording from the gastrocnemius/ soleus muscles. The H-response is the electrophysiological counterpart of the Achilles tendon reflex and evaluates S1 root fibers. As such, it has been suggested as a useful measure in patients with suspected S1 radiculopathies *(7)*. Although both the amplitude and latency of the H-reflex can be measured, it is the minimal latency that is most commonly used in clinical practice. The accuracy of a prolonged or absent H-reflex for the diagnosis of lumbosacral radiculopathy has been formally evaluated in a small number of studies with sensitivity ranging from 38% *(8)* to 89% *(6)* (Table 7.2). As for the studies examining F-waves, these estimates vary widely, which is likely attributable in large part to the variable patient populations included in these different studies. The studies estimating high sensitivity included only patients with both electromyographic and myelographic abnormalities *(6)*, whereas those studies including patients with only back or radicular pain with or without associated segmental neurological deficits provided substantially lower estimates of the diagnostic sensitivity of H-reflex abnormalities *(5,8)*. The overall impression, therefore, is that abnormalities of the H-reflex are quite sensitive for the diagnosis of S1 radiculopathy in the presence of other radiographic or electrophysiological evidence for an S1 radiculopathy.

2.3. What Is the Accuracy of Electromyography for the Diagnosis of Lumbosacral Radiculopathy?

Needle electromyography (EMG) provides a means to assess motor root fibers. The use of EMG to recognize and localize a radiculopathy requires that abnormalities be detected in at least two muscles of the same nerve root that are innervated by different peripheral nerves. Broadly speaking, two sorts of abnormalities may be detected: (1) fibrillations and

Table 7.2
Accuracy of H-Reflexes for the Diagnosis of Lumbosacral Radiculopathy

Reference	N	Patient population	Criteria for abnormality	Sensitivity	Comments
Aminoff (5)	20	S1 radicular pain and/or S1 segmental neurological deficit	>2 ms prolongation compared with the unaffected contralateral limb	45%	–
Kalyon (6)	55	"Clinical evidence of S1 root compression"	>1 ms prolongation compared with the unaffected contralateral limb	89%	Myelography & EMG abnormal in all patients
Fisher (8)	60	Back pain with or without radiculopathy	>2 ms prolongation compared with the unaffected contralateral limb	38%	Patients not specifically selected for S1 root disease
Albeck (37)	8	Patients with S1 radiculopathy, but no further details provided	Criteria for abnormal H-reflex latency not defined	(87.5%)	–
Wu (15)	98	Patients with lumbosacral radiculopathy (sciatica with segmental neurological deficit)	Absent H-reflex or prolongation by more than 2 standard deviations from normal in their laboratory	35%	Abnormal H-reflex in 24/25 (96%) of patients with S1 radiculopathy

Data from Sabbahi excluded because results not reported separately for upper and lower limb studies (38).

83

positive sharp waves and (2) neurogenic morphological changes of the motor unit potential (increased duration, increased amplitude and polyphasia). Following axonal injury of a nerve root, fibrillation potentials tend to develop in a proximal-to-distal sequence, appearing in parapsinal muscles within 6–7 days and in distal limb muscles in approximately 3 weeks. Chronic neurogenic changes may not develop for 2–3 months. The timing of the needle examination, therefore, will affect the frequency with which these various findings are detected. There is some controversy in the literature regarding whether only fibrillation potentials and positive sharp waves should be used as evidence for a radiculopathy, or whether chronic neurogenic changes in a myotomal distribution also constitute evidence for a radiculopathy. Another controversial issue is whether the finding of isolated parapsinal fibrillation potentials should constitute evidence for a radiculopathy.

Although needle EMG is commonly regarded as the most sensitive electrophysiological test for the diagnosis of radiculopathy (see reviews by Wilbourn [9] and by Fisher [10]), the evidence for this conclusion is relatively scant. As shown in Table 7.3, there are relatively few studies that have examined the sensitivity of EMG for the diagnosis of radiculopathy. Even these studies are methodologically flawed in that the criteria used to define a muscle as abnormal (i.e., whether reliance is placed only on fibrillations and positive sharp waves, or whether chronic neurogenic changes are also considered) are not always clearly specified, none of these studies have clearly specified the latency from symptom onset to needle examination, and some studies have included patients with back pain alone without requiring the presence of radicular symptoms or segmental neurological deficit. There is, therefore, substantial heterogeneity between the published studies which likely accounts for the wide variation in sensitivity of EMG that has been reported— 36% *(11)* to 86% *(1)*.

In study by Kuruoglu and colleagues, the sensitivity of EMG was found to be 62% when abnormalities were required in both limb and parapsinal muscles *(1)*. Sensitivity did not change significantly if the requirement for parapsinal abnormalities as well, was relaxed. By contrast, sensitivity increased to 82% if isolated parapsinal abnormalities were taken as evidence for a radiculopathy *(1)*.

From the available data, it seems that EMG has moderate sensitivity for the diagnosis of lumbosacral radiculopathy, with the caveat that there is a need for better studies in clearly defined patient populations with well defined disease duration and with clear articulation of the EMG abnormalities that will be construed as indicative of underlying radiculopathy.

2.4. What Is the Accuracy of Magnetic Resonance Imaging for the Diagnosis of Lumbosacral Radiculopathy?

An examination of the sensitivity and specificity of a particular test for the diagnosis of lumbosacral radiculopathy, like so many other clinical problems, raises the difficult question of what to use as the gold standard for the diagnosis against which the performance of the test in question should be compared. Evaluation of the sensitivity (true-positive rate) of a test requires that the gold standard identify the presence of the disease in question. In some respects, it is easier to evaluate the specificity (true-negative rate) of the test in question because this will only require that the gold standard be appropriate for identifying the absence of disease. For a condition like lumbosacral radiculopathy, it

Table 7.3

Accuracy of Electromyography for the Diagnosis of Lumbosacral Radiculopathy

Reference	n	Gold standard for diagnosis	Criteria for abnormality	Sensitivity
Aminoff (5)	28	Radicular pain and/or segmental neurological deficit	Unclear whether (1) fibs/PSWs, neurogenic MUPs or both were used for diagnosis, and (2) isolated paraspinal abnormalities were sufficient or if limb muscle involvement was also required	61%
Fisher (8)	60	Back pain with or without radiculopathy	Fibrillations and PSWs	48%
Kuruoglu (1)	100	Back pain with radiation to the leg and/or segmental neurological deficit	Unclear whether fibs/PSWs, neurogenic MUPs or both were used for diagnosis. Sensitivity falls to 62% if abnormalities in both limb and paraspinal muscles required	86%
Albeck (37)	24	Patients with S1 radiculopathy, but no further details provided	Fibrillations & PSWs in 2 muscles	48%
Nardin (16)	20	Back pain with radiation to the leg below the level of the buttock	Fibrillations/PSWs or chronic neurogenic changes in 2 muscles of the same myotome, innervated by different peripheral nerves with no abnormality in adjacent myotomes	60%
Khatri (14)	80	Back pain with radiation into the leg	Fibrillations and PSWs	64%
Haldeman (11)	100	Back pain with radiation into the leg	Either fibrillations/PSWs or chronic neurogenic changes were considered abnormal	36%
Wu (15)	98	Back pain with radiation to leg and segmental neurological deficit	Fibrillations/PSWs	73.5%

Data from Wilbourn (9) excluded as this study included in the denominator patients referred with the question of lumbosacral radiculopathy (i.e., not all patients were diagnosed with radiculopathy based on predefined criteria). PSW, positive sharp waves; MUP, motor unit potentials.

is intuitively meaningful to use the absence of clinical symptoms and signs as the gold standard for the absence of disease.

With this background, it is possible to consider the accuracy of magnetic resonance imaging (MRI) for the diagnosis of lumbosacral radiculopathy. In order to evaluate the specificity of abnormalities on lumbosacral MRI, a number of investigators have examined the frequency with which abnormalities are identified in asymptomatic people with no history of back pain or sciatica *(12,13)*.

Boden and colleagues evaluated 67 volunteers with no history of back pain, sciatica, or neurogenic claudication. Subjects were excluded if there was a history of any episode of nonradiating low-back pain lasting more than 24 hours or necessitating time off from work. The MRI scans from these 67 patients were mixed randomly with 33 scans from subjects with symptoms of a herniated disc or spinal stenosis and were presented to three neuroradiologists for review in a blinded fashion. The scans were interpreted according to the criteria outlined in Table 7.4. Some abnormality (disc bulge or extrusion) was present in 19 of 67 healthy volunteers (28%), with the frequency of such findings significantly greater among those over the age of 60 (~57%) compared with those younger than 60 (~20%) *(13)*.

In a study with a very similar design, Jensen and colleagues examined the MRI scans of 98 healthy volunteers with no history of either back pain lasting more than 48 hours or lumbosacral radiculopathy *(12)*. To reduce bias in the interpretation of the MRI scans, abnormal scans from 27 patients with back pain were randomly mixed in with the scans from the healthy volunteers before they were examined in a blinded fashion by two neuroradiologists according to the criteria outlined in Table 7.4. Fifty-two percent of healthy subjects had a bulging disc, 27% had a protrusion and 1% had an extrusion *(12)*.

These studies indicate that lumbosacral MRI is abnormal in a significant proportion of healthy subjects with no history of back pain or sciatica. The specificity of finding a disc bulge on MRI ranges from a low of 48% *(12)* to a maximum of 72% *(13)*. The study by Jensen and colleagues suggests that more extreme forms of disc herniation (i.e., "protrusion" and especially "extrusion"), however, may be more specific *(12)*.

2.5. How Well Do the Results of Electromyography and Neuroimaging Correlate With Each Other?

This question has been addressed by a limited number of studies (Tables 7.5 and 7.6). In two early studies, Khatri and Haldeman, respectively evaluated 85 and 100 patients with lower back pain that radiated into one leg (sciatica) using both computed tomography (CT) scan and EMG *(11,14)*. The results of both investigations (neuroimaging and EMG) were concordant in 72% *(11)* to 83% *(14)* of patients. Electromyographic abnormalities were unaccompanied by significant radiological findings in the minority of patients (4–11%) in both studies. Isolated radiological abnormalities (i.e., without accompanying EMG findings) were encountered in the minority of patients (6–35%). Wu and colleagues found concordance between CT and EMG in 76% of patients, isolated EMG findings in 9%, and isolated abnormalities on CT in 15% *(15)*. A more recent study by Nardin and colleagues using MRI rather than CT echoed these findings *(16)*. These investigators retrospectively examined 47 patients with either lumbosacral or cervical radiculopathy and found concordance between EMG and MRI in 60% of patients. Isolated electromyographc

Table 7.4
Radiographic Classification of Lumbosacral Disc Disease

	Boden (13)	Jensen (12) / Nardin (16)
Disc bulge	Diffuse extension of nonosseous material beyond the normal disc space	Circumferential symmetric extension of disc material beyond the inter-space
Disc protrusion	—	Focal or asymmetric extension of the disc beyond the interpsace with the base against the disc of origin broader than any other dimension of the protrusion
Disc extrusion	Focal extension of disc material beyond the osseous confines of the vertebral body, resulting in displacement of epidural fat, nerve root, or thecal sac	Base against the disc of origin narrower than the diameter of the extruding material itself or with no connection between the material and disc of origin
Stenosis	Nondiscogenic loss of signal in the epidural fat with compression of neural tissues within the canal	—

Table 7.5
Correlation Between Neuroimaging and Electromyography (EMG) (Study Design)

Reference	n	Methodology	Gold standard	Imaging	Criteria for abnormal EMG	Criteria for abnormal scan	Proportion abnormal EMG	Proportion abnormal scan
Nardin (16)	47	Retrospective Lumbosacral & cervical	Neck or back pain & radiation to arm or leg	MRI	Fibs/PSWs and chronic neurogenic changes	Bulge, protrusion, extrusion (see Table 7.4)	55%	57%
Haldeman (11)	100	Retrospective Lumbosacral	Back and leg pain (sciatica)	CT	Not specified	Herniation >3 mm or lateral stenosis	37%	68%
Khatri (14)	85	Retrospective Lumbosacral	Back and leg pain (sciatica)	CT	Fibs/PSW	Detailed description	64%	59%
Wu (15)	98	Retrospective Lumbosacral	Back pain with radiation to leg and segmental neurological deficit	CT	Fibs/PSW	Not specified	73.5%	87.8%

Fibs, fibrillation potentials; PSW, positive sharp waves; MRI, magnetic resonance imaging; CT, computed tomography.

Table 7.6
Correlation Between Neuroimaging and Electromyography (EMG)

Haldeman (11)	Normal CT	Abnormal CT	TOTAL
Normal EMG	28 (28%)	35 (35%)	63
Abnormal EMG	4 (4%)	44 (44%)	37
TOTAL	32	68	100

Khatri (14)	Normal CT	Abnormal CT	TOTAL
Normal EMG	24 (30%)	5 (6%)	29
Abnormal EMG	9 (11%)	42 (53%)	51
TOTAL	33	47	80

Nardin (16)	Normal CT	Abnormal CT	TOTAL
Normal EMG	11 (23%)	10 (21%)	24
Abnormal EMG	9 (19%)	17 (36%)	26
TOTAL	20	27	47

Wu (15)	Normal CT	Abnormal CT	TOTAL
Normal EMG	3 (3%)	15 (15%)	18
Abnormal EMG	9 (9%)	71 (72%)	80
TOTAL	12	86	98

CT, computed tomography.

abnormalities were detected in 19% of patients whereas isolated MRI findings were present in 21% of patients.

As discussed previously in this chapter, the specificity of neuroimaging appears to be relatively low, an impression supported by the data from Nardin and colleagues *(16)* (see also the accompanying editorial *[17]*). Practically nothing is known about the specificity of electromyographic abnormalities because there have been no EMG studies of asymptomatic subjects reporting the frequency with which findings indicative of radiculopathy are present. In the absence of evidence, intuition suggests that EMG abnormalities should have higher specificity when comparing patients with radiculopathy with healthy controls. The overall impression, therefore, is that there is discordance between EMG and neuroimaging findings in a significant minority of patients, and lesser weight should be given to isolated neuroimaging abnormalities given the relatively poor specificity of this finding.

3. TREATMENT

3.1. Is There a Role for Bed Rest in the Treatment of Sciatica?

Bed rest has been one of the traditional recommendations for patients with back pain and sciatica. Does the evidence, however, support such advice? There are, in fact, a number of randomized controlled studies that have addressed the utility of bed rest, but these have typically included patients with lower back pain, sciatica, or a combination of the two. There is only one randomized controlled trial that has compared bed rest with advice to stay active in a homogenous population of patients with sciatica. In this study from the Netherlands *(18)*, the authors recruited 183 patients from a population of 338 patients who were referred from their general practitioner with symptoms of back pain radiating into one leg below the gluteal fold. Only patients with sciatica (defined by at least two of the following: radicular pain distribution, increased leg pain on coughing, sneezing or straining, decreased muscle strength, sensory loss, reflex loss, or a positive straight leg raise test) were eligible for inclusion; radiographic evidence of nerve root compression was not required. This study did not specify the nature of the underlying disease causing sciatica, and so it is likely that the study population included patients with both "soft" disc disease and "hard" degenerative lumbar spine disease.

Patients randomized to bed rest were advised to stay in the supine or lateral recumbent position for 2 weeks. Patients in the control group were instructed to be up and about whenever possible, but to avoid straining the back or provoking pain. Concurrent therapy with simple analgesics, nonsteroidal anti-inflammatory agents and muscle relaxants was permitted. The primary outcome measures were the patient's and physician's perceptions of whether there had been any improvement. The investigators were blind to the treatment allocation. Secondary outcome measures included absenteeism from work, pain intensity, the need for subsequent surgical intervention, and scores on functional scales such as the Oswestry Low Back Pain Questionnaire and the modified Roland Disability Scale. Patient diaries indicated that those assigned to bed rest remained in bed for a mean of 21 hours per day, compared with a mean 10 hours per day in the control group. Despite good compliance with therapy, this study found no significant differences between the two groups in the primary or any of the secondary outcome measures. The results of this study are summarized in Table 7.7. Almost 90% of subjects in each group achieved satisfactory outcome (according to both patient and physician assessment). Seventeen percent of

Table 7.7
Primary Outcomes Among Patients in the Bed Rest and Control Groups at 12 Wk

Outcome measure	Bed rest (n = 92)	Control (n = 91)	Adjusted odds ratio (95% confidence interval)
Patient's assessment			
Improvement	87%	87%	1.0 (0.4–2.9)
Investigator's assessment			
Improvement	86%	89%	0.6 (0.2–1.7)

Data from ref. *18*.

patients in the bed-rest group and 19% in the control group eventually required surgery. This study, therefore, indicates that prolonged bed rest does not improve patient satisfaction with outcome, pain intensity, functional recovery, or the need for subsequent surgery.

3.2. What Is the Efficacy of Epidural Steroid Injections for the Treatment of Sciatica?

Although the mechanism of radicular pain due to a herniated lumbar disc is not entirely clear, inflammation and nerve root edema are proposed to play some role. The rationale for the use of epidural steroid injections for the treatment of sciatica lies in their anti-inflammatory effect. A number of studies have addressed the question of the efficacy of epidural steroid injections in the treatment of sciatica. The systematic review by Koes et al. (1995) *(19)* and the meta-analysis by Watts and Silagy *(20)* provide a very useful summary of the randomized controlled trials published prior to 1995. Koes and colleagues identified 12 studies and evaluated each based on predefined criteria for methodological quality, with the maximum score being 100 (highest-quality study). The results of the nine studies that included patients with sciatica are summarized in Table 7.8 (two studies have been excluded because inclusion criterion was lower back pain rather than radicular symptoms and one was excluded because the study population comprised only patients with postlaminectomy back pain). It is important to note the wide variation in the quality of the studies as well as the range of different outcome measures that were used. The study populations were also somewhat heterogeneous, although most studies tried to include patients with sciatica due to single level lumbar root compression that was likely caused by a herniated disc. Only the study by Cuckler et al. *(21)* specifically included patients with symptoms due to lumbar spinal stenosis. The most common methodological shortcomings included noncomparability of relevant baseline characteristics between the two study groups, the small sample size (ranging from 23 in the smallest to 99 in the largest study), failure to avoid co-interventions or to at least control for these between the two treatment groups, no attempt to evaluate patient blinding, and the absence of long-term follow-up.

The authors of five trials reported better results from epidural steroid injection compared with injection with placebo (*n* = 3) or local anesthetic (*n* = 2). In the remaining studies, the authors reported either no difference or worse outcome in the epidural steroid group. Of the four studies with the best methodological scores (>60 points), two reported favorable outcome. In general, there appeared to be no clear relationship between the methodological quality of the study and its outcome.

Table 7.8
Randomized Trials of the Efficacy of Epidural Steroid Injections in Patients With Sciatica

Indication	Methods score[a]	Outcome measure	Steroid	Control	Conclusion	Reference
Sciatica neurological signs (due to a herniated lumbar disc)	72	% Improving after 2 d (LBP)	33%	25%	NS	39
		% Improving after 2 d (radiating pain)	26%	13%	NS	
		% With subjective improvement	67%	42%	NS	
		% Undergoing surgery within 14 mo	58%	52%	NS	
Sciatica + 1-level neurological deficit	67	% Improving after 1 mo	67%	56%	NS	40
		% Pain-free at 3 mo	?	?	Significant	
Chronic LBP + sciatica	63	% With considerable pain relief	56%	26%	Significant	41
Sciatica (due to disc herniation or lumbar stenosis)	62	Subjective improvement after 24 hr	42%	44%	NS	21
Sciatica	59	Mean VAS at baseline, 4 and 52 wk	39,16,14	49,45,30	Significant	42
Acute sciatica	51	No. patients improved or cured according to the clinician	?	?	NS	43
Sciatica (due to herniated disc)	50	% Not returned to work at 3 mo	8%	40%	Significant	44
Sciatica + neurological signs	47	% Reporting improvement at 2 wk	90%	19%	Significant	45
Sciatica (due to herniated disc)	45	No. improved/cured during at 3 mo	18	16	NS	46

[a]Top score (best quality study) = 100
LBP, low back pain; VAS, visual analog scale.

Table 7.9
The Short-Term (<60 d) Efficacy of Epidural Steroid vs Placebo in Patients With Sciatica

Responders/sample size		Odds ratio	95% Confidence intervals	Log odds ratio (95% CI) (Treatment:control)	Reference
Treatment	Control				
8/27	5/24	1.57	0.45 – 5.49		39
14/21	18/32	1.53	0.50 – 4.67		40
9/16	5/19	3.36	0.88 – 12.80		41
12/42	8/31	1.15	0.41 – 3.22		21
8/12	2/11	6.60	1.31 – 33.16		42
15/19	32/44	1.38	0.41 – 4.71		43
21/35	11/36	3.23	1.28 – 8.17		44
17/19	3/16	16.53	4.40 – 62.17		45
18/24	16/24	1.48	0.43 – 5.09		46
140/243	108/267	2.61	1.89 - 3.77		TOTAL

0.3 0.5   1   2   4   10

Data from ref. 20.

In their meta-analysis, Watts and Silagy (20) included 11 placebo-controlled trials (some not published in the English literature) that involved a total of 907 patients with sciatica predominantly due to lumbar disc disease. They defined the main efficacy variable as relief of pain, with a clinically useful response considered to be at least a 75% improvement or reduction in pain. They calculated the odds ratio for each study to estimate the likelihood of a short-term beneficial effect being derived from epidural steroids. The odds ratios varied from 1.15 to 16.53 with a pooled odds ratio of 2.61 (95% confidence intervals 1.8 to 3.77) when compared with placebo, indicating that epidural steroids are more effective in reducing pain (Table 7.9). None of the trials summarized in this meta-analysis reported any major complications.

More recently (1997), Carette and colleagues (22) undertook a large (n = 158) randomized double-blind trial of epidural steroid injection in a homogenous population. All patients had sciatica, defined as the presence of constant or intermittent pain in one or both legs with radiation below the knee. Signs of nerve root irritation (positive straight leg raise) or nerve root compression (motor, sensory, or reflex deficit) or both had to be present as well as CT evidence of a herniated nucleus pulposus at a level corresponding to the symptoms and clinical findings. The study population, therefore, was well defined, with patients in the two treatment groups well balanced for relevant clinical features. Subjects were randomized to receive up to three epidural injections of methylprednisolone or saline. Patients were evaluated at 3 weeks, 6 weeks, and 3 months following randomization, with 156 patients (98.7%) completing the three follow-up visits. The primary outcome measure was the Oswestry Low Back Pain Disability Score. The results are summarized in Table 7.10. At 3 weeks, with the exception of there being fewer patients in the steroid group with residual sensory deficits, there were no significant differences in outcome between the two groups. At 6 weeks outcome variables improved in both groups to a similar extent; with the exception of significantly less severe leg pain in the steroid group (change in visual analog scale [VAS] score of –11.0 vs –21.1, p = 0.03), there were again no significant differences in outcome measures between the two groups. Similarly, at 3 months, although both groups

Table 7.10

Clinical and Functional Outcomes in a Randomized Controlled Trial of Epidural Steroids for Treatment of Sciatica

Outcome measure	3 wk after randomization		Change from baseline		p value
	MP (n = 77)	Placebo (n = 80)	MP (% ± SD)	Placebo (% ± SD)	
Oswestry score	41.6	44.5	−8.0 ± 15.3	−5.5 ± 14.3	NS
Oswestry score ≤20 (% of patients)	19.5	16.3	18.2 ± 38.8	15.0 ± 35.9	NS
VAS for previous week	44.9	49.1	−21 ± 29.2	−12.4 ± 27.3	NS
Positive straight leg raise (% of patients)	77.9	82.5	−13 ± 37.5	−10 ± 34.1	NS
Motor deficit (% of patients)	23.4	13.8	−6.5 ± 33.8	−15 ± 45.3	NS
Sensory deficit (% of patients)	32.5	41.3	−29.9 ± 48.8	−12.5 ± 48.7	0.03
Reflex change (% of patients)	26.0	32.5	−10.4 ± 34.7	−8.8 ± 32.7	NS

Adapted from ref. 22.
MP, methylprednisolone; VAS, visual analog scale of pain intensity; NS, not significant.

Table 7.11

Posttreatment Outcome Measure Following Transforaminal Epidural Steroid Injection

Outcome measure	TFESI	TPI
Change in Roland-Morris score[a]	+22.1	+18.3
Percent decrease in VAS score	82%	62%
Change in patient satisfaction score[a]	+2.1	+0.9
Proportion of patients with a successful outcome	84%	48%

[a]Increase in score indicates an improvement.

TFESI, transforaminal epidural steroid injection; TPI, trigger point injection; VAS, visual analog scale (pain intensity).

Data from ref. 23.

showed continued improvement in the outcome measures, there were no significant differences between the two groups. At 6 months after completion of the trial, there were no differences between the two groups in the cumulative probability of undergoing back surgery (25.8% in the steroid group and 24.8% in the placebo group, $p = 0.90$). Thus, despite surmounting many of the shortcomings of prior studies, these investigators failed to show any significant differences in functional outcome (Oswestry scores) or in the need for subsequent back surgery. This said, they did find evidence for mild-to-moderate improvement in leg pain and sensory deficits in the short-term. Of note is that this study included only patients with acute single-level disc herniation.

In considering the efficacy of a treatment modality such as epidural steroid injection, it is also necessary to know something about the adequacy of the injection technique. For example, none of the studies discussed until now have reported on the use of fluoroscopic guidance to ensure the accurate placement of the steroid being injected. As an alternative to the blind injection of steroids into the epidural space, fluoroscopy can be used to guide delivery of the steroid to the immediate vicinity of the affected nerve root. This procedure has variably been referred to as transforaminal epidural steroid injection (23) and selective nerve root injection (24).

The study by Vad and colleagues was a randomized controlled trial of the therapeutic value of transforaminal epidural steroid injection compared with saline trigger-point injections in patients with lumbosacral radiculopathy secondary to herniated nucleus pulposus that had failed other nonsurgical treatments (23). Patients were not blinded to the treatment that they received and outcome was measured by a patient satisfaction scale, with choice options of 0 (poor), 1 (fair), 2 (good), 3 (very good), and 4 (excellent) at 3 weeks, 6 weeks, 3 months, 6 months and 1 year. A successful outcome was defined as a patient satisfaction score of 2 or 3, improvement on the Roland-Morris score of ≥ 5 points, and pain reduction greater than 50% 1 year after treatment. The results (summarized in Table 7.11) are difficult to interpret because they are presented separately for each group in the format of a comparison between pre- and posttreatment status, and the timing of these measures is not clearly stated (i.e., are these outcomes at 3 weeks, 6 months, or 1 year?). The authors state that the difference in outcomes between the two groups was statistically significant ($p < 0.05$) and that these differences were maintained throughout the duration of the study, but the data to support these claims are not presented.

Riew et al. also included both patients with acute disc herniation and those with lumbar stenosis in their randomized, controlled, double-blind trial of selective nerve root injections of corticosteroid. Their aim was to determine whether such treatment might obviate the need for operative intervention in patients who would otherwise be surgical candidates (24). The study group included patients with degenerative lumbar radicular pain due to a (MRI- or CT-confirmed) herniated disc or spinal stenosis. All patients were considered operative candidates based on an inadequate response to at least 6 weeks of nonoperative management with anti-inflammatory medication, physical therapy, and activity modification. The North American Spine Society outcome instrument was the stated measure of treatment efficacy at a mean of 23 months (range 13–28 months) following randomization. Patients could request up to a total of four injections in an effort to relieve their symptoms; a decision on the part of the patient to proceed with surgery was used as a marker of the failure of injection treatment. Of the 28 patients injected with the combination of betamethasone and bupivicaine, only 8 opted for surgery; by comparison, of the 27 patients injected with bupivicaine alone, 18 opted for surgery ($p < 0.004$).

In summary, there have been many controlled trials of blind epidural steroid injection in patients with sciatica due to a herniated lumbar disc. The study by Carette et al. (22) of blind epidural steroid injection in patients with acute herniated discs showed no benefit, and in their systematic review Koes et al. (19) suggested that epidural steroids did not offer any clear benefit over placebo. The meta-analysis of largely the same group of studies by Watts and Silagy (20), however, suggested otherwise, with epidural steroids offering a small but significant advantage over placebo injection. What benefits there may be are limited and short-lived. A decision to utilize this form of treatment should be balanced against the relatively low risk of complications from this procedure. More recent studies (23) suggest that fluoroscopically guided epidural steroid injection (selective nerve root blockade or transforaminal epidural steroid injection) provides more consistent and meaningful improvement (e.g., decreased need for surgical intervention), but the quality of the studies supporting even this form of therapy do have their limitations.

3.3. What Is the Efficacy of Surgery (Discectomy) for Lumbar Radiculopathy Due to a Herniated Disc?

The study by Weber (25) included 126 patients with radiologically confirmed L5/S1 radiculopathy who had failed 2 weeks of conservative therapy. These patients were randomized to receive either inpatient physical therapy for 6 weeks ($n = 66$) or discectomy ($n = 60$). Follow-up was performed 1 year later. In addition to a full neurological examination with specific attention paid to the subjects' working capacity, the presence or absence of pain and the need for analgesics, and the patients' ability to engage in leisure activities, were assessed. Based on this assessment, the patients' outcomes were classified as good (patient completely satisfied), fair (patient satisfied, lesser complaints), poor (patient not satisfied, partly incapacitated), or bad (completely incapacitated for work as a result of chronic back pain or sciatica). Outcome was not assessed in a blinded fashion. Although 17 patients in the conservative treatment group failed therapy and were crossed over to the surgical group, the results reported were based on an intention-to-treat analysis (Table 7.12). The data support a short-term (1-year) benefit of surgery irrespective of whether the 17 patients who crossed over from the conservative group to the surgical group are included in the analysis. The results at 4 and 10 years show no significant

Table 7.12
Outcome of Physical Therapy vs Discectomy for Lumbosacral Radiculopathy

	Duration of follow-up since randomization					
	1 yr [a,b]		*4 yr* [b]		*10 yr* [b]	
Outcome assessment	*Medical*	*Surgical*	*Medical*	*Surgical*	*Medical*	*Surgical*
Good	36%	65%	52%	67%	56%	58%
Fair	42%	27%	36%	15%	38%	27%
Poor	20%	8%	8%	13%	6%	7%
Bad	2%	0	4%	0%	0%	0%
Died	–	–	–	2%	–	5%
Not examined	–	–	–	3%	–	3%

[a]Outcome statistically significantly better for surgery at 1 yr ($p = 0.0015$).

[b]Results are based on an intention-to-treat analysis (i.e., patients in the medical group who were crossed over to the surgical group are included in the medical group for this analysis); the results remain statistically significant even if these 17 patients are removed from the analysis.

Good (patient completely satisfied); Fair (patient satisfied with lesser complaints); Poor (patient not satisfied and partly incapacitated); Bad (patient completely incapacitated for work due to chronic back pain or sciatica).

Data from ref. *25*.

differences in outcome between the two treatment groups. Although it is true that the results of surgical treatment are superior to those of conservative therapy, it should be noted that 61% of patients who actually received conservative treatment achieved a satisfactory outcome (rated as good or fair).

Van Alphen et al. *(26)* performed a randomized controlled trial of chemonucleolysis (intradiscal injection of chymopapain) vs discectomy. All patients had a radicular syndrome due to an L4/5 or L5/S1 disc herniation confirmed with myelography, and all had failed to respond to 2 weeks of conservative therapy. Patients with severe neurological deficit and those with a history of prior lumbar disc surgery were excluded. Patients were randomized to one of the two treatment groups with a planned outcome analysis at 12 months. Those who were deemed to have failed treatment (because of failure to puncture or inject the disc, persistence or an increase in radicular signs and symptoms for more than 2 months, or because of recurrence of radicular symptoms and signs within the first 2 months) were referred for discectomy (repeat discectomy if this was the original treatment or first discectomy if the initial treatment had been chemonucleolysis). The planned outcome measures, therefore, were the proportion of patients who failed treatment (as defined previously), physician and patient assessment of outcome 1 year after the initial treatment, and the patient evaluation of outcome 1 year after the last treatment. Both physicians and patients rated outcome as satisfactory more often for the discectomy group, and in 25% of patients who underwent chemonucleolysis, the results were sufficiently unsatisfactory to require surgery within a year of the initial treatment (Table 7.13). The authors concluded that, in the short-term, the success rate of discectomy is superior to that of chemonucleolysis, but in the long-term, there is little difference between the two treatment modalities. Although the results are somewhat variable, most prior studies reported a benefit of chemonucleolysis over placebo *(27–30)*. The implication, therefore,

Table 7.13
Outcome of Chemonucleolysis vs Discectomy

Outcome measure	Chemonuleolysis (n = 73)	Discectomy (n = 78)	p value
Percentage who failed initial treatment	25%	3%	$p < 0.0001$
Physician assessment of outcome as satisfactory at 12 mo[a]	63%	85%	$p < 0.01$
Patient reporting satisfactory outcome at 12 mo[b]	60%	78%	–
Patient reporting satisfactory outcome 1 yr after last treatment[b,c]	73%	79%	NS

NS, not significant; –, p-value not provided

[a]Four grades: (1) no pain and no neurological deficit; (2) decreased pain and no neurological deficit, or no pain with neurological deficit; (3) pain not diminished together with a neurological deficit; (4) requirement for second treatment. Grades (1) and (2) classified as satisfactory with grades (3) and (4) classified as unsatisfactory.

[b]Score based on patient answer to the question, "Are you satisfied with the final result of treatment?". (1) yes; (2) largely; (3) barely; (4) no.

[c]This analysis was performed on an intention-to-treat basis (i.e., patients initially randomized to receive chemonucleolysis, but who failed treatment and subsequently underwent discectomy, are included in the chemonucleolysis group).

Data from ref. 26.

is that if chemonucleolysis is superior to placebo and surgery is superior to chemonucleolysis, then surgery provides the better outcome.

These are the only two prospective, randomized, controlled trials of surgery for the treatment of lumbar radiculopathy due to a herniated intervertebral disc. They show a short-term benefit (in terms of symptom relief and the degree of functional recovery) of surgery over both (1) conservative therapy with intensive physical therapy and (2) chemonucleolysis via the intradiscal injection of chymopapain. The two studies are also similar in that a significant proportion of patients in the nonsurgical treatment group achieved satisfactory outcome. The implication is that immediate referral for surgery would entail subjecting about 60% of patients to surgery who might otherwise have made a satisfactory recovery. Surgery, therefore, presents a tradeoff between (1) the desirable outcome of faster pain relief and functional recovery and (2) the risks and costs of poor outcomes, including persistent pain, disability, operative complications, and the need for reoperation. These data, therefore, support the contention that patients should not be referred immediately for surgery upon diagnosis of radiculopathy due to a herniated disc. Instead, a prolonged trial of conservative therapy is appropriate, with surgery reserved for those who fail to respond. Chemonucleolysis is perhaps best regarded as the final stage of conservative treatment. Its use remains controversial, however, in part because although there is strong evidence for its superior efficacy over other conservative measures, the final results of a policy of chemonucleolysis followed by surgery if chemonucleolysis fails may be poorer than the results of primary discectomy.

3.4. What Is the Efficacy of Epidural Steroid Injections in the Treatment of Spinal Stenosis?

The study by Cuckler and colleagues *(21)* was one of the few placebo-controlled trials of epidural steroid injection for the relief of sciatica that also included patients with lumbar stenosis. They recruited 73 patients with a clinical diagnosis of either acute herniated nucleus pulposus (those with acute unilateral sciatica) or spinal stenosis (those with neurogenic claudication, which was often bilateral and relieved by a change in posture). Patients were randomized in a double-blind fashion to receive either the combination of epidural steroid and local anesthetic (procaine) or procaine with saline. A short-term successful outcome was defined as subjective improvement of at least 75% as judged by the patient 24 hours after the procedure. The overall proportion of patients reporting subjective improvement irrespective of the clinical diagnosis (herniated disc or spinal stenosis) was 42% and 44% in the steroid and placebo groups, respectively. No significant differences emerged even after the data were segregated according to the underlying clinical diagnosis. Although this study showed no benefit of epidural steroid injections for the treatment of sciatica, the early (and probably premature) assessment of outcome at 24 hours may have precluded observing any response to the active treatment. The investigators did not raise the issue of the power of the study, but the heterogeneity of the study population and the small size of the subgroups (only 14–22 patients per diagnostic and treatment category) should lead to caution in the interpretation of these results.

As discussed previously, Riew et al. included patients with lumbar stenosis in their randomized, controlled, double-blind trial of selective nerve root injections of corticosteroid. Patients who were regarded as surgical candidates based on failure to respond to 6 weeks of nonoperative management were randomized to receive up to four selective nerve root injections of either steroid together with local anesthetic or local anesthetic alone. Of the 28 patients injected with the combination of betamethasone and bupivicaine, only 8 opted for surgery; by comparison, of the 27 patients injected with bupivicaine alone, 18 opted for surgery ($p < 0.004$).

Although limited, the available data suggest that blind epidural steroid injection is not beneficial for patients with lumbar spondylosis (lumbar stenosis). Data from a single study, however, suggest that fluoroscopically guided injection of steroid into the epidural space within which the affected nerve root is located (i.e., selective nerve root block) may be helpful. The utility of epidural steroid injection in patients with lumbar spondylosis, therefore, may hinge on the injection technique that is used.

3.5. What Is the Evidence Supporting the Use of Surgery in Patients With Degenerative Lumbar Spine Disease (Spinal Stenosis)?

Broadly speaking, the surgical options for the treatment of degenerative lumbar spine disease are fusion, decompression, or a combination of the two. Fusion is generally used for severe disc degeneration, misalignment, and spinal instability and aims to relieve discogenic and facet joint pain. Decompression is generally reserved for canal or lateral stenosis and aims to relieve the symptoms of intermittent neurogenic claudication. There are, however, no randomized controlled trials comparing any form of surgery for degenerative lumbar spine disease with natural history, placebo, or any form of conservative treatment.

Turner et al. attempted a meta-analysis of largely retrospective case series that reported the utility of decompressive laminectomy for lumbar spinal stenosis.*(31)*. They identified 74 studies meeting their inclusion and exclusion criteria. In general, clinical details were only reported in approximately 60% of studies. Based on the data reported, about 80% of subjects had back pain and leg pain, 60% had neurogenic claudication, and about 50% had neurologic deficits. The details of the surgical procedures, in terms of the number of levels subjected to laminectomy and whether discectomy or fusion was performed, were infrequently and incompletely described. Sample size varied from 6–473 patients. The authors of the meta-analysis developed their own definitions of outcome classified as good-to-excellent, fair, and poor, and where possible, they classified outcomes according to their own criteria so that they could compare outcomes across the various studies. The studies yielded widely differing results. The mean proportion of studies reporting "good-to-excellent" outcomes at long-term follow-up was 64%, with a range between 26% (three studies) and 100% (five studies). They were unable to identify any factors predictive of outcome. The nature and frequency of complications were incompletely reported, but included peri-operative death (0.32%), dural tears (~6%), deep infection (~1%), superficial infection (~2%), and deep venous thrombosis (~3%). The overall rate for any complication was ~13%. The re-operation rate was reported in only 25 papers and ranged from 0 to 21%.

There really is, therefore, no good-quality evidence to support surgical intervention in patients with lumbar spondylosis. Any decision to proceed with surgery (decompression, fusion, or a combination of the two), therefore, should be made in the context of what is known about the natural history of spinal stenosis, with the available evidence suggesting that approximately 40% of patients may improve spontaneously and a further 40% are likely to remain clinically unchanged (discussed in more detail in the following section).

4. PROGNOSIS

4.1. What Is the Natural History of Lumbar Disc Herniation?

The best data informing on the natural history of lumbar disc herniation are derived from the studies that have compared some active intervention (epidural steroid injection or surgery) with minimal or no active therapy. The details of these studies have already been outlined in the preceding sections. For the sake of clarifying what is known about the natural history of lumbar disc hernation, the data from the placebo and conservative-treatment groups are summarized in Table 7.14. It should be evident from these data that a significant proportion of patients with symptoms and disability due acute lumbar disc herniation improve with conservative treatment. The proportion of patients reporting satisfactory outcome rises from around 30% at 3 weeks to almost 80% at 1 year.

4.2. What Is the Natural History of Degenerative Lumbar Spinal Stenosis?

The inherent problem with the available natural history studies of degenerative lumbar spinal stenosis is that some bias has affected the way in which the subjects were selected for inclusion. Nevertheless, it is worth considering the available studies while recognizing their limitations.

Table 7.14
The Natural History of Lumbar Disc Herniation

Outcome measure	Proportion of patients	Reference
Marked or very marked improvement in symptoms 3 wk after receiving epidural injection of placebo[a]	30%	Carette (22)
Marked or very marked improvement in symptoms 3 mo after receiving epidural injection of placebo[a]	56%	Carette (22)
Fair to good outcome at 1 yr following an initial 6-wk course of intensive physical therapy[b]	78%	Weber (25)
Fair to good outcome at 4 yr following an initial 6-wk course of intensive physical therapy[b]	88%	Weber (25)

[a]In this study, patients rated their degree of overall improvement or deterioration on a descriptive seven-item scale that range from very marked improvement to very marked deterioration

[b]In this study, patients classified their response to treatment as good (completely satisfied), fair (satisfied with less complaints), poor (not satisfied and partially incapacitated), or bad (completely incapacitated for work due to chronic back pain or sciatica).

Porter and colleagues (32) selected patients whose clinical symptomatology indicated a nerve root entrapment syndrome. Criteria for inclusion included severe constant radicular pain in the leg (extending to at least the lower calf) that was not relieved by bedrest, minimal signs of root tension (straight leg raise to at least 70°), and age over 40. There was radiological evidence of degenerative changes in 80% of the 249 patients included in the study. Ninety percent of this cohort was managed expectantly (although 22% attended back school and 14% received epidural steroid injections). Outcome was assessed after 3 year via a questionnaire, with 78% reporting some persistence of root pain and 90% explaining that they were sufficiently satisfied with their condition that they had not sought further therapy.

Herno et al. (33) compared outcomes in 57 matched pairs of patients treated surgically and nonsurgically. They retrospectively identified 57 patients who had undergone myelography but had not been treated surgically. They then matched these patients for gender, age, myelographic findings, major symptom, and duration of symptoms, with 57 patients treated surgically (chosen from a database of 310 patients). The assessment of outcome was based on the Oswestry questionnaire (subjective disability) and functional status. In terms of subjective disability, there was no significant difference in excellent-to-good outcomes in the two groups. The functional status at follow-up was graded as good in 91% of the operative group and 94% of the nonoperative group. This study has many shortcomings, including its retrospective design, the lack of data on the starting level of pain and disability in each group, and the method used to select patients for conservative treatment.

Table 7.15
1-yr Outcome of Conservatively Treated Patients with Spinal Stenosis (The Maine
Lumbar Spine Study)

Symptoms	Worse	Unchanged	Improved
Low back pain compared with baseline	20%	38%	42%
Leg pain compared with baseline	12%	43%	45%

Data from ref. *34*.

The Maine Lumbar Spine Study *(34)* was a prospective cohort study of patients with lumbar spinal stenosis. The diagnosis of spinal stenosis was based on clinical and radiographic findings and also included patients with spinal stenosis secondary to a herniated lumbar disc. Patients were eligible for inclusion if they had failed 2 weeks of conservative therapy within the preceding 2 months. One hundred forty-eight patients were recruited. The decision to be treated surgically or conservatively was made by the patient and treating physician and did not affect eligibility for study inclusion. Laminectomy was the most common surgical procedure used and fusion was uncommon. One hundred thirty patients completed 1 year of follow-up, of whom 58 were treated nonsurgically. Outcome measures were based on health-related quality of life, including symptoms, functional status, and disability. The results of the conservatively treated group are summarized in Table 7.15. Approximately 40% of patients reported improvement in lower back and leg pain after 1 year.

Johnsson and colleagues described the outcome of nonsurgically treated patients with lumbar spinal stenosis *(35)*. This study included 32 patients with spinal stenosis who were thought to be require surgery, but were not treated surgically either because they refused surgery or because they were deemed unfit for anesthesia. Most patients had neurogenic claudication and a small proprortion had radicular pain either alone or in addition. All patients underwent myelography, and the mean anteroposterior diameter of the dural sac at its narrowest level was 7 mm, the most frequent stenotic levels were L3/4 and L4/5, multilevel stenosis was found in 11 patients, and complete block was found in four. The outcome after a mean follow-up of 49 months is summarized in Table 7.16. The results varied depending on the method used to assess outcome. Using a subjective VAS, 70% were unchanged and 15% improved. When examined by a nonblinded investigator, 41% were unchanged and 41% improved. These data suggest that approximately 85% of patients with lumbar spinal stenosis are unchanged or improved after prolonged follow-up. The strength of this report lies in the fact that the study subjects were patients who were referred for surgery, but were treated nonoperatively. It is, therefore, not subject to the criticism, as are many of the other natural history studies, that it is the patients with more mild disease who are not treated surgically *(33,34)*.

It should be clear from the studies described above that there remains some controversy about the natural history of lumbar spinal stenosis. The studies that have addressed this issue are each limited in various respects and have used different outcomes measures,

Table 7.16
Natural History of Lumbar Spinal Stenosis

Method of outcome assessment	Number of patients	Worse	Status unchanged	Improved
Visual analog scale[a]	27[b]	4 (15%)	19 (70%)	4 (15%)
Clinical examination	27[b]	5 (18%)	11 (41%)	11 (41%)

Data from ref. *35*.

[a]Patients asked to compare their situation prior to the myelogram and their present situation on a visual analog scale (ranging from 0 to 100 mm). A score of 0–45 mm was considered worse, 46–55 unchanged, and 56–100 improved.

[b]Three patients dead and two declined to participate, hence $n = 27$ rather than the original 32.

which makes comparison among them difficult. The essence, however, based on these limited data, is that only a minority of patients treated conservatively deteriorate over time, and that a significant minority might actually improve.

5. SUMMARY

- F-min, the most commonly measured parameter of the F-response, has a relatively low sensitivity and unknown specificity for the diagnosis of lumbosacral radiculopathy.
- The sensitivity of the F-response for the diagnosis of radiculopathy is slightly increased by measuring other F-wave parameters.
- The H-reflex is relatively insensitive for the diagnosis of S1 radiculopathy in the absence of other electrophysiological or radiographic evidence for radiculopathy.
- EMG has moderate sensitivity for the diagnosis of lumbosacral radiculopathy and is affected by the duration of symptoms as well as the specific nature and distribution of EMG abnormalities that are considered indicative of radiculopathy.
- The results of neuroimaging (MRI or CT) and EMG are concordant in approximately 60% of patients with suspected lumbosacral radiculopathy.
- Abnormal CT and MRI of the lumbosacral spine are frequently encountered in the absence of symptoms (especially in older age groups), indicating that the specificity of isolated abnormalities on neuroimaging is relatively low.
- There is no evidence that strict bed rest improves outcome (measured in terms of pain relief, functional recovery, and patient satisfaction) among patients with symptoms of sciatica.
- There is conflicting evidence about the efficacy of epidural steroid injections for the treatment of sciatica due to disc herniation and/or lumbar spondylosis, with the suggestion that fluroscopically guided injection provides more consistent and meaningful improvement (i.e., not just in symptoms, but also in the need for surgical intervention).
- Discectomy offers short-term benefit in terms of symptom relief and functional recovery for patients with lumbosacral radiculopathy due to a herniated disc, but approximately 60% of patients treated conservatively will have a satisfactory outcome without surgery.

- There is no good evidence to support surgical intervention in patients with lumbar spondylosis (spinal stenosis), and 40% of such patients may improve with conservative measures while a further 40% remain unchanged.
- The prognosis of lumbar disc herniation is good, with 30% of patients reporting satisfactory outcomes within 3 weeks and 80% achieving the same within 1 year.

REFERENCES

1. Kuruoglu R, Oh SJ, Thompson B. Clinical and electromyographic correlations of lumbosacral radiculopathy. Muscle Nerve 1994;17:250–251.
2. Mebrahtu S, Rubin M. The utility of F wave chronodispersion in lumbosacral radiculopathy. J Neurol 1993;240:427–429.
3. Aiello I, Patraskakis S, Sau GF, et al. Diagnostic value of extensor digitorum brevis F-wave in L5 root compression. Electromyogr Clin Neurophysiol 1990;30:73–76.
4. Toyokura M, Murakami K. F-wave study in patients with lumbosacral radiculopathies. Electromyogr Clin Neurophysiol 1997;37:19–26.
5. Aminoff MJ, Goodin DS, Parry GJ, Barbaro NM, Weinstein PR, Rosenblum ML. Electrophysiologic evaluation of lumbosacral radiculopathies: electromyography, late responses, and somatosensory evoked potentials. Neurology 1985;35:1514–1518.
6. Kalyon T, Bilgic F, Ertem O. The diagnostic value of late responses in radiculopathies due to disc herniation. Electromyogr Clin Neurophysiol 1983;23:183–186.
7. Schuchmann J. H reflex latency in radiculopathy. Arch Phys Med Rehabil 1978;59:185–187.
8. Fisher M, Shivde A, Teixera C, Grainer L. Clinical and electrophysiological appraisal of the significance of radicular injury in back pain. J Neurol Neurosurg Psychiatry 1978;41:303–306.
9. Wilbourn A, Aminoff M. AAEE minimonograph #32: the electrophysiologic examination in patients with radiculopathies. Muscle Nerve 1988;11:1099–1115.
10. Fisher M. Electrophysiology of radiculopathies. Clin Neurophysiol 2002;113:317–335.
11. Haldeman S, Shouka M, Robboy S. Computed tomography, electrodiagnostic and clinical findings in chronic workers' compensation patients with back and leg pain. Spine 1988;13:345–350.
12. Jensen M, Brant-Zawadzki M, Obuchowski N, Modic M, Malkasian D, Ross J. Magnetic resonance imaging of the lumbar spine in people without back pain. N Engl J Med 1994;331:69–73.
13. Boden SD, Davis DO, Dina TS, Patronas NJ, Wiesel SW. Abnormal magnetic-resonance scans of the lumbar spine in asymptomatic subjects. A prospective investigation. J Bone Joint Surg Am 1990;72:403–408.
14. Khatri B, Baruah J, McQuillen M. Correlation of electromyography with computed tomography in evaluation of lower back pain. Arch Neurol 1984;41:594–597.
15. Wu Z-A, Tsai C-P, Yang D-A, Chu F-L, Chang T. Electrophysiologic study and computed tomography in diagnosis of lumbosacral radiculopathy. Chinese Medical Journal 1987;39:119–125.
16. Nardin R, Patel M, Gudas T, Rutkove S, Raynor E. Electromyography and magnetic resonance imaging in the evaluation of radiculopathy. Muscle Nerve 1999;22:151–155.
17. Robinson L. Electromyography, magnetic resonance imaging, and radiculopathy: it's time to focus on specificity. Muscle Nerve 1999;22:149–150.
18. Vroomen PC, de Krom MC, Wilmink JT, Kester AD, Knottnerus JA. Lack of effectiveness of bed rest for sciatica. New Engl J Med 1999;340:418–423.
19. Koes BW, Scholten RJ, Mens JM, Bouter LM. Efficacy of epidural steroid injections for low-back pain and sciatica: a systematic review of randomized clinical trials. Pain 1995;63:279–288.
20. Watts R, Silagy C. A meta-analysis on the efficacy of epidural corticosteroids in the treatment of sciatica. Anaesthesiology and Intensive Care 1995;23:564–569.
21. Cuckler JM, Bernini PA, Wiesel SW, Booth RE, Rothman RH, Pickens GP. The use of steroids in the treatment of lumbar radicular pain. A prospective, randomized double-blind study. J Bone Joint Surg Am 1985;67:63–66.
22. Carette S, Leclaire R, Marcoux S, et al. Epidural corticosteroid injections for sciatica due to herniated nucleus pulposus. New Engl J Med 1997;336:1634–1640.

23. Vad VB, Bhat AL, Lutz GE, Cammisa F. Transforaminal epidural steroid injections in lumbosacral radiculopathy. A prospective randomized study. Spine 2002;27:11–16.

24. Riew KD, Yin Y, Gilula L, et al. The effect of nerve-root injections on the need for operative treatment of lumbar radicular pain. A prospective, randomized, double-blind study. J Bone Joint Surg Am 2000; 82-A:1589–1593.

25. Weber H. Lumbar disc herniation. A controlled, prospective study with ten years of observation. Spine 1983;8:131–140.

26. van Alphen HA, Braakman R, Bezemer PD, Broere G, Berfelo MW. Chemonucleolysis versus discectomy: a randomized multicenter trial. J Neurosurg 1989;70:869–875.

27. Dabezies E, Langford K, Morris J, Schields C, Wilkinson H. Safety and efficacy of chymopapain (Discase) in the treatment of sciatica due to a herniated nucleus pulposus. Results of a randomized, double-blind study. Spine 1988;13:561–565.

28. Fraser RD. Chymopapain for the treatment of intervertebral disc herniation. The final report of a double-blind study. Spine 1984;9:815–818.

29. Grogan W, Fraser R. Chymopapain. A 10-year, double-blind study. Spine 1992;17:388–394.

30. Javid MJ, Nordby EJ, Ford LT, et al. Safety and efficacy of chymopapain (Chymodiactin) in herniated nucleus pulposus with sciatica. Results of a randomized, double-blind study. JAMA 1983;249:2489–2494.

31. Turner JA, Ersek M, Herron L, Deyo R. Surgery for lumbar spinal stenosis. Attempted meta-analysis of the literature. Spine 1992;17:1–8.

32. Porter R, Hibbert C, Evans C. The natural history of root entrapment syndrome. Spine 1984; 9:418–421.

33. Herno A, Airaksinen O, Saari T, Luukkonen M. Lumbar spinal stenosis: a matched-pair study of operated and non-operated patients. Br J Neurosurg 1996;10:461–465.

34. Atlas SJ, Deyo RA, Keller RB, et al. The Maine Lumbar Spine Study, Part III. 1-year outcomes of surgical and non-surgical management of lumbar spinal stenosis. Spine 1996;21:1787–1794.

35. Johnsson K-E, Rosen I, Uden A. The natural course of lumbar spinal stenosis. Clin Orthop 1992; 279:82–86.

36. Toyokura M, Furukawa T. F wave duration in mild S1 radiculopathy: comparison between the affected and unaffected sides. Clin Neurophysiol 2002;113:1231–1235.

37. Albeck MJ, Taher G, Lauritzen M, Trojaborg W. Diagnostic value of electrophysiological tests in patients with sciatica. Acta Neurol Scand 2000;101:249–254.

38. Sabbahi M, Khalil M. Segmental H-reflex studies in upper and lower limbs of healthy subjects. Arch Phys Med Rehabil 1990;71:216–222.

39. Snoek W, Weber H, Jorgensen B. Double blind evaluation of extradural methyl prednisolone for herniated lumbar discs. Acta Orthop. Scand. 1977;48:635–641.

40. Mathews J, Mills S, Jenkins V, et al. Back pain and sciatica: controlled trials of manipulation, traction, sclerosant and epidural injections. Br J Rheumatol 1987;26:416–423.

41. Breivik H, Hesla P, Molnar I, Lind B. Treatment of chronic low back pain and sciatica: comparison of caudal epidural injections or bupivicaine and methylprednisolone with bupivicaine followed by saline. Adv Pain Res Ther 1976;1:927–932.

42. Bush K, Hillier S. A controlled study of caudal epidural injections of triamcinolone plus procaine for the management of intractable sciatica. Spine 1991;16:572–575.

43. Klenerman L, Greenwood R, Davenport H, White D, Peskett S. Lumbar epidural injections in the treatment of sciatica. Br J Rheumatol 1984;23:35–38.

44. Dilke T, Burry H, Grahame R. Extradural corticosteroid injection in management of lumbar nerve root compression. Br Med J 1973:635–637.

45. Ridley M, Kingsley G, Gibson T, Grahame R. Outpatient lumbar epidural corticosteroid injection in the management of sciatica. Br J Rheumatol 1988;27:295–299.

46. Beliveau P. A comparison between epidural anaesthesia with and without corticosteroid in the treatment of sciatica. Rheumatol Phys Med 1971;11:40–43.

III PERIPHERAL NERVE DISEASE

8 Polyneuropathy

1. INTRODUCTION

Peripheral neuropathies may be characterized as being focal, multifocal (asymmetric), or diffuse (symmetric). Polyneuropathy is the term used to describe a diffuse (symmetric) disorder of peripheral nerves. Polyneuropathy is typically considered a length-dependent or dying-back neuropathy in which symptoms begin in the feet and evolve symmetrically to affect more proximal aspects of the legs and eventually the hands as well. Most polyneuropathies affect sensory fibers earlier and more prominently than motor fibers, but this is certainly not uniformly so. Polyneuropathy is a disorder that is easily recognized by a neurologist when symptoms are accompanied by typical physical findings on examination (reduced or absent distal deep tendon reflexes, distal "stocking" pattern sensory loss, and/or distal muscle weakness and atrophy). Nerve conduction studies play an important role in defining the presence of a polyneuropathy and in terms of delineating the underlying pathophysiological process (i.e., primary axonal loss vs primary demyelination). Because nerve conduction studies only measure the activity of large fiber nerves, skin biopsy to determine the density of epidermal nerve fibers has been suggested as a useful test for the diagnosis of polyneuropathies that predominantly (or exclusively) affect small fiber nerve populations. Clinical examination and nerve conduction studies, however, will seldom facilitate an etiological diagnosis. Laboratory studies and nerve biopsy are the tests most commonly employed used to determine the cause of the polyneuropathy.

In this chapter, we will consider the role of nerve conduction studies in the diagnosis of polyneuropathy and will evaluate which electrophysiological parameters are most sensitive for the diagnosis. We shall also evaluate the evidence that supports the use of skin biopsy for the diagnosis of small fiber neuropathies and will consider the role of laboratory studies and peripheral nerve biopsy in determining etiology. We shall then consider the frequency with which no cause can be determined in patients who clearly have a polyneuropathy. Having considered these diagnostic issues, we shall turn to treatment. Focusing on diabetic neuropathy, the most common cause of polyneuropathy, we shall evaluate the evidence for the use of anti-depressants, anti-convulsants, and narcotic analgesics for the treatment of neuropathic pain. Finally, we shall consider a number of prognostic issues including identifying the risk factors for the development of diabetic neuropathy, asking whether intensive treatment of diabetes impacts on the risk of developing neuropathy and what the prognosis is (in terms of symptoms and disability) for patients with diabetic and idiopathic sensory-predominant polyneuropathy.

From: *Neuromuscular Disease: Evidence and Analysis in Clinical Neurology*
By: M. Benatar © Humana Press Inc., Totowa, NJ

2. DIAGNOSIS

2.1. What Is the Appropriate Work-Up to Determine the Etiology of a Sensory-Predominant Polyneuropathy and How Frequently Can No Cause Be Identified?

The diagnosis of idiopathic neuropathy is made when extensive investigations fail to reveal the cause of the neuropathy. Clearly, the frequency with which a neuropathy is labeled as idiopathic will depend on how aggressively the etiology is sought. A related question, therefore, is what investigations should reasonably be performed before labeling a neuropathy as idiopathic.

Given the tremendous range of disease processes that may cause neuropathy, the work-up will typically be dictated by the clinical context. Having said this, a frequently encountered clinical problem is that of a patient with a predominantly sensory polyneuropathy in whom there are no other known diseases or risk factors to suggest an etiology. The question then arises as to which investigations should be performed. There are limited published data that shed light on this issue. In one study, the authors reported the results of investigation of 138 consecutive patients seen in a tertiary referral center with a sensory neuropathy labeled as idiopathic based on no identifiable etiology following a detailed history, physical examination, and nerve conduction studies *(1,2)*. Having excluded patients with known diabetes, the oral glucose tolerance test still provided the highest diagnostic yield in that 53 of 87 (61%) patients tested were found to have an abnormal result based on the American Diabetic Association criteria. Diabetes was diagnosed in 13%, impaired glucose tolerance in 45% of patients, and abnormal fasting glucose in the remaining patients. Other commonly performed tests included anti-nuclear antibody (ANA), serum protein electrophoresis with immunofixation electrophoresis (SPEP/IFE), serum B_{12} concentration, erythrocyte sedimentation rate (ESR), folate, and thyroid-stimulating hormone (TSH). The results of ANA, SPEP/IFE, and B_{12} tests were abnormal in 2–3% of patients tested. ANA titers were uniformly low (<1:160) and the finding of an elevated titer did not change the diagnosis or management in any patient. ESR, folate, and TSH were normal in all patients tested (Table 8.1A). Based on this limited panel of investigations (with other tests such as serum B_6, Sjogren's antibodies, anti-ganglioside, and paraneoplastic antibodies performed very selectively), the prevalence of idiopathic polyneuropathy was found to be approximately 31% *(2)*.

These results suggest that abnormal glucose metabolism (impaired glucose tolerance or diabetes mellitus) is the most common underlying etiology in patients who present with sensory predominant polyneuropathy of unclear etiology and that other laboratory studies have limited diagnostic yield.

In a combined retrospective and prospective study of patients over the age of 65 with a clinical diagnosis polyneuropathy (based on the presence of distal, symmetric sensory symptoms or signs) as well as abnormal electrophysiological findings, Verghese and colleagues similarly found that diabetes was the single most common cause of neuropathy (accounting for ~40%) *(3)*. The next most common causes were hereditary (~8%), inflammatory-demyelinating (~5%), and alcoholic (~4%) neuropathy. Monoclonal gammopathy, cancer, uremia, B_{12} deficiency, hypothyroidism, and vasculitis each accounted for approximately 0.5–2% of cases (Table 8.1A). Approximately 19% of cases of neuropathy remained idiopathic despite extensive investigation *(3)*. The impli-

Table 8.1A
Diagnostic Yield of Laboratory Studies in Patients With Polyneuropathy

Investigation	Smith (2)	Verghese (3)
Serum protein electrophoresis/immunofixation electrophoresis	3%	2%
Serum B$_{12}$	2%	1%
Antinuclear antibody (ANA)	3%	–
Erythrocyte sedimentation rate (ESR)	0	–
Serum folate	0	–
Thyroid stimulating hormone (TSH)	0	0.7%
Renal function	–	2.2%

Table 8.1B
Prevalence of Abnormal Glucose Metabolism in Patients With "Idiopathic" Polyneuropathy

Reference	n	Patient population	IGT	Diabetes
Smith (2)	87	Patients thought on clinical grounds to have idiopathic peripheral neuropathy were included if no etiology was identified from the history, physical examination, and electrodiagnostic study. Those with a known history of diabetes were excluded.	45%	13%
Verghese (3)	402	Elderly (>65 yr) patients with symptoms and/or signs of neuropathy as well as electro-physiological evidence for neuropathy (at least two separate nerve responses abnormal in more than one limb) in 96% of patients	NR	40%
Novella (4)	48	Symptoms of decrease distal sensation and tendon hyporeflexia with normal serum B$_{12}$, and serum protein electrophoresis as well as the absence of other coexisting diseases or treatment that could cause neuropathy and no family history of neuropathy	27%	23%

IGT, impaired glucose tolerance; NR, not reported.

cation of this study is that testing for diabetes will unequivocally provide the highest diagnostic yield. Most other causes of neuropathy will be identified by a careful family history and a detailed history of exposure to alcohol in conjunction with a simple panel of laboratory studies including SPEP/IFE, renal function, B$_{12}$, and TSH.

Novella and colleagues similarly found evidence of abnormal glucose metabolism (either diabetes mellitus or impaired glucose tolerance) in 50% of the 48 patients they evaluated with otherwise idiopathic sensory polyneuropathy (4). Estimates, therefore, of the prevalence of abnormal glucose metabolism among patients with presumed idiopathic polyneuropathy have ranged from approximately 40 to approximately 60% (Table 8.1B).

Dyck and colleagues have emphasized the importance of a detailed family history as part of the evaluation of patients with apparently idiopathic sensory-predominant polyneuropathy *(5)*. They evaluated 205 patients with uncharacterized neuropathies, most of whom had been referred by neurologists. Remarkably, they found that 42% of these patients had inherited neuropathies. This conclusion was reached on the basis of careful enquiry about high-arched feet, curled-up toes, claw hands, wasting of muscles, kyphosis, scoliosis, plantar foot ulcers and subluxed hips, as well as polio and arthritis (conditions frequently mistaken for neuropathy). Family history, however, was insufficient in approximately 40% of the patients found to have inherited neuropathies, and in these instances the diagnosis was made only after relatives were examined clinically and with electrodiagnostic studies *(5)*.

Although the spectrum of causes of neuropathy will vary depending on the specific patient population, the available data suggest that the etiology of the majority of apparently idiopathic sensory-predominant neuropathies will be identified on the basis of a careful history with attention to risk factors for neuropathy (e.g., alcohol use, risk factors for HIV, and so on), a thorough family history to determine whether there are any affected family members (sometimes supplemented with examination of these relatives), and a simple battery of tests including a 2-hour glucose tolerance test, SPEP/IFE, serum B_{12} concentration, and renal and thyroid function. In a significant minority of patients with neuropathy, the cause will remain elusive despite these measures. Estimates from recently published studies of the frequency with which neuropathy remains truly idiopathic have ranged from 19% *(3)* to 31% *(2)*.

2.2. What Is the Accuracy of Nerve Conduction Studies for the Diagnosis of Polyneuropathy?

There has been surprisingly little formal investigation of the sensitivity and specificity of various electrodiagnostic findings for the diagnosis of polyneuropathy *(6–13)*. Most of these studies have only included patients with diabetic polyneuropathy *(6,9,10,12,13)*, although a few have also included patients with idiopathic axonal polyneuropathy as well as distal symmetric polyneuropathy due to various toxic and metabolic disorders *(7,8,11)*. One study also included patients with Guillain-Barre Syndrome and chronic inflammatory demyelinating polyradiculoneuropathy *(8)*. Because the role of electrodiagnostic testing in these disorders will be examined in the respective chapters devoted to each of these disorders, here we shall only consider the data that is relevant to diabetic and idiopathic axonal polyneuropathy.

These reports are extremely heterogeneous in terms of the patient populations studied, the variability (and inadequacy) of the gold standard used to define the presence of neuropathy (against which the performance of nerve conduction studies could be compared), and in terms of the control data used to distinguish normal from abnormal. In view of this heterogeneity, it is not possible to compare data from one study with the next, so instead we must rely on the internal comparisons made between different electrodiagnostic parameters within a given study. This heterogeneity is also likely responsible for the diversity of the results that have been reported and which are summarized in Table 8.2.

Estimates of the sensitivity of sural nerve conduction velocity have varied from as low as 30% *(13)* to as high as 87% *(7)* whereas the sensitivity of sural nerve response amplitude has ranged from 29% *(13)* to 62% *(6)*. The sensitivity of motor F-wave minimal latency has ranged from 36% *(13)* to 71% *(8)*. In those studies in which sural nerve conduction studies have been compared with motor F-wave minimal latencies *(10,12,13)*, the sensitivities have been quite similar in two studies *(10,13)* but in the third, motor F-wave minimal latencies were considerably more sensitive than measures of sural nerve function (~70% for the tibial nerve F-min compared with ~40% for the sural amplitude) *(12)*.

One study of the sural-to-radial response amplitude ratio (SRAR) reported a sensitivity of 90% *(11)*, but this was only compared with the sensitivity of the sural response amplitude alone and so comparison with F-wave minimal latency cannot be determined. A second study that examined SRAR also considered the tibial F-wave minimal latency and reported better sensitivity for SRAR (50% vs 30%).

Although, as noted before, it is extremely difficult to draw comparisons between the data presented in these studies, the weight of evidence seems to suggest that the SRAR is the most sensitive measure for diagnosing polyneuropathy, although the precise sensitivity will vary depending on the cut-off value used to define normality.

2.3. What Is the Utility of Quantitative Sensory Testing for the Diagnosis of Diabetic Polyneuropathy?

Quantitative sensory testing (QST) is a technique that is used to measure the detection threshold of accurately calibrated thermal, vibratory, and painful stimuli. It has been proposed as a sensitive measure of peripheral nerve dysfunction, with thermal stimuli being particularly helpful for the detection of small fiber nerve abnormalities given that traditional nerve conduction studies depend exclusively on the function of fast-conducting large-fiber nerves. Because QST requires the patient to report the subjective perception of these sensory stimuli, it is appropriately regarded as a psychophysical test. Abnormalities may reflect dysfunction of impulse transmission anywhere between the cutaneous sensory receptors on the one hand and the primary or association sensory cortex on the other. The interpretation of these tests, therefore, requires some caution.

The American Academy of Neurology Therapeutics and Technology Assessment Subcommittee recently published an evidence-based review of QST *(14)* in which it was concluded that QST measurement of "... vibration and thermal perception thresholds is probably an effective tool in the documentation of sensory abnormalities in patients with diabetic neuropathy (Level B recommendation)" and that "... QST is possibly useful in demonstrating thermal threshold abnormalities in patients with small fiber neuropathy (Level C recommendation)" *(14)*. In considering the validity of these conclusions it is helpful to evaluate some of the primary evidence upon which these recommendations were made. Table 8.3 summarizes the data categorized as class-II* presented in this report, although not all of these studies permit estimation of both sensitivity and specificity. These studies measured thermal and vibratory thresholds using a variety of different QST devices in patients either with diabetic or idiopathic small fiber polyneuropathy. Estimates of the sensitivity of QST ranged from approximately 28% to 86%, with specificity ranging from 83% to 100%. As would be expected for any diagnostic test, the higher specificity of 100% was obtained at the cost of a substantially reduced sensitivity (28%) *(15)*. One

---

*Class-II evidence is derived from prospective study of a narrow spectrum of people with the suspected condition, or a well designed retrospective study of a broad spectrum of persons with an established condition (by a gold standard) compared with a broad spectrum of controls, where the test is applied in a blinded evaluation, and enabling the assessment of appropriate tests of diagnostic accuracy.

Table 8.2
Accuracy of Nerve Conduction Studies for the Diagnosis of Polyneuropathy

Reference	n	Study population	Control data	Parameters studied	Sensitivity
Tackmann (6)	40	Patients with DM; most with signs of a predominantly sensorimotor polyneuropathy (weakness, wasting, impaired touch, pain & vibration, depressed or absent reflexes)	Normal values previously determined by the authors. Specific values not reported here	Sural AMP	**62%**
				Sural CV	46%
				Peroneal AMP	37%
				Peroneal CV	22%
				Tibial AMP	**68%**
				Tibial CV	14%
Kayser-Gatchalian (7)	187	Patients with mild symptoms and signs of polyneuropathy (paresthesia, numbness, cramps, heaviness, weakness, absent reflexes, diminished distal sensation). Included neuropathy due to DM, alcohol, B$_{12}$, and other causes	Normal value for sural CV derived from published regression equation: $57.4 - 0.05 \times age$. Supplemental data previously published by the authors.	Sural CV	**87%**
				Peroneal CV	21%
				Tibial CV	55%
Fraser (8)	75	Subjects seen in the EMG lab with clinical evidence for polyneuropathy and with the sural amplitude <5 µV. Results reported separately for diabetic & axonal neuropathies as well as for GBS and CIDP. Combined results for axonal/diabetes presented here.	Combination of normal volunteers and "normals" selected from patients seen in the EMG lab. Limits set at 2 SD above normal estimates using regression equations. 96th percentile used for F-dispersion and 2nd percentile for F-persistence	Motor AMP[a]	35%
				Motor DL [a]	38%
				Motor CV[a]	64%
				Sensory AMP[a]	**84%**
				Sensory CV[a]	18%
				F-min[a]	**71%**
				F-dispersion[a]	11%
				F-persistence[a]	24%
Claus (9)	46	Diabetics, all with sensory symptoms (numbness, paresthesia, burning feet)	101 healthy subjects with no evidence of neurological disease. Normal limits set as 2SD around the mean	Radial S. AMP	37%
				Radial S. CV	26%
				Median M. CV	**50%**
				Sural CV	**61%**
				Sural AMP	48%
				Peroneal CV	**61%**
				Peroneal AMP	39%

114

Study	N	Neuropathy definition	Normative/comparison	Measure	% abnormal
DCCT (10)	275	Diabetics with neuropathy, defined as the presence of two of the following: symptoms, signs, loss of reflexes. NCS performed at baseline prior to start of DCCT.	Abnormalities defined by centers participating in DCCT. Sural and Peroneal CV >40 m/s, Peroneal F-min ≥56 ms, Median CV >48 m/s	Peroneal F-min Peroneal CV Sural CV Median S. CV	50% 43% 51% 47%
Rutkove (11)	30	Polyneuropathy based on ≥2 of the following: (1) ↓ vibration, (2) ↓ light touch, (3) markedly ↓ ankle reflexes, (4) distal to proximal gradient reinnervation on EMG	Age-matched healthy controls selected prospectively	SRAR (0.4) Sural AMP	90% 66%
Andersen (12)	101	Diabetics referred to EMG lab, many with complaints of pain or paresthesia (but not clear how many were diagnosed with polyneuropathy)	All results corrected for age and height according to the authors' laboratory reference standards; results expressed as Z-scores	Sural AMP Sural CV Peroneal CV Peroneal AMP Peroneal F-min Tibial CV Tibial AMP Tibial F-min Median F-min Ulnar F-min	~40% ~33% ~48% ~13% ~66% ~35% ~18% ~70% ~48% ~60%
Pastore (13)	99	Diabetics with polyneuropathy defined as ≥2 of the following: (1) ↓ reflexes, (2) ↓ vibration below the knees, (3) ↓ light touch sensation in the legs	Normative data collected from 172 healthy controls studied in the EMG lab. Abnormal defined as >2 SD; height & age adjusted where needed	SRAR (0.34) Tibial F-min Sural AMP Sural CV	51% 36% 29% 30%

DM, diabetes mellitus; AMP, amplitude; CV, conduction velocity; F-min, minimal F-wave latency; S, sensory; NCS, nerve conduction studies; DCCT, diabetes control and complication trial; SRAR, sural/radial response amplitude ratio; M, motor.

[a] Median and ulnar nerves studied.

Table 8.3
Diagnostic Accuracy of Quantitative Sensory Testing

Reference	Population	Device	Sensory modality	Diagnostic accuracy
Guy (78)	50 Diabetic patients with neuropathy	Noncomputerized Marstock device	Thermal	Sensitivity 86% (thermal)
Masson (16)	90 Diabetic patients 35 without neuropathy 34 with neuropathy 21 with neuropathic foot ulcers	Neurometer	Vibration Current perception thresholds (where 2 kHz correlates with vibration & 5 Hz with warmth)	Sensitivity NR (vibration) "provides good discrimination between neuropathic and nonneuropathic groups." Scatter plots presented, but no data to calculate sensitivity or specificity
Navarro (79)	280 Diabetic patients with neuropathy	Thermal stimulator	Thermal	Sensitivity 79% (thermal) Sensitivity 39% (heat pain)
Dyck (15)	195 Diabetics—42 with poly-neuropathy (based on NIS(LL) scores	Case-IV	Vibration	Sensitivity 27.8% Specificity 100%
Holland (36)	20 patients with idiopathic small fiber neuropathy	Case-IV	Cold Vibration	Sensitivity 82% (cold) Sensitivity 60% (vibration) Specificity 83% (cold & vibration)

NR, not reported; NIS(LL), Neuropathy Impairment Score for the lower limbs study did not report sufficient data to calculate either sensitivity or specificity, but instead the data are presented as scatter plots and these seem to suggest substantial overlap in the thresholds measured for diabetic neuropathy and control patients, contrary to the conclusion reached by these authors that QST provides good discrimination between patients with neuropathy and those without *(16)*.

In view of the psychophysical nature of QST, concern has been raised that false-positive results may be obtained in subjects who are biased toward an abnormal test result. This question has been addressed by a number of investigators with conflicting results *(17,18)*. Some investigators have proposed that although healthy subjects who are asked to feign sensory loss may produce threshold values that are indistinguishable from those with peripheral neuropathy the variance of repeated measures of these threshold values is sufficiently greater than that in subjects with peripheral neuropathy, that the two may be distinguished *(18)*. Others have argued that such differences in the variance likely arise from the use of QST devices that incorporate subject response time and that discrimination between healthy subjects feigning sensory loss and those with peripheral neuropathy cannot be made using the more commonly employed Case-IV QST system, which is reaction-time exclusive *(17)*. Studies such as this do raise concerns about the specificity of QST.

The quality of the literature evaluating the diagnostic utility of QST, therefore, is extremely limited and the available evidence does not seem to support the conclusion that QST is probably useful for the diagnosis of diabetic and idiopathic small fiber polyneuropathy, respectively.

2.4. What Is the Role of Nerve Biopsy in the Diagnosis of Polyneuropathy?

There are a limited number of studies that have addressed the question of the diagnostic value of nerve biopsy in determining the etiology of polyneuropathy *(19–24)*. With two exceptions *(19,20)*, most of these studies are of limited quality, with the most common methodological shortcoming being inadequate description of the frequency with which the final diagnosis was made based on pathological findings. Nevertheless, the results of these studies are in agreement that peripheral nerve vasculitis is the most commonly identified etiological diagnosis. Other less common diagnoses include amyloid, hereditary neuropathy with liability to pressure palsies (HNPP), inflammatory neuropathy, and malignancy (Table 8.4).

Some have suggested that the diagnostic yield of sural nerve is highest among those with demyelinating physiology on nerve conduction studies *(19)*, but others have found no difference in yield between those with demyelinating and those with axonal physiology *(20)*.

The role of nerve (and muscle) biopsy in the diagnosis of peripheral nerve vasculitis is discussed in detail in Chapter 10 and will not be recapitulated here. The essence of this discussion (*see* pp. 176,178) is that nerve biopsy has a relatively high sensitivity for the diagnosis of vasculitis.

The diagnosis of amyloidosis requires histological demonstration of amyloid fibrils that characteristically show apple-green birefringence on polarized light-microscopy of Congo-red stained tissue samples. The sensitivity of nerve biopsy for the diagnosis of amyloidosis has been reported in a number of studies *(25–27)*, although the estimates of sensitivity in these studies have varied widely from 11% *(27)* to 100% *(25,26)*. The

Table 8.4
Value of Nerve Biopsy in the Etiological Diagnosis of Polyneuropathy

Reference	n	Study population	Diagnostic yield	Etiological diagnoses
Argov (19)	120	Retrospective evaluation of patients seen in the EMG laboratory with "electrophysiologically confirmed peripheral neuropathy." Biopsy in 42 patients in whom etiology unknown.	38%	Vasculitis—6 (11%) Amyloid—2 (4%) Inflammatory neuropathy—4 (8%) Hereditary ("onion bulbs")—6 (11%) Neoplasia—1 (2%) Other—1 (2%)
Midroni (20)	267	Retrospective review of consecutive series of nerve biopsies for which sufficient clinical information was available	21%	Vasculitis—20 (7.5%) Amyloid—4 (1.5%) Inflammatory neuropathy—4 (1.5%) HNPP—3 (1.1%) Amiodarone—3 (1.1%) Leprosy—2 (0.7%) Paraprotein—2 (0.7%) Granuloma (sarcoid)—2 (0.7%) Lymphoma (infiltrative)—2 (0.7%) Fabry's disease—1 (0.4%)
Oh (21)	385	Not specified	24%	Vasculitis—46 (12%) HNPP—27 (7%) Inflammatory neuropathy—12 (3%) Amyloid—2 (0.05%)
Rappaport (24)	60	Retrospective review of patients with suspected polyneuropathy who underwent nerve biopsy	? 15%	Vasculitis—6 (10%) Amyloid—1 (2%) Paraneoplastic—2 (3%)
Neundorfer (22)	80	Follow-up in 56 of 80 patients who had undergone sural nerve biopsy for the diagnosis of polyneuropathy	27%	Vasculitis—9 (16%) Amyloid—1 (2%) HNPP—2 (4%) CMT1A—3 (5%)

EMG, electromyography; HNPP, hereditary neuropathy with liability to pressure palsies; CMT1A, Charcot-Marie-Tooth type 1A.

reasons for this wide disparity are not entirely clear, although they likely relate in large part to the bias that may have been introduced via the methods used to select subjects for inclusion in the studies as well as the frequency with which nerve biopsy was used to obtain tissue for histological diagnosis. The studies reporting sensitivity of 100% are both retrospective case series of patients who were known to have amyloidosis, confirmed by biopsy of one tissue or another. One of these studies included 229 patients, but nerve biopsy was performed only in 12 cases *(26)*. Similarly, nerve biopsy was performed in only 10 of 31 patients in the second study *(25)*. In the study reporting a lower sensitivity, nerve biopsy was performed in all nine patients *(27)*. As a result of the variability of these results and the methodological limitations of each study, it is not possible to reliably estimate the sensitivity of nerve biopsy for the diagnosis of amyloidosis. Furthermore, none of these studies provide insight into the specificity of the staining techniques used to demonstrate the presence of amyloid, but data from the analysis of other tissue samples (discussed later) suggests that the specificity is high.

In evaluating the role of nerve biopsy for the diagnosis of amyloidosis, it is useful to consider the diagnostic utility of alternative sources of tissue such as abdominal fat aspiration *(28–33)*. Estimates of sensitivity range from 55% to 87.5%, with specificity of 100% in most studies (Table 8.5).

The available data do not permit reliable comparison of the diagnostic accuracy of nerve biopsy with that of tissue obtained from other sites such as abdominal fat pad, skin, rectum, and kidney. These data do, however, suggest that specificity is high and that sensitivity is incomplete. It is not clear whether the sensitivity of nerve biopsy is increased if there is clinical and/or electrophysiological evidence for involvement of the peripheral nervous system. However, based on these observations, it seems reasonable to conclude that negative immunohistochemisty of any single tissue sample should not be taken as evidence for the absence of amyloidosis if the clinical suspicion is high. Because fine needle aspiration biopsy of the abdominal fat pad is relatively noninvasive compared with nerve biopsy, it could be argued that the fat pad biopsy should be undertaken first, with nerve biopsy reserved for those in whom the clinical suspicion for amyloid remains high despite a negative abdominal fat pad biopsy.

In summary, therefore, nerve biopsy is most helpful for the diagnosis of vasculitis. Biopsy may also permit the diagnosis of amyloidosis, although fine needle aspiration biopsy of abdominal fat should probably be used for diagnosing amyloid before resorting to nerve biopsy. Rarely, nerve biopsy will lead to an alternate diagnosis such as hereditary or inflammatory neuropathy, sarcoidosis, or malignancy.

2.5. What Is the Role of Skin Biopsy in the Evaluation of Small Fiber Neuropathy?

A novel method for using skin biopsy specimens stained with antibodies to protein gene product 9.5 (PGP9.5) in order to estimate intra-epidermal nerve fiber (IENF) density was described McCarthy and colleagues in 1995 *(34)*. They performed skin biopsies in seven healthy controls, five HIV seropositive patients without evidence of neuropathy, five patients with HIV neuropathy, and eight patients with HIV seronegative sensory neuropathy and showed that the mean IENF density was significantly reduced in both the HIV-positive and -negative patients with neuropathy compared with healthy controls and the HIV seropositive individuals without neuropathy *(34)*. These data, although they

Table 8.5
Accuracy of Abdominal Fat Aspiration Biopsy for the Diagnosis of Amyloidosis

Reference	n	Study population	Gold standard for diagnosis	Sensitivity	Specificity
Masouye (32)	98	Subjects with symptoms suggestive of amyloid who were referred for FNAB	Clinical course ± biopsy of other tissue for histological confirmation	82%	100%
Guy (33)	45	Patients referred for FNAB	Clinical course ± biopsy of other tissue for histological confirmation	58%	100%
Ansari-Lari (31)	91	Patients referred for FNAB	Histological confirmation based on biopsy of alternate tissue	55%	74%
Duston (28)	17	Prospective study of abdominal fat aspiration samples sent to the laboratory	Histological confirmation based on biopsy of alternate tissue	57%	100%
Duston (29)	84	Abdominal fat aspirates of patients known to have amyloid	Histological confirmation based on biopsy of alternate tissue	84%	—
Libbey (30)	32	Patients with known amyloid	Histological confirmation based on biopsy of alternate tissue	87.5%	—

FNAB, fine needle aspiration biopsy.

provide proof of principle, do not permit estimation of the accuracy of skin biopsy for the diagnosis of small fiber neuropathy.

Any investigation of the accuracy of a test for the diagnosis of small fiber neuropathy will be confounded by the absence of a generally agreed upon gold standard against which the performance of the diagnostic test may be compared. In the absence of such a gold standard, it really is not possible to estimate the sensitivity and specificity of skin biopsy with determination of IENF density for the diagnosis of small fiber neuropathy. An alternative approach, which has been used to some extent in the literature, is to define the range of IENF density in healthy controls and to use this data to establish a normal range (e.g., less then the fifth percentile for age) and to then ask how frequently patients with symptoms suggestive of a small fiber neuropathy show reduced IENF density.

To establish normative reference values, McArthur and colleagues examined 98 carefully screened (by history and neurological examination) healthy controls who were then subjected to punch skin biopsy in the thigh and distal leg (35). Biopsy specimens were stained with the PGP9.5 antibody and the IENF density (number of nerves per millimeter) determined. Inter-observer and intra-observer variability were low, with the respective correlation coefficients ranging from 0.86 to 0.94 and 0.74 to 0.86. Percentiles were used to define the "normal" range. The fifth-percentile lower limit of normal for the thigh was 5.2 fibers per millimeter, and for distal part of the leg it was 3.8 per millimeter; age did not significantly affect nerve fiber density (35).

The same investigators selected 20 patients who had been diagnosed with painful sensory neuropathy on the basis of their clinical presentation, all of whom reported distally accentuated symptoms of dysesthesia and numbness without significant weakness or sensory ataxia. Using the fifth-percentile value in the distal leg from the healthy controls as the lower limit of normal, they estimated the sensitivity of skin biopsy for the diagnosis of small fiber neuropathy to be 45%, with a specificity of 97% (35,36). These data, therefore, seem to suggest either that the clinical criteria for diagnosing small fiber neuropathy are too loose or that skin biopsy with IENF density measurement is an insensitive test for this diagnosis. The results of this and other studies of the accuracy of IENF density for the diagnosis of small fiber neuropathy are summarized in Table 8.6. Substantially better sensitivity was reported in two subsequent studies (37,38), one of which was performed by the same investigators using the same reference values to define the normal range (37). The authors offer no explanation for why the sensitivity was so much better in the second group of patients they examined using the same biopsy technique, the same location for biopsy, and the same reference values. The disparity is not readily attributable to the patients included in each study because similar inclusion criteria were employed on each occasion. One possible explanation is that the pathologist was blinded to the origin of the skin biopsy specimen in the initial study but not in the second study, suggesting that the discrepant higher sensitivity may be due to investigator bias. Similarly, no mention is made of the investigator blinding in the study by Periquet et al. (38), again suggesting that the higher sensitivity may be due to bias.

In summary, therefore, the estimates of the sensitivity of IENF density estimation for the diagnosis of small fiber neuropathy vary widely, with the more reliable estimate being approximately 45% (with the judgement that this estimate is more reliable being based on the fact that the investigators were blinded to the source of the biopsies in this study). Specificity by definition is high (95%), because the fifth-percentile values derived from healthy controls were used to define the lower limit of normal. Notwithstanding the high specificity, the low sensitivity suggests that skin biopsy is not a useful screening test for patients with suspected small fiber neuropathy. The value of skin biopsy lies in ruling in (confirming) the diagnosis in that a postive test result is unlikely to be a false-positive given the high specificity of the test.

3. TREATMENT

3.1. What Is the Evidence for the Efficacy of the Tricyclic Antidepressants in the Treatment of Painful Diabetic Neuropathy?

A review of the literature reveals nine randomized placebo-controlled trials of tricyclic anti-depressants in the treatment of painful diabetic neuropathy. The details of design of these studies and their methodological quality as well as their results are summarized in Tables 8.7 and 8.8. They were all relatively small studies and were all cross-over in design, which means that each patient served as their own control, receiving either the active drug or placebo during one treatment period and the alternative drug during the second treatment period. Study design varied in that some included a washout period in between the two treatment periods in order to reduce the likelihood of a carry-over effect (i.e., active drug continuing to have an effect during the placebo treatment period). A number of different scales and scoring systems were used to evaluate the severity of

Table 8.6
Accuracy of Skin Biopsy and Intra-Epidermal Nerve Fiber Density Estimation for the Diagnosis of Small Fiber Neuropathy

Reference	n	Study population	Controls	LLN	Sensitivity	Specificity
McArthur (35,36)	20	Patients with painful sensory neuropathy diagnosed on the basis of distally predominant dysesthesia and numbness (2 DM, 5 HIV, 3 HIV + anti-retroviral, 11 idiopathic)	98 healthy controls screened by history and neurological examination	5th percentile (3.8/mm)	45%	97%[a]
Holland (37)	32	Patients with neuropathic limb pain, normal strength, JPS, reflexes & NCS with no known cause for small fiber neuropathy	98 healthy controls screened by history and neurological examination (same data from prior study by the same authors (35)	5th percentile (3.8/mm)	78%	Not stated, but should be 95%[a]
Periquet (38)	117	Patients with painful feet & normal strength were selected. Skin biopsy only performed in the 56 who had normal NCS	50 healthy volunteers with no neurological abnormalities on examination, normal NCS and QST	5th percentile (20/mm for age <60 and 11.8/mm for age >60)	79%	Not stated, but should be 95%[a]

LLN, lower limit of normal; DM, diabetes mellitus; HIV, human immunodeficiency virus; JPS, joint position sense; NCS, nerve conduction studies; QST, quantitative sensory testing.

[a]Use of the fifth percentile, by definition, implies that IENF density would be classified as abnormal in 5% of healthy subjects, which would mean that the specificity must be 95%. It is unclear how specificity could be 97% in the study by McArthur and colleagues.

symptoms at baseline and following each treatment period. These differences make it difficult to compare the results between the various studies.

In one study *(39)*, patients were asked to rate the severity of their pain and paresthesiae on a modified visual analog scale. The initial level of symptom intensity at the beginning of the study was assigned a value of 100% and subsequent scores were considered as positive or negative percent deviations. In other studies *(40,41)* patients were asked at follow-up to rate their pain relief (compared with baseline) as complete, a lot, moderate, slight, none, or worse. Finally, a number of investigators *(42–47)* used a six-item scale to evaluate the severity of the neuropathy symptoms. The six items include pain, paresthesia, dysesthesia, numbness, nightly aggravation, and sleep disturbance. Each item was scored as absent (0), very mild (0.5), mild (1), moderate (1.5), or severe (2), yielding a maximal (worst) possible score of 12 points. However, the way in which data from the "6-item neuropathy symptom scale" were used to define the final outcome varied between these studies. Some have simply compared neuropathy scale scores during treatment with placebo or with active drug *(43)*, whereas others have included a comparison of the median neuropathy scale scores in different treatment groups *(44–46)*. In their systematic review, McQuay et al. *(48)* defined a successful outcome as the attainment of a neuropathy scale score of ≤6, and this is the definition that has been used in the compilation of Table 8.8.

Of the tricyclic antidepressants, imipramine has been most frequently studied *(42,43,45,47)*. In the study by Kvinesdal et al. *(42)*, a fixed dose of imipramine was compared with placebo. The authors described the outcome of this study using a three-point global assessment scale, with 7 of 12 patients in the imipramine and no patients in the placebo group reporting a notable improvement in symptoms. They also evaluated outcome using the six-point neuropathy symptom scale. Using the definition of improvement, suggested by McQuay et al., of a neuropathy scale score of ≤6 *(48)*, 7 of 12 patients in the placebo group and 10 of 12 patients in the imipramine group would be classified as having a successful outcome. In their small study, Sindrup and colleagues also compared imipramine with placebo *(43)*. At the end of the study, patients were asked to indicate the treatment period during which they had felt the most relief from symptoms. Eight of the nine patients identified the imipramine treatment period as having provided the most relief from symptoms. Again, these authors also collected data using the six-item neuropathy scale. Seven patients in the placebo group attained a neuropathy scale score of ≤6, compared with eight patients in the imipramine group. In these two placebo-controlled studies, therefore, imipramine was taken to be superior to placebo based on one outcome measure, but the results are certainly less clear when described in terms of the second outcome measure. It is relevant to note that neither study prespecified which outcome measure would be used in the primary efficacy analysis. This shortcoming, together with the very small sample sizes, call into question the validity of the conclusion that imipramine has clearly been shown to be superior to placebo in the treatment of painful diabetic neuropathy.

In two separate studies, Sindrup and colleagues compared the efficacy of imipramine with paroxetine and placebo *(45)* and with mianserin and placebo *(47)*. These were slightly larger studies, and the dose of imipramine was adjusted in order to achieve a prespecified plasma drug concentration. In both, the results were primarily reported in terms of the neuropathy symptom score. As shown in Table 8.8, 18 of 19 patients attained

Table 8.7
Methodological Quality of Studies of Tricyclic Antidepressants for Painful Diabetic Neuropathy

Drug/reference	Method of randomization	Allocation concealment	Patient blinding	Observer blinding	Explicit inclusion/ exclusion criteria	Completeness of follow-up
Nortriptyline (39)	Unclear	Unclear	Adequate	Unclear	Adequate	25% drop-out rate
Imipramine (42)	Unclear	Unclear	Adequate	Unclear	Adequate	20% drop-out rate
Amitriptyline (40)	Unclear	Unclear	Adequate	Adequate	Adequate	21% drop-out rate
Amitriptyline/ Desipramine (41)	Unclear	Unclear	Unclear	Unclear	Adequate	15% drop-out rate
Imipramine (43)	Unclear	Unclear	Unclear	Unclear	Unclear	31% drop-out rate
Clomipramine/ Desipramine (44)	Unclear	Unclear	Adequate	Unclear	Adequate	27% drop-out rate
Imipramine (45)	Unclear	Unclear	Adequate	Unclear	Adequate	34% drop-out rate
Mianserin (47)	Unclear	Unclear	Unclear	Unclear	Unclear	18% drop-out rate

Table 8.8
Efficacy of Tricyclic Antidepressants in the Treatment of Painful Diabetic Neuropathy

Study design	Active treatment	Sample size (no. lost to follow-up)	Outcome measures	Proportion improving		Reference
				Active	Placebo	
Two 30-d periods; no washout	Nortriptyline 10 mg + fluphenazine 0.5 mg	24 (−6)	Modified visual analog scale (VAS)	13/18[a]	2/18[a]	Gomez-Perez (39)
Two 4-wk periods; no washout	Imipramine 50 mg/d × 1 wk then 100 mg × 4 wk	15 (−3)	6-item scale of symptoms 3-item global assessment	7/12[b]	0/12[b]	Kvinesdal (42)
Two 6-wk periods; no washout	Amitriptyline 25–100 mg/d	37 (−8)	6-point scale of degree of change in symptoms	15/29[c]	1/29[c]	Max (40)
Two 6-wk periods; 2-wk washout	Amitriptyline Desipramine	54 (−16) 54 (−16)	6-point scale of degree of change in symptoms	28/38[c] 23/38[c]	— —	Max (41)
Two 3-wk periods; no washout	Imipramine 12–225 mg/d	13 (−4)	6-item scale of symptoms 3-item global assessment	8/9[d]	1/9[d]	Sindrup (43)
Three 2-wk periods	Clomipramine 50–75 mg/d Desipramine 50–200 mg/d	26 (−7)	6-item scale of symptoms	14/18[e] 13/18[e]	10/18[e]	Sindrup (44)
Three 2-wk periods; 1–3-wk washout	Imipramine 25–350 mg/d Paroxetine 40 mg/d	29 (−10)	Mean VAS for diff. symptoms	18/20[e] 18/19[e]	14/20[e]	Sindrup (45)
Three 2-wk periods; 1-wk washout	Imipramine 25–350 mg/d Mianserin 60 mg/d	22 (−4)	6-item scale of symptoms	14/18[e] 11/18[e]	11/18[e]	Sindrup (47)

[a]Improvement defined as a >50% reduction in pain severity compared with baseline.

[b]Improvement defined as a "notable effect" on the 3-item (no effect, some/doubtful effect, notable effect) global assessment.

[c]Definition of improvement includes first 3 responses on 6-point scale (pain relief described as complete, a lot, moderate, slight, none, or worse).

[d]Improvement defined on a dichotomous basis with patients asked to indicate the treatment period during which they felt the most pain relief.

[e]Improvement defined as attainment of a neuropathy scale score of ≤ 6 (total of 12 points on the scale).

125

a score of ≤ 6 in the imipramine group compared with 14 of 20 in the placebo group *(45)*. Similarly, in the second study, 14 of 18 patients in the imipramine and 11 of 18 in the placebo group attained neuropathy scale scores of ≤ 6 *(47)*.

The generally accepted conclusion, therefore, that imipramine is effective in the treatment of neuropathic pain has been based on these four studies. In total, these studies report outcome data for 59 patients with diabetic neuropathy, 50 of whom showed a response to imipramine compared with 39 when treated with placebo. It should be noted, however, that the magnitude and clinical importance of the response is difficult to determine from these studies.

The magnitude of the clinical response to active drug was reported in the study of nortriptyline by Gomez-Perez et al. *(39)*. In this study, a significantly greater proportion of patients who received nortriptyline (72% compared with 11%) reported a ≥ 50% reduction in pain intensity (cf. data on anticonvulsants in Table 8.13). Of note is that a relatively low dose of nortriptyline (10 mg/day) was used, and the beneficial effect was noted at the end of the study period (30 days) but not midway through the study (15 days).

Max and colleagues examined the efficacy of amitriptyline in two separate placebo-controlled trials *(40,41)*. In the first study, the dose of amitriptyline was titrated according to clinical efficacy and side effects, with dosages varying from 25 to 150 mg per day. In an effort to ensure subject-blinding, the placebo group also received benztropine and diazepam in order to mimic the anticholinergic and sedative side effects of amitriptyline. After each treatment period, patients were asked to describe the relief from pain as complete, a lot, moderate, slight, none, or worse. Twenty-three of the 29 patients who completed the study reported less pain following treatment with amitriptyline; 10 described the response as "complete," 5 as "a lot" and 4 as "moderate." In contrast, only one patient reported less pain following treatment with placebo. Of note in this study was that the pain response to amitriptyline was independent of an effect on mood. It is also important to note that 28 of 29 patients reported side effects during treatment with amitriptyline, the most common being a dry mouth (26), sedation (19), and dizziness (8).

The second report by Max et al. *(41)* really included two studies: in the first, the efficacy of amitriptyline was compared with desipramine, and in the second, fluoxetine was compared with placebo. The dose of amitriptyline was again determined by titration to achieve a therapeutic plasma concentration. A response (defined, as in their prior study, as pain relief described as "complete," "a lot," or "moderate") to amitriptyline was observed in 28 of 38 patients. A response in the placebo group (of the fluoxetine-placebo study) was observed in 19 of 46 patients. The overall impression, therefore, from these two studies is that amitriptyline reduces the severity of pain in approximately 70% of patients. In these two studies, the placebo response rate varied from 3 to 40%.

Finally, there are two studies of desipramine for the treatment of painful diabetic neuropathy *(41,44)*. In the study by Max et al. *(41)* of amitriptyline vs desipramine, the response rate among those treated with desipramine was around 60%, only slightly lower (but not significantly so) from the response rate in the amitriptyline group. The study by Sindrup and colleagues *(44)* comparing desipramine, clomipramine, and placebo used the neuropathy symptoms scale score as a measure of outcome. They reported significantly better (lower) scores in the desipramine (and clomipramine) groups compared with placebo. As shown in Table 8.8 (using a neuropathy scale score ≤ 6 as a measure of treatment success), 72% of the desipramine group obtained relief of their pain, compared with 56% in the placebo group. Again, it is worth noting the small absolute number of patients on which this conclusion is based and the relatively small benefit over and above treatment with placebo.

In summary, therefore, data from a number of small randomized placebo-controlled trials support the use of nortriptyline, amitriptyline, desipramine, and clomipramine for the treatment of painful diabetic neuropathy. These studies were all limited by their small sample size and by the relatively small incremental benefit observed in the active treatment groups compared with those treated with placebo. Moreover, the incidence of side effects was substantial, a factor that will likely limit the usefulness of this group of drugs.

3.2. What Is the Efficacy of the Serotonin and Noradrenaline Reuptake Inhibitors in the Treatment of Painful Diabetic Neuropathy?

There have been four studies of nontricyclic anti-depressants for the treatment of painful diabetic neuropathy (41,45,46,49). Although all four studies were randomized controlled trials, they are lacking in a number of important respects (Table 8.9). Overall, however, the drop-out rates are lower than seen in studies of the tricyclic antidepressants (see Tables 8.9 and 8.10), suggesting that they are better tolerated. The results of these studies have been mixed. The study by Sindrup et al. (45) showed a beneficial response in patients treated with paroxetine, with the degree of improvement slightly less than that achieved with imipramine. In a separate study, Sindrup and colleagues (46) found a response rate of 87% among those treated with citalopram, compared with 53% among the placebo group. Max et al., by contrast, found there to be no significant difference in the response rates between fluoxetine and placebo treated patients (41). The more recent study by Rowbotham and colleagues of two doses of Venflaxaine (Effexor) "extended release'"showed improvement in pain intensity scores among those who received higher doses (150–225 mg/day) (49) (Table 8.10). Each of these studies reported mean or median changes in pain scores between active and placebo treated patients and none provided any measure of the proportion of patients achieving significant (e.g., 50%) reduction in pain scores.

The overall impression from these data is that some of the nontricyclic reuptake inhibitor antidepressants may provide a modest benefit for patients with painful diabetic neuropathy. Although the effects are generally less substantial than observed with the tricyclic antidepressants, they tend to be better tolerated.

3.3. What Is the Evidence for the Efficacy of Anticonvulsants in the Treatment of Neuropathic Pain?

A range of different anticonvulsants have been investigated in randomized controlled trials for their efficacy in treating painful diabetic neuropathy. Topiramate has been the subject of three studies (50–52) and Phenytoin has been studied twice (53,54) whereas Carbamazepine (55), Valproate (56), Lamotrigine (57), and Gabapentin (58) have each been the subject of a single randomized controlled trial. Pregabalin has recently been the subject of two trials (59,60). These studies have varied in methodological quality (Table 8.11) and in terms of their results (Table 8.12). Relatively high drop-out rates have plagued many of these studies, suggesting either that the drug under study is ineffective or that it is poorly tolerated at a dose that might be effective.

Table 8.9
Methodological Quality of Studies of Re-Uptake Inhibitors for Painful Diabetic Polyneuropathy

Drug/reference	Method of randomization	Allocation concealment	Patient blinding	Observer blinding	Explicit inclusion/ exclusion criteria	Completeness of follow-up
Paroxetine (45)	Unclear	Unclear	Adequate	Unclear	Adequate	Inadequate (31% drop-out rate)
Citalopram (46)	Unclear	Unclear	Adequate	Unclear	Adequate	Adequate (17% drop-out rate)
Fluoxetine (41)	Unclear	Unclear	Unclear	Unclear	Adequate	Adequate (15% drop-out rate)
Venlafaxine (49)	Unclear	Adequate	Adequate	Unclear	Adequate	Adequate (<1% drop-out rate)

Table 8.10
Re-Uptake Inhibitor for Painful Diabetic Neuropathy: Study Design and Results

Drug	Study design	Dosage	Outcome measure	Results
Paroxetine (& imipramine) (45)	Cross-over (n = 29) 3 × 2-wk periods with 1–3-wk washout in between Compared with placebo and imipramine	40 mg/d	VAS for each of the symptoms pain, paresthesia, dysesthesia, nightly aggravation, and sleep disturbance. Median VAS score for all 5 items used to measure outcome	↓ (improved) median 5-item VAS score in paroxetine group (81.5) compared with placebo (141.5)[a]; better scores for imipramine (37)
Citalopram (46)	Cross-over (n = 18) 2 × 3-wk periods with 1-wk washout in between Compared with placebo	40 mg/d	Scoring (0–2) of each of 6 items on a neuropathy symptom scale (pain, paresthesia, dysesthesia, numbness, nightly aggravation, and sleep disturbance); Median scores used to measure outcome	↓ (improved) median 6-item scores in citalopram group (4.0) compared with placebo group (6.0)
Fluoxetine (& desipramine & amitriptyline) (41)	Cross-over (n = 54) 2 × 6-wk periods with 2-wk washout in between Compared with placebo	20–40 mg/d	Subjective global rating of pain relief and self rating of pain intensity using a 13-point scale. No primary outcome measure specified.	No statistically significant differences between fluoxetine and placebo.
Venlafaxine (V) (49)	Parallel group (n = 244) 6-wk duration of therapy Compared with placebo	75 mg/d, 150–225 mg/d	Mean change in pain intensity VAS	↓ mean VAS scores of 18.7 (placebo), 22.4 (V-75 mg) and 33.8 (V-150/225 mg)

[a]Maximum visual analog scale (VAS) score of 500 (100 mm scale for each of five items). V, venlafaxine.

129

The two studies of Phenytoin yielded conflicting results *(53,54)*. One study reported no difference between phenytoin and placebo *(54)*, whereas the other reported improvement in symptoms more frequently in the phenytoin than in the placebo-treated group *(53)*. Both of these studies were conducted in the 1970s, and the methodological quality of each was limited (Table 8.11). Outcome was evaluated in the one study by means of postcards that were mailed to study subjects who were asked to "... cross a line between 'none' and 'severe', denoting symptomatology for that day" with the symptoms of pain, numbness, and pins and needles each represented by a line on the postcard *(54)*. In the second study, subjects were asked simply to rate the change in the severity of their pain and paresthesia on a five-point likert scale *(53)*. Both studies were small, and in neither was there any discussion of the power of the study to detect a clinical effect. It is difficult to draw firm conclusions regarding the efficacy of phenytoin from either of these studies.

The one study of Carbamazepine randomized 30 patients with various forms of diabetic neuropathy to receive either active drug or placebo in a cross-over study design *(55)*. The investigators reported the change in severity of symptoms during each treatment period, but no formal outcome measure was used to evaluate the response to therapy. Although the authors state that all but two patients treated with Carbamazepine improved, it is difficult to determine the real efficacy of the drug.

The study of Lamotrigine used a numerical pain scale as the primary measure of efficacy, with results reported as the change in mean pain scores from baseline, a measure which does not provide insight into the proportion of patients who achieved a clinically meaningful improvement in symptoms. As a secondary outcome measure, the authors reported that 12 of 29 (41%) of Lamotrigine-treated subjects achieved a 50% reduction in pain compared with only 5 of 30 (17%) in the control group (Table 8.13).

The study of Gabapentin employed an 11-point likert pain severity rating scale as the primary measure of efficacy, with the results also reported in terms of the differences in mean scores between the Gabapentin and placebo treated groups after the 8-week duration of the study *(58)*. As a secondary outcome measure, however, the authors did report that 26% of patients receiving Gabapentin reported being pain free at the end of the study, compared with 15% of placebo-treated patients *(58)* (Table 8.13).

Pain severity was estimated with the short form of the McGill pain questionnaire (SF-MPQ) in the study of the efficacy of Valproate *(56)*. This outcome measure, like those used in the studies of Lamotrigine and Gabapentin, was reported in terms of the mean change in pain score from baseline in the placebo and valproate treated groups (Table 8.12). The authors do not report the proportion of patients in each group who achieved a greater than 50% reduction in pain severity, but do indicate that the proportion of patients with MPQ score ≥ 5 (indicative of excruciating pain) fell from 71% to 39% in the valproate group while remaining constant at 50% in the placebo group *(56)*.

Topiramate has been the subject of three reports (five studies) *(50–52)* with the methodological quality of these studies being somewhat variable (Table 8.11). The major limitation of each study is the high drop-out rate in the Topiramate treated patients, ranging from 28% to 58%, and also in the placebo group, ranging from 27 to 41%. Two of these studies found no significant benefit from Topiramate *(50,51)*, whereas a third did show improved pain control *(52)*. The authors of the latter study argue that the reasons for their detecting an effect whereas prior studies did not related to their use of a 100-mm visual analog scale (VAS) both for determining eligibility for the study and for measuring

Table 8.11
Methodological Quality of Anticonvulsant Trials

	Method of randomization	Allocation concealment	Patient blinding	Observer blinding	Explicit inclusion/ exclusion criteria	Completeness of follow-up
Rull (55)	Unclear	Unclear	Adequate	Adequate	Unclear	Adequate. Drop-out rate of 10%.
Chadda (53)	Unclear	Unclear	Unclear	Unclear	Adequate	Adequate. Drop-out rate of 5%.
Saudek (54)	Unclear	Unclear	Adequate	Adequate	Adequate	Unclear
Eisenberg (57)	Adequate	Unclear	Adequate	Unclear	Adequate	Adequate. Drop-out rates: 17% (L), 27% (placebo). No ITT analysis.
Edwards (50)	Unclear	Unclear	Unclear	Unclear	Inadequate	Inadequate. 28% drop-out rate for Topiramate with no ITT analysis
Thienel (51)	Adequate	Unclear	Unclear	Unclear	Adequate	Inadequate. Drop-out rates: 41% (P), 46% (T-100) 53% (T-200), 58% (T-400) ITT analysis
Raskin (52)	Adequate	Unclear	Adequate	Unclear	Adequate	Inadequate. Drop-out rates: 27% (P), 53% (T). ITT analysis
Backonja (58)	Adequate	Unclear	Adequate	Adequate	Adequate	Adequate. Drop-out rates: 17% (G), 20% (placebo) ITT analysis
Kochar (56)	Unclear	Unclear	Unclear	Unclear	Inadequate	Adequate. Drop-out rates: 6.7% (V), 20% (placebo). No ITT analysis
Rosenstock (59)	Adequate	Unclear	Adequate	Unclear	Adequate	Adequate. Drop-out rates: 14% (pregabalin), 11% (placebo)
Lesser (60)	Adequate	Adequate	Adequate	Adequate	Adequate	Adequate: Drop-out rates: 4–15% (pregabalin), 2% (placebo)

P, placebo; T-100, topiramate 100 mg/d; T-200, Topiramate 200 mg/d; T-400, Topiramate 400 mg/d; ITT, intention to treat; L, lamotrigine; G, gabapentin; V, valproate.

Table 8.12
Anticonvulsants for the Treatment of Painful Diabetic Neuropathy

Reference	n	Design	Drug	Dose	Outcome measure	Results
Rull (55)	30	Cross-over 2 × 3-wk periods	Carbamazepine	Titration 200–600 mg/d	Pain intensity	28/30 improved (C) vs 19/30 (P).
Chadda (53)	40	Cross-over 2 × 2-wk periods 1-wk washout	Phenytoin	Fixed 300 mg/d	Pain intensity Paresthesias	28/38 moderate improvement (Ph) vs 10/38 (P)
Saudek (54)	12	Cross over 2 × 23-wk	Phenytoin	100 mg tid after 600 mg load	Pain intensity using a visual analog scale	No difference between the two groups
Eisenberg (57)	59	Parallel group 8-wk duration	Lamotrigine	Dose titration from 25 mg/d to 200 mg bid	Numerical pain scale	↓ mean pain intensity 6.4–4.2 (L) 6.5–5.3 (P)
Edwards (50)	27	Parallel group 13-wk (9-wk dose titration)	Topiramate	Dose titration to max tolerated dose (200 mg bid)	McGill Pain Questionnaire & visual analog pain scale	MPQ: 14.3–11.1 (T) 22.7–25.1 (P) VAS: 69–40.7 (T) 64.6–70.4 (P)
Theniel (51)	524	Parallel group 18–22 wk	Topiramate	Dose ranging 100–400 mg/d in different groups	Visual analog scale	VAS: 57.7–43.1 (P) 60.1–36.1 (T-100) 55.8–38.3 (T-200) 56.3–39.7 (T-400)
Raskin (52)	323	Parallel group 12 wk	Topiramate	Dose titration to max tolerated (400 mg qd)	Visual analog scale	VAS: 68.0–46.2 (T) 69.1–54.0 (P)
Backonja (58)	165	Parallel group 8-wk (4-wk dose titration)	Gabapentin	Dose titration to max tolerated (1200 mg tid)	Pain severity on an 11-point likert scale	Mean pain scores 6.4 –3.9 (G) 6.5–5.1 (P)
Kochar (56)	60	Parallel group 1 mo	Valproate	200 mg tid	McGill Pain Questionnaire	MPQ: 5.0–3.1 (V) 4.9–4.6 (P)
Rosenstock (59)	146	Parallel group 8 wk	Pregabalin	300 mg/d	Pain severity on an 11-point likert scale	Mean pain scores 6.5–4.0 (pregabalin) 6.1–5.3 (placebo)
Lesser (60)	338	Parallel group 5 wk	Pregabalin	75 mg/d, 300 mg/d & 600 mg/d	Pain severity on an 11-point likert scale	Change in mean pain score compared to placebo: –1.26 (75 mg), –1.45 (600 mg)

P, placebo; Ph, phenytoin; C, carbamazepine; L, lamotrigine; T, topiramate; O, oxcarbazepine; G, gabapentin; V, valproate; MPQ, McGill Pain Questionnaire.

Table 8.13
Clinically Meaningful Reduction in Pain

Anticonvulsant	Proportion of patients with 50% reduction in pain intensity		Reference
	Active drug	*Placebo*	
Lamotrigine	41%	17%	57
Topiramate	36%	21%	52
Gabapentin	26%[a]	15%[a]	58
Valproate	Not reported	Not reported	56
Pregabalin	40%	15%	59
Pregabalin	~47%	18%	60

[a]The proportion of patients with 50% reduction in pain intensity is not reported in this study, but these data represent the proportion of patients reporting no pain at the end of the study.

outcome, as well as the nature of the outcome measures that they used. Patients were asked to "please rate the intensity of the pain that you are currently feeling in lower extremities" rather than the more general question, "how would you rate your pain" without specifying the time or location of the pain. It is difficult to believe that these subtleties were responsible for the effects observed in this study, and the result should be treated with caution given the high proportion of patients who did not complete the study. In the one study that showed a benefit, 36% of patients treated with Topiramate achieved a 50% improvement in pain severity compared to 21% in the placebo-treated group *(52)* (Table 8.13).

Pregabalin has been the subject of two recent, well designed, randomized controlled trials *(59,60)*. Both were parallel group studies. In the one study, pregabalin was used at a fixed dose of 300 mg/day *(59)* whereas in the second study, subjects were randomized to receive either placebo or one of three doses of pregabalin—75 mg/day, 300 mg/day, or 600 mg/day *(60)*. Both studies used as the primary outcome measure an 11-point likert scale on which patients were asked to grade the severity of their pain, and both used a range of secondary outcome measures including the McGill Pain Questionnaire, SF-36, the Patient Global Impression of Change, the Clinician Global Impression of Change, and the Profile of Mood States. The pregabalin-treated patients (at a dose of at least 300 mg/day) achieved better outcomes than the placebo-treated patients on all measures of outcome, with approximately 40% of pregabalin-treated patients achieving at least a 50% reduction in pain severity scores (Table 8.13).

The overall impression from the data on the efficacy of anticonvulsants for the treatment of painful diabetic neuropathy is that each of a number of agents may yield some benefit, but that improvement in pain severity tends to be modest. With one exception (a study that compared amitriptyline with gabapentin), there is no information comparing the relative efficacy of these different agents and whether failure to respond to one agent is of any value in predicting response (or lack thereof) to another agent. Tolerance for the drug will likely be an important determinant of therapy.

3.4. What Is the Evidence for the Efficacy of Opiates in the Treatment of Painful Peripheral Neuropathy?

There are a limited number of studies that have examined the efficacy of opiate analgesics for painful diabetic polyneuropathy *(61–63)*, but the available data do indicate that this class of drugs may be beneficial.

Gimbel and colleagues *(61)* examined the efficacy of controlled-release oxycodone (Oxycontin) in patients with painful diabetic peripheral neuropathy in a randomized, double-blind, placebo-controlled trial. Adjuvant analgesics were permitted at stable prestudy dosages, but the use of such therapy was well balanced between the two groups. The primary efficacy analysis was based on the average daily pain intensity between days 28 and 42 of the study, with pain intensity rated on an 11-point scale ranging from 0 (no pain) to 10 (worst pain imaginable). These results were reported as the "least squares mean" scores, a measure of group means adjusted for covariates and other terms in the statistical model. A total of 159 subjects were randomized and received at least one dose of study medication. There were 82 and 77 patients in the OxyContin and placebo groups, respectively. The average daily dose of Oxycontin was 27 mg between study days 15 and 42. The results of the primary analysis are summarized Table 8.14. In addition to showing a benefit in terms of reduced pain intensity, subjects receiving Oxycontin showed improvement on a range of secondary outcome measures including average pain intensity, worst pain intensity, and sleep quality *(61)*.

The authors conclude that these results show that controlled release oxycodone was significantly more effective than placebo on a wide variety of measures of pain relief. It is noteworthy that pain relief was achieved relatively quickly (within the first week of therapy) and that relatively low doses of oxycodone were required (mean daily dose of 27 mg) compared with the maximum allowable daily dose of 120 mg.

Notwithstanding these results demonstrating efficacy, many neurologists remain uncomfortable using narcotic analgesics, in part because of the high risk for dependence and abuse. Tramadol, on the other hand, is a synthetic nonnarcotic analgesic that exerts its effects via binding to μ-opioid receptors and exerts a weak inhibitory effect on norepinephrine and serotonin uptake. Because the development of tolerance and dependence appear to be low, it has been suggested that Tramadol may be a useful agent with low potential for abuse. Its efficacy in patients with painful diabetic neuropathy has been examined in a double-blind, randomized, placebo-controlled trial *(62)*. The design of this study was such that subjects first entered a screening/washout phase during which other analgesic agents were discontinued. Patients were then randomized to one of two treatment groups, Tramadol or placebo. Tramadol was started at a dose of 50 mg/day and titrated over 10 days in 50 mg increments every 3 days to 200 mg/day (the dose could subsequently be modified to obtain optimal pain relief, to a maximum of 400 mg/day). A total of 131 patients participated in the study, and the analysis is based on data from 127 patients (data from two patients in each group were omitted). The results are summarized in Table 8.14. Tramadol, at an average daily dose of 210 mg/day, was more effective than placebo in alleviating the pain of diabetic polyneuropathy *(62)*. The benefits of Tramdol were also apparent on a variety of secondary outcome measures including physical and social functioning. The number of patients needed to treat (NNT) in order to provide one patient with a greater than 50% reduction in pain intensity was 3.1

Table 8.14
The Efficacy of Opiate Analgesics in Painful Diabetic Polyneuropathy (DPN)

Reference	Drug	Dosage	Outcome measure	n	Results (pre→post)
Gimbel (61)	Oxycontin	Start 10 mg bid, titrate as needed and tolerated to max. 60 mg bid	Average daily pain intensity	157	Mean score: 6.8 → 5.3 (placebo) 6.9 → 4.2 (Oxycontin)
Harati (62)	Tramadol	Start 50 mg/d, titrate as needed and tolerated to max. 400 mg/d	Pain intensity scale (0–4)	131	Mean score: 2.5 → 2.2 (placebo) 2.6 → 1.4 (Tramadol)
Sindrup (63)	Tramadol	Titrated to maximum dose of 200 mg bid	Pain intensity scale (0–10)	34 (15 with DPN)	Median score: 6.0 → 6.0 (placebo) 6.0 → 4.0 (Tramadol)

(62). In a study of patients with painful neuropathy of various etiologies (including subjects with diabetic polyneuropathy), the NNT for Tramadol was similar (4.5) (63).

The results suggest that Oxycontin and Tramadol are effective in alleviating the pain of diabetic polyneuropathy, but their efficacy relative to the tricyclics and anticonvulsants remains unclear.

4. PROGNOSIS

4.1. Are There Any Factors That Are Useful in Predicting Which Patients With Diabetes Will Develop Polyneuropathy?

There are a number of studies that help to answer this question (15,64–66). On January 1, 1986, the Rochester Diabetic Neuropathy Study (RDNS) investigators identified all patients with diabetes who were resident in Rochester. Of the 870 patients identified in this way, 380 agreed to participate in a cross-sectional study and, of these, 264 were included in a longitudinal cohort study. These patients were followed over time using the NIS(LL)+7 scale. The NIS(LL)+7 is the Neuropathy Impairment Scale for the lower limbs that has been modified by the inclusion of results for five nerve conduction study parameters, heartbeat variation with deep breathing, and vibration detection threshold. NIS(LL)+7 values greater than the 97.5th percentile for healthy control subjects were used to define the presence of polyneuropathy. As shown in Table 8.15, the initial multivariate analysis showed that foot vessel calcification and severity of retinopathy were risk factors for neuropathy in type I diabetes, that mean glycosylated hemoglobin concentration was the only risk factor among type II diabetics, and that the severity of retinopathy, and the natural log of the interaction between duration of diabetes and mean 24-proteinuria, as well as the mean glycosylated hemoglobin concentration, were risk factors for neuropathy among the type I and type II diabetics combined. Retinopathy, foot vessel calcification, and 24-hour proteinuria are indicators of the presence of microvascular disease. Because microvascular disease was regarded as a comorbidity rather than a risk factors for neuropathy, the multivariate analysis was repeated excluding these variables. As shown in Table 8.15, this analysis showed that the variables duration-of-diabetes and glycosylated hemoglobin concentration (and the interaction between the two) were the most important risk factors for the development of neuropathy. These results suggest that it is the duration of exposure to chronic hyperglycemia that is the most important risk factor for neuropathy.

The Seattle Prospective Diabetic Foot Study (65) recruited US veterans with diabetes who were followed prospectively using insensitivity to the 5.07 g monofilament to define the presence of neuropathy. Of the 387 patients without neuropathy at the time of entry into the study, follow-up information was available in 288 (74%), of whom 58 (20%) developed neuropathy. As shown in Table 8.15, multivariate analysis for the risk of developing neuropathy showed that height, history of foot ulceration, age, and glycosylated hemoglobin concentration as well as low serum albumin were all important predictors. Low serum albumin and foot ulceration likely reflect comorbid microvascular disease but, unlike the RDNS described previously, the analysis was not repeated after these factors were excluded. Although this study was in agreement with the RDNS that glycosylated hemoglobin concentration is an important risk factor for neuropathy, it identified age and height as risk factors that had not been identified in the RDNS (65).

A prospective multicenter longitudinal study in the Netherlands of 486 patients with type-II diabetes, using the clinical neuropathy examination (CNE) to definite the presence of neuropathy, identified age, height, duration of diabetes, glycosylated hemoglobin concentration, body mass index, and the ankle-arm index as risk factors for progression of CNE scores. This study did not provide a separate analysis for patients who developed neuropathy (i.e., patients who crossed the threshold of a CNE score of 4 for the diagnosis of neuropathy). The ankle-arm index likely represents the presence of comorbid microvascular disease. Like the Settle and RDNS, chronic exposure to hyperglycemia was identified as important risk factors for neuropathy. The identification of age and height as risk factors buttresses the findings of the Seattle study.

In summary, therefore, chronic exposure to high concentrations of glucose is the most consistently identified risk factor for the development of neuropathy. This risk factor represents the combined effects of long duration of diabetes and the degree of elevation of blood sugar concentration. Advancing age and increasing height have been identified as risk factors in two independent studies. The presence of other microvascular complications such as retinopathy and nephropathy are likely markers for the presence of neuropathy rather than risk factors *per se*.

4.2. Does Treatment of Diabetes Have an Effect on the Development and Progression of Polyneuropathy?

The recognition that chronic exposure to hyperglycemia is an important risk factor for the develop of diabetic neuropathy raises the question of whether aggressive treatment of hyperglycemia will reduce the risk of developing neuropathy. The Diabetes Control and Complications Trial (DCCT) was a large multicenter study that was designed to answer the question whether intensive treatment of diabetes, with the goal of maintaining blood glucose concentrations close to the normal range, would have the effect of reducing the frequency and severity of the long-term microvascular complications of diabetes (67,68). The DCCT involved 1441 patients with insulin-dependent diabetes mellitus who

Table 8.15
Risk Factors for Diabetic Polyneuropathy

Study (reference)	n	Design	Outcome measure used to define neuropathy	Risk factors
Rochester Diabetic Neuropathy Study (15,64)	264	Prospective Included type I & type II DM Multivariate analysis	NIS(LL)+7	Type I DM—foot vessel calcification & retinopathy severity level Type II DM—mean GhB Type I and type II DM—ln (duration diabetes × mean 24 h proteinuria), mean GhB Type I diabetes—ln (GHb × duration of diabetes) Type II diabetes—mean GHb
Seattle Prospective Diabetic Foot Study (65)	387	Prospective Included type I & type II DM Multivariate analysis	Neuropathy defined on the basis of insensitivity to the 5.07 g monofilament at ≥1 of 9 sites on either foot.	Height History of foot ulcer before study onset Age at entry into the study GHb concentration at study entry Current smoker Low serum albumin
Netherlands (66)	486	Prospective Included type II DM only Multivariate analysis Modeled change in CNE score rather than neuropathy	Neuropathy defined on the basis of a CNE score >4	Age Duration of diabetes $HBA1_c$ Height BMI Ankle-arm index

NIS(LL+7), neuropathy impairment score (lower limbs)+7; ln, natural log; GHb, glycosylated hemoglobin; $HBA1_c$, hemoglobin A1; CNE, clinical neuropathy examination; BMI, body mass index.

had not yet developed severe microvascular complications. Diabetic retinopathy was used as the primary outcome measure in this study, and the presence or absence of retinopathy at the time of entry into the study determined whether subjects were included in the primary or secondary prevention cohorts. Although the occurrence of neuropathy is reported separately for each of these two cohorts, the distinction seems less relevant given that the presence or absence of neuropathy was not used to guide inclusion in the primary or secondary prevention cohorts. Study subjects were randomized to either conventional therapy (1–2 daily injections of insulin, daily self-monitoring of blood glucose, and education about diet and exercise) or intensive therapy (3–4 daily injections of insulin with the dose adjusted according to the results of self-monitored blood glucose performed at least four times per day, dietary intake, and anticipated exercise). At baseline, neuropathy was present in approximately 6% of the combined primary and secondary prevention cohorts. Follow-up data was available in 99% of patients with a mean duration of 6.5 years (range 3.5 to 9 years).

The main neurological end point for the study was the development of confirmed clinical neuropathy, which was defined as clinical neuropathy (definite abnormal neurological examination) confirmed by abnormal nerve conduction or autonomic nervous system testing or both (Table 8.16). As shown in Table 8.17, intensive diabetes therapy reduced the risk of all almost all neurological outcome measures including clinical neuropathy, confirmed clinical neuropathy as well as isolated abnormalities of nerve conduction studies and/or autonomic function testing *(68)*.

It might be argued that the clinical criteria used to define neuropathy are somewhat vague, and that the electrophysiological parameters and values used to define abnormality are not without controversy. It is not clear, for example, that mild slowing of conduction velocity in isolation should be taken as evidence of an early peripheral neuropathy (see the discussion earlier in this chapter on the electrodiagnosis of polyneuropathy). Nevertheless, the impact of intensive diabetes therapy on such a wide range of clinical and electrophysiological measures is convincing—aggressive therapy is effective in reducing the risk of developing neuropathy.

4.3. What Is the Prognosis for Diabetic Polyneuropathy?

In view of the high prevalence of this condition, there are remarkably few published data on the prognosis for patients with diabetic polyneuropathy. One small study of patients with diabetic neuropathy reported follow-up in 36 patients after a mean duration of 4.7 years *(69)*. The investigators used a VAS to record the severity of symptoms (pain, paresthesia, numbness, and so on) and also performed nerve conduction studies at study entry and again at follow-up. They found that there was no overall change in symptom scores over the approximately 4-year duration of the study. Some improvement was noted in 11 patients and no subject experienced complete resolution of symptoms. There was no change in peroneal nerve conduction velocity, although there was a small, but significant, decline in median motor nerve conduction velocity *(69)*. It is not really possible to draw any firm conclusions from a small study of this nature with a relatively short duration of follow-up.

Some idea of the natural history of diabetic polyneuropathy may be obtained by examining the outcome of placebo-treated patients in studies of various treatments for diabetic neuropathy. The recombinant human nerve growth factor study, for example, recruited more than 1000 patients with diabetic neuropathy, with 515 subjects random-

Table 8.16
Diabetes Control and Complications Trial Neurological Endpoints

Confirmed clinical neuropathy—a finding of definite clinical neuropathy by physical examination and history confirmed by unequivocal abnormality of either nerve conduction or autonomic nervous system response as defined below.

Clinical neuropathy—a definite diagnosis of peripheral diabetic neuropathy by clinical examination based on the presence of at least two of the following:
   –Physical symptoms
   –Abnormalities on sensory examination
   –Absent or decreased deep tendon reflexes

Abnormal nerve conduction—at least one abnormal conduction attribute on each of at least two anatomically distinct peripheral nerves according to the following standards:
   Median motor nerve
      Amplitude <4.2 mV
      Velocity <49 m/s
      F-wave latency >31.8 ms
   Median sensory nerve
      Amplitude <10 µV
      Conduction velocity <48 m/s
   Peroneal nerve
      Amplitude <2.5 mV
      Velocity <40 m/s
      F-wave latency >56 ms
   Sural nerve
      Amplitude <5 µV
      Velocity <40 m/s

Abnormal autonomic response—any of the following indications of cardiac autonomic neuropathy:
      R-R- variation (mean resultant) <15
      R-R variation <20 in combination with valsalva ratio <1.5
      Orthostatic hypotension caused by autonomic neuropathy as indicated by a decrease of at least 10 mmHg in diastolic blood pressure in postural studies confirmed by blunted norepinephrine response in plasma catecholamine specimens

Subclinical neuropathy—abnormal nerve conduction, autonomic nervous system response, or both without definite diagnosis of peripheral neuropathy by clinical examination

Data from ref. *68*.

ized to receive placebo *(70)*. The primary outcome measure was the NIS(LL) and secondary outcome measures included the Neuropathy Symptoms and Change (NSC) score, the Patient Benefit Questionnaire (PBQ), a measure of quality of life (QOL), and independence with activities of daily living (ADL) well as a subjective global symptom assessment (a seven-point likert scale). Follow-up using the NIS(LL) after 1 year of treatment showed that 34% of placebo treated patients were improved, 41% were unchanged and 25% were worse. Comparison of baseline and posttreatment scores on the NSC, the PBQ, and the global assessment scale showed no differences. Admittedly, the duration of follow-up was relatively short (i.e., only 1 year), but these results suggest that the neuropathy improves or remains stable in approximately 75% of patients and deteriorates in approximately 25% *(70)*. Some confounding may have resulted from the fact that treat-

Table 8.17
Neurological Endpoints of the Diabetes Control and Complication Trial

	Primary prevention cohort			Secondary prevention cohort			Combined cohorts
	Conventional therapy	Intensive therapy	Risk reduction (95% CI)	Conventional therapy	Intensive therapy	Risk reduction (95% CI)	Risk reduction (95% CI)
Patients (n)	291	248	–	307	315	–	–
Confirmed clinical neuropathy	9.6%	2.8%	71 (34–87)	16.9%	6.7%	61 (36–76)	64 (45–76)
Clinical neuropathy	15.2%	6.9%	54 (22–73)	21.2%	11.8%	45 (20–62)	48 (29–62)
Subclinical neuropathy							
ANS *and* NCS abnormal	0.7%	0	–	4.2%	2.2%	–	–
ANS *or* NCS abnormal	33.4%	15.4%	54 (35–67)	40.2%	29%	28 (10–42)	37 (24–48)
Abnormal nerve conduction	40.2%	16.5%	59 (44–70)	52.4%	32.7%	38 (25-48)	44 (34-53)
Abnormal autonomic nervous system function	5.5%	2.4%	–	11.8%	5.7%	51 (16-72)	53 (24-70)

CI, confidence interval; ANS, autonomic nervous system; NCS, nerve conduction studies.
Data from ref. 68.

ment of diabetes is likely more intensive in treatment trials such as this than among diabetics not participating in a randomized controlled trial.

There are very limited data, therefore, on which to base a discussion of the prognosis of diabetic neuropathy. At least in the short-term (a period of a few years), the available data seem to suggest that the neuropathy remains stable or even improves. There are no published data that inform on the long-term prognosis for patients with diabetic neuropathy.

4.4. What Is the Prognosis for Idiopathic Sensory-Predominant Polyneuropathy?

Although the outcome of patients with idiopathic sensory-predominant polyneuropathy has been reported in a number of studies (71–77), the quality of the published data is limited, with only three of these studies using a formal disability scale to evaluate the functional impact of disease progression (73,74,76). Substantial bias was also likely introduced into some of these studies because the inclusion criteria specified that the neuropathy had either not progressed or progressed slowly over a defined period prior to entry into the study (75,76) (Table 8.18).

McLeod's early series of patients suggested that there was little progression over a median follow-up period of 5 years but this study did not use any formal outcome measure to quantify disease severity and/or disability (71). More recently, Jann and colleagues similarly reported little progression of disease, but similarly did not employ any formal outcome measure to quantify disease progression or disability (75).

Of the 50 patients with cryptogenic sensorimotor polyneuropathy studied by Notermans and colleagues, 23 required a cane for ambulation at follow-up compared with only one of 21 patients with a purely sensory neuropathy, suggesting that the absence of motor symptoms/signs portends a better prognosis (73). The study by Grahmann and colleagues differs from the others summarized in Table 8.18 in that it included patients with asymmetric neuropathies and mononeuritis multiplex in addition to patients with the more typical cryptogenic symmetric sensorimotor polyneuropathy (74). This study does not provide a breakdown of the proportion of patients with progressive disease and simply states that the mean disability after 24 months of follow-up was mild-to-moderate (74).

Finally, the study by Vrancken seems to capture disability at one point in time in that no follow-up is recorded (76). The data from this study suggest a benign outcome, with modified Rankin disability scale scores of 1–2 in 95% of patients with onset over the age of 6 and Rankin scores of 1–2 in 78% of younger onset patients. These results should be interpreted cautiously, given the selection bias that resulted from inclusion only of patients with slowly progressing or nonprogressive disease over a period of at least 6 months (76).

The theme that emerges from these studies is that idiopathic predominantly sensory polyneuropathy is generally a slowly progressing disease. Disability does accumulate over time, although it tends to be mild-to-moderate in severity. There is some suggestion that motor involvement (73) and younger age of onset (76) may portend a slightly worse prognosis.

5. SUMMARY

- The etiology of a polyneuropathy can usually be determined on the basis of a careful history with attention to risk factors for neuropathy (e.g., alcohol use, HIV risk factors), a thorough family history, and a simple battery of laboratory tests including fasting blood

Table 8.18
Prognosis of Idiopathic Sensory-Predominant Polyneuropathy

Reference	n	Population	Prognosis
McLeod (71)	47	Symmetrical polyneuropathy for at least 1 yr with no identifiable cause.	Little change in mean disability over time" with median "follow-up of 5 yr. Nine patients deteriorated, four improved and the remaining 34 were unchanged.
Notermans (72,73)	75	Chronic symmetrical polyneuropathy presenting in middle or old age with no known etiology after extensive investigation	Disease was progressive in all patients over 5 yr: Distribution of mRS scores changed as follows: 35% → 5% (mRS = 1), 35% → 63% (mRS = 2); 1% → 3% (mRS = 3)
Grahmann (74)	29	Polyneuropathy of undetermined cause—mixed population with 45% symmetric sensorimotor, 38% symmetric sensory, 14% asymmetric, and 3% mononeuritis multiplex	After median follow-up of 2 years, average disability grade 2.4 on the McLeod scale where grade 2 is mild motor and/or sensory symptoms and grade 3 is moderately disabled by motor or sensory symptoms
Wolfe (77)	66	Cryptogenic sensory neuropathy (slight motor findings permitted, but no motor symptoms)	After a mean follow-up of 12.5 mo, there was progression in 14 patients (although no formal scale used to measure disease severity). Worse prognosis correlated with longer duration of follow-up
Jann (75)	67	Neuropathy of more than 1-yr duration without progression over ≥2 mo	Most showed slight progression, but no change in 6 patients (although no formal scale used to measure disease severity)
Vrancken (76)	127	Symptomatic sensory/sensorimotor neuropathy physical signs; insidious onset; slow or no progression over 6 months; no identifiable cause; axonal physiology	Lesser disability in those over the age of 65 with short duration disease compared to younger age of onset with short duration disease. Late vs early onset mRS scores: 44% vs 25% mRS = 1; 51% vs 53% mRS = 2; 5% vs 22% mRS = 3

mRS, modified Rankin score.

glucose with a 2-hour glucose tolerance test, serum protein electrophoresis/immuno-fixation electrophoresis, serum B_{12}, and thyroid and renal function.

- Sural nerve biopsy may be required for the diagnosis of vasculitis and will also facilitate diagnosis of amyloidosis (although fine needle aspiration of abdominal fat may be preferable for the diagnosis of amyloid as it is less invasive).
- Approximately 20–30% of polyneuropathies will remain idiopathic despite these investigations.
- The SRAR is probably the most sensitive electrophysiological measure for the diagnosis of polyneuropathy; prolongation of minimal F-wave latencies and reduction in sural response amplitude also play an important role in the diagnosis.
- QST has variable (although probably reasonable) sensitivity, but specificity is poor. It is, therefore, useful for "ruling out" the diagnosis of small fiber neuropathy in that normal test results are less likely to be false negatives.
- Skin biopsy with estimation of epidermal nerve fiber density has relatively poor sensitivity, but specificity is high. It is, therefore, useful for "ruling in" the diagnosis of small fiber neuropathy in that abnormal test results are unlikely to be false positives.
- Data from a number of small randomized controlled trials support the use of the tricyclic antidepressants nortriptyline, amitriptyline, and clomipramine as well as the reuptake inhibitors paroxetine, citalopram, and venlafaxine for the treatment of painful diabetic neuropathy.
- Data from a number of randomized controlled trials support the use of the anticonvulsants carbamazepine, valproate, gabapentin, topiramate, lamotrigine, and pregabalin for the treatment of painful diabetic neuropathy.
- Data from a small number of randomized controlled trials support the use of Oxycontin and Tramadol for the treatment of painful diabetic neuropathy.
- There are barely any data on the comparative efficacy of antidepressants, anti-convulsants and opiate analgesics for the treatment of painful diabetic neuropathy.
- Chronic hyperglycemia is the most important risk factors for the development of diabetic polyneuropathy.
- Intensive treatment to keep blood glucose concentrations as close to normal as possible has the effect of reducing the occurrence of diabetic polyneuropathy.
- There are limited published data on the prognosis of diabetic neuropathy, but the available data suggest that the neuropathy does not progress over the short term (period of 1–4 years) among patients whose diabetes is adequately treated.
- The progression of idiopathic, predominantly sensory polyneuropathy is generally slow, although mild-to-moderate disability may accumulate over time.

REFERENCES

1. Singleton JR, Smith AG, Bromberg MB. Increased prevalence of impaired glucose tolerance in patients with painful sensory neuropathy. Diabetes Care 2001;24:1448–1453.
2. Smith AG, Singleton JR. The diagnostic yield of a standardized approach to idiopathic sensory-predominant neuropathy. Arch Intern Med 2004;164:1021–1025.
3. Verghese J, Bieri PL, Gellido C, Schaumburg HH, Herskovitz S. Peripheral neuropathy in young-old and old-old patients. Muscle Nerve 2001;24:1476–1481.
4. Novella SP, Inzucchi SE, Goldstein JM. The frequency of undiagnosed diabetes and impaired glucose tolerance in patients with idiopathic sensory neuropathy. Muscle Nerve 2001;24:1229–1231.
5. Dyck PJ, Oviatt KF, Lambert EH. Intensive evaluation of referred unclassified neuropathies yields improved diagnosis. Ann Neurol 1981;10:222–226.

6. Tackmann W, Kaeser HE, Berger W, Rueger AN. Sensory and motor parameters in leg nerves of diabetics: intercorrelations and relationships to clinical symptoms. Eur Neurol 1981;20:344–350.

7. Kayser-Gatchalian MC, Neundorfer B. Sural nerve conduction in mild polyneuropathy. J Neurol 1984;231:122–125.

8. Fraser JL, Olney RK. The relative diagnostic sensitivity of different F-wave parameters in various polyneuropathies. Muscle Nerve 1992;15:912–918.

9. Claus D, Mustafa C, Vogel W, Herz M, Neundorfer B. Assessment of diabetic neuropathy: definition of norm and discrimination of abnormal nerve function. Muscle Nerve 1993;16:757–768.

10. Effect of intensive diabetes treatment on nerve conduction in the Diabetes Control and Complications Trial. Ann Neurol 1995;38:869–880.

11. Rutkove SB, Kothari MJ, Raynor EM, Levy ML, Fadic R, Nardin RA. Sural/radial amplitude ratio in the diagnosis of mild axonal polyneuropathy. Muscle Nerve 1997;20:1236–1241.

12. Andersen H, Stalberg E, Falck B. F-wave latency, the most sensitive nerve conduction parameter in patients with diabetes mellitus. Muscle Nerve 1997;20:1296–1302.

13. Pastore C, Izura V, Geijo-Barrientos E, Dominguez JR. A comparison of electrophysiological tests for the early diagnosis of diabetic neuropathy. Muscle Nerve 1999;22:1667–1673.

14. Shy ME, Frohman EM, So YT, et al. Quantitative sensory testing. Report of the Therapeutics and Technology Assessment Subcommittee of the American Academy of Neurology. Neurology 2003;60:898–904.

15. Dyck PJ, Davies JL, Litchy WJ, O'Brien PC. Longitudinal assessment of diabetic polyneuropathy using a composite score in the Rochester Diabetic Neuropathy Study cohort. Neurology 1997;49:229–239.

16. Masson EA, Veves A, Fernando D, Boulton AJ. Current perception thresholds: a new, quick, and reproducible method for the assessment of peripheral neuropathy in diabetes mellitus. Diabetologica 1989;32:724–728.

17. Freeman R, Chase KP, Risk MR. Quantitative sensory testing cannot differentiate simulated sensory loss from sensory neuropathy. Neurology 2003;60:465–470.

18. Yarnitsky D, Sprecher E, Tamir A, Zaslansky R, Hemli JA. Variance of sensory threshold measurements: discrimination of feigners from trustworthy performers. J Neurol Sci 1994;125:186–189.

19. Argov Z, Steiner I, Soffer D. The yield of sural nerve biopsy in the evaluation of peripheral neuropathies. Acta Neurol Scand 1989;79:243–245.

20. Midroni G, Bilbao JM. Peripheral Neuropathy and the role of nerve biopsy. Biopsy diagnosis of peripheral neuropathy. Butterworth-Heinemann, Boston: 1995: pp. 1–11.

21. Oh SJ. Diagnostic usefulness and limitations of the sural nerve biopsy. Yonsei Medical Journal 1990;31:1–26.

22. Neundorfer B, Grahmann F, Engelhardt A, Harte U. Postoperative effects and value of sural nerve biopsies: a retrospective study. Eur Neurol 1990;30:350–352.

23. Chia L, Fernandez A, Lacroix C, Adams D, Plante V, Said G. Contribution of nerve biopsy findings to the diagnosis of disabling neuropathy in the elderly. A retrospective review of 100 consecutive patients. Brain 1996;119:1091–1098.

24. Rappaport WD, Valente J, Hunter GC, et al. Clinical utilization and complications of sural nerve biopsy. Am J Surg 1993;166:252–256.

25. Kelly JJ, Kyle RA, O'Brien PC, Dyck PJ. The natural history of peripheral neuropathy in primary systemic amyloidosis. Ann Neurol 1979;6:1–7.

26. Kyle RA, Greipp PR. Amyloidosis (AL). Clinical and laboratory features in 229 cases. Mayo Clin Proc 1983;58:665–683.

27. Simmons Z, Blaivas M, Aguilera AJ, Feldman EL, Bromberg MB, Towfighi J. Low diagnostic yield of sural nerve biopsy in patients with peripheral neuropathy and primary amyloidosis. J Neurol Sci 1993;120:60–63.

28. Duston MA, Skinner M, Meenan RF, Cohen AS. Sensitivity, specificity, and predictive value of abdominal fat aspiration for the diagnosis of amylodosis. Arthritis Rheum 1989;32:82–85.

29. Duston MA, Skinner M, Shirahama T, Cohen AS. Diagnosis of amyloidosis by abdominal fat aspiration. Analysis of four years' experience. Am J Med 1987;82:412–414.

30. Libbey CA, Skinner M, Cohen AS. Use of abdominal fat tissue aspirate in the diagnosis of systemic amyloidosis. Arch Intern Med 1983;143:1549–1552.

31. Ansari-Lari MA, Ali SZ. Fine-needle aspiration of abdominal fat pad for amyloid detection. A clinically useful test? Diagn Cytopathol 2004;30:178–181.

32. Masouye I. Diagnostic screening of systemic amyloidosis by abdominal fat aspiration: an analysis of 100 cases. Am J Dermatopathol 1997;19:41–45.

33. Guy CD, Jones CK. Abdominal fat pad aspiration biopsy for tissue confirmation of systemic amyloidosis: specificity, positive predictive value, and diagnostic pitfalls. Diagn Cytopathol 2001;24:181–185.

34. McCarthy BG, Hsieh ST, Stocks A, et al. Cutaneous innervation in sensory neuropathies: evaluation by skin biopsy. Neurology 1995;45:1848–1855.

35. McArthur JC, Stocks EA, Hauer P, Cornblath DR, Griffin JW. Epidermal nerve fiber density. Normative reference range and diagnostic efficiecy. Arch Neurol 1998;55:1513–1520.

36. Holland N, Stocks A, Hauer P, Cornblath D, Griffin J, McArthur J. Intraepidermal nerve fiber density in patients with painful sensory neuropathy. Ann Neurol 1997;48:708–711.

37. Holland NR, Crawford TO, Hauer P, Cornblath DR, Griffin JW, McArthur JC. Small-fiber sensory neuropathies: clinical course and neuropathology of idiopathic cases. Ann Neurol 1998;44:47–59.

38. Periquet M, Novak V, Collins M, et al. Painful sensory neuropathy. Prospective evaluation using skin biopsy. Neurology 1999;53:1641–1647.

39. Gomez-Perez FJ, Rull JA, Dies H, Rodriguez-Rivera JG, Gonzalez-Barranco J, Lozano-Castañeda O. Nortriptyline and Fluphenazine in the symptomatic treatment of diabetic neuropathy. A double-blind cross-over study. Pain 1985;23:395–400.

40. Max M, Culnane M, Schafer S, et al. Amitriptyline relieves diabetic neuropathy pain in patients with normal or depressed mood. Neurology 1987;37:589–596.

41. Max MB, Lynch SA, Muir J, Shoaf SE, Smoller B, Dubner R. Effects of desipramine, amitriptyline and fluoxetine on pain in diabetic neuropathy. N Engl J Med 1992;326:1250–1256.

42. Kvinesdal B, Molin J, Frøland A, Gram LF. Imipramine treatment of painful diabetic neuropathy. JAMA 1984;251:1727–1730.

43. Sindrup S, Ejlertsen B, Frøland A, Sindrup E, Brøsen K, Gram L. Imipramine treatment in diabetic neuropathy: relief of subjective symptoms without changes in peripheral and autonomic nerve function. Eur J Clin Pharm 1989;37:151–153.

44. Sindrup S, Gram L, Skjold T, Grodum E, Brøsen K, Beck-Nielsen H. Clomipramine vs desipramine vs placebo in the treatment of diabetic neuropathy symptoms. A double-blind cross-over study. Br J Clin Pharmacol 1990;30:683–691.

45. Sindrup SH, Gram LF, Brøsen K, Eshøj O, Mogensen EF. The selective serotonin reuptake inhibitor paroxetine is effective in the treatment of diabetic neuropathy symptoms. Pain 1990;42:135–144.

46. Sindrup SH, Bjerre U, Dejgaard A, Brøsen K, Aaes-Jørgensen T, Gram LF. The selective serotonin reuptake inhibitor citalopram relieves the symptoms of diabetic neuropathy. Clin Pharmacol Ther 1992;52:547–552.

47. Sindrup S, Tuxen C, Gram L, et al. Lack of effect of mianserin on the symptoms of diabetic neuropathy. Eur J Clin Pharmacol 1992;43:251–255.

48. McQuay H, Tramèr M, Nye B, Carroll D, Wiffen P, Moore R. A systematic review of antidepressants in neuropathic pain. Pain 1996;68:217–227.

49. Rowbotham MC, Goli V, Kunz NR, Lei D. Venlafaxine extended release in the treatment of painful diabetic neuropathy: a double-blind, placebo-controlled trial. Pain 2004;110:697–706.

50. Edwards KR, Glantz MJ, Button J, Norton JA, Whittaker T, Cross N. Efficacy and safety of Topiramate in the treatment of painful diabetic neuropathy: a double-blind, placebo-controlled study. Neurology 2000;54:A81.

51. Thienel U, Neto W, Schwabe S, Vijapurkar U. Topirmate in painful diabetic polyneuropathy: findings from three double-blind placebo controlled trials. Acta Neurol Scand 2004;110:221–231.

52. Raskin P, Donofrio P, Rosenthal N, et al. Topiramate vs Placebo in painful diabetic neuropathy. Analgesic and metabolic effects. Neurology 2004;63:865–873.

53. Chadda V, Mathur M. Double blind study of the effects of diphenylhydantoin sodium on diabetic neuropathy. J Assoc Physicians India 1978;26:403–406.

54. Saudek CD, Werns S, Reidenberg MM. Phenytoin in the treatment of diabetic symmetrical polyneuropathy. Clin Pharmacol Ther 1977;22:196–199.

55. Rull JA, Quibrera R, Gonzalez-Millan H, Lozano-Castañeda O. Symptomatic treatment of peripheral diabetic neuropathy with carbamazepine (Tegretol): double-blind crossover study. Diabetologia 1969;5:215–218.

56. Kochar D, Jain N, Agarwal R, Srivastava T, Agarwal P, Gupta S. Sodium valproate in the management of painful neuropathy in type 2 diabetes — a randomized placebo contolled trial. Acta Neurol Scand 2002;106:248–252.

57. Eisenberg E, Lurie Y, Braker C, Daoud D, Ishay A. Lamotrigine reduces painful diabetic neuropathy. A randomized, controlled study. Neurology 2001;57:505–509.

58. Backonja M, Beydoun A, Edwards KR, et al. Gabapentin for the symptomatic treatment of painful neuropathy in patients with diabetes mellitus. A randomized controlled trial. JAMA 1998;280:1831–1836.

59. Rosenstock J, Tuchman M, LaMoreaux L, Sharma U. Pregabalin for the treatment of painful diabetic peripheral neuropathy: a double-blind, placebo-controlled trial. Pain 2004;110:628–638.

60. Lesser H, Sharma U, LaMoreaux L, Poole R. Pregabalin relieves symptoms of painful diabetic neuropathy: A randomized controlled trial. Neurology 2004;63:2104–2110.

61. Gimbel JS, Richards P, Portenoy RK. Controlled-release oxycodone for pain in diabetic neuroapthy. A randomized controlled trial. Neurology 2003;60:927–934.

62. Harati Y, Gooch C, Swenson M, et al. Double-blind randomized trial of tramadol for the treatment of the pain of diabetic neuropathy. Neurology 1998;50:1842–1846.

63. Sindrup SH, Andersen G, Madsen C, Smith T, Brosen K, Jensen TS. Tramadol relieves pain and allodynia in polyneuropathy: a randomized double-blind, controlled trial. Pain 1999;83:85–90.

64. Dyck PJ, Davies JL, Wilson DM, Service FJ, Melton LJ, O'Brien PC. Risk factors for severity of diabetic polyneuropathy. Intensive longitudinal assessment of the Rochester Diabetic Neuropathy Study Cohort. Diabetes Care 1999;22:1479–1486.

65. Adler AI, Boyko EJ, Ahroni JH, Stensel V, Forsberg RC, Smith DC. Risk factors for diabetic peripheral sensory neuropathy. Results of the Seattle Prospective Diabetic Foot Study. Diabetes Care 1997; 20:1162–1167.

66. van de Poll-Franse L, Valk G, Renders C, Heine R, van Eijk J. Longitudinal assessment of the development of diabetic polyneuropathy and associated risk factors. Diabet Med 2002;19:771–776.

67. The effect of intensive treatment of diabetes on the development and progresion of long-term complications in insulin-dependent diabetes mellitus. The Diabetes Control and Complications Trial Research Group, N Engl J Med 1993;329:977–986.

68. The effect of intensive diabetes therapy on the development and progression of neuropathy. The Diabetes Control and Complications Trial Research Group. Ann Intern Med 1995;122:561–568.

69. Boulton A, Armstrong W, Scarpello J, Ward J. The natural history of painful diabetic neuropathy—a 4 year study. Postgrad Med J 1983;59:556–559.

70. Apfel SC, Schwartz S, Adornato BT, et al. Efficacy and safety of recombinant human nerve growth factor in patients with diabetic polyneuropathy: a randomized controlled trial. rhNGF Clincal Investigator Group. JAMA 2000;284:2215–2221.

71. McLeod J, Tuck R, Pollard J, Cameron J, Walsh J. Chronic polyneuropathy of undetermined cause. J Neurol, Neurosurg Psychiatry 1984;47:530–535.

72. Notermans NC, Wokke JH, Franssen H, et al. Chronic idiopathic polyneuropathy presenting in middle or old age: a clinical and electrophysiological study of 75 patients. J Neurol, Neurosurg Psychiatry 1993;56:1066–1071.

73. Notermans N, Wokke J, van der Graaf Y, Franssen H, van Dijk G, Jennekens F. Chronic idiopathic axonal polyneuropathy: a five year follow-up. J Neurol, Neurosurg Psychiatry 1994;57:1525–1527.

74. Grahmann F, Winterholler M, Neundorfer B. Cryptogenic polyneuropathies: an out-patient follow-up study. Acta Neurol Scand 1991;84:221–225.

75. Jann S, Beretta S, Bramerio M, Defanti CA. Prospective follow-up study of chronic polyneuropathy of undetermined cause. Muscle Nerve 2001;24:1197–1201.

76. Vrancken AF, Franssen H, Wokke JH, Teunissen LL, Notermans NC. Chronic idiopathic axonal polyneuropathy and successful aging of the peripheral nervous system in elderly people. Arch Neurol 2002;59:533–540.

77. Wolfe GI, Baker NS, Amato AA, et al. Chronic cryptogenic sensory polyneuropathy: Clinical and laboratory characteristics. Arch Neurol 1999;56:540–547.

78. Guy R, Clark CA, Malcolm P, Watkins P. Evaluation of thermal and vibration sensation in diabetic neuropathy. Diabetologica 1985;28:131–137.

79. Navarro X, Kennedy WR. Evaluation of thermal and pain sensitivity in type I diabetic patients. J Neurol, Neurosurg Psychiatry 1991;54:60–64.

9 Paraproteinemic Neuropathies

1. INTRODUCTION

The detection of a monoclonal protein (gammopathy) in the serum of a patient with a peripheral neuropathy is important for two reasons. First, it may provide information about the prognosis and likelihood of response to immunosuppressive therapy. Second, it may indicate the presence of an underlying plasma cell proliferative disorder, such as multiple myeloma, osteosclerotic myeloma, Waldenstrom's macroglobulinemia, or primary systemic amyloidosis. The term monoclonal gammopathy of undetermined significance (MGUS) has been used when no specific hematological diagnosis is forthcoming.

There are a number of different ways to think about the neuropathies associated with monoclonal gammopathies. Because it is important to be aware of the specific underlying hematological diagnosis, it is helpful, in part, to think in these terms. Are the neuropathies associated with multiple myeloma, osteosclerotic myeloma, or amyloidosis, for example, sufficiently characteristic in their presentation, response to treatment, or prognosis? What is the spectrum of polyneuropathy encountered in patients with an MGUS? Does it matter whether the MGUS is of the IgG or IgM isotype? Does the presence of anti-myelin associated glycoprotein (MAG) antibodies impact on the response to treatment? Is it more useful to think about the gammopathy associated neuropathies in terms of the underlying electrophysiology rather than the isotype and reactivity of the monoclonal protein? These and other questions are the focus of this chapter.

2. DIAGNOSIS

2.1. What Is the Most Sensitive Technique for the Detection of an M-Protein?

A variety of techniques are available for the detection, characterization, and quantification of monoclonal immunoglobulin peaks. These techniques differ in terms of their methodology as well as their sensitivity for the detection of monoclonal proteins present in a low concentration. There are limited data to guide the choice of electrophoretic assay, but an understanding of their respective methodologies facilitates a common-sense approach.

Serum protein electrophoresis (SPEP) entails the separation of proteins based on their patterns of migration under the influence of an electric field. Following electrophoresis, the proteins are visualized by staining with a dye. SPEP may be performed using either a low- or high-resolution technique. In a survey conducted by the College of America Pathologists, specimens with a subtle but distinct M-protein were sent to multiple laboratories for evaluation. Those laboratories using high-resolution techniques detected the

From: *Neuromuscular Disease: Evidence and Analysis in Clinical Neurology*
By: M. Benatar © Humana Press Inc., Totowa, NJ

M-protein in 96% of the samples, compared with a detection rate of 28% among the laboratories using low-resolution techniques *(1)*. Routine high-resolution SPEP is appropriate for the detection of large monoclonal spikes that are present in most cases of multiple myeloma or Waldenstrom's macroglobulinemia. The M-protein associated with polyneuropathy (frequently an MGUS) is more often smaller, and may require the use of an even more sensitive technique for its demonstration. Immunofixation electrophoresis involves the separation of proteins under the influence of an electric field, but is followed by immunoprecipitation with antibodies directed against the various heavy and light chains of immunoglobulins. This technique will demonstrate even very small quantities of a monoclonal protein.

The diagnostic evaluation for a monoclonal protein should also involve urine protein electrophoresis in order to demonstrate the presence and type of monoclonal free light chains. Because these may be entirely filtered by the glomerulus and excreted in the urine, they may elude detection if only serum proteins are subject to electrophoresis.

Based on these principles as well as published guidelines, the appropriate evaluation of patients suspected of having a monoclonal gammopathy as the cause of their polyneuropathy should include high-resolution serum protein electrophoresis and immunofixation electrophoresis as well as urine protein electrophoresis *(2)*.

2.2. What Is the Nature of the Polyneuropathy Associated With Multiple Myeloma?

Although one prospective study suggested a high incidence of subclinical polyneuropathy in a group of patients with multiple myeloma, symptomatic peripheral neuropathy is rarely encountered. Perhaps the largest series was reported by Kelly et al. from their experience at the Mayo clinic *(3)*. They identified 10 patients with multiple myeloma and peripheral neuropathy, 4 of whom had evidence of (secondary) amyloidosis on rectal biopsy. The polyneuropathy was clinically heterogeneous among the six patients without amyloid deposition. Four presented with a relatively mild sensorimotor neuropathy that had progressed slowly over many months or even years. Motor involvement was mild compared with the sensory findings, and all sensory modalities were equally affected. Electrodiagnostic evaluation showed mildly slowed conduction velocities and mildly reduced response amplitudes. One of the patients in this group presented with a slowly progressive purely sensory neuropathy and the other with a subacute, severe, predominantly motor neuropathy. Electrodiagnostic evaluation in these two patients similarly showed changes that were considered most consistent with primary axonal degeneration. The four patients with amyloid were more homogenous, presenting with a slowly progressing distal, axonal sensorimotor polyneuropathy, with small fiber function more severely affected and pain frequently reported. These data suggest that multiple myeloma may be associated with a purely sensory, sensorimotor, and pure motor neuropathy, each with axonal physiology.

2.3. What Is the Nature of the Polyneuropathy Associated With Osteosclerotic Myeloma?

Osteosclerotic myeloma is a rare variant of multiple myeloma in which the malignant proliferation of plasma cells occurs in a focus (plasmacytoma) outside of the bone marrow. In contrast with the lytic or diffuse osteoporotic skeletal lesions of multiple myeloma, the bony lesions in osteosclerotic myeloma are typically sclerotic. They may be single or multiple. In contrast with multiple myeloma patients, who usually present with systemic symptoms and in whom polyneuropathy is uncommon, osteoslcerotic myeloma is often recognized as the result of investigations initiated following presentation with a polyneuropathy. Although osteosclerotic myeloma is not always associated with an M-protein, a small M-protein is present in about 75–80% of cases *(4)*.

Kelly and colleagues were the first to describe a reasonably sized series of patients with osteosclerotic myeloma and polyneuropathy *(5)*. They reported their experience with 16 such patients, all of whom presented with longstanding neuropathic symptoms (median duration of 20 months). Paraesthesiae were the most commonly reported symptom, and pain was rare. Motor symptoms followed later and began with distal symmetrical weakness that gradually spread more proximally. By the time of evaluation, motor symptoms were more prominent and disabling than the sensory symptoms. Examination confirmed the presence of predominantly large fiber sensory loss as well as significant weakness. Cranial nerve involvement was rare. Electrodiagnostic testing showed significantly slowed conduction velocity and prolongation of distal slowing in the face of relatively preserved response amplitudes. Needle electromyography (EMG) showed mild distal ongoing denervation and chronic reinnervation changes. These findings were interpreted as showing evidence for a predominantly demyelinating process with secondary axonal loss. Cerebrospinal fluid (CSF) protein was elevated in all of the patients.

A proportion of patients with osteosclerotic myeloma may exhibit any of a number of systemic features including hepatosplenomegaly, gynecomastia, hyperpigmentation, edema, lymphadenopathy, digital clubbing, and testicular atrophy. A variety of terms have been used to describe this disorder including the polyneuropathy, organomegaly, endocrinopathy, M-protein, and skin changes (POEMS) syndrome and the Crow-Fukase syndrome *(6)*. In their large retrospective series, Nakanishi et al. did not provide the results of detailed electrophysiological testing, but the available data suggest that the neuropathy was most likely demyelinating in nature. The clinical and electrophysiological characteristics of the neuropathy that accompanies osteosclerotic myeloma, therefore, are those of a demyelinating neuropathy that clinically resembles chronic inflammatory demyelinating polyneuropathy (CIDP). Sung and colleagues have suggested that there may be subtle electrophysiological differences between POEMS neuropathy and CIDP *(7)*. They compared 8 patients with POEMS to 42 patients with CIDP and 7 patients with Charcot-Marie-Tooth disease (CMT)1A. They found that distal latency was not as prolonged, that conduction block was less frequent, and that distal compound muscle action potential (CMAP) amplitudes were more reduced in the POEMS patients than in the other two groups of patients. But it seems unlikely that any of these features are sufficiently distinctive to permit identification of a POEMS neuropathy purely on the basis of the electrophysiological features.

2.4. What Is the Nature of the Polyneuropathy Associated With Primary Systemic Amyloidosis?

Primary systemic amyloidosis is a multisystem disease characterized by the deposition of amyloid in various tissues throughout the body. Peripheral neuropathy develops in about 15% of patients and may either be the presenting symptom or be eclipsed by the systemic manifestations of the disorder. The clinical and electrophysiological features of the neuropathy are well characterized by the retrospective study from the Mayo clinic *(8)*. In this study, Kelly and colleagues identified 31 patients with peripheral neuropathy due to primary systemic amyloidosis. One-third presented with symptoms primarily related to the neuropathy and one-fifth had symptoms of carpal tunnel syndrome. A monoclonal spike was evident on serum protein electrophoresis in only 20% of patients, but serum and urine immunoelectrophoresis showed an M-protein in 40% of patients so studied. Those whose illness was dominated by neurological symptoms presented primarily with a sensorimotor and/or autonomic neuropathy. Sensory symptoms were most prominent, with most patients reporting dysesthesia in the feet and hands. Examination confirmed the disproportionate affectation of pain and temperature sensation. Most patients reported symptoms of autonomic dysfunction, including postural hypotension, impotence, diarrhea, constipation, and bladder dysfunction. Weakness was generally mild and distally predominant. CSF protein was elevated in 8 of the 10 patients in whom it was examined and two patients had a mild pleocytosis. Neurophysiological evaluation showed evidence of a primarily axonal process.

The prototypic neuropathy of primary systemic amyloidosis, therefore, is that of a slowly progressive, often painful, polyneuropathy characterized predominantly by (small fiber) sensory and autonomic involvement and axonal physiology. A superimposed carpal tunnel syndrome may also be present.

2.5. What Is the Spectrum of Neuropathy Encountered in Patients With MGUS?

The literature relevant to MGUS neuropathy is a complex and often contradictory one. With even a superficial perusal of this literature, it is clear that the MGUS neuropathies are not a homogenous group. One of the difficulties encountered when reading this literature is that it includes descriptions of IgG- and IgM-associated neuropathies without sufficient attention to the observation that more than one clinico-electrophysiological syndrome may be encountered in association with both IgG and IgM MGUS. In their retrospective case series, Gorson and Ropper *(9)*, for example, described the clinical and electrophysiological properties of 36 patients with an MGUS neuropathy. They divided patients into two groups based on the dominant underlying physiology—axonal (16 patients) or demyelinating (20 patients). The clinical presentation of patients in the axonal group was that of insidious onset and slowly progressing distal numbness and paresthesiae, with one-third of the patients reporting pain. Mild distal weakness was commonly found on examination although it was not always subjectively reported. Twelve of the 16 patients in this group had an IgG gammopathy (three had IgM and one had IgA). CSF protein was elevated in only two patients. By contrast, the clinical presentation of patients in the demyelinating group was that of combined distal sensory loss (mostly large fiber) with symmetric generalized weakness. About one-third of patients reported pain. Sixteen of the 20 patients had an IgM gammopathy and CSF protein was usually elevated. Although this is a useful distinction in a very broad sense, a more careful reading of the literature suggests that it is an oversimplification to regard IgM MGUS as synonymous with a demyelinating neuropathy and IgG MGUS as indicative of an axonal process (Table 9.1).

Table 9.1

Spectrum of Neuropathy Associated With IgG and IgM Monoclonal Gammopathy
of Undertermined Significance (MGUS)

MGUS	Neuropathy
IgM (anti-MAG positive)	1. Sensorimotor neuropathy with prominent large fiber involvement and distal demyelination *(10–13)*
IgM (anti-MAG negative)	1. Syndrome that is clinically and electrophysiologically indistinguishable from the anti-MAG neuropathy *(11,18,19)* 2. Axonal sensorimotor polyneuropathy *(19,20)* 3. Sensory neuronopathy *(11)* 4. CIDP-like syndrome *(11)*
IgG	1. CIDP-like syndrome *(22)* 2. Axonal sensorimotor polyneuropathy *(18,19)*

2.6. Is There a Specific Syndrome Associated With Monoclonal IgM Antibodies Directed Against Myelin-Associated Glycoprotein?

Perhaps the most distinctive and well recognized syndrome is that of the anti-MAG neuropathy. In their retrospective review of nine patients with neuropathy and an IgM gammopathy, Hafler and colleagues *(10)* identified six patients in whom the antibody showed reactivity to MAG. All six patients presented with slowly progressing distal paresthesiae and all but one had diminished distal vibration and joint position sense with absent ankle reflexes. Mild distal weakness was common, but weakness was never severe enough to impair walking. Very limited electrophysiological data were reported, with the mean median nerve motor conduction velocity markedly slowed at 27 m/s (normal >50 m/s). CSF protein was elevated (mean 118 mg/dL) and nerve biopsy in four patients confirmed the presence of extensive demyelination. Kelly's report of seven patients with anti-MAG reactive IgM monoclonal gammopathy *(11)* confirmed the clinical syndrome as described by Hafler and provided a slightly more detailed electrophysiological description of the syndrome. He reported a mean median motor nerve conduction velocity of 35 m/s, a mean distal latency of 7.9 ms (normal <4.5), and a normal compound muscle action potential response amplitude of 5.4 mV (normal >4). Needle EMG was performed in all seven patients and showed mild ongoing denervation and chronic reinnervation changes in a distal-to-proximal gradient.

Kaku and colleagues subsequently drew attention to a specific electrophysiological characteristics of this syndrome *(12)*. They described four patients with slowly progressing, predominantly large fiber sensory polyneuropathy in association with IgM antibodies reactive against MAG and sulphated glucuronyl paragloboside (SGPG). They noted that distal latency was disproportionately prolonged relative to the degree of more proximal conduction velocity slowing. They used the terminal latency index (TLI), a value calculated using the formula TLI = distal distance/(distal latency × conduction velocity), to describe this feature of the anti-MAG neuropathy syndrome. They found the terminal latency indices to be ≤ 0.25 in 16 of 21 (76%) nerves studied in these four patients. By comparison, a TLI ≤ 0.25 was only found in 3 of 49 (6%) nerves in patients with CIDP and 11 of 195 (6%) in patients with CMT1A. Moreover, in only one patient with CMT or CIDP was the TLI ≤ 0.25 in more than one nerve, whereas it was found in the majority of nerves in every patient with the anti-MAG neuropathy. These findings have since been confirmed in a larger group of patients with anti-MAG neuropathy (*n* = 15) in whom a correlation between the anti-MAG antibody titer and the degree of distal slowing of conduction velocity was shown (*13*).

The characteristic clinical syndrome, therefore, is that of the insidious onset of a predominantly sensory, distal polyneuropathy. Although large fiber function is particularly impaired in the typical syndrome, all sensory modalities may be equally affected. Some investigators have commented on the presence of a postural tremor in the upper extremities. Kaku et al., for example, observed a mild postural tremor in two of their four patients (*12*) although Kelly had made particular note of the absence of a tremor in his seven patients (*11*). Subsequent investigators have commented on the presence of a postural tremor in the hands in 30% (*14*) to 50% (*15*) of patients with the anti-MAG neuropathy. The presence of the tremor does not seem to correlate with the degree of proprioceptive loss in the upper limbs (*14*).

As noted before, the typical electrophysiological finding is that of demyelination that particularly affects distal nerve segments (*12*). This may be evidenced by a short terminal latency index. Not all authors have found such prominent distal demyelination. Ellie et al., for example, found a mean TLI of 0.33 ms and noted a TLI less than 0.25 ms in at least one nerve in less than one-half of their patients (*15*). It has been noted that the distally predominant demyelination may be a feature early in the course of the polyneuropathy but that with progression of the disease, the slowing of conduction velocity becomes more uniform (*16*). This change in the distribution of conduction velocity along the nerve segment over time may provide a partial explanation for why this particular physiology has not been reported by all investigators (*17*).

2.7. What Are the Clinical and Electrophysiological Manifestations of IgM MGUS Neuropathy That Is Not Associated With MAG Reactivity?

Patients with an IgM gammopathy that is not reactive to MAG have a more varied clinical presentation. In some patients, the clinical syndrome and electrophysiological findings are indistinguishable from those seen in patients with the anti-MAG reactive neuropathy. In Kelly's series of 14 patients (*11*), for example, 5 of the 7 patients in the MAG nonreactive group presented with clinical symptomatology that was indistinguishable from the MAG reactive group, and 4 of these patients had similar electrodiagnostic findings. Suarez and Kelly similarly found that their 15 MAG-reactive and 8 MAG nonreactive patients with IgM gammopathy were not distinguishable on clinical grounds (*18*). Electrophysiological testing showed a trend toward longer distal latency and slower conduction velocity in the MAG-reactive group, but these differences were only significant for the median nerve (*18*). Finally, in the prospective study by Notermans and colleagues, four of the MAG nonreactive patients were clinically and electrophysiologically indistinguishable from the seven MAG reactive patients (*19*).

In most case series of patients with IgM gammopathy and neuropathy in which anti-MAG testing was done, a small proportion of patients in the MAG nonreactive group present with a clinical syndrome indistinguishable from the MAG reactive patients, but with different electrodiagnostic findings. Four of 8 MAG-negative patients in one series presented with a clinical syndrome characterized predominantly by sensory symptoms (numbness, paresthesiae, and gait unsteadiness) more marked in the legs than the arms, and with relatively mild distal muscle weakness (indistinguishable from the MAG-positive group). Electrodiagnostic testing, however, showed changes indicative of a primarily axonal process *(19)*. Nobile-Orazio and colleagues similarly found axonal physiology in 76% of their 26 MAG-negative patients (whereas a similar proportion of MAG-positive patients showed demyelinating physiology) *(20)*. For the most part, the MAG-positive and -negative patients were clinically indistinguishable, presenting with a distal symmetrical sensorimotor polyneuropathy. The only difference was that proprioceptive loss and sensory ataxia occurred more commonly in the MAG-positive group ($p < 0.0001$). These and other studies support the existence of an insidious, symmetric, distal sensorimotor polyneuropathy with axonal physiology in patients with IgM MGUS neuropathy.

Finally, there are a few MAG-nonreactive patients with IgM MGUS who present with a different clinical syndrome. In Kelly's series, for example, one of the MAG-nonreactive patients had a relapsing and remitting polyradiculoneuropathy that resembled CIDP *(11)*. Another, who presented with slowly progressive distal sensory symptoms, was found electrophysiologically to have no motor involvement and was thus thought to have a sensory neuronopathy syndrome *(11)*. Presumably, although it is not explicitly stated, the electrophysiological features were those of reduced sensory nerve action potential amplitudes with normal conduction velocities. Reports such as these suggest that an even more variegated clinical and electrophysiological phenotype may be encountered in the population of patients with MAG nonreactive IgM MGUS (Table 9.1).

2.8. What Is the Nature of the Polyneuropathy Associated With an IgG MGUS?

Dalakas and Engel were among the first to report an association between polyneuropathy and an IgG monoclonal gammopathy *(21)*. They described 11 patients with a clinical syndrome characterized by insidious onset of symmetrical distal muscle weakness with or without paresthesiae, and (mostly large fiber) sensory loss. The monoclonal protein was of the IgG isotype in seven of these patients. The degree of distal weakness varied from Medical Research Council (MRC) grade 0/5 to 4/5, and two patients presented with exclusively proximal muscle weakness. CSF protein was elevated in four of the seven patients with the IgG gammopathy. The results of detailed electrophysiological testing were not reported, but it seems that two of these patients showed conduction velocity slowing in the demyelinating range *(21)*. This report was important in part because of the description of a polyneuropathy in association with an IgG gammopathy, but also because it hinted at the heterogeneity of the clinico-electrophysiological characteristics of the polyneuroapthy that might occur in this context.

Bleasel and colleagues subsequently reported a small case series comprising five patients with an IgG gammopathy who presented with a clinical syndrome and electrophysiological findings that were similar to those of patients with CIDP *(22)*. In all five patients, the earliest symptoms were sensory and took the form of distal limb paresthesiae and numbness that ascended over a period of several weeks to months. There was considerable variation in the degree of weakness present, but three of the five patients had sufficiently severe weakness that they were bed-bound at some stage in the course of their illness. Cranial nerves were affected in two patients—one patient reported facial paraesthesiae and the other was noted to have vocal cord paresis. CSF protein was elevated in all five patients, although to a variable degree. The electrophysiological findings included marked slowing of motor conduction velocity, conduction block, temporal dispersion, and absent sural sensory responses. Needle EMG showed relatively mild denervation and chronic (neurogenic) reinnervation changes *(22)*. This report confirmed previous observations that patients with an IgG gammopathy may present with a CIDP-like illness with typical demyelinating physiology.

The association between an IgG gammpathy and an axonal polyneuropathy has been recognized by a number of investigators. In their retrospective series of 39 patients with MGUS neuropathies, Suarez and Kelly included 13 patients with an IgG gammopathy *(18)*. Ten of these patients presented with a clinical syndrome dominated by distal sensory symptoms (mostly numbness; some had tingling, and only two had pain). All sensory modalities were affected, although large fibers perhaps more severely so. Weakness, when present, was distal and mild. The electrophysiological findings in these patients were mild and did not meet criteria for demyelination *(18)*. The prospective study by Notermans and colleagues similarly included 17 patients with an IgG gammopathy who presented with a slowly progressive, distal, symmetric sensorimotor polyneuropathy. In eight of these patients, the physiology was purely axonal, and in seven it showed a mixture of axonal and demyelinating features *(19)*.

In conclusion, therefore, IgG gammopathy may be associated with two different types of neuropathy—one demyelinating and one axonal. Some patients present with a subacute syndrome characterized by sensory and motor features, often with moderate-to-severe muscle weakness, an elevated CSF protein, and unequivocal demyelinating physiology. For obvious reasons, this has been designated a CIDP-like syndrome. On the other hand, some patients present with a syndrome characterized by the insidious onset of predominantly sensory symptoms and signs with relatively mild weakness and axonal or mixed axonal and demyelinating physiology. Of note is that this latter syndrome is clinically and electrophysiologically indistinguishable from the subset of MAG-nonreactive IgM gammopathy patients with axonal physiology (described above).

2.9. What Sort of Work-Up Is Needed in Patients With Monoclonal Gammopathy Associated Neuropathy in Order to Evaluate for the Presence of an Underlying Plasma Cell Proliferative Disorder?

The typical scenario is that of a patient with a polyneuropathy who, in the course of the work-up for the etiology of the neuropathy, is found to have a monoclonal gammopathy. The question that arises is whether this represents an MGUS or whether it is a sign of an underlying hematological malignancy such as Waldenstrom's macroglobulinemia, multiple myeloma, osteoslcerotic myeloma, or B-cell lymphoma. Should such patients undergo a skeletal radiographic survey (to detect lytic and/or sclerotic bony lesions) and should they be subject to a bone marrow biopsy? Unfortunately, there are limited data available to assist in providing a clear answer to this question.

In trying to answer these questions, it is useful to note the hematological criteria for the diagnosis of an MGUS. It is defined by the presence of an M-protein level less than 30g/L; a bone marrow plasma cell infiltration of less than 10%; the absence of lytic bone lesions, anemia, or other laboratory or clinical abnormalities; and stability of the M-

Table 9.2
Hematological Malignancies in Patients With Gammopathy-Associated Neuropathy

Malignancy	No. patients	M-protein	Clinical symptoms
Multiple myeloma	8	<1 to 30 g/L	Fatigue, weight loss, bone pain, infections, night sweats
NHL	10	<1 to 18 g/L	Fatigue, weight loss, bone pain, infections, night sweats
Plasmacytoma	3	<1 to 8 g/L	Fatigue, weight loss, bone pain, infections, night sweats
POEMS syndrome	1	3 g/L	Fatigue, weight loss
Castleman's disease	1	<1g/L	Fatigue, weight loss, bone pain

NHL, non-Hodgkin's lymphoma; POEMS, polyneuropathy, organomegaly, endocrinopathy, M-protein, and skin changes. Data from ref. *23*.

protein level. Because the level of the serum M-protein is an important component of the differentiation between MGUS and M-proteins associated with hematological malignancies, one approach is to base the decision to investigate further on serum concentration of the M-protein. One problem that immediately emerges is that the diagnosis of MGUS cannot really be made without knowing whether lytic bone lesions are present and the extent of plasma cell infiltration in the bone marrow.

The study by Eurelings and colleagues provides some useful information *(23)*. Within a population of 1100 patients with polyneuropathy who were screened for the cause of the neuropathy over a 12-year period, they identified a monoclonal gammopathy in 104 patients. Further investigations in those in whom an M-protein was identified included skeletal X-ray, chest X-ray, abdominal ultrasound, and bone marrow examination in addition to clinical examination and routine biochemical evaluation. A hematological malignancy was identified in 23 patients (22%), the details of which are outlined in Table 9.2. Of note is that in all of these patients (except in three with non-Hodgkin's lymphoma [NHL]), the polyneuropathy was progressive over a period of weeks to months. In multivariate analysis comparing those with and without a hematological malignancy, weight loss, more rapid progression of the polyneuropathy, and M-protein level >1g/L were the factors that emerged as independent predictors of patients likely to have a hematological malignancy.

This is an important paper for a few reasons. It suggests that among those patients with a monoclonal gammopathy that is recognized following presentation with a neuropathy, the proportion with an underlying hematological malignancy is relatively high (~20%). The authors do acknowledge that this figure is likely to be an overestimate as a result of selection bias due to their being a tertiary referral center. Nevertheless, had they followed traditional recommendations and performed a bone marrow biopsy only when the M-protein level was greater than 10 g/L, then an underlying hematological malignancy would have been missed in 15 patients. It is worth emphasizing that they found an M-protein level >1 g/L as being predictive of the risk of an underlying hematological malignancy. These data, therefore, would suggest that one cannot rely solely on the concentration of the M-protein to decide whether to perform a skeletal survey and bone marrow biopsy, and that these investigations should be part of the routine work-up of patients with gammopathy-associated neuropathy.

3. TREATMENT

3.1. Is Immunosuppressive Therapy Effective in the Treatment of IgM Gammopathy-Associated Neuropathy?

The question of treatment for polyneuropathy associated with anti-MAG IgM gammopathy has been the subject of a number of randomized controlled trials. One difficulty with interpreting the data from these studies is that the inclusion criteria varied somewhat. Only two studies explicitly stated that the neuropathy was of the demyelinating variety *(24,25)* with only one of these specifying the electrophysiological criteria for demyelination *(25)*. Anti-MAG reactivity was determined in all of the studies, but in only two of these did all of the patients have demonstrable anti-MAG antibodies. In the remaining studies, the results were not reported separately for those with and without anti-MAG reactivity.

Dalakas and colleagues studied 11 patients with a demyelinating neuropathy associated with an IgM gammopathy (9 of which showed reactivity to MAG) *(24)*. Patients were randomized to receive monthly infusions for 3 months of either placebo or IVIg, administered at a dose of 1 g/kg/day for 2 days. The study had a cross-over design, and after a washout period, patients received the alternate treatment. A variety of measures were used to evaluate outcome including manual muscle strength testing using the MRC scale, a neuromuscular symptom index, and a score of sensory symptoms. No patients improved during treatment with placebo, and two patients showed a significant, albeit temporary, improvement in strength during the IVIg phase. The authors concluded that IVIg may exert a modest and short-lived benefit in a small number of patients with IgM-associated demyelinating polyneuropathy.

In a larger prospective controlled trial of IVIg, Comi and colleagues *(25)* randomized 22 patients in a cross-over design to receive 2 days of either placebo or IVIg (1 g/kg/day). All patients had a demyelinating polyneuropathy associated with an IgM MGUS. MAG reactivity was positive in 11 of the 19 patients tested. The primary endpoint of the study was the difference in disability grade, assessed using the Inflammatory Neuropathy Cause and Treatment (INCAT) disability scale, 2 weeks after treatment. The disability score decreased by a mean of 0.18 points during the IVIg treatment period and by 0.14 points in the placebo period, neither change being significant. At 4 weeks, the disability score decreased (improved) by 0.55 points in the IVIg group, whereas there was no significant change in the placebo group. Although the improvement was statistically significant, the clinical relevance of a half point improvement on a 10-point scale is not clear. Secondary outcome measures at 2 weeks, however, suggested some small degree of benefit from IVIg based on improvement in the modified Rankin scale score, the 10-m walking time, and strength of hand grip. The authors concluded that IVIg "... improves nerve function in some patients with IgM paraproteinemic demyelinating neuropathy *(25)*." The study did not address whether even this small benefit was sustained over more a prolonged period of follow-up.

Chlorambucil has been used in the treatment of IgM MGUS neuropathy, with the rationale being that it is effective in other chronic B-cell lymphoproliferative disorders. Oksenhendler and colleagues compared the efficacy of chlorambucil alone with the combination of chlorambucil and plasma exchange in a randomized controlled study *(26)*. Thirty-nine patients were randomized to one of the two treatment groups—chlorambucil (1 mg/kg/day) for 12 months with or without a 4-month course of plasma exchange. Outcome was evaluated in a nonblinded fashion. The primary endpoint was the clinical neuropathy disability score (CNDS) following 12 months of treatment. CNDS is a 72-point scale that includes measure of muscle strength, reflex changes, and sensory function. The mean CNDS score improved by 2.1 and 1.8 points in the chlorambucil and plasma exchange groups, respectively, a nonsignificant difference ($p = 0.7$). The authors concluded that plasma exchange offers no additional benefit, but this study leaves open the question of whether chlorambucil alone has any effect. Based on the changes in CNDS scores, it would seem not.

Two studies have examined the effects of interferon (IFN)-α (27,28). In the first, a randomized, controlled, but open (i.e., nonblinded) study, Mariette and colleagues (27) randomly assigned patients to 6 months of treatment with either IVIg or IFN-α. The main endpoint was the change in CNDS score between the time of randomization and the 6-month follow-up visit. The study was terminated prematurely after 10 patients had been assigned to each treatment group because of an apparent benefit from IFN-α. Whereas only 1 of 10 patients in the IVIg group showed signs of improvement, 8 of 10 patients in the IFN-α group improved by ≥ 20 points on the CNDS score (27). These results prompted a second study by the same group, this time with outcome determined in a blinded fashion (28). This study was also terminated prematurely (for business reasons) after 24 patients had been randomized. The mean CNDS did not change significantly in either group over the 6 months of treatment.

Other treatments that have been examined in nonrandomized open studies include fludarabine (29) and rituximab (30), but the efficacy of these agents awaits demonstration in randomized controlled trials.

In summary, therefore, although variable in design and inclusion criteria, the available literature suggests that, with the possible exception of IVIg, which may exert a small beneficial effect for a limited period, there are no proven effective immunosuppressive therapies for the treatment of IgM MGUS MAG-reactive demyelinating polyneuropathy.

3.2. Is CIDP–MGUS Responsive to Immunosuppressive Therapy?

A CIDP-like syndrome has been reported in association with both an IgG and an IgM MGUS, but these patients were excluded from the major randomized controlled trials of steroids, plasmapheresis, and IVIg in CIDP (refer to Chapter 12 for references and a discussion of these studies). The data supporting the use of various forms of immunosuppressive therapy in CIDP-MGUS, therefore, derive more from retrospective case series and by inference from the studies of idiopathic CIDP. Bleasel et al., for example, reported their experience of five patients with IgG MGUS in association with CIDP. All five responded to the combination of prednisone and azathioprine and/or plasmapheresis (22). Di Troia's retrospective series of patients with IgG gammopathy and neuropathy included 10 patients with a CIDP-like illness, 8 of whom were treated. Sustained improvement was evident in six patients following plasmapheresis ($n = 1$), steroids ([$n = 2$], and IVIg [$n = 3$]). The largest series was reported in the case–control study reported by Simmons and colleagues (31). These authors reviewed their experience with 103 CIDP patients, 77 with idiopathic CIDP (CIDP-I) and 26 with CIDP associated with a gammopathy (CIDP–MGUS). Ninety and 80% of CIDP-I and CIDP–MGUS patients, respectively, were treated at the time of first presentation. Treatment usually comprised prednisone (60 mg/kg/day) for 1–3 months followed by a gradual taper and/or plasmapheresis (five exchanges over 10–14 days). Eighty-one percent of the CIDP-I patients responded to treatment compared with only 52% in the CIDP–MGUS group. The CIDP–MGUS group included 13 patients with an IgM gammopathy and 13 with an IgG or IgA gammopathy. Subgroup analysis indicated no difference between these two groups in terms of response to immunosuppressive therapy. The available data, therefore, suggest that patients with CIDP-MGUS do respond to immunosuppressive therapy. Although the degree of response may be less than that encountered in idiopathic CIDP, so is the initial degree of disability (31). The net result is that the functional level attained following treatment is similar in the two groups.

3.3. Is Immunosuppressive Therapy Effective in the Treatment of MGUS-Associated Axonal Neuropathy?

There are no randomized controlled trials of patients with axonal MGUS and neuropathy, and the available data are derived from small retrospective case series. Gorson and Ropper described a series of 16 patients with an axonal neuropathy and MGUS, 12 of whom had an IgG gammopathy (9). Seven patients received plasmapheresis, five were treated with IVIg, and seven with steroids. Clinical improvement was seen in one patient (who had received steroids). The retrospective study by Di Troia et al. included seven patients with an IgG gammopathy and an axonal polyneuropathy (32). Three of these patients were treated with steroids and one reported consistent improvement. The published data on the treatment and outcome of this group of patients are grossly inadequate and insufficient to permit recommendations about treatment.

3.4. What Is the Appropriate Therapy for Patients With Neuropathy and Osteosclerotic Myeloma?

There is a genuine lack of data that inform on the best approach to the management of these patients. There are no controlled trials, and the available data are derived from single case reports and relatively small case series. The Mayo Clinic experience, reported by Kelly and colleagues (5), is one of the largest series. Six of their patients had been treated as though they had an idiopathic demyelinating neuropathy before the diagnosis of osteoblastic myeloma was made. These patients received high-dose steroids and/or azathioprine for 2–3 months, with no sustained clinical response, suggesting that immunosuppressive therapy targeting the neuropathy is of limited value. Treatment directed toward the osteoblastic myeloma itself is contingent upon whether the lesions are single or multiple. In Kelly's series, those with multiple lesions were treated with prednisone (60 mg per day) and melphalan (0.15 mg/kg/day) for seven days every 6 weeks, but there was no sustained improvement in the neuropathy in any of these patients (5). On the other hand, there are case reports suggesting that a similar approach may occasionally produce a substantial improvement in the neuropathy (33,34). Kelly et al. suggested that those with solitary bony lesions treated with local irradiation showed some improvement in the neuropathy. This improvement was significant and sustained in three patients, moderate in two and only slight in one. The improvement was apparent within 6 months and was sustained even 1–2 years after treatment (5).

Based on the available data, therefore, it is extremely difficult to know how best to treat patients with osteosclerotic myeloma and peripheral neuropathy. It is not clear that they do (or do not) respond to immunosuppressive therapy as do patients with idiopathic CIDP. Treatment is generally directed toward the underlying myeloma and differs depending on whether the skeletal lesions are solitary or multiple. Whether improvement in the neuropathy should be expected with treatment of the myeloma is simply not well established.

3.5. Is Amyloid Neuropathy Responsive to Any Form of Treatment?

Although the combination of melphalan and prednisone has been shown in randomized controlled trials to prolong survival in patients with primary systemic amyloid *(35)*, no form of treatment has been shown to impact on the progression of the associated polyneuropathy.

4. PROGNOSIS

In considering the prognosis of patients with gammopathy-associated polyneuropathy, there are a number of issues to address. A distinction should be made between those neuropathies diagnosed in the context of an underlying hematological disorder (e.g., multiple myeloma, osterosclerotic myeloma, Waldenstrom's macroglobulinemia, or primary systemic amyloidosis) and those associated with a monoclonal gammopathy of undeterminted significance. For the first group, because treatment is directed primarily toward the underlying malignancy, it seems intuitively more appropriate to consider the prognosis of the neuropathy and the malignancy together. For those neuropathies associated with an MGUS, it is helpful to make a distinction between the prognosis of the neuropathy itself on the one hand and the risk of developing a hematological malignancy on the other.

4.1. What Degree of Disability Can Be Expected in MGUS Associated Neuropathy?

There are relatively few studies that provide helpful information about the long-term prognosis for the polyneuropathy associated with gammopathy. One reason for the paucity of data relates to the way in which patients have been grouped. For example, most studies have grouped together all patients with polyneuropathy in association with a MGUS of a particular isotype (either IgM or IgG/A). The problem with this approach, as should be evident from the foregoing discussions, is that neither IgM nor IgG MGUS-associated neuropathy is a homogenous clinical entity. Within each group, there are patients with a CIDP-like illness and others with an axonal sensorimotor polyneuropathy; and within the IgM group, there is a subset of patients (mostly those with reactivity against MAG) with a particular clinical phenotype and electrophysiological evidence of predominantly distal demyelination. Classification of the neuropathies associated with monoclonal gammopathies into these three groups—(1) CIDP-like, (2) distal demyelinating with predominant large fiber involvement and frequent MAG positivity, and (3) axonal sensorimotor—seems appropriate given the relative homogeneity within each group in terms of clinical presentation, electrodiagnostic features, and response to therapy. The prognosis for each is discussed separately.

4.1.1. CIDP-Like Polyneuropathy

Simmons and colleagues reported their experience with the long-term follow-up of a cohort of patients with CIDP–MGUS *(36)*.This was not a natural history study, in that most patients were treated with various forms of immunosuppressive therapy. However, it does provide an indication of the course and prognosis of the neuropathy given the best available treatment. The clinical course was relapsing in 24%, monophasic in 28%, and progressive in 48%. They used the modified Rankin disability score to describe the functional level reached by the 25 patients in their cohort. At last follow-up, three (12%) were grade 0 (asymptomatic), eight (32%) were grade 1 (nondisabling symptoms), seven (28%) were grade 2 (minor symptoms with some restriction of lifestyle), four (16%) were grade 3 (moderate symptoms significantly interfering with lifestyle), two (8%) were grade 4 (moderately severe symptoms clearly preventing independent existence), and one had died of CIDP. Mild disability or less (mRS ≤ 2), therefore, was noted in 72% of patients.

4.1.2. Distally Predominant Demyelinating Neuropathy With Anti-MAG Reactivity

Smith described the long term prognosis of a cohort of patients with IgM anti-MAG associated polyneuropathy *(14)*. Symptom onset was gradual in most patients. Sensory symptoms began first and were followed weeks to years later with weakness. Tremor, incoordination, and gait unsteadiness followed the weakness. Symptoms usually progressed slowly over the first 1–5 years and then either stabilized or progressed extremely slowly. In many (14 of 18) patients, paresthesiae subsequently improved spontaneously, although numbness typically persisted. Weakness was slowly progressive in approximately one-half of the patients in this study. Overall, the disability produced by the neuropathy was very variable. Most patients had very little disability even after more than 15 years of follow-up. Two patients (11%) in this group had severe sensory ataxia and required assistance with activities of daily living. Four patients (22%) were disabled, primarily by tremor and gait unsteadiness.

4.1.3. Axonal Sensorimotor Polyneuropathy

There are no good studies that provide reliable information about the natural history of the neuropathy in this group of patients.

4.2. What Is the Risk of Hematological Malignancy in Patients With an MGUS-Associated Neuropathy?

There are a number of studies that have addressed the long-term risk of progression of MGUS to the development of a hematological malignancy *(37–39)*. It should be noted, however, that most of these series included all patients with MGUS rather than patients with MGUS and a neuropathy. Sample sizes in these studies ranged from 128 to 335 and patients were followed for periods of up to 10 years. The risk of malignant transformation (i.e., development of multiple myeloma, Waldenstrom's macroglobulinemia, amyloidosis or another malignant lymphoproliferative disorder) was 7% *(39)* to 11% *(37)* at 5 years and 16% *(37)* to 19% *(38)* at 10 years.

A recent prospective study examined the risk of developing a hematological malignancy in a large series of patients with MGUS-associated polyneuropathy *(40)*. After a mean follow-up of 3 years, malignancy was diagnosed in 17 of 176 patients (~10%), suggesting that the risk of malignant transformation is higher among those with MGUS-associated neuropathy than among patients with MGUS without neuropathy. Multivariate analysis identified unexplained weight loss, progression of the neuropathy, unexplained fever or night sweats, and the higher M-protein level as independent prognostic variables significantly associated with malignant transformation (40).

4.3. What Is the Prognosis of Patients With Polyneuropathy and Multiple Myeloma?

The available limited data suggest that the prognosis for these patients is poor. Slow progression of the neuropathy is most often encountered, although a minority may stabilize (3).

4.4. What Is the Prognosis of Patients With Polyneuropathy and Osteosclerotic Myeloma?

The available data, although limited, suggest that the prognosis is better for solitary skeletal lesions than it is when there are multiple lesions. In the series of 16 patients described by Kelly (5), 9 had multiple lesions and 7 had solitary lesions. Seven of the nine with multiple lesions were treated with melphalan and prednisone. Three of these improved slightly (but remained wheelchair-bound) but subsequently deteriorated despite continued therapy; two stabilized on chemotherapy; and two continued to worsen. On the other hand, all six patients with solitary lesions who were treated with localized irradiation showed signs of improvement. The extent of improvement and functional level achieved were not reported (5).

4.5. What Is the Prognosis of Patients With Polyneuropathy and Primary Systemic Amyloidosis?

There are two separate prognostic issues, one relating to the neuropathy itself and the other to the patient survival. Most of the data on the natural history of the polyneuropathy associated with primary systemic amyloidosis are derived from the Mayo Clinic. In their early series, Kelly et al. reported their experience with 31 patients with primary systemic amyloidosis (PSA) and peripheral neuropathy (8). The neuropathy was the dominant clinical feature in 13 (42%) patients. Eleven patients were treated (with melphalan and prednisone). In all patients, the neuropathy was relentlessly progressive despite treatment. Spontaneous stabilization or improvement was not noted in any patients. A subsequent series, also from the Mayo Clinic, included 26 patients with PSA in whom neuropathy was the dominant initial manifestation (41). Sixteen of these patients were treated (typically with melphalan and prednisone). The neuropathy was relentlessly progressive in all the patients and was debilitating in most.

The prognosis for survival in PSA is generally poor, as a result of the effects of the systemic deposition of the amyloid protein. The kidneys (nephrotic syndrome), heart (congestive cardiac failure), and bowel (malabsorption) are commonly affected. There are some data to suggest that those in whom the neuropathy is the dominant clinical manifestation have a slightly better prognosis. In one of the randomized controlled trials of chemotherapy for PSA, median survival was 34 months among those presenting primarily with neuropathy. This was significantly more favorable than the 16-month median survival of those presenting with nephrotic syndrome and the 5-month survival of those presenting with congestive cardiac failure *(35)*.

5. SUMMARY

- Although there is limited evidence to support this recommendation, basic principles and published recommendations suggest that patients with suspected paraproteinemic neuropathy should undergo high-resolution serum protein electrophoresis and immunofixation electrophoresis as well as urine protein electrophoresis.
- Clinically overt peripheral neuropathy appears to be uncommon among patients with multiple myeloma, and the neuropathy that does occur, although clinically heterogeneous, is usually axonal in nature.
- Osteosclerotic myeloma is most commonly associated with a demyelinating neuropathy that resembles CIDP.
- Peripheral neuropathy is present in approximately 15% of patients with primary systemic amyloidosis; the neuropathy is axonal in nature and is characterized by small fiber sensory loss, pain, and autonomic dysfunction.
- The neuropathy associated with an MGUS is clinically and electrophysiologically heterogeneous; a useful, although somewhat simplistic, classification suggests an association between demyelinating neuropathy and IgM MGUS on one hand, and axonal neuropathy and IgG MGUS on the other.
- IgM anti-MAG antibodies are usually associated with a demyelinating neuropathy that is characterized clinically by large fiber sensory loss; distal nerve segments bear the brunt of the disease with disproportionate prolongation of distal latencies.
- The neuropathies associated with IgM gammopathy without MAG reactivity are clinically and electrophysiologically more heterogeneous—the neuropathy may be clinically and electrophysiologically indistinguishable from the anti-MAG neuropathy, but may also manifest as a more typical distally predominant sensorimotor axonal polyneuropathy.
- IgG gammopathy may be associated with two different types of neuropathy—one demyelinating and one axonal.
- Among those patients with a monoclonal gammopathy that is recognized following presentation with a neuropathy, the proportion with an underlying hematological malignancy is relatively high (~20%).
- The available literature suggests that, with the possible exception of IVIg, which may exert a small beneficial effect for a limited period, there are no proven effective immunosuppressive therapies for the treatment of IgM MGUS MAG reactive demyelinating polyneuropathy.
- Patients with CIDP associated with an MGUS do respond to immunosuppressive therapy.
- There are insufficient published data from which to draw any firm conclusions as to whether IgG MGUS-associated neuropathies respond to immunosuppressive therapy.
- It is not clear whether patients with osteosclerotic myeloma and peripheral neuropathy respond to immunosuppressive therapy as do patients with idiopathic CIDP; treatment is generally directed toward the underlying myeloma and differs depending on whether the skeletal lesions are solitary or multiple.

- There is no proven effective therapy for the neuropathy associated with primary systemic amyloidosis.
- The prognosis for CIDP associated with an MGUS is generally good, with mild disability (Rankin score ≤2) in approximately 70% of patients.
- Disability in most patients with anti-MAG associated neuropathy is usually mild, even after prolonged follow-up.
- There are no data on the natural history of MGUS-associated axonal neuropathy.
- The available data are very limited, but suggest that the prognosis for myeloma-associated neuropathy is generally poor
- The prognosis for neuropathy associated with osteosclerotic myeloma is not well established, but is generally more favorable for those with solitary skeletal lesions.
- The prognosis for neuropathy associated with primary systemic amyloidosis is generally poor.

REFERENCES

1. Keren DF. Procedures for the evaluation of monoclonal immunoglobulins. Arch Pathol Lab Med 1999;123:126–132.
2. Keren DF, Alexanian R, Goeken JA, Gorevic PD, Kyle RD, Tomar RH. Guidelines for clinical and laboratory evaluation of patients with monoclonal gammopathies. Arch Pathol Lab Med 1999;123:106–107.
3. Kelly JJ, Kyle RA, Miles JM, O'Brien PC, Dyck PJ. The spectrum of peripheral neuropathy in myeloma. Neurology 1981;31:24–31.
4. Miralles GD, O'Fallon JR, Talley NJ. Plasma-cell dyscrasia with polyneuropathy. The spectrum of POEMS syndrome. N Engl J Med 1992;327:1919–1923.
5. Kelly J, Kyle R, Miles J, Dyck P. Osteosclerotic myeloma and peripheral neuropathy. Neurology 1983;33:202–210.
6. Nakanishi T, Sobue I, Toyokura Y, et al. The Crow-Fukase syndrome: a study of 102 cases in Japan. Neurology 1984;34:712–720.
7. Sung J-Y, Kuwabara S, Ogawara K, Kanai K, Hattori T. Patterns of nerve conduction abnormalities in POEMS syndrome. Muscle Nerve 2002;26:189–193.
8. Kelly JJ, Kyle RA, O'Brien PC, Dyck PJ. The natural history of peripheral neuropathy in primary systemic amyloidosis. Ann Neurol 1979;6:1–7.
9. Gorson KC, Ropper AH. Axonal neuropathy associated with monoclonal gammopathy of undetermined significance. J Neurol, Neurosurg Psychiatry 1997;63:163–168.
10. Hafler DA, Johnson D, Kelly JJ, Panitch H, Kyle R, Weiner HL. Monoclonal gammopathy and neuropathy: myelin-associated glycoprotein reactivity and clinical characteristics. Neurology 1986;36:75–78.
11. Kelly JJ. The electrodiagnostic findings in polyneuropathies associated with IgM monoclonal gammopathies. Muscle Nerve 1990;13:1113–1117.
12. Kaku DA, England JD, Sumner AJ. Distal accentuation of conduction slowing in polyneuropathy associated with antibodies to myelin-associated glycoprotein and sulphated glucuronyl paragloboside. Brain 1994;117:941–947.
13. Trojaborg W, Hays A, van den Berg L, Younger D, Latov N. Motor conduction parameters in neuropathies associated with anti-MAG antibodies and other types of demyelinating and axonal neuropathies. Muscle Nerve 1995;18:730–735.
14. Smith I. The natural history of chronic demyelinating neuropathy associated with benign IgM paraproteinaemia. A clinical and neurophysiological study. Brain 1994;117:949–957.
15. Ellie E, Vital A, Steck A, Boiron J-M, Vital C, Julien J. Neuropathy associated with "benign" anti-myelin associated glycoprotein IgM gammopathy: clinical, immunological, neurophysiological pathological findings and response to treatment in 33 cases. J Neurol 1996;243:34–43.

16. Ponsford S, Willison H, Veitch J, Morris R, Thomas P. Long-term clinical and neurophysiological follow-up of patients with peripheral neuropathy associated with benign monoclonal gammopathy. Muscle Nerve 2000;23:164–174.
17. Yeung K, Thomas P, King R, et al. The clinical spectrum of peripheral neuroapthies associated with benign monoclonal IgM, IgG and IgA paraproteinaemia. Comparative clinical, immunological and nerve biopsy findings. J Neurol 1991;238:383–391.
18. Suarez G, Kelly JJ. Polyneuropathy associated with monoclonal gammopathy of undetermined significance: Further evidence that IgM MGUS neuropathies are different than IgG-MGUS. Neurology 1993;43:1304–1308.
19. Notermans N, Wokke J, Lokhorst H, Franssen H, van der Graaf Y, Jennekens F. Polyneuropathy associated with monoclonal gammopathy of undetermined significance. A prospective study of the prognostic value of clinical and laboratory abnormalities. Brain 1994;117:1385–1393.
20. Nobile-Orazio E, Manfredini E, Carpo M, et al. Frequency and clinical correlates of anti-neural IgM antibodies in neuropathy associated with IgM monoclonal gammopathy. Ann Neurol 1994;36:416–424.
21. Dalakas MC, Engel WK. Polyneuropathy with monoclonal gammopathy: studies of 11 patients. Ann Neurol 1981;10:45–52.
22. Bleasel A, Hawke S, Pollard J, McLeod J. IgG monoclonal paraproteinaemia and peripheral neuropathy. J Neurol, Neurosurg Psychiatry 1993;56:52–57.
23. Eurelings M, Notermans NC, van de Donk NW, Lokhorst HM. Risk factors for hematological malignancy in polyneuropathy associated with monoclonal gammopathy. Muscle Nerve 2001;24:1295–1302.
24. Dalakas MC, Quarles RH, Farrer RG, et al. A controlled study of intravenous immunoglobulin in demyelinating neuropathy with IgM gammopathy. Ann Neurol 1996;40:792–795.
25. Comi G, Roveri L, Swan A, et al. A randomised controlled trial of intravenous immunoglobulin in IgM paraprotein associated demyelinating neuropathy. J Neurol 2002;249:1370–1377.
26. Oksenhendler E, Chevret S, Leger JM, et al. Plasma exchange and chlorambucil in polyneuropathy associated with monoclonal IgM gammopathy. J Neurol Neurosurg Psychiatry 1995;59:243–247.
27. Mariette X, Chastang C, Clavelou P. et al. A randomised clinical trial comparing interferon-alpha and intravenous immungloublin in polyneuropathy associated with monoclonal IgM. J Neurol Neurosurg Psychiatry 1997;63:28–34.
28. Mariette X, Brouet J-C, Chevret S, et al. A randomised double-blind trial versus placebo does not confirm the benefit of alpha-interferon in polyneuropathy associated with monoclonal IgM'. J Neurol Neurosurg Psychiatry 2000;69:279–280.
29. Sherman WH, Latov N, Lange D, Heyes R, Younger D. Fludarabine for IgM antibody-mediated neuropathies. Ann Neurol 1994;36:326–327.
30. Pestronk A, Florence J, Miller T, Choksi R, Al-Lozi M, Levine T. Treatment of IgM antibody associated polyneuropathies using rituximab. J Neurol Neurosurg Psychiatry 2003;74:485–489.
31. Simmons Z, Albers JW, Bromberg MB, Feldman EL. Presentation and initial clinical course in patients with chronic inflammatory demyelinating polyradiculoneuropathy: Comparison of patients without and with monoclonal gammopathy. Neurology 1993;43:2202–2209.
32. Di Troia A, Carpo M, Meucci N, et al. Clinical features and anti-neural reactivity in neuropathy associated with IgG monoclonal gammopathy of undetermined significance. J Neurol Sci 1999;164:64–71.
33. Parra R, Fernandez JM, Garcia-Bragado F, Bueno J, Biosca M. Successful treatment of peripheral neuropathy with chemotherapy in osteoslcerotic myeloma. J Neurol 1987;234:261–263.
34. Donofrio P, Albers J, Greenberg H, Mitchell B. Peripheral neuropathy in osteosclerotic myeloma: clinical and electrodiagnostic improvement with chemotherapy. Muscle Nerve 1984;7:137–141.
35. Kyle RA, Gertz MA, Greipp PR, et al. A trial of three regimens for primary amyloidosis: colchicine alone, melphalan and prednisone, and melphalan, prednisone and colchicine. N Engl J Med 1997;336:1202–1207.
36. Simmons Z, Albers JW, Bromberg MB, Feldman EL. Long-term follow-up of patients with chronic inflammatory demyelinating polyradiculoneuropathy, without and with monoclonal gammopathy. Brain 1995;118:359–368.
37. Kyle RA. 'Benign' monoclonal gammopathy. A misnomer? JAMA 1984;251:1849–1854.
38. Blade J, Lopez-Guillermo A, Rozman C, et al. Malignant transformation and life expectancy in monoclonal gammopathy of undetermined significance. Br J Haematol 1992;81:391–394.

39. Baldini L, Guffanti A, Cesana B, et al. Role of different hematologic variables in defining the risk of malignant transformation in monoclonal gammopathy. Blood 1996;87:912–918.
40. Eurelings M, Lokhorst H, Kalmijn S, Wokke J, Notermans N. Malignant transformation in polyneuropathy associated with monoclonal gammopathy. Neurology 2005;64:2079–2084.
41. Rajkumar SV, Gertz MA, Kyle RA. Prognosis of patients with primary systemic amyloidosis who present with dominant neuropathy. Am J Med 1998;104:232–237.

10 Vasculitic Neuropathy

1. INTRODUCTION

The term "vasculitis" is used to describe a group of disorders that are characterized by the presence of a specific pathological finding—namely, inflammation and necrosis of blood vessel walls. Broadly speaking, this group of disorders may be classified into the systemic and nonsystemic (or localized) vasculitides. The systemic vasculitides encompass a broad range of diseases including (a) the vasculitides that result from direct infection of the blood vessel wall (e.g., syphilis, tuberculosis, and HIV infection), (b) the necrotizing vasculitides (e.g., polyarteritis nodosa, Churg-Strauss syndrome, Wegener's granulomatosis, and the connective tissue disorders rheumatoid arthritis, systemic lupus erythematosis, and Sjogren's syndrome), (c) the hypersensitivity vasculitides (e.g., drug-induced cryoglobulinemia and malignancy) and (d) the giant cell arteritides (temporal arteritis and Takayasu's arteritis). The nonsystemic vasculitides may affect either the central or the peripheral nervous system exclusively. In this chapter, we are concerned with the form of nonsystemic vasculitis that is confined to the peripheral nervous system as well as the systemic vasculitides in which the peripheral nervous system is also affected.

How frequently is vasculitis that affects the peripheral nervous system part of a broader systemic disease process and how frequently is the vasculitis confined to the peripheral nervous system? What types of neuropathies may result from vasculitis and which nerves are most commonly affected? How should vasculitis of the peripheral nervous system be treated and what is the long-term outcome for patients with this disorder? These and other questions are the focus of this chapter.

2. DIAGNOSIS

2.1. Is Vasculitis of the Peripheral Nervous System Usually an Isolated Problem or Does It Typically Occur in the Context of Systemic Vasculitis?

Most, if not all, of the available literature on vasculitis of peripheral nerves comprises retrospective case series. Investigators have typically searched either a discharge diagnosis or nerve biopsy database to identify patients with the diagnosis of vasculitis. Clinical records have then been examined to determine whether the vasculitis is confined to the peripheral nervous system (nonsystemic vasculitis) or whether other organ systems are also affected (systemic vasculitis). As shown in Table 10.1, estimates of the relative frequencies of systemic and nonsystemic vasculitis have varied widely among different studies, with nonsystemic vasculitis accounting for between 0 and 64% of all cases. This variability is likely due to the retrospective nature of all of these studies with the potential for substantial selection bias. Overall, these studies included 470 patients with vasculitis

From: *Neuromuscular Disease: Evidence and Analysis in Clinical Neurology*
By: M. Benatar © Humana Press Inc., Totowa, NJ

Table 10.1
Peripheral Nerve Involvement in Systemic and Nonsystemic Vasculitis

Study	Patient selection	n	Clinical context	Systemic disease
Chang (14)	Discharge & biopsy databases searched for "systemic vasculitis"	19	Nonsystemic—2 Systemic—17	PAN (8), RA (9), hypereosinophilic syndrome (1), "arteritis" (1)
Kissel (4)	Neuromuscular database search to identify patients with necrotizing angiopathy	16	Nonsystemic—7 Systemic—9	SLE (1), PAN (1), undifferentiated CTD (5)
Harati (16)	Biopsy database search to identify patients with necrotizing angiopathy	33	Nonsystemic—21 Systemic—12	PAN (2), RA (2), undifferentiated CTD (4), scleroderma (1), other—malignancy (3)
Bouche (17)	Retrospective series of patients with vasculitis and neuropathy	22	Nonsystemic—0 Systemic—22	PAN (16), Churg-Strauss (6)
Dyck (7)	Retrospective series of patients with neuropathy and vasculitis	65	Nonsystemic—20 Systemic—45	PAN (32), Churg-Strauss (4), Sjogren's (3), RA (2), Wegeners (1), scleroderma (1), SLE (1), HIV (1)
Said (18)	Retrospective review of patients with biopsy proven necrotizing arteritis	100	Nonsystemic—32 Systemic—68	RA (25), PAN (19), Sjogren's (2), Mixed CTD (3), SLE (1), Systemic sclerosis (1), other —HIV, sarcoid, GCA, CLL, asthma, mastocytosis (13)
Hawke (5)	Review of nerve biopsies to identify those with vasculitis	34	Nonsystemic—2 Systemic—32	PAN (11), Churg-Strauss (3), RA (7), undifferentiated CTD (8), Sjogren's (1), Wegeners (1), other—CLL + cryoglobulins (1)
Wees (6)	Review of consecutive patients	17	Systemic—17	PAN (11), RA (5), SLE (1)
Collins (8)	Case series of patients with vasculitic neuropathy	36	Systemic—25 Nonsystemic—11	RA (8), PAN (4), microscopic polyangiitis (2), Wegeners (2), hypersensitivity vasculitis (2), SLE (1), other—MGUS, zoster infection, malignancy (6)
Singhal (19)	Retrospective series of patients with vasculitic neuropathy	20	Systemic—13 Nonsystemic—7	PAN (6), SLE (4), Churg-Strauss (2), Wegeners (1)
Collins (3)	Review of biopsy database to identify patients with vasculitis	48	Nonsystemic—48	None
Hattori (12)	Retrospective series	28	Systemic—28	Churg-Strauss (28)
Puechal (20)	Retrospective series	32	Systemic—32	RA (32)

PAN, polyarteritis nodosa; RA, rheumatoid arthritis; SLE, systemic lupus erythematosis; CTD, connective tissue disease; GCA, giant cell arteritis; CLL, chronic lymphoid leukemia, HIV, human immunodeficiency virus; MGUS, monoclonal gammopathy of undetermined significance.

affecting the peripheral nervous system. In 150 of these patients (32%), the vasculitic process was confined to the peripheral nervous system (i.e., nonsystemic).

2.2. Which Are the Most Common Systemic Vasculitides in Which the Peripheral Nervous System is Involved?

Systemic vasculitis occurs most frequently in the context of a connective tissue disorder, but may also arise in association with a variety of other diseases including malignancies, HIV infection, sarcoidosis, and cryoglobulinemia. Of the connective tissue disorders, peripheral nerve vasculitis is most commonly associated with polyarteritis nodosa and rheumatoid arthritis. These two disorders account for more than 70% of cases of peripheral nerve involvement in systemic vasculitis. Other, less common collagen disorders include undifferentiated or mixed connective tissue disease, Churg-Strauss syndrome, Sjogren's, systemic lupus erythematosis (SLE), Wegener's granulomatosis, and scleroderma (summarized in Table 10.1).

2.3. What Is the Pattern of Nerve Involvement in Vasculitis of the Peripheral Nervous System?

A variety of different patterns of peripheral nerve involvement have been described in association with vasculitis. Most neuropathies are sensorimotor, but purely sensory neuropathies have been reported *(1,2)*. As shown in Table 10.2A, mononeuritis multiplex is the most common pattern of peripheral nerve involvement by vasculitis, with distal symmetric sensorimotor polyneuropathy the next most frequent. Other, less common patterns include mononeuropathies, brachial plexopathy, lumbosacral plexopathy, cutaneous sensory neuropathy, and asymmetric polyneuropathy (which represents an overlapping mononeuritis multiplex). Although the data comparing the frequency of these patterns of neuropathy among those with systemic and nonsystemic vasculitis are limited, the available data do not suggest any obvious differences—mononeuritis multiplex remains the most frequently encountered presentation (Table 10.2B).

2.4. Are There Any Clinical Features That Are Particularly Suggestive of Vasculitis as the Cause of a Peripheral Neuropathy?

Apart from the nature of the peripheral neuropathy (e.g., mononeuritis multiplex vs distal symmetric polyneuropathy), the clinical presentation of patients with vasculitic neuropathy has not been reported in substantial detail in most of the published case series. As shown in Table 10.3, the available data permit limited conclusions. The age of onset varies widely, although most patients are over the age of 50. Duration of neuropathic symptoms also varies, with less than 25% of patients reporting symptoms of less than 1 month and the majority reporting symptoms of less than 6 months' duration. In some series, pain has been extremely common *(3)*, and other authors have emphasized that vasculitis may be the cause of apparently idiopathic, predominantly small fiber neuropathy *(1)*. Overall, however, pain is insufficiently frequent to be of diagnostic use. Similarly, the presence or absence of systemic symptoms does not seem to be helpful in predicting whether a neuropathy is likely to be vasculitic in origin.

Because mononeuritis multiplex is the most frequent pattern of peripheral nerve involvement due to vasculitis, this pattern of neuropathy should prompt a nerve biopsy in search of vasculitis. Apart from the pattern of involvement (i.e. mononeuritis multiplex), it is

Table 10.2A
Patterns of Peripheral Nerve Involvement in Vasculitis

Study	Type of neuropathy — number of subjects
Kissel (4)	Mononeuritis multiplex—10
	Distal symmetric sensorimotor polyneuropathy—6
Harati (16)	Mononeuritis multiplex—8
	Distal symmetric sensorimotor polyneuropathy—25
Said (18)	Mononeuritis multiplex—62
	Distal symmetric sensorimotor polyneuropathy—19
	Mononeuropathy—13
Hawke (5)	Mononeuritis multiplex—16
	Distal symmetric sensorimotor polyneuropathy—8
	Asymmetric neuropathy—10
Wees (6)	Mononeuritis multiplex—6[a]
	Distal symmetric sensorimotor polyneuropathy—11[a]
Collins (8)	Asymmetric polyneuropathy (overlapping mononeuritis multiplex)—27
	Mononeuritis multiplex—5
	Lumbosacral plexopathy—3
	Distal symmetric sensorimotor polyneuropathy—1
Singhal (19)	Mononeuritis multiplex—11
	Asymmetric polyneuropathy (overlapping mononeuritis multiplex)—5
	Distal symmetric sensorimotor polyneuropathy—4
Collins (3)[b]	Asymmetric polyneuropathy (overlapping mononeuritis multiplex)—37
	Mononeuritis Multiplex—6
	Lumbosacral plexopathy—4
	Distal symmetric sensorimotor polyneuropathy—1
Seo (2)[c]	Symmetric sensory polyneuropathy—10
	Asymmetric sensory polyneuropathy—3
	Sensory mononeuropathy—3
	Sensory mononeuritis multiplex—1

[a]Authors' classification is somewhat unclear; the results shown here are the best approximation based on the published data.

[b]Fourteen of the patients with nonsystemic vasculitis were reported previously (4,8).

[c]Although all patients in this series presented with purely sensory symptoms and did not develop motor weakness during follow-up, motor abnormalities were present in all patients on nerve conduction studies.

extremely difficult to build a clinical profile that should suggest vasculitis as the cause of the neuropathy. Neither the duration of symptoms nor the presence of systemic symptoms (e.g., fever and weight loss) and pain help to distinguish vasculitic neuropathy from other causes of peripheral neuropathy, although it is expected that systemic symptoms would be more common in systemic rather than nonsystemic vasculitis. One caveat to this conclusion is that there really have been no large scale studies that have formally examined the sensitivity and specificity of various clinical symptoms and signs for the diagnosis of vasculitis.

Table 10.2B
Differences in Peripheral Nerve Involvement in Systemic and Nonsystemic Vasculitis

Study	Systemic vasculitis	Nonsystemic vasculitis
Dyck (7)	–	Mononeuritis multiplex—12
		Asymmetric neuropathy—4
		DSMP—3
		Sensory polyneuropathy—1
Davies (13)	–	Mononeuritis multiplex—11
		DSMP—10
		Asymmetric neuropathy—4
Bouche (17)	–	Mononeuritis multiplex—11
		Mononeuropathy—3
		Distal symmetric sensorimotor polyneuropathy—3
		Brachial plexopathy—3
		Unspecified—3
Moore (15)	Mononeuritis multiplex—8	–
	DSMP—3	
	Cutaneous neuropathy—2	
Hattori (12)	Mononeuritis multiplex—20	–
	Asymmetrical polyneuropathy (overlapping mononeuritis)—8	
Collins (3)	–	Asymmetric polyneuropathy (overlapping mononeuritis multiplex)—37
		Mononeuritis multiplex—6
		Lumbosacral plexopathy—4
		Distal symmetric sensorimotor polyneuropathy—1
Puechal (20)	Mononeuritis multiplex—17	–
	Mononeuropathy—3	
	DSMP—12	

DSMP, distal symmetric sensorimotor polyneuropathy.

2.5. What Are the Most Common Neurophysiological Findings in Patients With Vasculitic Neuropathy?

The results of detailed neurophysiological testing have been reported in only a limited number of studies. Kissel and colleagues, for example, described the results of nerve conduction studies and electromyography (EMG) for most of the patients included in their series of 16 patients (4). These results provide evidence for an axonal process that affects both sensory and motor nerves (Table 10.4A). The most frequent finding was an absent sural response, with upper limb sensory responses absent in a smaller proportion of patients. Peroneal motor responses were absent in almost 50% of patients with median and ulnar motor responses almost invariably present. Considering other published series,

Table 10.3
Clinical Presentation of Vasculitic Neuropathy

Study	Age	Duration of symptoms	Pain	Systemic symptoms	Patient population
Kissel (4)	Median: 65 Range: 21–76	<1 mo: 19% 1–6 mo: 56% >6 mo: 25%	69%	75%	Mixed systemic and nonsystemic
Dyck (7)	Median: 53.5 Range: 23–74	≤ 6 mo: 30% >6 mo: 70%	NR	NR	Nonsystemic
Prayson (21)	Mean: 72.5 Range: 19–94	NR	40%	Fever: 12% Weight loss:21% Skin lesions:5%	Mixed systemic and nonsystemic
Hawke (5)	Mean: 61 Range: 23–79	<1 mo: 24% 1–6 mo: 47% >6 mo: 29%	53%	NR	Mixed systemic and nonsystemic
Martinez (22)	Median: 42.5 Range 17–68	≤ 6 mo: 80% >6 mo: 20%	NR	100%	Polyarteritis nodosa
Collins (8)	Mean: 62.1 Range: 12–86	NR	83%	64%	Mixed systemic and nonsystemic
Hattori (12)	Median: 52 Range: 22–78	<1 mo: 100%	32%	100%	Churg-Strauss
Collins (3)	Median: 66.5 Range: 21–88	Median: 5 mo Range: 2 wk– 8 yr	96%	Weight loss: 35% Fevers: 15%	Nonsystemic
Puechal (20)	Mean: 59 Range: 30–86	NR	NR	Weight loss: 40% Fever: 40%	Rheumatoid arthritis

NR, not reported.

the peroneal nerve is most frequently affected, followed by the tibial and ulnar nerves (Table 10.4B).

In the study by Kissel and colleagues, needle EMG showed neurogenic (reduced) recruitment of motor units in the arms and legs in almost all patients, with proximal and distal muscles equally affected. Fibrillation potentials and positive sharp waves were present in a smaller proportion of patients, also without obvious predilection for distal or proximal muscles (4). In their series of 34 patients with vasculitic neuropathy, Hawke and colleagues found absent motor responses in 25 of 86 nerves studied in the legs and 5 of 47 nerves studied in the arms; sensory responses were absent in 46 of 78 nerves tested (5). Finally, Wees and colleagues demonstrated absent sural sensory responses in 13 of 15 patients who underwent neurophysiological testing (6). Although not described in detail, other investigators have commented that neurophysiological studies were consistent with an axonal process (5,7).

In one study, moderate-to-severe slowing of conduction velocity was noted in only 3 of 52 nerves in which responses were elicited (6%) (4). In another study, marked slowing of motor conduction velocity was found in a single nerve in one patient (5). A number of

Table 10.4A
Neurophysiological Findings in Peripheral Nerve Vasculitis

Sensory nerve conduction studies	
Absent sural response	7/14 (50%)
Absent median response	5/13 (38%)
Absent ulnar response	4/9 (44%)
Motor nerve conduction studies	
Absent peroneal response	8/17 (47%)
Absent median response	1/13 (8%)
Absent ulnar response	1/12 (8%)
Neurogenic recruitment of motor units	
Distal leg	12/12 (100%)
Proximal leg	10/12 (83%)
Distal arm	11/12 (92%)
Proximal arm	11/12 (92%)
Fibrillations/positive sharp waves	
Distal leg	8/12 (67%)
Proximal leg	5/12 (42%)
Distal arm	7/12 (58%)
Proximal arm	6/12 (50%)

Data from ref. *4*.

Table 10.4B
Motor Nerve Involvement in Vasculitic Neuropathy

	Frequency of involvement (percentage)	
Nerve	*Collins* (3)	*Other series (combined)* (4–6)
Peroneal	90	91
Tibial	81	42
Ulnar	65	41
Femoral	63	7
Superior gluteal	52	–
Median	48	29
Radial	44	18
Musculucutaneous	40	–
Axillary	40	–

Percentages represent the proportion of patients with a particular nerve affected.

reports have drawn attention to the occasional finding of conduction block *(5,7–10)* in patients with vasculitic neuropathy, but these clearly represent the minority of patients.

The overall impression, therefore, is that the most common electrophysiological findings in patients with vasculitic neuropathy are absent sensory and motor responses and the presence of fibrillations/positive sharp waves and neurogenic recruitment of motor unit potentials distally and proximally in both the arms and legs. Conduction block may occasionally be demonstrated, but this is usually a transient finding.

2.6. How Useful Are Serological Markers of Inflammation and Collagen-Vascular Disorders for the Diagnosis of Vasculitic Neuropathy?

The results of laboratory studies have been reported in a patchy fashion throughout the literature for both systemic and nonsystemic vasculitis. The available data come from retrospective case series in which the proportion of patients with vasculitis who show positive test results are reported. Such data provide an estimate of the sensitivity of these tests, but do not inform on their specificity. The available data, summarized in Table 10.5, permit a few general conclusions. Serological markers tend to be abnormal more frequently among patients with systemic compared with nonsystemic vasculitis. The frequency with which abnormal serological markers are detected varies widely. Elevation of erythrocyte sedimentation rate (ESR) above 50 mm/hour, for example, was reported in 77% of patients with systemic vasculitis in one study *(8)* but in no patients in another study *(4)*. In general the sensitivity of these tests (elevated ESR, raised anti-nuclear antibody [ANA] titer, positive rheumatoid factor [RF], anemia, leukocytosis, decreased serum complement, and the presence of anti-hepatitis-B surface-antigen antibodies) is relatively low. Specificity is likely also to be low because there is no reason to suspect that these tests would be abnormal selectively in patients with vasculitis of the peripheral nervous system but not in patients with vasculitis not affecting the peripheral nerves or among patients with other systemic inflammatory disorders. One caveat is that the specificity may be adequate in the appropriate clinical context. For example, in a patient with mononeuritis multiplex of uncertain etiology, an elevated ESR and ANA might be interpreted as providing supportive evidence for an underlying collagen-vascular disorder.

2.7. How Useful Is Nerve and Muscle Biopsy for the Diagnosis of Peripheral Nerve Vasculitis?

There are a limited number of studies that have been adequately designed to evaluate the accuracy of nerve and muscle biopsy for the diagnosis of vasculitis. In each of the retrospective series discussed in this chapter thus far, patients have been selected on the basis of abnormal neuropathological findings. The implication is that they provide no information about the diagnostic accuracy of biopsy.

In one of the few studies that evaluated the diagnostic utility of sural nerve biopsy for the diagnosis of vasculitis, Rappaport and colleagues retrospectively reviewed their experience with sural nerve biopsy in patients with suspected peripheral neuropathy *(11)*. Their cohort of 60 patients included 29 in whom the diagnosis of vasculitis was suspected clinically. Sural nerve biopsy confirmed the diagnosis in only 6 (20%). This study suffered from a number of methodological limitations including the relatively small number of patients who had nerve conduction studies performed prior to biopsy (22% of patients) and the inclusion of patients with clinical diagnoses of myasthenia gravis, multiple sclerosis, and myopathy, suggesting that the inclusion criteria were somewhat lax. Furthermore, no clear gold standard for the diagnosis of vasculitic neuropathy was specified, making it difficult to know whether vasculitis was the correct diagnosis in the remaining 23 patients in whom this diagnosis was suspected but whose biopsies were nondiagnostic. These limitations should lead to caution in placing too much emphasis on the low diagnostic sensitivity of nerve biopsy in this study.

The retrospective case series of Collins and colleagues is of a substantially better quality *(8)*. These investigators evaluated all patients with suspected peripheral nerve

Table 10.5
Laboratory Studies in Patients With Peripheral Nerve Vasculitis

Study	↑ ESR	ANA	RF	Anemia	Leukocytosis	↓ Complement	Hep B-S-Ag
Collins (8)	77/27/61[a]	33/10/27	55/13/42	64/45/58	61/27/50	21/0/15	NR
Wees (6)[d]	82/-/82[b]	NR	53/-/53	53/-/53	35/-/35	50/-/50	20/-/20
Bouche (17)[f]	23/-/23	NR	18/-/18	NR	64/-/64	NR	33/-/33
Dyck (7)[f]	-/15/15[a] -/30/30[c]	-/36/36	-/33/33	-/0/0	-/0/0	NR	NR
Hawke (5)[e]	78/-/78[c]	NR	NR	25/-/25	NR	NR	33/-/33
Kissel (4)	0/0/0[a]	33/0/19	44/0/25	NR	NR	NR	NR
Chang (14)[d]	NR	NR	63/-/63	NR	NR	32/-/32	NR
Singhal (19)	-/-/90	-/-/70	-/-/46	NR	NR	NR	NR
Hattori (12)	42/-/42[a]	0/-/0	86/-/86	NR	90/-/90	NR	0/-/0
Collins (3)[f]	-/25/25[a]	-/39/39	-/20/20	-/31/31	-/23/23	-/11/11	NR
Puechal (20)	NR	27/-/27	97/-/97	NR	NR	62/-/62	0/-/0

Values are percent of abnormal results expressed as proportion of subjects in whom the test was performed. Not all tests were performed on every patient in any particular study.

Three values are presented in each column, representing the sensitivity of the individual test for patients with systemic vasculitis/nonsystemic vasculitis/the entire cohort. If the first or second number is the same as the third, this indicates that all of the patients in the study had either systemic (first and third numbers the same) or nonsystemic (second and third numbers the same) vasculitis.

NR, not reported; ESR, erythrocyte sedimentation rate; ANA, anti-nuclear antigen; RF, rheumatoid factor; Hep B-S-Ag, Hepatitis B surface antigen.

[a]Defined as ESR >50 mm/h.
[b]Definition of increased ESR not specified.
[c]Defined as ESR >30 mm/h.
[d]All patients with systemic vasculitis.
[e]All but two patients with systemic vasculitis.
[f]All patients with nonsystemic vasculitis.

vasculitis who had undergone biopsy of the superficial peroneal nerve and peroneus brevis muscle (SPN/PBM). In order to evaluate the diagnostic performance of biopsy, it was necessary to establish alternate criteria that might serve as the gold standard for the diagnosis. These investigators used a combination of clinical, laboratory, and pathological features to construct such criteria. Incorporation bias was not eliminated completely in that pathological evidence of definite or probable vasculitis was still taken as evidence for vasculitis (thus potentially inflating the sensitivity of the test). They included 70 patients with suspected vasculitis who underwent biopsy, of which 36 were subsequently diagnosed with vasculitis and 34 with diagnoses other than vasculitis. Biopsy showed evidence of definite/probable vasculitis in 22 patients, yielding a sensitivity of 61%. Parenthetically, the sensitivity was similar for patients with systemic (60%) and nonsystemic (64%) vasculitis. Specificity of 100% is implied although not directly stated. If biopsies with features that were suspicious for vasculitis were regarded as indicating vasculitis, then the sensitivity increased to 86%, but at the expense of specificity falling to 85%.

Muscle biopsy did not provide additional diagnostic accuracy in patients with nonsystemic vasculitis because pathological abnormalities in nerve indicating definite or probable vasculitis were present in all seven of these patients (100%). For patients with systemic vasculitis in whom nerve biopsy was normal, muscle biopsy permitted the diagnosis of vasculitis in two additional patients, thus increasing sensitivity from 60% to 68%. These findings suggest that muscle biopsy cannot replace nerve biopsy, but that the combination of nerve and muscle biopsy improves diagnostic accuracy.

In a retrospective cohort study, Collins and colleagues reviewed their experience with nerve (with or without muscle) biopsy in patients with nonsystemic vasculitis *(3)*. Of the 48 patients with nonsystemic vasculitis in this study, 11 had been included in a prior publication by the same group *(8)*. They again used as the gold standard for the diagnosis of vasculitis a combination of clinical, laboratory, and pathological features. The sensitivities of sural nerve and SPN/PBM biopsies for definite vasculitis were 47% and 58%, respectively (not significantly different, $p = 0.56$). If pathological features indicating probably (rather then definite) vasculitis were used, sensitivities increase to 80% and 74%, respectively.

The overall impression, therefore, is that nerve biopsy has a relatively high sensitivity for the diagnosis of vasculitis. Sensitivities are similar for sural and superficial peroneal nerve biopsies and may be increased slightly by performing a muscle biopsy as well.

3. TREATMENT

3.1. What Is the Evidence for the Efficacy of Corticosteroids and Cyclophosphamide in Patients With Vasculitic Peripheral Neuropathy?

There are no randomized controlled trials that have evaluated any therapeutic strategy for patients with vasculitis, systemic or nonsystemic. All of the available data are derived from retrospective cohort studies, with the quality of the treatment data reported in these series varying considerably.

In their series of 48 patients with nonsystemic vasculitis, Collins and colleagues *(3)* treated 28 patients with steroids alone and 20 patients received corticosteroids together with adjunctive immunosuppressive therapy (cyclophosphamide in 18 and IVIg in 2).

The dose of steroids used was not uniform throughout the study. The most common regimen comprised 100 mg prednisone per day for 1–2 weeks, followed by 100 mg/day every other day with a median duration of treatment being 12.5 months (range 2–45 months). Cyclophosphamide was typically administered orally at a dose of 100–150 mg/day with the median duration of therapy being 5 months (range 1–30 months). Patients in each treatment group were comparable with respect to relevant baseline parameters (age, duration of symptoms, disability score, and so on). The presence or absence of long-term response was used as the primary outcome measure, with long-term response defined as present if at least one variable (pain, sensory loss, objective weakness, composite Medical Research Council [MRC] score, or disability score) improved for ≥ 6 months, or absent if any variable worsened or all variables remained unchanged. Long-term response was observed in 17/28 (61%) patients treated initially with steroids alone and 19/20 (95%) patients treated with steroids and adjunctive immunosuppresion (cyclophosphamide in all but two cases). The relapse rate was higher among those treated with steroids alone (59%) compared with those receiving combination therapy (29%). A significant proportion of those who failed to response to steroids alone or who relapsed following initial therapy with steroids alone were subsequently treated with the combination of steroids and cyclophosphamide. Of the 25 patients who were treated with this combination at any stage during the illness, a long-term response was observed in 23 (92%). Seven of these 23 responders relapsed; four of five who were then treated with steroids responded and both of those re-treated with combination steroids and cyclophosphamide achieved a long-term response *(3)*. These data suggest (but do not prove) that combination therapy with steroids and cyclophosphamide for a median duration of 5 months offers an excellent chance of clinical improvement for patients with nonsystemic vasculitis.

Hattori and colleagues reported their experience with 28 Churg-Strauss syndrome patients with vasculitic neuropathy *(12)*. All patients were initially treated with corticosteroids, usually at a dose of 1 mg/kg/day for 1 month. A therapeutic response was defined as an improvement on the modified Rankin Scale (mRS) score of at least one point after 4 weeks of treatment. Such a response was observed in 12 patients (43%). Long-term outcome was regarded as favorable for those with mRS scores ≤2 at final follow-up, with 15 of 28 patients (54%) reaching this endpoint. Only two of the patients who initially responded relapsed. Both were treated with oral cyclophosphamide with "apparent improvement in neurological symptoms" in both *(12)*.

4. PROGNOSIS

4.1. What Is the Long-Term Prognosis for Patients With Nonsystemic Vasculitis?

Three studies, including a total of 98 patients, reported outcome of patients with nonsystemic vasculitis, most of whom were treated with some form of immunosuppressive therapy (Table 10.6A) *(3,7,13)*. The mortality rate from complications associated with active vasculitis ranged from 4% to 15%. Among the survivors, most patients (67–87%) are left with some disability, but are able to ambulate independently. A significant minority of patients (9–24%) requires assistance with ambulation and the small minority either achieves full remission or is severely disabled and unable to ambulate even with

Table 10.6A
Prognosis for Nonsystemic Vasculitis

Study	Follow-up duration	Final disability (among survivors)				Relapse rate	Mortality
		Asymptomatic	Ambulation without assistance	Requires assistance for ambulation	Nonambulatory		
Dyck (7)	Median: 11.5 yr Range: 1–35 yr	Not reported	12/17 (70.5%)	4/17 (23.5%)	1/17 (6%)	–	3/20 (15%)
Davies (13)	Median: 14.7 yr Range: 1–36 yr	Not reported	20/23 (87%)	2/23 (9%)	1/23 (4%)	32%	1/25 (4%)
Collins (3)	Median: 6.3 yr Range: 0.5–22 yr	5/40 (12.5%)	27/40 (67.5%)	7/40 (17.5%)	1/140 (2.5%)	46%	5/48 (10%)

Table 10.6B
Prognosis for Systemic Vasculitis

Study	Follow-up duration	Final disability (among survivors)				Relapse rate	Mortality
		Asymptomatic	Ambulation without assistance	Requires assistance for ambulation	Nonambulatory		
Moore (15)	8 mo	4/11 (36%)	7/13 (64%)[a]	–	–	–	2/13 (15%)
Chang (14)	Mean: 4.3 yr Range: 0.3–10 yr	4/14 (29%)	7/14 (50%)	–	–	36%	5/19 (26%)
Hawke (5)[c]	Mean: 3 yr Range: 0.1–8 yr	9/18 (50%)	5/18 (28%)[b]	3/18 (17%)	1/18 (6%)	0	6/34 (18%)
Puechal (20)	Mean: 7.2 yr Range: 1–22 yr	17/18 (94%)	–	–	–	25%	14/32 (44%)

Percentages do not always total 100% because patients lost to follow-up and those who died from unrelated diseases are excluded.
[a]Objective signs of weakness and/or sensory deficits that interfere with routine functioning.
[b]Moderate disability, but able to ambulate independently.
[c]All but 2 of the 34 patients in this series had systemic vasculitis, but prognosis was not reported separately for systemic and nonsystemic vasculitis.

assistance. Nonsystemic vasculitis, therefore, is not a benign disease even when treated with aggressive immunosuppressive therapy. The mortality rate is not insignificant and the majority of patients have residual functional deficits.

4.2. What Is the Long-Term Prognosis for Patients With Systemic Vasculitis?

The long term prognosis of 56 patients with systemic vasculitis can be gleaned from four retrospective studies (Table 10.6B) *(5,14,15)*. The vast majority of these patients were aggressively treated with some form of immunosuppressive therapy. The mortality rate was slightly higher than that reported for nonsystemic vasculits, ranging from 15 to 26%. Of the survivors, a relatively small proportion requires assistance with ambulation (17%) or become nonambulatory (6%). A significant proportion has residual functional deficits while retaining the ability to ambulate independently (28–64%), with the remainder recovering completely (29–50%). Like nonsystemic vasculitis, systemic vasculitis is not a benign disease. The mortality rate is not insignificant and the majority of patients have residual functional deficits.

4.3. Are There Any Prognostic Factors That Predict Outcome in Patients With Vasculitis?

There has been very little investigation into the question of whether any parameters present at the time of initial presentation might be predictive of the long-term prognosis. In one retrospective cohort study, the investigators examined a number of clinical and laboratory parameters including age, gender, duration of disease, MRC composite muscle strength score, disability score, ESR, the presence of leukocytosis, anemia, elevated ANA, and a positive rheumatoid factor. None of these were found to have any prognostic value *(3)*. In another study, investigators considered the type of neuropathy, age, gender, and the duration of symptoms and found that only age held some prognostic value, but further details are not given *(5)*. Therefore, based on the available published literature to date, there is no reliable evidence to indicate whether any clinical features or laboratory findings are predictive of response to therapy or ultimate disability.

5. SUMMARY

- Vasculitis of the peripheral nervous system may occur in isolation (nonsystemic vasculitis) or in conjunction with a systemic disorder (systemic vasculitis); the latter accounts for about 70% of cases of peripheral nerve vasculitis.
- Rheumatoid arthritis and polyarteritis nodosa are the two most common causes of systemic vasculitis.
- Mononeuritis multiplex is the most common pattern of peripheral nerve involvement in vasculitis of the peripheral nerve system, both systemic and nonsystemic, although other patterns including a distal symmetric sensorimotor polyneuropathy and an asymmetric polyneuropathy (overlapping mononeuritis multiplex) also occur with reasonably high frequency.
- Other than the pattern of mononeuritis multiple, there is no typical profile or clinical presentation that should suggest vasculitis as a cause of peripheral neuropathy.
- The peroneal nerve is most commonly affected in vasculitc mononeuritis multiplex, occurring in approximately 90% of patients.

- The neurophysiology of vasculitic neuropathy is usually that of an axonal process, although conduction block may occasionally be encountered.
- Serological markers tend to be abnormal more frequently among patients with systemic compared with nonsystemic vasculitis.
- In general, both the sensitivity and specificity of tests like the ESR, ANA, and rheumatoid factor are relatively low.
- Nerve biopsy has a relatively high sensitivity for the diagnosis of vasculitis, with similar diagnostic accuracy obtained with sural and superficial peroneal nerve biopsies; sensitivity may be increased slightly by performing a muscle biopsy as well.
- There are no randomized controlled trials of the treatment of vasculitic neuropathy.
- Data from a single retrospective series suggest that outcome is more favorable among patients treated with both cyclophosphamide and high-dose steroids (95%) compared with those treated with steroids alone (61%), and that the rate of relapse is also lower (29%) for combination therapy compared with steroids alone (59%).
- Prognosis is similar for patients with systemic and nonsystemic vasculitis. Neither is a benign disease, with each having a median mortality rate of 15% (range 4–44%) and a majority of patients being left with residual functional deficits.

REFERENCES

1. Kelkar P, McDermott WR, Parry GJ. Sensory-predominant, painful, idiopathic neuropathy: inflammatory changes in sural nerves. Muscle Nerve 2002;26:413–416.
2. Seo J, Ryan H, Claussen G, Thomas T, Oh S. Sensory neuropathy in vasculitis. A clinical, pathologic and electrophysiologic study. Neurology 2004;63:874–878.
3. Collins M, Periquet M, Mendell J, Sahenk Z, Nagaraja H, Kissel J. Nonsystemic vasculitic neuropathy. Insights from a clinical cohort. Neurology 2003;61:623–630.
4. Kissel JT, Slivka AP, Warmolts JR, Mendell JR. The clinical spectrum of necrotizing angiopathy of the peripheral nervous system. Ann Neurol 1985;18:251–257.
5. Hawke S, Davies L, Pamphlett R, Guo Y, Pollard J, McLeod J. Vasculitic Neuropathy. A clinical and pathological study. Brain 1991;114:2175–2190.
6. Wees SJ, Sunwoo IN, Oh SJ. Sural nerve biopsy in systemic necrotizing vasculitis. Am J Med 1981;71:525–532.
7. Dyck PJ, Benstead TJ, Conn DL, Stevens JC, Windebank AJ, Low PA. Nonsystemic vasculitic neuropathy. Brain 1987;110:843–854.
8. Collins M, Mendell J, Periquet M, et al. Superficial peroneal nerve/peroneus brevis muscle biopsy in vasculitic neuropathy. Neurology 2000;55:636–643.
9. Jamieson PW, Giuliani MJ, Martinez AJ. Necrotizing angiopathy presenting with multifocal conduction blocks. Neurology 1991;41:442–444.
10. McCluskey L, Feinberg D, Cantor C, Bird S. "Pseudo-conduction block" in vasculitic neuropathy. Muscle Nerve 1999;22:1361–1366.
11. Rappaport WD, Valente J, Hunter GC, et al. Clinical utilization and complications of sural nerve biopsy. Am J Surg 1993;166:252–256.
12. Hattori N, Ichimura M, Nagamatsu M, et al. Clinicopathological features of Churg-Strauss syndrome-associated neuropathy. Brain 1999;122:427–439.
13. Davies L, Spies J, Pollard J, McLeod J. Vasculitis confined to peripheral nerves. Brain 1996;119:1441–1448.
14. Chang RW, Bell CL, Hallett M. Clinical characteristics and prognosis of vasculitic mononeuropathy multiplex. Arch Neurol 1984;41:618–621.
15. Moore PM, Fauci AS. Neurologic manifestatinos of systemic vasculitis. A retrospective and prospective study of the clinicopathologic features and responses to therapy in 25 patients. Am J Med 1981;71:517–524.

16. Harati Y, Niakan E. The clinical spectrum of inflammatory-angiopathic neuropathy. J Neurol Neurosurg Psychiatry 1986;49:1313–1316.

17. Bouche P, Leger J, Travers M, Cathala H, Castaigne P. Peripheral neuropathy in systemic vasculitis: clinical and electrophysiologic study of 22 patients. Neurology 1986;36:1598–1602.

18. Said G, Lacroix-Ciaudo C, Fujimura H, Blas C, Faux N. The peripheral neuropathy of necrotizing arteritis: A clinicopathological study. Ann Neurol 1988;23:461–465.

19. Singhal B, Khadilkar S, Gursahani R, Surya N. Vasculitic neuropathy: profile of twenty patients. J Assoc Physicians India 1995;43:459–461.

20. Puechal X, Said G, Hilliquin P, et al. Peripheral neuropathy with necrotizing vasculitis in rheumatoid arthritis. A clinicopathologic and prognostic study of thirty-two patients. Arthritis and Rheumatism 1995;38:1618–1629.

21. Prayson RA, Sedlock DJ. Cliniopathologic study of 43 patients with sural nerve vasculitis. Human Pathology 2003;34:484–490.

22. Cruz Martinez A, Barbado FJ, Ferrer MT, Vazquez JJ, Perez Conde MC, Gil Aquado A. Electrophysiological study in systemic necrotizing vasculitis of the polyarteritis nodosa group. Electromyogr Clin Neurophysiol 1988;28:167–173.

11   Guillain-Barré Syndrome

1. INTRODUCTION

The Guillain-Barré Syndrome (GBS) is the most common cause of acute neuromuscular paralysis in developed countries, affecting 1–2 people per 100,000 annually. The mortality is about 10%, and approximately 20% of patients are left with significant motor disability. Our understanding of GBS has evolved since Landry's description of the clinical features of "acute ascending paralysis" in the late 1800s and Guillain and Barré's recognition of the albuminocytological dissociation in the cerebrospinal fluid in the early 1900s. It is classically regarded an acute demyelinating polyradiculoneuropathy, characterized clinically by the acute onset of symmetric weakness and arreflexia with relatively minor sensory impairment. Cerebrospinal fluid (CSF) analysis characteristically yields an elevated protein concentration but little or no pleocytosis, and the electrophysiology reveals evidence of demyelination. Over the years, however, unusual variants of this syndrome have been recognized, including an axonal form. Plasmapheresis and intravenous immunoglobulin (IVIg) have become the mainstay of therapy and steroids are thought not to be beneficial.

What is the diagnostic accuracy of particular clinical symptoms and signs for the diagnosis of GBS? What is the diagnostic utility of the albuminocytological dissociation? What are the electrodiagnostic features that characterize GBS and how accurate are the diagnostic criteria that have been proposed? What is the evidence that plasmapheresis and IVIg are beneficial to patients with GBS and what is the nature of this benefit? Do these forms of treatment affect the ultimate degree of disability or do they simply hasten recovery? Are there any clinical or electrophysiological parameters that may be used to predict prognosis? These and other questions are the subject of this chapter.

2. DIAGNOSIS

2.1. What Are the Clinical Features of GBS?

There are relatively few large studies that have collected and clearly reported the clinical features of patients with GBS. Even among the available studies, the data are frequently presented in such a way that any effort to synthesize and summarize the findings of these various studies is difficult. One study, for example, might report the frequency of particular symptoms or signs at the time of hospital admission, whereas another might describe the initial symptoms and signs and yet another might report the clinical features at the time of maximum severity of the illness. Furthermore, efforts to determine the diagnostic accuracy of various clinical symptoms and signs are hindered by the lack of any studies that have included patients who were thought to have GBS, but

From: *Neuromuscular Disease: Evidence and Analysis in Clinical Neurology*
By: M. Benatar © Humana Press Inc., Totowa, NJ

were subsequently found to have an alternative diagnosis. This precludes estimation of the specificity of any clinical feature. Finally, any discussion of the diagnostic accuracy (i.e., sensitivity and specificity) of symptoms and signs is hindered by the use of clinical criteria as the gold standard for the diagnosis of GBS, leaving such a study susceptible to incorporation bias.

In view of these difficulties, the best approach seems to be to simply describe the results of the few studies that have examined large number of patients with GBS and which reported the frequency with which various symptoms and signs were present (1–3).

In 1973, Masucci and Kurtzke described their experience with 50 consecutive male patients seen at one Veterans Administration hospital (1). Muscle weakness was the initial symptom in 36 patients, occurring alone in 16 patients and together with sensory symptoms in 20 patients. Isolated sensory symptoms were the initial symptom in 14 patients, 8 of whom complained only of paresthesia with the other 6 reporting only pain (1) (Table 11.1). Ropper and colleagues reported similar results in their retrospective series from the Masscahusetts General Hospital (MGH) published in 1991 (2) (Table 11.1). In each of these series, the symptoms most commonly progressed in an "ascending" pattern, with spread from the lower limbs to the upper limbs and cranial nerves (38–54%). In a smaller minority of patients, the progression was "descending," with spread from the cranial nerves or upper limbs to the lower limbs (6–14%). In the remaining patients, there was no spatial progression of symptoms over time.

The patterns of weakness at initial presentation and at the time of maximal severity of symptoms are summarized in Table 11.2. There are conflicting data regarding whether weakness is predominantly proximal or distal, but most studies agree that weakness is most frequently more severe in the legs than in the arms and that isolated weakness in the arms is extremely unusual (if it ever occurs). Ropper and colleagues note that although weakness is typically said to be symmetric, some degree of asymmetry is usually present. They do not, however, estimate the frequency with which this occurs, but do report that only two patients had monoplegia affecting an arm at the time of symptom onset (2). A single patient in the series by Masucci and Kurtzke had isolated weakness in one leg (1).

Most studies seem to agree that the facial nerve is the most commonly affected cranial nerve, with facial weakness usually bilateral (even if somewhat asymmetric) (1–3) (Table 11.3). The extent to which cranial nerve involvement has been reported in these series is quite variable. Although these studies do indicate that the extra-ocular muscles, tongue, and pharyngeal muscles may also be affected, it is difficult to reliably estimate the frequency of these findings (Table 11.3).

Sensory symptoms are present in the majority of patients (58%–72%), and pain is also a frequent complaint (32%–71%) (1–3). The details of the findings on sensory examination are not well described in most studies, although one study indicates that the sensory loss usually affects multiple modalities with a distal predominance (1). The relevant studies are summarized in Table 11.4.

Changes in deep tendon reflexes are summarized in Table 11.5. These data vary somewhat but seem to suggest that the majority of patients are areflexic at the time of initial presentation and the most patients loose all deep tendon reflexes during the course of the disease. Of note, however, is that a significant minority of patients retain at least some deep tendon reflexes (1–3).

Table 11.1
Initial Symptoms in the Guillain-Barré Syndrome

	Masucci (n = 50)	Ropper (n = 169)
Weakness	36 (72%)	108 (64%)
Weakness alone	16 (32%)	20 (12%)
Weakness with paresthesia	13 (26%)	44 (26%)
Weakness with pain	3 (6%)	24 (14%)
Weakness with paresthesia & pain	4 (8%)	20 (12%)
Sensory symptoms alone	14 (28%)	Not reported
Pain alone	6 (12%)	Not reported
Paresthesia alone	8 (16%)	Not reported

Data from refs. 1,2.

Table 11.2
Pattern of Weakness in the Guillain-Barré Syndrome

	Ropper (n = 169)[a]	Winer (n = 100)[b]	Masucci (n = 50)[a]
Legs > arms	91 (54%)	–	–
Legs alone	–	–	11 (22%)
Arms > legs	24 (14%)	"Occasionally"	–
Arms alone	–	0	0
Legs = arms	54 (32%)	–	–
Proximal > distal	98 (58%)	49 (49%)	9 (18%)
Distal > proximal	44 (26%)	27 (27%)	11 (22%)
Proximal = distal	27 (16%)	–	30 (60%)

[a]Pattern at the time of maximal weakness.
[b]Pattern at the time of initial examination.
Data from refs. 1–3.

Table 11.3
Cranial Nerve Involvement in the Guillain-Barré Syndrome

	Ropper (n = 169)	Winer (n = 100)	Masucci (n = 50)
Ptosis	14 (8%)	–	1 (2%)
Extra-ocular muscle weakness/diplopia	21 (13%)	13 (13%)	1 (2%)
Facial weakness	> 60%[a]	53 (53%)	13 (26%)[b]
Pharyngeal weakness	–	–	8 (16%)

[a]Markedly asymmetric (but not unilateral) in 12%.
[b]Bilateral in nine patients and unilateral in four patients.
Data from refs. 1–3.

2.2. What Are the Typical CSF Findings in Patients With GBS?

A major difficulty in interpreting the literature with regard to the typical CSF findings in patients with GBS is the varying time interval from symptom onset to the time of lumbar puncture. The results of the available studies are summarized in Table 11.6.

Table 11.4
Sensory Symptoms and Signs in the Guillain-Barré Syndrome[a]

	Masucci (n = 50)	Winer (n = 100)	Ropper (n = 169)
Symptoms			
Paresthesias	29 (58%)	75 (75%)	122 (72%)
Pain	16 (32%)	50 (50%)	120 (71%)
Signs			
↓ pain sensation	25 (50%)	22 (22%)	–
↓ proprioception	23 (46%)	52 (52%)	–
↓ vibration sense	25 (50%)	59 (59%)	–
↓ temperature	17 (34%)	–	–
None	11 (22%)	–	–
Pattern			
Distal	36 (78%)[b]	–	–

[a]Numbers (percentages) are cumulative over the course of the illness.
[b]Result expressed as the percent of 46 patients with sensory symptoms.
Data from refs. 1–3.

Table 11.5
Reflex Changes in Patients With the Guillain-Barré Syndrome

	Ropper (n = 168)[a]	Masucci (n = 50)[b]	Winer (n = 100)[b]
Areflexia (4 limbs)	109 (65%)	29 (58%)	83 (83%)
Hyporeflexia (4 limbs)	–	5 (10%)	–
Absent ankle reflexes	151 (90%)	–	–
Absent knee reflexes	134 (80%)	–	–

[a]At the time of initial presentation.
[b]At some stage during the course of the illness or at the time of maximal impairment.
Data from refs. 1–3.

Table 11.6
Cerebrospinal Fluid Findings in Patients With Guillain-Barré Syndrome

	Masucci (n = 50)	Winer (n = 100)	Ropper Retrospective (n= 164)	Ropper Prospective (n = 111)
↑ Cerebrospinal fluid protein	40 (80%)	80 (80%)	155 (91%)	81 (73%)
Pleocytosis	3 (6%)	11 (11%)	39 (24%)	16 (14%)

Data from refs. 1–3.

In their series of 50 patients Masucci and Kurtzke did not specify the latency from symptom onset to the time of CSF analysis. They found CSF protein to be normal in 10 (20%) of patients and made note of the fact that the CSF protein remained normal in three patients at the nadir of their illness (1). They obtained serial CSF samples from 36 patients and could discern no particular pattern because CSF protein concentration either increased or decreased over time in some patients and fluctuated widely in the others *(1)*. Overall, they found no correlation between the severity of symptoms and the degree of elevation of CSF protein *(1)*. No CSF specimen contained more than eight cells *(1)*. Winer and colleagues similarly did not present their CSF data based on latency from symptom onset in reporting an elevated CSF protein concentration in 80% of patients, but they did observe that CSF protein was more commonly elevated when the sample was collected after the first week of the illness *(3)*. Pleocytosis (cell count exceeding 5/μL) was noted in 11 patients with a median cell count of 8 (range 6 to 103/μL) *(3)*. Ropper and colleagues reported the results of both their retrospective and prospective series of patients at the MGH *(2)*. The proportion of patients with normal CSF protein declined from 34% in the first week to 18% in the second week of the illness. They also observed a CSF pleocytosis in a larger proportion of patients, in part because of their stricter definition of what constituted a pleocytosis (greater than 4 cells/mm^3) *(2)*. Significant pleocytosis (cell count greater than 30 cells/mm^3) was present in only 1–2% of patients *(2)*.

The overall impression from these data is that the majority of (but not all) patients with GBS show an increased CSF protein concentration, and that this finding becomes more likely (but not inevitable) as the disease progresses. The frequency of a pleocytosis was somewhat variable, ranging from 6 to 24%, and was very rarely greater than 30 cells/mm^3.

2.3. What Are the Earliest Electrodiagnostic Findings in Patients With GBS?

This question has been the subject of a number of studies, but for the most part, study design has been poor and reporting of results unclear. The study by Gordon and Wilbourn is the exception *(4)*. These investigators retrospectively reviewed the medical records of all patients with GBS who underwent electrodiagnostic studies within the first 7 days of the onset of motor symptoms, with the intention of determining the most common early electrical findings *(4)*. One problem with this study was that the gold standard employed for determining that GBS was the correct diagnosis included a combination of clinical, laboratory, and electrophysiological data, thus leaving the study susceptible to the problem of incorporation bias. They included 31 patients (ranging in age from 4 to 76 years), all of whom had motor weakness and 29 of whom (94%) had loss of deep tendon reflexes. The results are summarized in Table 11.7. Abnormalities of the H-reflex were the most frequent finding, being absent in 97% of patients and being the only electrodiagnostic abnormality in five (16%) patients *(4)*. F-wave abnormalities were also frequently encountered, but in no patients did the F-wave latency exceed 150% of the upper limit of normal, a finding that would clearly indicate the presence of demyelination. Sural sparing (absent upper extremity sensory nerve action potential responses in the face of normal sural responses) was present in nine (29%) patients *(4)*. Findings on motor nerve conduction studies indicated demyelinating physiology (distal latency prolonged by more than 150% or conduction velocity slowed by more than 70%) in the minority of patients (42% and 16%, respectively).

2.4. What Is the Diagnostic Accuracy of Electrodiagnostic Studies in GBS?

Although there have been a number of studies reporting the electrophysiological findings in patients with GBS, relatively few provide useful information about the sensitivity of electrodiagnostic tests and even fewer about their specificity.

Table 11.7
Early Electrodiagnostic Findings in the Guillain-Barré Syndrome

Electrodiagnostic parameter	Any abnormality	Abnormality indicating demyelinating physiology
H-reflexes	Absent in 30 (97%)	–
F-waves	Absent/prolonged latency in 26 (84%)	In no patients was F-wave latency >150% of ULN
SNAP amplitude	Abnormal in the upper extremity in 19 (61%) Abnormal sural response in 7 (16%)	–
CMAP amplitude	Reduced in 22 (71%)	–
Distal latency	Prolonged in 20 (65%)	Prolonged >150% ULN in 13 (42%)
Conduction velocity	Slowed in 16 (52%)	Slowed to <70% LLN in 5 (16%)
Conduction block[a]	–	Present in 4 (13%)
Temporal dispersion[a]	–	Present in 18 (58%)

ULN, upper limit of normal; LLN, lower limit of normal; SNAP, sensory nerve action potential; CMAP, compound muscle action potential.

[a]The criteria used for conduction block and temporal dispersion are not clearly defined.
Data from ref. 4.

Ropper and colleagues, for example, reported their experience with 113 patients with GBS who were evaluated prospectively (5). In all patients, the diagnosis was based on the clinical criteria of progressive limb weakness, distal limb paresthesiae, and absent tendon reflexes. Most of these patients (n = 103) underwent electrodiagnostic testing within the first 3 weeks of the illness. One difficulty with this study relates to the criteria used to identify electrodiagnostic abnormalities as being indicative of demyelination. For example, a distal nerve lesion was defined by the presence of a greater than 15% increase in the duration of the distal compound muscle action potential (CMAP) or a prolongation of the distal latency (without specifying the degree of distal latency prolongation that was required). Similarly, distal conduction block was defined on the basis of specific response amplitudes, seemingly ignoring the possibility that reduced response amplitudes might represent axonal loss. Finally, proximal conduction block was defined by absent F-responses or reduced F-response persistence (5). Given these limitations, it is difficult to know how to interpret their report of finding both proximal conduction block and distal lesions in 27% of patients, isolated proximal conduction block in a further 27%, and both distal and proximal conduction blocks in 10% of patients. Only their finding of generalized slowing (more than 80% below the lower limit of normal) in 22% of patients is readily interpretable. This study, therefore, really does not provide much useful information about the sensitivity of electrodiagnostic abnormalities for the diagnosis of GBS.

Albers et al. retrospectively reported their experience of 70 patients with GBS who underwent sequential electrodiagnostic studies (6). In all patients, the diagnosis was based on clinical criteria that required the presence of weakness in multiple limbs as well as areflexia. All patients had CSF analysis, and those with a pleocytosis exceeding 40 cells/mm^3 were excluded, as were those with coexisting medical problems that might be associated with peripheral neuropathy. Importantly, the results of electrodiagnostic studies were not used to determine the diagnosis of GBS. In general, motor nerve conduction abnormalities preceded changes in sensory nerve conductions. The frequency with which individual parameters (conduction velocity, distal latency, and so on) were abnormal, and sufficiently so to indicate demyelinating physiology, is not reported. However, the authors do indicate that 50 patients (71%) fulfilled their prespecified criteria for demyelination in multiple nerves (see Table 11.8) and that a further 11 patients (16%) fulfilled criteria for demyelination in a single nerve (6). The authors do not indicate the time frame to which these results apply. That is to say, they do not specify whether these 87% of patients met criteria for demyelination within the first week, 2 weeks, etc. of the onset of symptoms. In summary, therefore, these data indicate a sensitivity of 71–87% (depending on the stringency with which the criteria are applied) for the diagnosis of GBS, but this figure is probably artificially high because of the inclusion of patients with more advanced disease.

Various authors have suggested different sets of electrodiagnostic criteria for GBS (see Table 11.8), but there is no widespread agreement regarding which provide the best combination of sensitivity and specificity. Many studies have simply specified a new set of criteria without providing any empirical data to substantiate the proposed criteria (6–8). Relatively few studies have compared the diagnostic accuracy of different sets of criteria (9,10). Meulstee and colleagues, for example, used data from the Dutch Guillain-Barré Study of intravenous immunoglobulin vs plasma exchange (PE) as well as 45 healthy controls, to compare their criteria (see Table 11.8) with those proposed by Albers (6), Albers and Kelly (7), and Asbury and Cornblath (11). In so doing, they also compared the sensitivity of these various sets of criteria at three different time points during the course of GBS—6 days, 13 days, and 34 days (time points representing the median intervals from symptom onset to date on which the electromyography was performed). They found that their own criteria displayed sensitivities of 60%, 66%, and 72% at the three respective time points, superior at each time point with respect to the other criteria (9). Specificity was 100%, which is perhaps not surprising given the choice of healthy subjects as a control group.

Van den Bergh and colleagues examined the sensitivity and specificity of 10 published sets of diagnostic criteria for demyelinating polyneuropathy (including both GBS and chronic inflammatory demyelinating polyradiculoneuropathy [CIDP]) in their series of patients with GBS (n = 52), CIDP (n = 28), amyotrophic lateral sclerosis (n = 40), and diabetic polyneuropathy (DPN) (n = 32) (10). Overall, combining sensitivity and specificity, the best results were obtained using the criteria of the Dutch GBS Study Group (sensitivity 68%, specificity 94% for DPN, and 100% for motor neuron disease). They then performed a sensitivity analysis in order to determine what combination of stringency of abnormalities and number of abnormal nerves would be required to maximize sensitivity while preserving specificity. The criteria that they developed (summarized in Table 11.8) yielded a sensitivity of 75% and a specificity (for amyotrophic lateral sclerosis and diabetic polyneuropathy) of 100% when applied to their population of patients (10).

The most recently proposed criteria by Van den Bergh and colleagues, therefore, seem to offer the best combination of sensitivity and specificity (and simplicity). As indicated in Table 11.8, these criteria require the presence of slowed conduction velocity (less than 70% the lower limit of normal), prolonged distal motor latency (more than 150% the

Table 11.8
Electrodiagnostic Criteria for the Guillain-Barré Syndrome

Study	Conduction velocity	Distal latency	Conduction block	F-response
Albers *(6)*				
parameter	<95% LLN or <85% (amp < 50%)	>110% ULN or >120% (if ↓ amp)	30% or evidence for TD	>120% ULN
criteria	≥2 nerves	≥2 nerves	≥2 nerves	≥2 nerves
diagnosis	Requires at least one of the above criteria in two different nerves			
Albers & Kelly *(7)*				
parameter	<95% LLN or <80% (amp < 50%)	>115% ULN or >125% (if ↓ amp)	30% or evidence for TD	>125% ULN
criteria	≥2 nerves	≥2 nerves	≥1 nerve	≥1 nerve
diagnosis	Requires at least three of these criteria			
Asbury & Cornblath *(11)*				
parameter	<80% LLN or <70% (amp < 80%)	>125% ULM or >150% (amp < 80%)	20% (with <15% change in duration)	>120% ULN or >150% (amp < 80%) OR absent response
criteria	≥2 nerves	≥2 nerves	≥1 nerve	≥2 nerves
diagnosis	Requires at least three of these criteria			
Dutch GBS *(9)*				
parameter	<70% LLN	>150% ULN	"CMAP decay"[a]	>150% ULN
criteria	≥1 nerve	≥1 nerve	≥1 nerve	≥1 nerve
diagnosis	Requires at least two criteria in two different nerves			
Italian GBS *(39)*				
parameter	<80% LLN or <70% (amp < 80%)	>125% ULN or >150% (amp < 80%)	20%	>120% ULN or >150% (amp < 80%)
criteria	≥2 nerves	≥2 nerves	≥1 nerve	≥2 nerves
diagnosis	Requires at least two abnormal criteria			
Ho *(8)*				
parameter	<90% LLN or <85% (amp < 50%)	>100% ULN or >120% (↓ amp)	Evidence of unequivocal TD	>120% ULN
criteria	≥1 nerve	≥ 1 nerve	≥ 1 nerve	≥ 1 nerve
diagnosis	Requires at least one criterion in two or more nerves			
Van den Bergh *(10)*				
parameter	<70% LLN	>150% ULN	30–50%[b]	>120% (150%)[c] OR absent F with CMAP ≥20%
criteria	≥2 nerves	≥2 nerves	≥2 nerves	≥2 nerves
diagnosis	Any single criterion is sufficient for the diagnosis of AIDP. May also meet criteria with conduction block in one nerve and one other abnormality.			

[a]CMAP decay defined as any abnormal proximal CMAP if distal CMAP normal or proximal CMAP greater than 1 mV smaller than distal CMAP when distal CMAP >5 mV in the arm and >3 mV in the leg.

[b]50% required for *definite* diagnosis of CIDP and 30% for *probable* diagnosis of CIDP

[c]F-wave prolongation of 150% required if distal negative-peak CMAP is <50% of normal.

ULN, upper limit of normal; LLN, lower limit of normal.

upper limit of normal), prolonged F-responses (greater than 120% of the upper limit of normal or 150% if the CMAP amplitude is reduced) and conduction block of 50%. The requirements for demyelination are met if at least two nerves show any of these changes. Conduction block together with any other single abnormality is also sufficient for the diagnosis of demyelination. One caveat is that these criteria have not yet been tested by other investigators in a population of patients other than those from whom the criteria were developed.

3. TREATMENT

3.1. Is There a Role for Corticosteroids in the Treatment of GBS?

A role for corticosteroids in the treatment of GBS might be expected on the basis of their propensity to reduce the inflammation that plays an important role in the pathophysiology of this neuropathy. The efficacy of corticosteroids in GBS has been the subject of a number of randomized (and quasi-randomized) controlled studies *(12–17)*, the results of which have been summarized in a systematic review by the Cochrane Collaboration *(18)*. The study by the Guillain-Barré Syndrome Steroid Trial Group was by far the largest of these studies *(19)*, and its effects dominate the systematic review *(18)*.

The Guillain-Barré Syndrome Steroid Trial Group study was a double-blind placebo-controlled trial in which 240 patients were randomized to receive either placebo or intravenous methylprednisolone (500 mg) per day for 5 days. Patients were eligible for inclusion if disease was of sufficient severity to preclude running and if neurological symptoms had begun within the preceding 15 days. Disease severity was scored on a seven-point functional disability scale (reproduced in Table 11.9). The predefined primary outcome measure was a 0.5-grade difference in disability grade between the steroid and placebo groups at 4 weeks. The Cochrane systematic review similarly used the difference in disability grades between the steroid and control groups as the primary outcome measure. These data are summarized using the "weighted mean difference" (WMD) in Table 11.10. The WMD is obtained by determining the difference in mean scores between the steroid and control groups in each study and then calculating a weighted average of these means, with the weights determined primarily by the relative size of each study. A value of zero indicates no difference between the two treatment groups. As illustrated in Table 11.10, neither the individual studies nor the systematic review found a significant difference between the steroid- and control-treated patients.

The GBS Steroid Trial Group considered a variety of secondary outcome measures, including the duration of mechanical ventilation and the time taken to recover the ability to ambulate independently. These outcomes were also considered in the Cochrane systematic review. No significant differences between the steroid- and control-treated patients were found for any of these outcome measures.

Although the largest of the steroid studies in GBS (performed by the GBS Steroid Trial Study Group) was, for the most part, a well designed study, it did have one important shortcoming. Fifty-three percent of patients in the steroid group and 65% of patients in the placebo group also received plasmapheresis. It is at least theoretically possible that the greater use of plasmapheresis in the placebo group may have biased the study against a therapeutic benefit of steroids. The investigators dismiss this possibility based on their multiple regression analysis, which failed to reveal a significant beneficial effect of

Table 11.9
Functional Disability Scale Used in Guillain-Barré Syndrome Treatment Trials

Grade	Description
0	Healthy
1	Minor symptoms or signs and capable of running or manual work
2	Able to walk 5 m across an open space without assistance, walking frame or stick, but unable to run or incapable of manual work
3	Able to walk 5 m across an open space with the help of one person and waist-level walking frame, stick or sticks
4	Chair-bound or bed-bound, unable to walk as in (3)
5	Assisted ventilation required (for at least part of the day)
6	Death

Table 11.10
Effects of Steroids on Outcome in the Guillain-Barré Syndrome

	Steroids		Placebo		WMD
Study	n	Mean FDS score	n	Mean FDS score	(±95% CI)[a]
GBS Steroid Trial Group (19)	124	0.8	118	0.73	0.07 (−0.23,0.37)
Hughes (13)	21	0.24	19	0.74	−0.50 (−1.04, 0.04)
Shukla (16)	6	0.67	8	0.88	−0.21 (−1.81, 1.39)
Summary	–	–	–	–	**−0.06 (−0.32, 1.39)**

WMD, weighted mean difference; CI, confidence interval; FDS, functional disability scale
[a]Positive values indicate an effect in favor of steroids and negative values an effect in favor of the placebo. Data from ref. 18.

plasmapheresis, although subsequent studies demonstrating the efficacy of plasmapheresis should lead to this conclusion being treated with some degree of skepticism.

Most recently, van Koningsveld and colleagues examined the efficacy of corticosteroids when used in conjunction with intravenous immunoglobulin (20). Using the same steroid protocol as the Dutch GBS Steroid Trial Group, they randomized 223 patients to receive either placebo or intravenous methylprednisolone at a dose of 500 mg daily for 5 days. All patients also received IVIg at a dose of 0.4 g/kg/day for 5 days. The primary outcome measure was the proportion of patients in each group who improved by at least one grade (on the seven-point disability score; Table 11.9). The primary endpoint was achieved by 63 of 113 (56%) controls and 76 of 112 (68%) of patients treated with steroids (odds ratio [OR] 1.68, 95% confidence interval [CI] 0.97–2.88, $p = 0.06$) (20). After controlling for various prognostic factors (age, disability score at randomization, number of days between onset of symptoms and randomization, compound muscle action potential amplitude, and preceding infection with cytomegalovirus) in a multivariate analysis, the OR (favoring treatment with steroids) increased to 2.96 (95% CI 1.26–6.94, $p = 0.01$). The authors justified this analysis on the basis of unequal distribution of some of these prognostic factors between the two treatment groups at baseline, and interpreted these adjusted results to indicate a small benefit from the addition of methylprednisolone to IVIg in the treatment of patients with GBS *(20)*.

This conclusion has not been uniformly accepted. Hughes, for example, incorporated data from the study by van Koningsveld into a meta-analysis and found that it did not change the overall estimation of the steroid treatment effect *(21)*. Van Koningsveld and colleagues have retorted that it is inappropriate to combine data from their study, which examined the effect of steroids used in conjunction with intravenous immunoglublin, with data from studies that evaluated the effects of steroids alone. Irrespective of the validity of these arguments, it would seem that any treatment effect (if indeed it is present at all) is extremely small and of questionable clinical significance. The overall impression, therefore, is that there is no role for steroids in the treatment of GBS.

3.2. Is Plasma Exchange Effective in Patients With Guillain-Barré Syndrome?

There are six published randomized controlled trials that have compared the efficacy of PE with supportive care *(22–27)*. The characteristics of these studies are summarized in Table 11.11. The results of these studies have been summarized in a Cochrane Systematic Review *(28)*. The largest two prospective randomized studies that compared plasmapheresis with best supportive care in patients with GBS were performed by the American Guillain-Barré Syndrome Study Group *(12)* and the French Cooperative Study *(26)*.

The American study randomized 245 patients to plasmapheresis vs best conventional therapy. Patients with mild disease or those under the age of 12 years were excluded. Clinical evaluation comprised assessment on a seven-point scale, with grade 2 representing the ability to walk without assistance (*see* Table 11.9). Primary outcome measures were specified in advance as (1) the number of patients who improved one grade 4 weeks after randomization, (2) the time taken to improve by one grade, and (3) the time taken to reach grade 2. The intention to evaluate clinical outcome at 6 months was planned in advance, but the nature of the measures to be used at this time point were not specified. Neither patients nor physicians were blinded to the treatment used. Both groups were equivalent in terms of demographic profile. The results are summarized in Table 11.12.

This study clearly demonstrated that plasmapheresis increases the rate of clinical recovery, and this effect was particularly marked in patients who were treated within 7 days of the onset of symptoms and in those who required a ventilator after randomization. The outcome measures at 6 months, however, are more difficult to interpret, with results reported in terms of the number of patients who failed to improve one clinical grade, occurring in a smaller proportion (3% vs 13%) of those who received plasmapheresis. However, closer inspection reveals that a similar proportion (75% vs 74%) in each group did improve by one clinical grade. The difference between those who did improve by one grade in the conventional treatment group and those who did not comprises those patients who are listed as "treatment failures" in the plasmapheresis group. These "treatment failures" represent those patients who did not complete the course of plasmapheresis. The second outcome measure reported at 6 months was the number of patients who failed to reach grade 2 (i.e., able to ambulate without assistance). Here the percentages were 18% and 29% for plasmapheresis and conventional therapy, respectively, a difference that is statistically significant ($P < 0.05$). It is perhaps surprising that the results were not

Table 11.11
Studies of Plasma Exchange (PE) in Guillain-Barré Syndrome (GBS)

Study	n	Entry criteria: disease severity	PE Schedule	Primary endpoint	Methodology	Results (end-point achieved)
Greenwood (23)	29	Unable to walk without assistance	5 exchanges over 5 d	Improvement in disability grade after 1 mo	No patient blinding	7/14 (PE) vs 6/15 (control)
Osterman (25)	38	Unable to walk without assistance	5–8 exchanges over 7–10 d	Improvement in functional dis-ability grade ≥ 1 point after 1 mo	No patient blinding Effort made to keep observer unaware of treatment assigned Inadequate allocation concealment	14/18 (PE) vs 6/20 (control)
American GBS Study Group (12)	245	Unable to walk without assistance	3–5 exchanges over 7–14 d	Proportion of patients improved ≥ 1 grade after 1 mo	No patient blinding Effort made to keep observer unaware of treatment assigned	59% (PE) vs 39% (control)
Farkkila (22)	29	Any motor deficit	3–5 exchanges	Rate of improvement of isometric hand grip force	No patient blinding Inadequate allocation concealment	More rapid rate of improvement in the PE group
French Cooperative Group (26)	220	Any motor deficit	4 exchanges over 8 d	Time to recover walking with assistance	No patient blinding Effort made to keep observer unaware of treatment assigned	Median time to endpoint 44 d (control) vs 30 d (PE)
French Cooperative Group (27)	91	Able to stand alone or walk with assistance	2 exchanges over 3 d	Time to onset of motor recovery (defined by ≥2-point improvement in functional muscular score)	No patient blinding Effort made to keep observer unaware of treatment assigned	Median time to endpoint 8 d (control) vs 4 d (PE)

Table 11.12
Efficacy of Plasma Exchange in the Guillain-Barré Syndrome (GBS) in the American GBS Study

Outcome measure	Conventional	Plasmapheresis	p value
Number of patients improving 1 grade at 4 wk	39%	59%	<0.01
Time to improve 1 grade (days)	40	19	<0.001
Time to reach grade 2 (days)	85	53	<0.001
Duration of ventilation (days)[a]	23	9	<0.05
Failure to improve 1 clinical grade by 6 mo	13%	3%	<0.01
Improved by one clinical grade at 6 mo	75%	74%	NS
Unable to walk without assistance at 6 mo (i.e., failing to reach grade 2)	29%	18%	<0.05

[a]In patients who required ventilation only after randomization. NS, not significant.
Data from ref. 12.

expressed as the number of patients who *did* reach grade 2, but these numbers cannot be calculated from the data provided. The overall impression is that the data for better final outcome in those treated with plasmapheresis are not very convincing.

The French Cooperative Study randomized 220 patients to treatment with or without plasmapheresis. Patients with disease of any severity were included (although as it happens, there was a tendency to recruit patients with more severe disease), provided that age was greater than 16 years and motor symptoms had begun within the preceding 17 days. Neither patients nor physicians were blinded. Clinical assessment was made using binary measures on 28 tests of motor function (converted to a score from 0 to 100). The primary outcome measure was the time to recover the ability to walk with assistance. Secondary outcome measures included (1) change in score, (2) the number of patients requiring ventilation after randomization, (3) time to onset of motor recovery (defined as a gain of two items on the functional score), (4) time to begin ventilatory wean, and (5) time to walk without assistance. There were no differences in patient demographics between the treatment and control groups. The results are summarized in Table 11.13. The results of 1-year follow-up of the patients from the French Cooperative Study were subsequently published *(29)* (Table 11.14).

This study also provided clear evidence of an increased rate of recovery in patients treated with plasmapheresis. The evidence for improved final outcome, however, is again less convincing, in part because there was no clear explanation for the difference between the percentage of patients who made a complete recovery and the percentage who were able to return to work. It is possible that failure to make a complete recovery might simply have entailed an absent reflex or mild sensory disturbance, which might not represent a clinically important difference. This, however, is purely speculative because sufficient data are not provided.

The results of the Cochrane systematic review of the six randomized controlled studies comparing PE with supportive care are summarized in Tables 11.15A (dichotomous outcomes) and 11.15B (continuous outcomes). These results indicate a beneficial effect of PE on a range of outcome measures including walking without assistance, improve-

Table 11.13
Efficacy of Plasma Exchange in the Guillain-Barré Syndrome (GBS) in the French Cooperative
GBS Study

Outcome measure	Control	Plasmapheresis	p value
Time to recover walking with assistance (days)[a]	44	30	< 0.011
Time to onset of motor recovery (days)	13	6	< 0.005
Time to begin ventilatory wean (days)	31	18	< 0.01
Time to recover walking without assistance (days)	111	70	< 0.001

[a]Primary outcome measure.
Data From ref. 26.

Table 11.14
Long-Term Effects of Plasma Exchange in Guillain-Barré Syndrome

Outcome measure at 1 yr	Control	Plasmapheresis	p value
Complete recovery	37%	60%	0.001
Return to work	67%	76%	NS
Full muscular strength recovery	52%	71%	0.007
Severe disability	11%	11%	NS

NS, not significant.
Data from ref. 29.

ment by at least one grade on the functional disability scale (Table 11.9), mean improvement in functional disability scale score, requirement for mechanical ventilation, recovery of full muscle strength at 1 year and the presence of severe motor sequelae at 1 year.

Finally, it should be noted that PE is effective at all ages above 12 years (having not been adequately tested in younger patients) and is effective irrespective of the severity of disability at the time treatment is initiated (27,28). The available data also support the contention that PE is effective whether therapy is initiated within or beyond 7 days of the onset of symptoms (12,26,28). It appears that a course of four exchanges is superior to two exchanges, but that no further benefit is derived from increasing the number of exchanges to six (27). Continuous flow PE appears to be superior to intermittent flow, and the cell separation and filtration techniques offer equivalent efficacy (12,26,28). The type of replacement fluid used does not seem to impact the efficacy of PE (26,28).

In summary, therefore, a course of four PEs (using the continuous cycle technique) is effective in improving both the rate of recovery as well as the degree of motor recovery achieved within the first year.

3.3. Is Intravenous Immunoglobulin Effective in Patients With Guillain-Barré Syndrome?

Most studies of intravenous immunoglobulin (IVIg) in the treatment of patients with GBS have compared IVIg with PE (30–33) (summarized in Table 11.16) although two studies in the pediatric population have compared IVIg with placebo or no treatment (34,35). The results of these studies have also been summarized in a Cochrane Collaboration systematic review (36).

Table 11.15A
Systematic Review of Plasma Exchange Studies in Guillain-Barré Syndrome:
Dichotomous Outcomes

Outcome	Treatment	Control	OR (95% CI)
Walking or not with assistance	31/172	32/177	1.02 (0.58, 1.77)
Improved or not by one grade	176/308	110/315	2.49 (1.8, 3.44)
Walking or not without assistance	35/172	21/177	1.97 (1.07, 3.61)
Ventilated or not	44/308	85/315	0.45 (0.3, 0.67)
Recovery of full strength at 1 yr or not	135/199	112/205	1.83 (1.2, 2.8)
Death or not at 1 yr	15/321	18/328	0.85 (0.42, 1.72)
Severe motor sequelae at 1 yr or not	35/321	55/328	0.59 (0.37, 0.94)
Relapses within 1 yr or not	13/321	4/328	2.98 (1.06, 8.39)

OR, odds ratio; CI, confidence interval. Data from ref. 28.

Table 11.15B
Systematic Review of Plasma Exchange Studies in Guillain-Barré Syndrome:
Continuous Outcomes

Outcome	Treatment		Control		WMD (95% CI)[a]
	n	Mean	n	Mean	
Mean improvement (number of grades)	290	−1	295	+0.1	−1.1 (−1.55, −0.65)
Duration of mechanical ventilation (days)	57		75		−5.09 (−12.94, 2.76)

[a]Negative value indicates an effect in favor of treatment with plasma exchange.
WMD, weighted mean difference; CI, confidence intervals.
Data from ref. 28.

The evidence for the benefit of IVIg is primarily derived from two large prospective randomized studies that compared plasmapheresis and IVIg. The first of these was published by the Dutch Guillain-Barré Study Group (31). This trial randomized 150 patients to receive either plasmapheresis or IVIg. Only patients who were unable to walk without assistance and whose symptoms had begun within the preceding two weeks were eligible for randomization. Children younger than 4 years were excluded. Clinical assessment was made using the same seven-point scale used by the American Guillain-Barré Study Group (Table 11.9), supplemented by a 60-point Medical Research Council grading system (six muscles on each side, with strength graded from 0 to 5). The last follow-up was performed 6 months after randomization. Physicians were partially blinded (i.e., one of two physicians were blinded at the time of evaluation and the blinded and nonblinded scores were compared). The primary outcome measure was improvement of at least one grade on the seven-point functional scale 4 weeks after randomization. Secondary outcome measures included (1) time required to improve at least one functional grade and (2) time required to recover independent ambulation (these outcomes measures were all also used by the American Guillain-Barré Study Group) (Table 11.17).

Table 11.16
Studies of Intravenous Immunoglobulin in Guillain-Barré Syndrome

Study	n	Entry criteria: disease severity	Treatment	Primary endpoint	Methodology	Results (end-point achieved)
PSGBS Group (30)	383	Unable to walk 5 m without assistance	0.4 g/kg/d × 4 d vs 5–6 PE over 8–13 d	Mean improvement in disability grade	Inadequate patient blinding	0.8 (IVIg) vs 0.9 (PE)
Van der Meche (31)	150	Unable to walk 10 m without assistance	0.4 g/kg/d × 5 d vs 5 PE over 7–14 d	Proportion improved by ≥1 grade on disability scale at 4 wk	Patient blinding was inadequate with potential for bias in observer blinding	53% (IVIg) vs 34% (PE)
Bril (32)	50	Unable to perform manual work	0.5 g/kg/d × 4 d vs 5 PE over 7–10 d	Time to improve ≥1 disability grade	Patient and observer blinding were inadequate ITT analysis was not performed	39 d (IVIg) vs 39 d (PE)
Diener (33)	25	Moderate to severe disease	0.4 g/kg/d × 5 d vs PE or immune adsorption × 5 d	Proportion of patients improved by ≥1 grade at 4 wk	Patient and observer blinding were inadequate Excess follow-up loss Baseline differences	16/20 (IVIg) vs 15/21 (PE) & 7/14 (immune adsorption)

PE, plasma exchange; ITT, intention to treat; PSGBS, Plasma Exchange/Sandoglobulin Guillain-Barré Syndrome.

200

Table 11.17
Effect of IVIg in Guillain-Barré Syndrome (GBS) (The Dutch GBS Study Group)

Outcome measure	PE	IVIg	p value
Number improved by 1 grade at 4 wk	34%	53%	0.024
Time to improve 1 grade	41 d	27 d	0.05
Time to recover independent ambulation	69 d	55 d	0.07
Number requiring assisted ventilation	42%	27%	<0.05

IVIg, intravenous immunoglubulin; PE, plasma exchange.

This study clearly demonstrated the efficacy of IVIg in the treatment of patients with severe GBS. Furthermore, the data suggested that IVIg might be even more efficacious than PE. The nature of the benefit, however, is explicit in terms of rate of recovery, but not in terms of whether treatment alters the ultimate outcome or degree of recovery.

It is interesting to note that only 34% of patients treated with PE had improved by one grade at 4 weeks after randomization. In comparison, in the American Guillain-Barré Syndrome Study Group, 59% of patients treated with PE improved by one grade at 4 weeks. The authors of this study suggest that this discrepancy might have been due to their enrolling patients sooner after the onset of their illness. The implication is that patients in the early stages of the disease may still deteriorate further and therefore take longer to recover to an equivalent functional grade.

The other large study was performed by the Plasma Exchange/Sandoglobulin Guillain-Barré Syndrome Trial Group *(30)*. Investigators randomized 383 patients to receive PE, IVIg, or a combination of the two (PE followed by IVIg) (the results of the combination therapy are discussed in the section "Is there a Role for Combining Plasmapheresis and IVIg?"). Only patients older than 16 years and with severe disease (unable to walk without assistance) were eligible for inclusion in the study. The seven-point disability scale used by the American and Dutch GBS Study Groups were used to evaluate patients clinically (Table 11.9). Patient demographics at randomization were similar in all treatment groups, with average duration of illness prior to randomization being 1 week. The aim of the study was to determine whether IVIg was equivalent or superior to PE, and whether PE followed by IVIg was superior to either treatment alone. A difference of 0.5 grades at 4 weeks between two treatment groups was specified in advance as being indicative of a difference in treatment-related outcome. Secondary outcome measures included time to walking unaided, time to discontinuation of ventilatory support, and the average rate of recovery (Table 11.18).

There were no significant differences in any of the outcome measures between the plasmapheresis and the IVIg treatment groups. As in the Dutch study, patients with a longer duration of disease prior to randomization had a better outcome at 4 weeks. The explanation offered is that these patients were further along the natural history of the disease and hence more likely to show spontaneous recovery. In addition, patients with more severe disease would be expected to present early (and hence be randomized sooner in the course of the disease).

The results of these two large studies as well as of a number of smaller studies have been analyzed in a systematic review published by the Cochrane Collaboration *(36)*.

Table 11.18

Plasma Exchange/Sandoglobulin Guillain-Barré Syndrome Trial Group

Outcome measure	PE	IVIg	PE + IVIg
Mean change in disability grade at 4 wk	0.9	0.8	1.1
Time to discontinuation of ventilation	29 d	26 d	18 d
Time to walk unaided	49 d	51 d	40 d

PE, plasma exchange; IVIg, intravenous immunoglubulin.

Table 11.19A

Systematic Review of Intravenous Immunoglobulin (IVIg) Studies
in Guillain-Barré Syndrome: Continuous Measures

Outcome	IVIg (n)	Plasma exchange (n)	WMD (95% CI)
Change in disability grade 4 wk after randomization	273	263	−0.04 (−0.26, 0.19)
Change in disability grade in patients ventilated at the time of randomization	15	12	1.38 (0.69, 2.07)

WMD, weighted mean difference; CI, confidence interval.

Table 11.19B

Systematic Review of Intravenous Immunoglobulin (IVIg) Studies
in Guillain-Barré Syndrome: Dichotomous Measures

Outcome	IVIg (n/N)	Plasma exchange (n/N)	Relative risk (95% CI)
Death	7/296	9/286	0.78 (0.31, 1.95)
Death or disabled after 12 mo	21/129	19/114	0.98 (0.55, 1.72)
Relapse/treatment-related fluctuation	12/227	13/218	0.89 (0.42, 1.89)

n, number of subjects with outcome; N, number of subjects at risk for the outcome.

These results are summarized in Tables 11.19A (continuous measures) and 11.19B (dichotomous measures). As explained previously, the weighted mean difference (WMD) is obtained by determining the difference in mean scores between the IVIg and PE groups in each study, and then calculating a weighted average of these means with the weights determined primarily by the relative size of each study. A value of zero indicates no difference between the two treatment groups. The finding of a WMD of −0.04 indicates a 0.04-grade greater improvement among patients treated with IVIg (with the CIs interpreted as consistent with a 0.26-grade greater improvement for patients receiving IVIg as well as a 0.19-grade improvement for patients treated with PE). In essence, there is no meaningful difference in outcomes between the two treatment groups. For the dichotomous outcomes considered (Table 11.19B), the 95% CIs of the risk ratios for death, death or disability at 12 months, and the occurrence of relapses/treated-related fluctuations all span unity, indicating no difference between the two treatment modalities.

3.4. Is There a Role for Combining Plasmapheresis and IVIg?

The Plasma Exchange/Sandoglobulin Guillain-Barré Syndrome Trial Group Study (30) included three treatment arms, with some patients receiving only plasmapheresis, others IVIg alone, and yet others receiving plasmapheresis followed by IVIg. The more complete results of this study are summarized in Table 11.18.

Considering the outcomes of change in disability grade 4 weeks after randomization, death as well as death/disability at 1 year, there were no significant differences between any of the different treatment groups. These results indicate that the combination of IVIg and PE offers no benefit over IVIg alone.

4. PROGNOSIS

4.1. Which Clinical and Electrodiagnostic Factors Predict Outcome in Patients With the Guillain-Barré Syndrome?

The question of prognosis in GBS has been addressed by a number of studies (37–39). For the most part, there is broad agreement between these studies regarding the clinical and electrodiagnostic findings that predict recovery.

McKhann et al. performed a multivariate analysis on the data obtained from the American Guillain-Barré Syndrome Study Group's prospective randomized investigation of plasmapheresis in GBS (37). Cornblath and colleagues examined the prognostic value of motor nerve conduction studies from patients in the same trial (40). These studies identified severely reduced mean distal compound muscle action potential amplitude (<20% of normal) as the most important prognostic factor, with the requirement for mechanical ventilation at the time of randomization, shorter duration of illness prior to randomization (<7 days), and older age also independently predictive of a worse outcome. The impact of the combination of these variables on the probability of recovery to ambulate independently is shown in Table 11.20 for those patients treated with continuous-cycle plasma exchange. Mean distal CMAP amplitude is determined by expressing the CMAP amplitude of each motor nerve studied as a percentage of the lower limit of normal, summing these values, and then dividing by the number of nerves studies (i.e., an average of the percentage reduction in response amplitudes of the motor nerves studied).

Visser et al. (38) examined the data from the Dutch GBS Trial (31) to identify prognostic factors. Potential factors identified in a univariate analysis were then tested in a multivariate analysis in rank order according to the sequence in which they became available in the clinical setting. Using this novel approach, they identified a preceding gastrointestinal illness, older age (>50 years), more severe disease, and a recent cytomegalovirus infection as predictive of a poor early (8-week) outcome. The same clinical features were identified at the 6-month end point, with the additional factor of a rapid onset of weakness (i.e., patients presenting within 4 days of the onset of symptoms).

The results of these two studies are largely in agreement with each other, identifying older age, the rapidity of progression of symptoms, and the presence of more severe disease (measured by the requirement for mechanical ventilation in the American study) as poor prognostic indicators. These studies differed, however, in that distal compound

Table 11.20
Cumulative Probability of Recovery to Independent Ambulation

	Distal CMAP	1 mo	3 mo	6 mo
Not ventilated				
Illness > 7 d				
Age 30	>80% normal	0.55	0.95	1.00
	≤80% normal	0.25	0.67	0.86
Age 60	>80% normal	0.43	0.89	0.98
	≤80% normal	0.18	0.54	0.74
Illness ≤7 d				
Age 30	>80% normal	0.39	0.85	0.96
	≤80% normal	0.16	0.49	0.70
Age 60	>80% normal	0.29	0.74	0.90
	≤80% normal	0.12	0.38	0.57
Ventilated				
Illness >7 d				
Age 30	>80% normal	0.26	0.84	0.96
	≤80% normal	0.10	0.48	0.68
Age 60	>80% normal	0.19	0.72	0.89
	≤80% normal	0.07	0.37	0.55
Illness ≤7 d				
Age 30	>80% normal	0.17	0.67	0.86
	≤80% normal	0.06	0.33	0.50
Age 60	>80% normal	0.12	0.54	0.75
	≤80% normal	0.05	0.24	0.39

Data for those receiving continuous cycle plasma exchange. CMAP, compound muscle action potential. Data derived from ref. 37.

muscle action potential amplitude was identified as an important prognostic indicator in the American, but not in the Dutch, study. Similarly, the nature of the antecedent infectious illness appeared to be significant in the Dutch study.

Prognostic factors were also studied by the Italian Guillain-Barré Study Group (39). In a multivariate analysis, they also identified older age, preceding gastrointestinal infection, severity of disability at nadir of the illness, and electrodiagnostic evidence of axonal loss as adversely predictive of clinical recovery (defined as the absence of symptoms or signs potentially interfering with daily living activities) (39). This report includes some conflicting data. The tabulated data suggest that longer latency to nadir of the illness is associated with a worse outcome, but the text summary of the results indicates the opposite.

Taken together, therefore, factors adversely predictive of recovery include older age, greater severity of the illness (including the requirement for mechanical ventilation), preceding gastrointestinal infection, and mean distal CMAP amplitude below 20% of normal.

5. SUMMARY

- Muscle weakness, either alone or in combination with sensory symptoms (paresthesias, pain or both), is the most common symptom in patients with GBS.

Table 11.21
Summary of the Effects of Plasmapheresis in Guillain-Barré Syndrome

Outcome measure	American (2)	French (3,4)	Dutch (5)
No. of patients improved 1 grade at 4 wk	59%	N/A	34%
Time to independent ambulation	53 d	70 d	69 d

- Weakness in the legs is most prominent, and may be more severe either proximally or distally.
- Symptoms most commonly progress in an "ascending" fashion, spreading from the legs to the arms and cranial nerves.
- The majority of patients with GBS are areflexic at the time of initial presentation, with most of those with retained reflexes losing them during the course of the illness; a small minority of patients may retain at least some deep tendon reflexes.
- Most patients (70–90%) with GBS show an elevated CSF protein concentration at some stage during the course of their illness. A minor pleocytosis may be seen in as many as 24% of patients, although counts greater than 30 cells/mm^3 are extremely rare.
- The most frequently encountered early electrodiagnostic changes in GBS are absent H-reflexes and absent/prolonged F-responses. Changes indicative of demyelinating physiology may seen in the minority (16–42%) of patients within the first 7 days.
- There is no widespread agreement regarding the most accurate electrodiagnostic criteria for GBS. The criteria proposed by the Dutch GBS Group seem to offer the highest sensitivity (60%, 66%, and 72% at 1, 2, and 5 weeks, respectively) without compromising specificity (100%). More recently, Van den Bergh and colleagues proposed criteria that may increase sensitivity to 75%, but these still require independent confirmation.
- The available evidence suggests that intravenous methylprednisolone is ineffective in the treatment of patients with GBS, even when used in combination with IVIg (although the latter claim is disputed).
- There is good evidence that PE and IVIg are each effective forms of therapy in patients with GBS, as measured by the rate of clinical recovery.
- There is no good evidence that the combination of PE and IVIg is superior to either treatment alone.
- In some of the studies, the complication rate associated with IVIg was lower than that associated with PE, suggesting that this should be the first line of treatment.
- Outcome measures and methods of clinical evaluation have differed among the studies, but their results are summarized in Table 11.21.
- The evidence that final outcome is improved by any form of treatment is less clear. The follow-up data from the French Cooperative Study suggests that this is the case, but the outcome measures used are a little dubious. The Systematic Reviews by the Cochrane Collaboration indicate that long-term outcome is improved by both plasma exchange and IVIg.
- There is no clear advantage to the use of one type of replacement fluid (albumin or fresh frozen plasma) during PE, but continuous cycle exchange is superior to intermittent cycle.
- Adverse clinical prognostic factors include advancing age, greater degree of disability at the time treatment is initiated, and preceding gastrointestinal infection.

- Reduced (by 80% or more) distal compound muscle action potential may be the best early predictor of adverse outcome, measured in terms of recovery of the ability to walk without assistance.

REFERENCES

1. Masucci E, Kurtzke J. Diagnostic criteria for the Guillain-Barre Syndrome. An analysis of 50 cases. J Neurol Sci 1971;13:483–501.
2. Ropper AH, Wijdicks EF, Truax B. Guillain-Barre Syndrome. In: Plum F, ed. Contemporary Neurology Series. FA Davis Company, Philadelphia: 1991.
3. Winer J, Hughes R, Osmond C. A prospective study of acute idiopathic neuropathy. I. Clinical features and their prognostic value. J Neurol Neurosurg Psychiatry 1988;51:605–612.
4. Gordon PH, Wilbourn AJ. Early electrodiagnostic findings in Guillain-Barre Syndrome. Arch Neurol 2001;58:913–917.
5. Ropper AH, Wijdicks EF, Shahani BT. Electrodiagnostic abnormalities in 113 consecutive patients with Guillain-Barre Syndrome. Arch Neurol 1990;47:881–887.
6. Albers JW, Donofrio PD, McGonagle TK. Sequential electrodiagnostic abnormalities in acute inflammatory demyelinating polyradiculoneuropathy. Muscle Nerve 1985;8:528–539.
7. Albers JW, Kelly JJ. Acquired inflammatory demyelinating polyneuropathies: clinical and electrodiagnostic features. Muscle Nerve 1989;12:435–451.
8. Ho T, Mishu B, Li C, et al. Guillain-Barre Syndrome in Northern China. Relationship to Campylobacter jejuni infection and anti-glycolipid antibodies. Brain 1995;118:597–605.
9. Meulstee J, van der Meche F. Electrodiagnostic criteria for polyneuropathy and demyelination: application in 135 patients with Guillain-Barre Syndrome. The Dutch Guillain-Barré Study Group. J Neurol Neurosurg Psychiatry 1995;59:482–486.
10. Van den Bergh PY, Pieret F. Electrodiagnostic criteria for acute and chronic inflammatory demyelinating polyradiculoneuropathy. Muscle Nerve 2004;29:565–574.
11. Asbury A, Cornblath D. Assessment of current diagnostic criteria for Guillain-Barre Syndrome. Ann Neurol 1990;27(Suppl):S21–S24.
12. Plasmapheresis and acute Guillain-Barre syndrome. The Guillain-Barre syndrome study Group. Neurology 1985;35:1096–1104.
13. Hughes R, Newsom-Davis J, Perkin G, Pierce J. Controlled trial of prednisolone in acute polyneuropathy. Lancet 1978;2:750–752.
14. Mendell J, Kissel J, Kennedy M, et al. Plasma exchange and prednisone in Guillain-Barre syndrome: a controlled randomized trial. Neurology 1985;35:1551–1555.
15. Swick HM, McQuillen MP. The use of steroids in the treatment of idiopathic polyneuritis. Neurology 1976;26:205–215.
16. Shukla S, Agarwal R, Gupta OR, Pande G, Mamta S. Double blind controlled trial of prednisolone in Guillain-Barre syndrome—a clinical study. Clinician - India 1988;52:128–134.
17. Singh N, Gupta A. Do corticosteroids influence the disease course or mortality in Guillain-Barre syndrome? J Assoc Physicians India 1996;44:22–24.
18. Hughes R, van der Meche F. Corticosteroids for Guillain-Barre syndrome. Cochrane Database Systematic Reviews 2000;3,CD001446.
19. Guillain-Barré Syndrome Steroid Trial Group. Double-blind trial of intravenous methylprednisolone in Guillain-Barré syndrome. Lancet 1993;341:586–590.
20. van Koningsveld R, Schmitz P, van der Meche F, Visser L, Meulstee J, van Doorn P. Effect of methylprednisolone when added to standard treatment with intravenous immunoglobulin for Guillain-Barre syndrome: randomised trial. Lancet 2004;363:192–196.
21. Hughes R. Treatment of Guillain-Barre syndrome with corticosteroids: lack of benefit? Lancet 2004;363:181–182.
22. Farkkila M, Kinnunen E, Haapanen E, Livanainen M. Guillain Barre syndrome: quantitative measures of plasma exchange therapy. Neurology 1987;38:837–840.
23. Greenwood R, Newsom-Davis J, Hughes R, et al. Controlled trial of plasma exchange in acute inflammatory polyradiculoneuropathy. Lancet 1984;1:877–879.

24. Plasmapheresis and acute Guillain-Barré syndrome. The Guillain-Barré Sydrome Study Group. Neurology 1985;35:1096–1104.
25. Osterman P, Fagius J, Lundemo G, et al. Beneficial effects of plasma exchange in acute inflammatory polyradiculoneuropathy. Lancet 1984;2:1296–1299.
26. Efficiency of plasma exchange in Guillain-Barre syndrome: role of replacement fluids. French Cooperative Group on Plasma Exchange in Guillain-Barre Syndrome. Ann Neurol 1987;22:753–761.
27. Appropriate number of plasma exchanges in Guillain-Barre Syndrome. French Cooperative Group on Plasma Exchange in Guillain-Barré Syndrome. Ann Neurol 1997;41:298–306.
28. Raphael J, Chevret S, Hughes R, Annane D. Plasma exchange for Guillain-Barre Syndrome. Cochrane Database Systematic Reviews 2004; 3:CD001798.
29. Plasma Exchange in Guillain-Barré Syndrome: one-year follow-up. French Cooperative Group on Plasma Exchange in Guillain-Barré Syndrome. Ann Neurol 1992;32:94–97.
30. Randomised trial of plasma exchange, intravenous immunoglobulin, and combined treatments in Guillain-Barre syndrome. Plasma exchange/Sandoglobulin Guillain-Barre Trial Group. Lancet 1997;349:225–230.
31. van der Meche F, Schmitz P. A randomized trial comparing intravenous immune globulin and plasma exchange in Guillain-Barré syndrome. Dutch Guillain-Barre Study Group. N Engl J Med 1992;326:1123–1129.
32. Bril V, Ilse W, Pearce R, Dhanani A, Sutton D, Kong K. Pilot trial of immunoglublin versus plasma exchange in patients with Guillain-Barre syndrome. Neurology 1996;46:100–103.
33. Diener H-C, Haupt WF, Kloss TM, et al. A preliminary, randomized, multicenter study comparing intravenous immunoglobulin, plasma exchange, and immune adsorption in Guillain-Barre syndrome. Eur Neurol 2001;46:107–109.
34. Gurses N, Uysal S, Cetinkaya F, Islek I, Kalayci A. Intravenous immunoglobulin treatment in children with Guillain-Barre syndome. Scand J Infect Dis 1995;27:241–243.
35. Wang R, Feng A, Sun W, Wen Z. Intravenous immunoglobulin in children with Guillain-Barre syndrome. Journal of Applied Clinical Pediatrics 2001;16:223–224.
36. Hughes R, Raphael J, Swan A, van Doorn P. Intravenous immunoglobulin for Guillain-Barre syndrome. Cochrane Database Systematic Reviews 2004; 3:CD002063.
37. McKhann G, Griffin J, Cornblath D, et al. Plasmapheresis and Guillain-Barre Syndrome: analysis of prognostic factors and the effect of plasmapheresis. Ann Neurol 1988;23:347–353.
38. Visser L, Schmitz P, Meulstee J, van Doorn P, van der Meche F. Prognostic factors of Guillain-Barré syndrome after intravenous immunoglobulin or plasma exchange. The Dutch Guillain-Barre Study Group. Neurology 1999;53:598–604.
39. The prognosis and main prognostic indicators of Guillain-Barre syndrome. A multicenter prospective study of 297 patients. The Italian Guillain-Barre Study Group. Brain 1996;119:2053–2061.
40. Cornblath DR, Mellits ED, Griffin JW, et al. Motor conduction studies in Guillain-Barré Syndrome: description and prognostic value. Ann Neurol 1988;23:354–359.

12 Chronic Inflammatory Demyelinating Polyradiculoneuropathy

1. INTRODUCTION

Chronic inflammatory demyelinating polyradiculoneuropathy (CIDP) is an acquired demyelinating neuropathy in which motor symptoms generally predominate over sensory symptoms and large fiber sensory dysfunction is more common than small fiber loss. The course may either be relapsing and remitting or chronically progressive. CIDP may occur in isolation or in the context of a number of systemic disorders, including HIV and hepatitis C infection, inflammatory bowel disease, lymphoproliferative disorders and osteosclerotic myeloma. The importance of distinguishing CIDP from among other causes of peripheral neuropathy lies in the observation that a significant proportion of patients with CIDP may respond to immune-modifying therapy. In this chapter, we consider important diagnostic questions that relate to the optimal electrophysiological criteria that should be used to define the disorder and the relative diagnostic utility of sural nerve biopsy. Many different forms of immunosuppressive therapy have been proposed for the treatment of CIDP, and although some of these therapeutic modalities have been studied in randomized controlled trials, many have not. We shall also consider the evidence supporting the use of these various immunosuppressive agents as well as the prognosis for patients who are treated in this manner.

2. DIAGNOSIS

2.1. Which Electrophysiological Criteria Should Be Used for the Diagnosis of CIDP?

Over the last 15 years, a number of criteria for the electrodiagnosis of CIDP have been proposed (1–7). Each of these are based on the same pattern of abnormalities, namely slowing of conduction velocity, prolongation of the distal latency, prolongation of the F-response and the presence of conduction block or temporal dispersion. The criteria vary, however, in the magnitude of change required for each of these parameters as well as the required number of affected nerves in order for the diagnosis to be made (Table 12.1).

Remarkably, there have been relatively few empirical data published in support of these criteria. Only the revisions proposed by a limited number of authors (3,6–8) in fact, have been based on application of the existing criteria to a novel data set, with the revised criteria suggested on the basis of improved diagnostic accuracy of the new criteria (Table 12.2).

From: *Neuromuscular Disease: Evidence and Analysis in Clinical Neurology*
By: M. Benatar © Humana Press Inc., Totowa, NJ

Table 12.1

Electrophysiological Criteria for the Diagnosis of Chronic Inflammatory Demyelinating Polyradiculoneuropathy (CIDP)

Study	Conduction velocity (CV)	Distal latency (DL)	Conduction block (CB)	F-response
Albers & Kelly *(1)*				
parameter	<75% LLN	>130% ULN	30%	>130% ULN
criteria	≥2 nerves	≥2 nerve	≥1 nerve	≥1 nerve
diagnosis	Requires at least three criteria for the diagnosis of CIDP			
Bromberg (Albers & Kelly) *(3)*	As for the Albers & Kelly criteria except that the CV and DL parameters may be met with only one nerve being abnormal			
AAN *(2)*				
parameter	<80% LLN or <70% (amp < 80%)	>125% ULN or >150% (amp < 80%)	20%	>120% ULN or >150% (amp < 80%)
criteria	≥2 nerves	≥2 nerves	≥1 nerve	≥2 nerves
diagnosis	Requires at least three criteria for the diagnosis of CIDP			
Barohn *(4)*				
parameter	<70% LLN			
criteria	≥2 nerves			
diagnosis	Requires that two nerves are abnormal for this single criterion to be met for the diagnosis of CIDP			
Bromberg (Barohn) *(3)*	As for Barohn criteria except that CV parameter may be met with only one nerve being abnormal			
INCAT *(5)*				
parameter	<80% LLN or <70% (amp < 80%)	>125% ULN or >150% (amp < 80%)	20%	>120% ULN or >150% (amp < 80%)
criteria	≥1 nerve	≥1 nerve	≥2 nerves	≥2 nerves
diagnosis	Requires (1) CB criterion and one other criterion OR (2) CV, DL or F criteria in ≥3 nerves OR (3) CV, DL or F criteria in two nerves with histological evidence for demyelination			
Saperstein *(29)*				
parameter	<80% LLN or <70% (amp < 80%)	>125% ULN or >150% (amp < 80%)	50–60%[a]	>120% ULN or >150% (amp < 80%)
criteria	≥2 nerves	≥2 nerves	≥1 nerve	≥2 nerves
diagnosis	Requires two criteria for the diagnosis of CIDP			
Van den Bergh *(6)*				
parameter	<70% LLN	>150% ULN	30–50%[b]	>120% (150%)[c] OR absent F with CMAP ≥20%
criteria	≥2 nerves	≥2 nerves	≥2 nerves	≥2 nerves
diagnosis	Any single single criterion is sufficient for the diagnosis of CIDP. May also meet criteria with CB in one nerve and one other abnormality.			

[a]50% for median and ulnar nerves; 60% for tibial and peroneal nerves.

[b]50% require for definite diagnosis of CIDP and 30% for probable diagnosis of CIDP.

[c]F-wave prolongation of 150% required if distal negative-peak CMAP < 50% of normal.

LLN, lower limit of normal; ULN, upper limit of normal; CMAP, compound muscle action potential.

Table 12.2

Accuracy of Electrophysiological Criteria for the Diagnosis of Chronic Inflammatory
Demyelinating Polyradiculoneuropathy (CIDP)

Study	Dx of CIDP	Controls	Criteria (see Table 12.1)	Sens.	Specificity	
Bromberg (3)	Clinical[a]	MND, DPN	Albers & Kelly	50%	100%	
			Bromberg (A&K)	66%	100%	
			AAN	46%	100%	
			Barohn	43%	100%	
			Bromberg (Barohn)	66%	100%	
Haq (8)	Clinical[b] & EDX	DPN	Albers & Kelly	33%	100%	
			AAN	33%	100%	
			Barohn	29%	100%	
Nicolas (7)	Clinical[b]	Axonal PN	AAN	62%	–	
			Nicolas	90%	97%	
Van den Bergh (6)	Clinical[a]	MND, DPN			ALS	DPN
			AAN	35%	100%	100%
			INCAT	43%	97%	91%
			Saperstein	57%	100%	97%
			Nicolas	50%	100%	91%
			Van den Bergh	75%	100%	100%

[a]Sensorimotor disturbance, CSF albuminocytological dissociation and response to immunosuppressive therapy.

[b]Sensorimotor disturbance, CSF albuminocytological dissociation and no requirement for therapeutic response.

MND, motor neuron disease; DPN, diabetic polyneuroapthy; PN, polyneuropathy; AAN, American Academy of Neurology; INCAT, inflammatory neuropathy cause and treatment.

The highest combination of sensitivity and specificity was reported by Nicolas and colleagues (7), using their own data. However, when these criteria were applied to another dataset, the sensitivity was significantly reduced to 50%, which is more consistent with the sensitivity of all other published criteria (6).

Based on the quality of their methodology, it is worth considering two of these papers in more detail (3,6). Bromberg examined the diagnostic accuracy of three sets of criteria—those proposed by Albers and Kelly (1), those published by the American Academy of Neurology (AAN) (2) and those proposed by Barohn and colleagues (4)—in three groups of patients, those with CIDP (n = 70), those with motor neuron disease (MND) (n = 47), and those with diabetic polyneuropathy (DPN) (n = 63) (3). The diagnosis of CIDP was (appropriately) based on clinical criteria, thus avoiding the problem of incorporation bias. The clinical criteria included a progressive, relapsing, or stepwise course characterized by weakness and sensory symptoms, cerebrospinal fluid albumino-cytological dissociation, and a response to either steroids or plasma exchange. The sensitivity and specificity are shown in Table 12.2.

Using the data from his study, Bromberg showed that the sensitivity of the Albers and Kelly and Barohn criteria could be improved by reducing the number of abnormal nerves required in order for criteria to be met. He modified the Barohn criteria such that only one nerve (rather than two) with conduction velocity less than 70% of the lower limit of normal would be required for the diagnosis of CIDP. He similarly modified the Albers and Kelly criteria such that only a single nerve (rather than two) with conduction velocity less than 75% of the lower limit of normal or distal latency more than 130% of the upper limit of normal would be required for the diagnosis of CIDP. Using these modified criteria, the sensitivity for each increased to 66% (3). This improvement in sensitivity was accomplished without compromising specificity at all.

Finally, he used his data set to determine the effect on specificity of increasing the sensitivity even further. This was accomplished by changing each nerve conduction value such that the requirement for demyelination was made less stringent. He found that there was substantial overlap in the distributions of nerve conduction values for each measurement (conduction velocity, distal latency, and so on) among the three disorders (CIDP, MND and DPN). If the threshold for defining demyelination was reduced in order to increase sensitivity to 75%, specificity plummeted to nearly 0%. His overall conclusion was that the sensitivity of 66% accomplished by the strategy outlined above was the best that could be achieved without significantly reducing specificity. The revised criteria that he suggested are summarized in Table 12.1.

Van den Bergh and colleagues examined the sensitivity and specificity of 10 published sets of diagnostic criteria for demyelinating polyneuropathy (including both Guillain-Barré syndrome [GBS] and CIDP) in their series of patients with GBS ($n = 52$), CIDP ($n = 28$), amyotrophic lateral sclerosis [ALS] ($n = 40$), and DPN ($n = 32$) (6). The sensitivity of these sets of criteria for the diagnosis of CIDP varied from 39% to 89%, with the highest sensitivities being achieved with the criteria proposed by Albers, Donofrio, and McGonagle (89%), the American GBS group criteria (82%), and the British GBS group (82%). Specificity was generally extremely good (100%) for patients with MND and more variable for patients with DPN. Overall, combining sensitivity and specificity, the best results were obtained using the criteria of the Dutch GBS Study Group (sensitivity 68%, specificity 94% for DPN and 100% for MND). The results are essentially identical to those reported by Bromberg using his modification of the AAN and Barohn criteria (these criteria were not evaluated in the Van den Bergh study). In the Van den Bergh study, sensitivity could be increased to 71%, but at the expense of reducing specificity for DPN to 91% using the Italian GBS Study Group criteria.

Van den Bergh and colleagues undertook a sensitivity analysis in order to determine what combination of stringency of abnormalities and number of abnormal nerves would be required to maximize sensitivity while preserving specificity. The criteria that they developed (summarized in Table 12.1) yielded a sensitivity of 75% and a specificity (for MND and DPN) of 100% when applied to their population of patients (6).

2.2. What Is the Utility of Nerve Biopsy in the Diagnosis of CIDP?

The utility of sural nerve biopsy as an aid to the diagnosis of CIDP remains somewhat controversial because there are conflicting published data.

In one retrospective cohort study, Molennar and colleagues recruited 64 patients in whom the diagnosis of CIDP had been considered clinically (9). These patients were subsequently categorized into those with CIDP ($n = 23$) and those without ($n = 31$), with the gold standard for the diagnosis of CIDP being made at follow-up on the basis of a relapsing-remitting neuropathy with beneficial response to immunosuppressive therapy. They collected data about six clinical variables from all patients including (1) relapsing course, (2) symmetric sensorimotor polyneuropathy in the arms and legs, (3) absent reflexes in all four limbs, (4) increased cerebrospinal fluid (CSF) protein, (5) results of neurophysiological studies, and (6) relevant clinical or laboratory features that were sufficient to attribute the neuropathy to another cause. Neurophysiological studies were taken to be indicative of demyelination based on a modification of the Albers and Kelly criteria. Sural nerve biopsy specimens were then reviewed by an investigator blinded to the clinical details. For each clinical parameter, they were able to calculate the sensitivity and specificity for the diagnosis of CIDP. The results of neurophysiological studies were found to have the highest combination of sensitivity (0.87) and specificity (0.85). These six variables were then entered into a multivariate logistic regression model, with a positive diagnosis of CIDP used as the dependent variable. This model indicated that elevated CSF protein, neurophysiological evidence for demyelination, and the absence of an alternative etiology for the neuropathy were the three factors that most strongly predicted the diagnosis of CIDP. These three variables, together with the results of sural nerve biopsy, were then entered into a second logistic regression model to determine the predictive value of sural nerve biopsy given these other clinical findings. The results of the biopsy were found to have no significant additional predictive value.

These data from the logistic regression models were buttressed by the results of a clinical test of the utility of sural nerve biopsy. A neurologist was provided with the relevant clinical details (except for the results of the biopsy) and asked to indicate their degree of certainty regarding the diagnosis of CIDP. The neurologist was able to correctly make the diagnosis of CIDP (while avoiding misdiagnoses) in 95% of cases. The biopsy results were then provided, and the investigators examined the effect of the neurologist's knowledge of the biopsy results on the final diagnosis. Diagnostic performance was not improved by the additional information provided by the biopsy.

The study by Haq and colleagues also set out to examine the diagnostic utility of sural nerve biopsy, although the study design was quite different. These investigators selected 24 patients who were known to have CIDP and who had undergone sural nerve biopsy, as well as 12 patients who were known to have DPN who had also had a sural nerve biopsy. The diagnosis of CIDP was made on the basis of the criteria proposed by Dyck, which included symmetric distal and/or proximal limb involvement (sensory or motor), mainly large fiber sensory loss when present, progressive or relapsing course lasting at least 8 weeks, CSF albumino-cytological dissociation, and electrodiagnostic features of a demyelinating neuropathy. There was no requirement for a response to immunosuppressive therapy. The biopsies were then reviewed in a blinded fashion by three investigators who were asked to determine whether the pathological criteria for demyelination (as defined by the AAN Ad Hoc Subcommittee) were met. Separate determinations were made based on the results of teased fiber preparation and the results of electron microscopy. They were then able to determine the sensitivity and specificity of the biopsy results for the diagnosis of CIDP. The results of teased fiber preparations showed a sensitivity of 50% and a specificity of 83%. The results of electron microscropy showed improved sensitivity and specificity of 79% and 91%, respectively. The authors argued that the relatively greater sensitivity of nerve biopsy findings compared with published electrodiagnostic criteria argues in favor of the utility of sural nerve biopsy in the diagnostic evaluation of patients who may have CIDP.

Haq and colleagues offered two explanations for the improved sensitivity and speci-ficity of sural nerve biopsy in their study compared with the study by Molenaar et al. The first is that they used electron microscopy much more frequently than did the prior study, in which almost one-half of the biopsies were not examined using this technique. The second explanation provided is that the study by Molennar and colleagues employed electrophysiological criteria with already high sensitivity and that biopsy would not, therefore, be expected to add much more diagnostically under such circumstances. The strength, however, of the study by Molenaar lies in the choice of the study population. These authors included all patients with possible diagnosis of CIDP rather than employ-ing the approach adopted by Haq and colleagues, which was to select two very different populations—those with definite CIDP and those definitely without CIDP. In part for this reason and in part because sural nerve biopsy is appropriately used only after the results of clinical evaluation and electrodiagnostic studies have been performed, the study by Molenaar and colleagues more accurately reflects the clinical scenario. Thus, although limited by not having used electron microscopy very frequently, the study by Molenaar and colleagues is of better quality and supports the idea that sural nerve biopsy has relatively little predictive value for the diagnosis of CIDP over and above the clinical evaluation and results of routine electrophysiological testing.

3. TREATMENT

3.1. What Is the Evidence That Steroids Are of Benefit to Patients With CIDP?

The utility of prednisolone in the treatment of CIDP has been examined in a single quasi-randomized trial (10). Patients with CIDP who had not previously received immu-nosuppressive therapy were eligible for inclusion in this study. Patients who fulfilled entry criteria were well matched for age, duration of symptoms, and initial neurology disability scale scores. Subjects were randomized to receive either prednisolone or no treatment. Prednisolone was initiated at 120 mg every other day with 5 mg per day on the alternate days, and was tapered over a period of 13 weeks. Forty patients were enrolled, but only 28 patients completed the trial, with 14 in each group. The neurological disability score (a summed score of muscle strength, reflexes and sensory loss) was used as a measure of outcome, with patients evaluated at 6 weeks and then at 3 months. The results are summarized in Table 12.3.

In the no-treatment group, the mean neurological disability score (NDS) change was −1.5 (worsening), compared with +10 points (improvement) in the prednisolone group.

There are a number of methodological flaws in this study. First, the technique used for randomization was inadequate in that the first patient of each pair was randomized and the second patient of each pair simply received the alternative treatment. The implication is that treatment allocation was not concealed. Second, patients could not have been blinded because there was no placebo, and no mention is made of whether the investiga-tors were blinded to the treatment group to which patients were assigned. Third, the final analysis included only those patients who completed the study, i.e., an intention-to-treat analysis was not performed. This may have introduced significant bias because the drop-out rate was 30% (i.e., only 28 of 40 randomized subjects completed the study). When the subject of corticosteroids for the treatment of CIDP was reviewed by the Cochrane

Table 12.3

Efficacy of Prednisolone in the Treatment of Chronic Inflammatory Demyelinating
Polyradiculoneuropathy

Change in neurological disability score	No-treatment group[a]	Prednisone group[a]
Worse	8 (57%)	2 (14%)
Unchanged	1 (7%)	0
Improved	5 (36%)	12 (86%)

[a]Values refer to numbers of patients.
Data from ref. *10*

Collaboration, the authors undertook a sensitivity analysis in order to determine the
extent to which the results of this study might have differed if all randomized patients had
been included in the final analysis *(11)*. In this analysis, the authors imputed the worst
outcome for all patients excluded from the original analysis. In doing so, they found that
the results indicated a trend in favor of prednisolone, but the results were no longer
significant.

Apart from the data from this single randomized study, there are data from a number
of large uncontrolled case series that suggest a beneficial effect from steroids *(4,12,13)*.

Considering the results of the single randomized study as well as the data from the
uncontrolled case series, the conclusion seems to be that prednisolone leads to a small but
significant improvement in disability in previously untreated patients with CIDP. The
latency from the start of treatment to the onset of improvement is unclear, with the
available data suggesting that the norm is 4–8 weeks, but that it may take as long as 5
months *(4,12)*.

3.2. Is Intravenous Immunoglobulin Effective in the Treatment of Patients With CIDP?

The efficacy of intravenous immunoglobulin (IVIg) in the treatment of patients with
CIDP has been the subject of four randomized placebo-controlled trials *(14–17)*. IVIg has
also been compared with plasmapheresis in one study *(18)* and with oral prednisolone in
another *(5)*. The four placebo-controlled trials will be examined here. Two of these
employed a cross-over design *(14,16)* and two used a parallel group design *(15,17)*.
Details of the dosing and duration of IVIg use in these trials as well as the outcome
measures used and an assessment of study quality are summarized in Table 12.4.

In the individual studies, a clinical response (defined as a significant improvement in
disability) was observed in as few as 27% *(17)* and as many as 63% *(14)* of IVIg-treated
patients. Although each trial used a different scoring system to evaluate outcome, which
makes it difficult to provide an overall summary of the effect of IVIg, a significant
improvement in disability (as determined by each study) was reported in 37 of the 82
patients (45%) who received IVIg compared with 10 of 67 (15%) placebo-treated patients
(pooled relative risk of 3.17 with 95% confidence interval ranging from 1.74 to 5.75). In
a recent systematic review by the Cochrane Collaboration, the authors used the modified
Rankin scale (mRS) to compare treatment effects across studies *(19)*. One trial reported
outcome using the mRS *(17)*, and data from two other studies could be transformed to

Table 12.4
Trials of IVIg in the Treatment of CIDP

	Hahn (14)	Mendell (15)	Thompson (16)	Vermuelen (17)	Dyck (18)	Hughes (5)
Treatment Study design	IVIg vs placebo Double-blind, cross-over	IVIg vs placebo Double-blind, parallel group	IVIg vs placebo Double-blind, cross-over	IVIg vs placebo Double-blind, parallel group	IVIg vs PE Single blind, cross-over	IVIg vs steroids Double-blind, cross-over
Sample size	$n = 30$ IVIg (25) Placebo (25)	$n = 53$ IVIg (30) Placebo (23)	$n = 7$ IVIg (7) Placebo (7)	$n = 28$ IVIg (15) Placebo (13)	$n = 20$ IVIg (15) PE (17)	$n = 32$ IVIg (24) Steroids (24)
Intervention	0.4 g/kg/d × 5 d	1 g/kg/d × 2 d	0.4 g/kg/d × 5 d	0.4 g/kg/d × 5 d	0.4 g/kg/wk × 3 wk, 0.2 g/kg/wk × 3 wk vs PE 2/wk × 3 wk, PE 1/wk × 3 wk	Equivalent of 1 g/kg/d × 2 d vs 60 mg/d × 2 wk, 40 mg/d × 1 wk, 30 mg/d × 1 wk, 20 mg/d × 1 wk, 10 mg/d × 1 wk
Primary outcome	Neurological disability score	Average muscle score	Hammersmith motor ability score	modified Rankin scale	Neurological disability score	INCAT disability scale
Secondary outcomes	Clinical grade, hand grip, electrophysiology	Hughes functional disability scale, FVC, electrophysiology	Timed 10 m walk, MRC sum score, myometry		Summed CMAP of ulnar, median & peroneal nerves, summed SNAP of median & sural, vibration detection threshold	Timed 10 m walk, modified Rankin scale, SF-36, MRC sum score, grip strength and others
Study quality	Adequate concealment of allocation	Adequate concealment of allocation; no ITT analysis	Unclear allocation concealment	Adequate allocation concealment	Unclear allocation concealment; investigators & patients not blinded	Adequate allocation of concealment

INCAT, inflammatory neuropathy cause and treatment; PE, plasma exchange; FVC, forced vital capacity; CMAP, compound muscle action potential; SNAP, sensory nerve action potential; MRC, Medical Research Council; ITT, intention-to-treat.

produce an mRS score *(15,16)*. Summarizing the data from these three studies, an improvement of at least one point on the mRS was noted in 16/51 patients treated with IVIg and 5/42 patients receiving placebo (pooled relative risk of 2.47 with 95% confidence interval ranging from 1.02 to 6.01) *(19)*. The mean improvement in disability was 0.17–0.4 points in patients treated with IVIg and 0.00–0.23 points in those receiving placebo *(19)*.

Open follow-up was available for all but one patient following completion of one of the controlled trials *(14)*. It became apparent that patients with relapsing CIDP obtained only temporary benefit from any single course of IVIg. A response to repeat courses of IVIg, however, was consistently observed. Although the duration of treatment benefit varied considerably, it could be fairly reliably predicted for each patient. In this way, nine patients were maintained on long term IVIg pulse therapy, with infusions administered either at the earliest sign of relapse or just before the anticipated relapse. The dose of IVIg could usually be tapered down to ≤ 1 g/kg body weight and administered as a single-day infusion. A few patients required the addition of a small dose of prednisolone to their regular IVIg infusions.

These data, therefore, suggest that IVIg is effective in the treatment of patients with CIDP, although fewer than one-half of patients treated with IVIg will show a significant improvement in their level of disability. Furthermore, the effect of IVIg is often not lasting in patients with relapsing-remitting disease, and these patients may require regular infusions in order to maintain a clinical response.

3.3. How Does IVIg Compare With Plasma Exchange in the Treatment of Patients With CIDP?

IVIg and plasma exchange (PE) were compared head-to-head in a single (observer)-blinded study *(18)* (Table 12.4). This trial included patients with static or worsening disability who had not received PE or IVIg in the preceding 6 weeks and in whom there had been no change in their maintenance immunotherapy within the same time period. PE was performed twice weekly for the first 3 weeks and once weekly for the second 3 weeks. IVIg was administered at a dose of 0.4 g/kg once per week for the first three weeks and 0.2 g/kg once per week for the second 3 weeks. The 6-week course of PE or IVIg was followed by a washout period of variable duration. Those who failed to respond to the initial therapy or who relapsed (to their original level of disability) were then crossed over to receive the alternative therapy. In total, 17 patients were treated with PE and 15 received IVIg. Primary end-points included NDS, the weakness subset of the NDS, and the summated compound muscle action potential (CMAP) of ulnar, median, and peroneal nerves. Secondary end-points were the summated sensory nerve action potential (SNAP) of median and sural nerves and vibratory detection threshold of the great toe. Endpoints were examined at the end of each 6-week study period. Patients who received either PE or IVIg (as either the first or second treatment) showed significant and comparable improvement from baseline in all three primary end-points. Of the 17 patients who received PE in either phase, the mean NDS improvement was 38.3 points. Of the 15 patients who received IVIg in either phase, the mean NDS improvement was 36.1 points. The similar degree of improvement observed with each treatment modality suggests that they are of equal efficacy.

3.4. How Does IVIg Compare With Corticosteroids for the Treatment of CIDP?

IVIg and oral prednisolone have been compared head-to-head in a single randomized controlled trial with a cross-over design *(5)* (Table 12.4). Patients were randomized to receive a single treatment with IVIg (2 g/kg administered over 1–2 days) or oral corticosteroids for 2 weeks (*see* Table 12.4), with outcome evaluated after 2 weeks. The intention was to allow a 4-week washout period before patients were crossed over to receive the second treatment. Thirty-two patients were randomized, with only 24 completing both treatment periods. Although not available from the published paper, the number of patients who showed an improvement of at least one Inflammatory Neuropathy Cause and Treatment (INCAT) disability grade was reported in 9 of 16 IVIg treatments and 8 of 13 prednisolone treatments in a Cochrane systematic review *(19)*. These results confirm the efficacy of both oral steroids and IVIg, but the study was not adequately powered to detect a difference in efficacy between the two treatment modalities.

3.5. Is Plasmapheresis Effective in the Treatment of Patients With CIDP?

The role of plasmapheresis has been examined in two prospective placebo-controlled trials *(20,21)*. In the first, Dyck et al. *(20)* randomized 34 patients with CIDP to receive plasma exchange or sham exchange. Randomization was stratified according to age (<50 or ≥50), gender, and (<100 or ≥100). The controlled trial lasted 3 weeks, whereafter those who received sham exchange were offered PE (open trial). Neurological evaluation was performed at weekly intervals for the duration of the controlled and open trials. Evaluation included measurement of NDS, dynamometer measurement of maximal handgrip, maximal finger pinch, and maximal inspiratory and expiratory pressures as well as sensory thresholds. Nerve conduction studies were performed both before and after PE. Twenty-nine patients completed the controlled study—15 assigned to PE and 14 to sham exchange. No subjective differences were reported between patients randomized to the two treatment groups. At 3 weeks, five patients receiving PE had an improvement in NDS compared with baseline (Δ NDS) that exceeded the largest improvement attained by any patient who received sham exchange. The authors describe these results as "striking differences ... between the two treatment groups," but it should be noted that there was significant overlap in the ΔNDS between the two treatment groups, and results for mean ΔNDS for the two treatment groups are not reported. Improvement in nerve conduction indexes favored PE, but this observation is tempered by the observation of almost significant differences in these indexes between the treatment groups at baseline.

Building on these results, Hahn et al. *(21)* designed a double-blind placebo-controlled trial of PE in patients with CIDP. They recruited only patients who had not previously and were not currently receiving other forms of immunosuppressive therapy. Eighteen patients were randomized to receive either plasma or sham exchange (10 exchanges over a 4-week period) followed by a washout phase, cross-over for a month of the alternate therapy, and then a second washout phase. The outcome measures employed were similar to those used in the Mayo study *(20)*, in order to facilitate comparison of the results of the two studies. Three of the 18 patients failed to complete the trial, but the results are reported using an intention-to-treat analysis. With PE, significant improvement was observed on all outcome measures. A substantial improvement in neurological function was found in 12 of 15 (80%) patients, with a mean NDS change of 38 points for the group as a whole.

This improvement was typically evident within days of starting treatment. Significant improvements in electrophysiological measures (motor nerve conduction velocity, distal latency, and CMAP amplitude) were also found. Eight of the 12 patients (66%) who improved with PE, subsequently relapsed after stopping PE with the deterioration occurring within 7–14 days of the last exchange. The authors conclude that a beneficial effect from PE could be expected early in the course of CIDP provided that the clinical, electrophysiological, and histological features were those of primary demyelination without secondary axonal loss.

The results of this study were more impressive than those of the initial study of PE by Dyck et al. *(20)* (80% vs 33% rate of improvement). This difference may relate, at least in part, to the more aggressive schedule of PE employed in this study.

3.6. Is There Evidence to Support the Use of Cytotoxic Drugs in the Treatment of CIDP?

The body of literature relevant to the use of cytotoxic drugs for the treatment of CIDP is a small one, mostly comprised of case reports and small case series. In a recent systematic review on the subject published by the Cochrane collaboration *(22)*, the authors identified one randomized controlled trial comparing the combination of azathioprine and prednisolone with prednisolone alone *(23)* as well as a randomized, placebo-controlled, cross-over study of β-interferon-1a in patients with treatment-resistant CIDP *(24)*. Neither study showed a beneficial effect on any of the outcome measures used.

4. PROGNOSIS

4.1. What Is the Long-Term Outcome of Patients With CIDP Who Are Treated With Aggressive Immunosuppressive Therapy?

The only studies to have addressed long-term outcome of sizable cohorts of patients with CIDP are retrospective *(25–28)*. Most have used the mRS as a measure of functional outcome *(25,27,28)*. Each study included both patients with idiopathic CIDP and patients with CIDP associated with a monoclonal gammopathy of undetermined significance, although the outcomes were not always reported separately for these two groups. In none of these papers was outcome classified according to the treatment received. The overwhelming majority of patients in each study had been treated with aggressive immunosuppressive therapy usually comprising prednisolone, IVIg and/or PE. The outcomes at final follow-up are shown in Table 12.5.

As shown in Table 12.5, approximately 70–75% of patients with CIDP will have only slight or no residual disability following appropriate therapy.

A few of these studies tried to determine which factors, if any, were most predictive of a favorable outcome, although there is little agreement between these studies. Choudhary and Hughes suggested that female gender was the only factor associated with a better outcome, finding no association with younger age of onset, mean duration of disease, and pretreatment disability grade *(26)*. Sghirlanzoni and colleagues, on the other hand, suggested that younger age and relapsing-remitting disease (rather than monophasic progressive disease) as well as the presence of demyelinating electrophysiology without secondary axonal loss were predictive of a better outcome *(25)*. Two studies have shown that the outcome is no different between those with idiopathic CIDP and those with

Table 12.5

Prognosis for Chronic Inflammatory Demyelinating Polyradiculoneuropathy (CIDP) Patients
Treated With Aggressive Immunotherapy

Modified Rankin scale score	*Gorson* (27) (n = 60)	*Simmons* (28) (n = 94)	*Sghirlanzoni* (25) (n = 60)
0—no symptoms at all	4 (6.7%)	29 (30.9%)	15 (25%)
1—no significant disability carry out all previous activities, 2—slight disability (unable to but otherwise independent)	38 (63.3%)	49 (52.1%)	30 (50%)
3—moderate disability (requires some help, but able to walk without assistance) 4—moderately severe disability (requires assistance for bodily needs) 5—severe disability (requiring constant nursing)	18 (30%)	12 (12.8%)	12 (20%)
Death due to CIDP	–	*4 (4.3%)*	*3 (5%)*

monoclonal gammopathy of undetermined significance (MGUS)-associated CIDP
(27,28).

5. SUMMARY

- There are numerous published criteria that have been used to define the presence of an acquired demyelinating neuropathy, many of which have simply been suggested without adequate supportive experimental data.
- Most criteria rely on some combination of slowed conduction velocity, prolonged distal latency, prolonged or absent F-responses, conduction block, and temporal dispersion.
- Maximum sensitivity of 66–75% has been reported for the criteria published by Bromberg and Van den Bergh, respectively.
- Specificities as high as 100% have been reported, but these are almost certainly overestimates given the nature of the populations that have been studied (i.e., inappropriate choice of control groups).
- The available evidence suggests that sural nerve biopsy has relatively low predictive value for the diagnosis of CIDP given the results of clinical evaluation and electrophysiological testing.
- The results of a single randomized study as well as the data from the uncontrolled case series support the conclusion that prednisolone leads to a small but significant improvement in disability in previously untreated patients with CIDP; the latency from treatment to improvement is typically 4–8 weeks, but may be even longer.
- IVIg is effective in the treatment of patients with CIDP, although fewer than one-half of patients treated with IVIg will show a significant improvement in their level of disability; furthermore, the effect is often relatively short-lived and patients may require regular infusions in order to maintain a clinical response.
- Response rates for patients with CIDP following plasmapheresis have ranged from 33% to 80%, depending on the frequency with which exchanges are administered.

- The available evidence suggests that IVIg and plasmapheresis have equivalent efficacy in patients with CIDP.
- The body of literature relevant to the use of cytotoxic drugs for the treatment of CIDP is a small one, mostly comprised of case reports and small case series; there are no data from randomized controlled trials to support the use of these agents.
- Approximately 70–75% of patients with CIDP will have only slight or no residual disability following appropriate therapy.

REFERENCES

1. Albers JW, Kelly JJ. Acquired inflammatory demyelinating polyneuropathies: clinical and electrodiagnostic features. Muscle Nerve 1989;12:435–451.
2. Research criteria for diagnosis of chronic inflammatory demyelinating polyneuropathy (CIDP). Report from an Ad Hoc Subcommittee of the American Academy of Neurology AIDS Task Force. Neurology 1991;41:617–618.
3. Bromberg MB, Feldman EL, Albers JW. Chronic inflammatory demyelinating polyradiculoneuropathy: Comparison of patients with and without an associated monoclonal gammopathy. Neurology 1992;42:1157–1163.
4. Barohn RJ, Kissel JT, Warmolts JR, Mendell JR. Chronic inflammatory demyelinating polyradiculoneuropathy. Clinical characteristics, course, and recommendations for diagnostic criteria. Arch Neurol 1989;46:878–884.
5. Hughes R, Bensa S, Willison H, et al. Randomized controlled trial of intravenous immunoglobulin versus oral prednisone in chronic inflammatory demyelinating polyradiculoneuropathy. Ann Neurol 2001;50:195–201.
6. Van den Bergh PY, Pieret F. Electrodiagnostic criteria for acute and chronic inflammatory demyelinating polyradiculoneuropathy. Muscle Nerve 2004;29:565–574.
7. Nicolas G, Maisonobe T, Le Forestier N, Leger J-M, Bouche P. Proposed revised electrophysiological criteria for chronic inflammatory demyelinating polyradiculoneuropathy. Muscle Nerve 2002;25:26–30.
8. Haq RU, Fries TJ, Pendlebury WW, Kenny MJ, Badger GJ, Tandan R. Chronic inflammatory demyelinating polyradiculoneuropathy. A study of proposed electrodiagnostic and histologic criteria. Arch Neurol 2000;57:1745–1750.
9. Molenaar DS, Vermuelen M, de Haan R. Diagnostic value of sural nerve biopsy in chronic inflammatory demyelinating polyneuropathy. J Neurol Neurosurg Psychiatry 1998;64:84–89.
10. Dyck P, O'Brien P, Oviatt K, Dinapoli R, Daube J, Barleston J. Prednisone improves chronic inflammatory demyelinating polyradiculoneuropathy more than no treatment. Ann Neurol 1982;11:136–141.
11. Mehndiratta M, Hughes R. Corticosteroids for chronic inflammatory demyelinating polyradiculoneuropathy. Cochrane Database Systematic Reviews 2004; 2:CD002062.
12. Dalakas M, Engel W. Chronic relapsing (dysimmune) polyneuropathy: pathogenesis and treatment. Ann Neurol 1981;9(Suppl):134–145.
13. McCombe P, Pollard J, McLeod J. Chronic inflammatory demyelinating polyradiculoneuropathy. A clinical and electrophysiological study of 92 cases. Brain 1987;110:1617–1630.
14. Hahn A, Bolton C, Zochodne D, Feasby T. Intravenous immunoglobulin treatment in chronic inflammatory demyelinating polyneuropathy. A double-blind, placebo-controlled, cross-over study. Brain 1996;119:1067–1077.
15. Mendell J, Barohn R, Freimer M, et al. Randomized controlled trial of IVIg in untreated chronic inflammatory demyelinating polyradiculoneuropathy. Neurology 2001;56:445–449.
16. Thompson N, Choudhary P, Hughes R, Quinlivan R. A novel trial design to study the effect of intravenous immunoglobulin in chronic inflammatory demyelinating polyradiculoneuropathy. J Neurol 1996;243:280–285.
17. Vermeulen M, van Doorn P, Brand A, Strengers P, Jennekens F, Busch H. Intravenous immunoglobulin treatment in patients with chronic inflammatory demyelinating polyneuropathy: a double-blind, placebo-controlled study. J Neurol Neurosurg Psychiatry 1993;56:36–39.
18. Dyck P, Litchy W, Kratz K, et al. A plasma exchange versus immune globulin infusion trial in chronic inflammatory demyelinating polyradiculoneuropathy. Ann Neurol 1994;36:838–845.

19. Van Schaik I, Winer J, De Haan R, Vermeulen M. Intravenous immunoglobulin for chronic inflammatory demyelinating polyradiculoneuropathy. Cochrane Database Systematic Reviews 2004; 2:CD001797.

20. Dyck P, Daube J, O'Brien P, et al. Plasma exchange in chronic inflammatory demyelinating polyradiculoneuropathy. N Engl J Med 1986;314:461–465.

21. Hahn A, Bolton C, Pillay N, et al. Plasma-exchange therapy in chronic inflammatory demyelinating polyneuropathy. A double-blind, sham-controlled, cross-over study. Brain 1996;119:1055–1066.

22. Hughes R, Swan A, van Doorn P. Cytotoxic drugs and interferons for chronic inflammatory demyelinating polyradiculoneuropathy. Cochrane Database Systematic Reviews 2004;2:CD003280.

23. Dyck P, O'Brien P, Swanson C, Low P, Daube J. Combined azathioprine and prednisone in chronic inflammatory-demyelinating polyneuropathy. Neurology 1985;35.

24. Hadden R, Sharrack B, Bensa S, Soudain S, Hughes R. Randomized trial of interferon-beta-1a in chronic inflammatory demyelinating polyradiculoneuropathy. Neurology 1999;53:57–61.

25. Sghirlanzoni A, Solari A, Ciano C, Mariotti C, Fallica E, Pareyson D. Chronic inflammatory demyelinating polyradiculoneuropathy: long-term course and treatment of 60 patients. Neurol Sci 2000;21:31–37.

26. Choudhary P, Hughes R. Long-term treatment of chronic inflammatory demyelinating polyradiculoneuropathy with plasma exchange or intravenous immunoglobulin. QJM 1995;88:493–502.

27. Gorson KC, Allam G, Ropper AH. Chronic inflammatory demyelinating polyneuropathy: Clinical features and response to treatment in 67 consecutive patients with and without a monoclonal gammopathy. Neurology 1997;48:321–328.

28. Simmons Z, Albers JW, Bromberg MB, Feldman EL. Long-term follow-up of patients with chronic inflammatory demyelinating polyradiculoneuropathy, without and with monoclonal gammopathy. Brain 1995;118:359–368.

29. Saperstein DS, Katz JJ, Amato AA, Barohn RJ. Clinical spectrum of chronic acquired demyelinating polyneuropathies. Muscle Nerve 2001;24:311–324.

13 Multifocal Motor Neuropathy

1. INTRODUCTION

Multifocal motor neuropathy (MMN) is a relatively recently recognized clinical entity that was formally described by Parry and Clark in the mid-1980s (1,2). The clinical presentation in each of the patients in this original series had suggested a diagnosis of motor neuron disease, but nerve conduction studies showed multifocal conduction block in motor nerves. The recognition that this syndrome represented a form of a chronic demyelinating neuropathy has spawned much debate regarding its relationship to other chronic demyelinating neuropathies such as chronic inflammatory demyelinating polyradiculoneuropathy (CIDP) and the Lewis-Sumner syndrome, and has also raised the possibility that patients with the disorder might respond to immunosuppressive therapy. What are the clinical and electrophysiological features of MMN, and how does it differ from other chronic demyelinating neuropathies? What is the diagnostic accuracy of anti-GM1 antibodies? Do patients with MMN respond to immunosuppressive therapy, and what is the long term prognosis for patients with this disorder? These and other questions are the focus of this chapter.

2. DIAGNOSIS

2.1. What Are the Typical Clinical Manifestations of MMN?

MMN is a syndrome first described in detail by Parry and Clark in the mid 1980s (1,2) and since recognized and reported by a number of other investigators (3–9). The literature on MMN largely comprises case series in which patients were included based on the presence of particular clinical symptoms and findings on examination, with or without the presence of specific electrophysiological features—typically, conduction block in motor nerves with normal sensory nerve conduction studies.

Because the clinical features have been used to define the syndrome (i.e., have served as the gold standard for the diagnosis), there is no objective way of determining the range of clinical manifestations that may be seen in this disorder. Many case series have described the clinical features of a group of patients, but estimation of the spectrum of clinical manifestations that may be encountered is constrained by the clinical criteria that were used to select patients for inclusion in the study. For example, because most case series only included patients with no or minimal sensory symptoms, it is not surprising that sensory symptoms and signs have been reported to occur very infrequently in patients with MMN. A few studies have included patients on the basis of electrophysiological criteria alone (6), and these provide more meaningful characterization of the clinical manifestations of the disorder.

From: *Neuromuscular Disease: Evidence and Analysis in Clinical Neurology*
By: M. Benatar © Humana Press Inc., Totowa, NJ

In their original report, Parry and Clark described five patients who were initially erroneously diagnosed with motor neuron disease *(2)*. The descriptions since then *(3,5–9)* have, for the most part, reiterated the clinical features described in the original case series (Table 13.1). One subtle refinement of the clinical syndrome was recognized by Krarup and colleagues in their description of three patients with this syndrome who had relatively little atrophy in muscles with marked weakness *(4)*. The larger case series have consistently shown that men are more commonly affected than women, and that disease onset is typically in the fifth decade of life. Weakness is most commonly distal, with the hands affected more frequently than the feet. Atrophy is common, although less marked than might be expected on the basis of the severity of weakness. Cramps and fasciculations are variable. Minor sensory symptoms may be present, but sensory findings on examination are minimal or absent (Table 13.1).

2.2. How Frequently Does Conduction Block Occur in MMN, and Is There a Predilection for Involvement of Proximal or Distal Nerve Segments?

Whether conduction block is always found in MMN depends in part on how the disorder is defined. If the diagnostic criteria require the presence of conduction block, then it will, by definition, be present in all patients. The question is more meaningful, however, if the syndrome is defined clinically. Before considering the evidence, it is helpful to clarify a few concepts. Conduction block is typically defined as a reduction in response amplitude following proximal stimulation relative to the response amplitude following distal stimulation. Although there is general agreement that an amplitude reduction of 50% or more is sufficient to define conduction block, controversy persists as to whether 20–49% reductions should also be taken to imply the presence of conduction block. One approach has been to define amplitude reduction of $\geq 50\%$ as definite conduction block and amplitude reduction of 20–49% as partial conduction block. In defining the presence of conduction block it is also necessary to consider the degree of temporal dispersion—that is, the extent to which the duration of the proximal response is increased relative to that of the distal response. Because the amplitude of a response will decline as a function of increasing temporal dispersion (because of phase cancellation), amplitude reduction should only be used to define conduction block when there is little temporal dispersion (typically less than 15%). In the presence of more marked temporal dispersion, conduction block should rather be defined in terms of a reduction in the area of the response between distal and proximal sites of stimulation.

It should also be recalled that routine nerve conduction studies only examine relatively distal segments of nerves. Median and ulnar nerve studies do not evaluate nerve segments more proximal to just above the elbow, and peroneal and tibial conduction studies do not examine nerve segments more proximal than the popliteal fossa. In order to evaluate more proximal nerve segments in the upper limbs, for example, it is necessary to stimulate nerves in the axilla, at Erb's point, and/or at the level of the spinal roots. If conduction blocks occur exclusively in proximal nerve segments, they will not be detected by routine nerve conduction studies. In considering studies that have incorporated such proximal stimulation, it is important to be aware of the technical difficulties inherent to proximal nerve segment stimulation. Because it is difficult to administer supramaximal stimuli to proximal nerve segments, reductions in response amplitude may reflect submaximal stimulation rather than true conduction block. One approach to ensuring that a stimulus

Table 13.1
Clinical Features of Multifocal Motor Neuropathy

Reference	n	Inclusion criteria	Mean age (range)	M:F	Initial symptoms	Atrophy	Reflexes	Sensation
Pestronk (7)	25	Nonfamilial, asymmetric, LMN weakness & wasting with CB	46 (24–69)	17:8	Hand (21) Foot (2)	25	Present—9 Absent—13	No symptoms or signs
Chaudhry (9)	9	Chronic progressive, distal weakness with evidence of CB	44 (26–59)	7:2	Hand (6) Foot (3)	Not stated	Asymmetric reduction in reflexes	None—patients with senory symptoms were excluded
Bouche (6)	24	Persistent multifocal CB in motor nerves	50	20:4	Hand (21) Foot (3)	15	↓/absent (17) normal (6) brisk (1)	No symptoms or signs
Katz (8)	16	Weakness in distribution of ≥ 2 peripheral nerves (excluded bulbar, facial, & respiratory weakness as well as pain or sensory deficits)	48	12:4	Hand (48) Legs (8)	Not stated	Not stated	None by definition (see inclusion criteria)
Federico (26)	16	Asymmetric lower motor neuron syndrome without sensory or bulbar signs and CB (>30%) in motor nerves	44 (26–64)	15:1	Hand (14) Arm (1) Foot (1)	Mild (4) Moderate (5) Severe (7)	Asymmetric reduction reduction in areas of weakness in all patients	Normal sensory examination in all by definition (see inclusion criteria)
Nobile-Orazio (40)	23	Asymmetric limb weakness affecting muscles of ≥2 nerves & without sensory or upper motor neuron signs	40 (21–62)	14:9	Arm (15) Leg (3) Arm + Leg (5)	Not stated	Not stated	Mild sensory signs (2)

LMN, lower motor neuron; CB, conduction block.

225

of adequate intensity has been delivered is only to accept a fall in response amplitude as being due to conduction block if a response of normal amplitude can be elicited with contralateral stimulation.

Finally, it should be remembered that routine nerve conduction studies will not readily detect conduction block in nerve segments that lie distal to the most distal site of stimulation during the study. For example, the most distal site of stimulation during routine median and ulnar nerve conduction studies is the wrist. Conduction block distal to the wrist will yield small response amplitudes that do not decrease further following more proximal stimulation. Such a pattern of diffusely reduced response amplitude along the length of a nerve is usually taken to imply an axonal process, but this is not necessarily the case. It is, therefore, at least theoretically possible that conduction block may be responsible for the electrophysiological finding of diffusely reduced response amplitudes.

In the light of these considerations, we turn now to the evidence that informs on the questions posed at the beginning of this section. The study by Katz and colleagues is one of the few that defined patients with MMN on purely clinical grounds (i.e., did not require the presence of conduction block for the diagnosis) *(8)*. Of the 16 patients included in this study, conduction block was present in 15 (94%). Pakiam and Parry described five patients with the clinical syndrome of MMN in whom careful electrophysiological testing showed other features of demyelination, but no conduction block *(10)*. Interestingly, rapid clinical and electrical improvement was noted in three of the four patients in this series who were treated with intravenous immunoglobulin (IVIg), suggesting that conduction block rather than axonal degeneration was responsible for the responses that had initially been either absent or markedly reduced in amplitude.

The relative frequencies with which blocks are identified in proximal and distal nerve segments are summarized in Table 13.2A. These estimates vary substantially, but seem to suggest that proximal and distal conduction block occur with approximately equal frequency. Perhaps more important is the observation that proximal conduction block in the absence of distal conduction block in at least one other nerve within the same patient may occur, although the frequency with which it does has varied between 12.5% *(8)* and 80% *(11)* in different studies. The reasons for this wide variation are unclear, and from the available data it cannot be concluded that the finding of isolated conduction block is a function of testing insufficient number of nerves. Although this may be true in some of the studies *(8,11,12)*, it is not true of others *(2,4)* (*see* Table 13.2B).

In conclusion, therefore, conduction block is the most commonly encountered electrophysiological abnormality in patients with MMN and is typically, although not always, present in both proximal and more distal nerve segments. In a significant minority of patients, conduction block may only be present in more proximal nerve segments, with the implication that this electrophysiological feature may be missed if more proximal nerve segments are not examined.

2.3. Is Conduction Block the Only Electrophysiological Finding in Patients With MMN?

The published data suggest that nerve conduction studies in patients with MMN frequently show other signs of demyelination in addition to the finding of multifocal motor conduction block. With one exception *(8)* most studies suggest that conduction velocity slowing is encountered in 40% *(2,13)* to 100% *(4)*, F-wave abnormalities in 50 *(3,8)* to

Table 13.2A
Electrophysiological Features of Multifocal Motor Neuropathy

Reference	n	Distal CB	Proximal CB	CV slowing	DL prolongation	F prolongation
Parry (2)	5	4 (80%)	4 (80%)	2 (40%)	not reported	not reported
Pestronk (3)	2	Both with block, but site not specified		1 (50%)	0	1 (50%)
Krarup (4)	3	3 (100%)	not reported	3 (100%)	1 (33%)	not reported
Comi (11)	5	1 (20%)	4 (80%)	0	not reported	Absent in 3 (60%)
Chaudhry (12)	9	6 (67%)	6 (67%)	7 (78%)[a]	4 (44%)[b]	9 (100%)[b]
Katz (8)	16	9 (56%)	4 (25%)	12 (75%)[a]	7 (44%)[c]	8 (50%)[c]
Nobile-Orazio (13)	5	5 (100%)	2 (40%)	2 (40%)[a]	not reported	not reported
Pestronk (7)	76	25 (33%) but site not specified	Detailed electrophysiological results not reported			

CB, conduction block; CV, conduction velocity; DL, distal latency.

[a]Slowing to less than 70% of the lower limit of normal.

[b]Distal latency/F-response prolonged by ≥125%.

[c]Distal latency/F-response prolonged by ≥120%.

Table 13.2B
Proximal Conduction Block (CB) in Multifocal Motor Neuropathy

Reference	n	Number of patients with isolated proximal CB	Number of nerves studied
Parry (2)	5	2	6–7
Krarup (4)	3	0	4
Comi (11)	5	4	2–4
Chaudhry (12)	9	3	1–2
Katz (8)	16	2	1–2
Nobile-Orazio (13)	5	0	–

227

100% *(12)*, and prolongation of distal latency is present in 33% *(4)* to 44% *(8,12)* of patients with MMN (Table 13.2A). Most patients with MMN, therefore, also manifest other electrophysiological features that suggest the presence of a demyelinating neuropathy.

2.4. What Are the Typical Cerebrospinal Fluid Findings in MMN?

Cerebrospinal fluid (CSF) protein concentration has been reported in many, but not all, series of patients with MMN. As shown in Table 13.3. CSF protein is normal in the majority of patients and, when CSF protein concentration is increased, the elevation is typically mild. Very few studies have explicitly reported the CSF cell count *(13)*, but for those studies in which the results of lumbar puncture were reported, it seems reasonable to conclude that failure to mention the presence of a pleocytosis implies its absence. The overall impression, therefore, is that the CSF is usually normal in MMN, with the occasional exception of a mild increase in protein concentration.

2.5. What Is the Accuracy of Anti-GM1 Antibodies for the Diagnosis of MMN?

Following the initial description of the clinical syndrome of MMN by Parry and Clark, Pestronk and colleagues reported two patients with this disorder in whom they had detected antibodies directed against GM1 and other gangliosides *(3)*. Since then, there have been numerous reports of low affinity and low titer anti-GM1 ganglioside antibodies in association with a variety of neurological disorders, notably amyotrophic lateral sclerosis (ALS), as well as in healthy controls. In trying to discern the significance of these antibodies with respect to the diagnosis of MMN, it has become apparent that it is necessary to consider only high-titer anti-GM1 antibodies, although with the caveat that there has not been widespread agreement on the cut-off value that should be used to distinguish low from high titers. Although many case series have reported the frequency with which anti-GM1 ganglioside antibodies are encountered among patients with MMN, the more useful studies are those that have examined the frequency with which these antibodies are present in patients with MMN as well as in patients with a variety of other neurological and nonneurological disorders and among healthy controls *(14–16)*. These studies included patients with a variety of neurological disorders, including ALS, the Guillain-Barré syndrome, chronic inflammatory demyelinating polyradiculoneuropathy and idiopathic sensorimotor polyneuropathy as well as patients with systemic nonneurological disorders and healthy controls. As discussed elsewhere in this book, the ideal study population should resemble the population in which the diagnostic test will be used. As shown in Tables 13.4A and 13.4B, high-titer anti-GM1 antibodies are encountered most frequently in patients with MMN, although they do occur in a small minority of patients with other neurological diseases. In these studies the sensitivity has ranged from 60% *(14)* to 85% *(16)* with somewhat better specificity ranging from 92% *(16)* to 99% *(15)*. One further issue to be aware of is the anti-GM1 antibody isotype, because both immunoglobulin (IgG) and IgM antibodies have been reported in patients with various neurological diseases. The studies by Pestronk et al. *(16)* and by Taylor et al *(15)* considered only IgM anti-GM1 antibodies, whereas the study by Adams et al reported the results of both IgM and IgG antibodies *(14)*. The conclusion seems to be that

Table 13.3
Cerebrospinal Fluid Protein in Multifocal Motor Neuropathy

Reference	Number of patients with LP	Number of patients with normal CSF protein	Number of patients with abnormal CSF protein	CSF protein concentration in patients with increased protein
Parry (2)	5	5 (100%)	0	–
Pestronk (3)	2	1 (50%)	1 (50%)	Max 69mg/dL
Krarup (4)	3	3 (100%)	0	–
Bouche (6)	19	19 (100%)	0	–
Chaudhry (9)	8	7 (87.5%)	1 (12.5%)	Max 54mg/dL
Nobile–Orazio (13)	4	2 (50%)	2 (50%)	Max 72mg/dL

LP , lumbar puncture; CSF, cerebrospinal fluid

Table 13.4A
High-Titer Anti-GM1 Ganglioside Antibodies in Multifocal Motor Neuropathy

	Taylor (15)[a]			Adams (14)[b]			Pestronk (16)[c]		
	Ab +	Ab –	Total	Ab +	Ab –	Total	Ab +	Ab –	Total
MMN	10	6	16	6	4	10	23	4	27
CIDP	3	7	10	–	–		0	22	22
ALS	0	121	121	5	38	43	0	89	89
SMA	1	7	8	0	5	5	–	–	
OND	–	–		2	44	46	–	–	
NND	–	–		3	34	37	0	22	22
GBS	–	–					0	22	22
Idiopathic SMPN	–	–					0	19	19
MN without CB	–	–					3	7	10
Chinese immune neuropathies	–	–					15	28	43
Healthy controls	1	361	362	0	41	41	–	–	

Ab+, antibody positive; Ab-, antibody negative; MMN, multifocal motor neuropathy; CIDP, chronic inflammatory demyelinating polyradiculoneuropathy; ALS, amyotrophic lateral sclerosis; SMA, spinal muscular atrophy; OND, other neurological disorders; NND, nonneurological disease; GBS, Guillain-Barre syndrome; SMPN, sensorimotor polyneuropathy; MN, motor neuropathy; CB, conduction block.

[a]High-titer defined as > 1:4000.
[b]High-titer defined as > 1:1000.
[c]High-titer defined as > 1:1800.

Table 13.4B
Sensitivity and Specificity of High-Titer Anti-GM1 Antibodies

Antibodies	Sensitivity	Specificity[a]
Taylor (15)	62.5%	99%
Adams (14)	60%	94%
Pestronk (16)	85%	92%

[a]All non-multifocal motor neuropathy patients from Table 13.4A combined.

the finding of high-titer IgM anti-GM1 antibodies has reasonably good sensitivity and high specificity for the diagnosis of MMN.

2.6. Is MMN a Disorder Distinct From the Lewis-Sumner Syndrome?

In 1982, Lewis and colleagues described five patients with a chronic asymmetric sensorimotor neuropathy that was most prominent in the arms and with focal involvement of individual peripheral nerves (usually the median or ulnar nerve). These patients all displayed electrophysiological features of multifocal conduction block (17). They distinguished these patients from CIDP primarily because of their presentation with a clinical picture of mononeuritis multiplex. What appears to be the same disorder has since been described under a range of different names, including multifocal acquired demyelinating sensory motor (MADSAM) neuropathy (18), upper limb predominant multifocal chronic inflammatory demyelinating polyneuropathy (19), multifocal inflammatory demyelinating neuropathy (20), and multifocal motor and sensory demyelinating neuropathy (MMSDM) (21). The obvious difference between the Lewis-Sumner syndrome and MMN is the presence of prominent sensory symptoms and signs as well as abnormalities of sensory nerve conduction studies in the former, but because MMN has been defined in terms of the absence of such sensory abnormalities, the question arises whether MMN and the Lewis-Sumner syndrome are distinct entities or variants of the same disease.

The clinical features of patients described in studies that included at least five patients with this syndrome are summarized in Table 13.5A. The mean ages of patients in these studies have ranged from 38 to 57 years, with a male preponderance in all (18–20,22) except the original report by Lewis and colleagues (17). The vast majority of patients present with sensory or sensorimotor symptoms, and the upper extremity is involved more commonly than the lower extremity, with distal hand musculature most severely affected. Muscle atrophy has been variably reported but does not appear to be a prominent feature. Deep tendon reflexes are usually depressed in areas affected clinically and complete areflexia is less common. Cranial neuropathies are encountered in a significant minority of patients with involvement of the optic (17), occulomotor (18), trigeminal (22), facial (22,23), glossopharyngeal (23) and vagus nerves (23) reported. There are, therefore, many similarities between the Lewis-Sumner syndrome and MMN, including the multifocal nature of the nature of the disease with clinical presentation of mononeuropathy multiplex, the predilection for each to involve distal hand musculature, and the focal depression or absence of reflexes. The major clinical differences include the presence of sensory symptoms and signs as well as the occurrence of cranial neuropathy in the Lewis-Sumner syndrome (Table 13.5B).

With regard to the results of laboratory investigations, CSF protein is elevated in approximately 54% of patients (Table 13.5B), compared with only 13% of patients with MMN (Table 13.3). Sensory nerve conduction studies are normal in MMN, whereas abnormalities are common and prominent in patients with the Lewis-Sumner syndrome (17–20,22,23). Electrophysiological abnormalities of motor nerves in the Lewis-Sumner syndrome include distal and proximal conduction block, slowing of conduction velocity, and prolongation of both distal motor latency and F-responses (17–20,22,23), although these abnormalities seem to occur slightly less frequently outside of nerves with conduction block than amongst patients with MMN (Table 13.2A). Anti-GM1 antibodies are

Table 13.5A
Clinical Features of the Lewis-Sumner Syndrome

Reference	n	Mean age (range)	M:F	Initial symptoms	Symptom location	CN palsy	Reflexes	Atrophy	Comments
Lewis (17)	5	45 (23–67)	1:4	Sensory (5) SM (1)	Hand (5)	2 (II)	Not reported	1	—
Saperstein (18)	11	57 (43–73)	10:1	?	Arms (6) Legs (5)	2 (III)	↓/absent in most	?	Sensory symptoms always conformed to discrete sensory nerve distribution
Viala (22)	23	44 (22–72)	17:6	SM (15) Sensory (8)	Hand (16) Foot (7)	5 (III, IV, V, VII)	—	13	Ulnar nerve most commonly affected
Verschueren (23)	13	47	7:6	Sensory (8) Motor (4) SM(1)	Arms (5) Legs (7)	4 (VII, IX, X)	Normal (1) Absent or decreased focally (9)	2	Median & ulnar nerves most commonly affected Predominantly large-fiber sensory involvement
Gorson (19)	10	54 (25–75)	6:4	Sensory (10)	Arms (9)[a] Arm/leg (1)[a]	None reported	None reported	Not reported	—
Van den Berg-Vos (20)	6	38 (28–58)	5:1	Sensory (3) Motor (2) SM (1)	Hand (4) Arm (1) Leg (1)	1	Absent or decreased focally (4) Areflexia (2)	3	—
Oh (21)	16	52 (18–77)	13:3	Sensory (5) Motor (11)	Arm (9) Leg (5)	2 (V, VII)	↓/ absent (15) ↑(2)	6	—

SM, sensorimotor.
[a]Patients were selected on the basis of arm involvement.

Table 13.5B
Differences Between MMN and the Lewis-Sumner Syndrome

	Lewis-Sumner[a]	MMN[b]
Symptoms		
Distribution	Asymmetric	Asymmetric
Arms > legs	Yes	Yes
Prominent sensory symptoms	Yes	No
Generalized areflexia	Rare	No
Laboratory Features		
Elevated CSF protein	Common	Rare
Elevated GM1 antibodies	No	Yes (~50–60%)
Electrophysiological findings		
Conduction block	~86%	~98%[c]
Conduction velocity slowing	~ 27%	~60%
Distal latency prolongation	~ 25%	~40%
F-wave prolongation	~26%	~66%
Abnormal sensory responses	Majority	Almost never

[a]Data from *17,19,20,22,41*
[b]Data from *2-4,8,11-13*
[c]There are a few exceptions. *See* refs. *8,10*

Table 13.5C
Cerebrospinal Fluid (CSF) Protein in Lewis-Sumner Syndrome

Reference	No. patients with LP	No. normal CSF protein	No. abnormal CSF protein	↑ CSF protein concentration
Lewis (17)	4	2	2 (50%)	Max 90mg/dL
Saperstein (18)	11	2	9 (81%)	Max 84mg/dL
Viala (22)	18	12	6 (33%)	Max 100mg/dL
Vershueren (23)	12	6	6 (50%)	Max 99mg/dL
Gorson (19)	7	2	5 (71%)	Max 128mg/dL
Van den Berg-Vos (20)	6	3	3 (50%)	Max 82mg/dL
Oh (21)	12	5	7 (58%)	Max 459mg/dL

present in a significant minority of patients with MMN, but are not present in patients with the Lewis-Sumner syndrome.

MMN and the Lewis-Sumner syndrome, therefore, share a number of similarities. Both are forms of mononeuropathy multiplex in which the physiology is that of demyelination. The clinical presentation in each disorder is with unilateral or asymmetric symptoms in the hands, and conduction block is the most frequently encountered electrophysiological abnormality in both disorders. The primary differences between MMN and the Lewis-Sumner syndrome, therefore, are the presence of sensory symptoms, signs, and electrophysiological abnormalities in the latter, as well as the presence of anti-GM1 antibodies in a significant minority of patients with MMN. The difference in sensory findings between the two disorders is a function of how the syndrome of MMN has been defined. Taking the cue from the original report by Parry and Clark, in which patients with this syndrome did not report sensory symptoms, other investigators have actively excluded patients with sensory findings. The presence of a biological marker—antibodies directed against GM1 ganglioside—in one disorder but not the other provides the strongest evidence for drawing a distinction between the two conditions.

Finally, it has been suggested that MMN and the Lewis-Sumner syndrome differ with respect to their responsiveness to various forms of immunosuppressive therapy. One of the frequently voiced claims is that patients with MMN, in contrast with those with the Lewis-Sumner syndrome, do not respond to steroids or plasmapheresis, and that these therapies may even be harmful to patients with MMN. The evidence for the claim that steroids and plasma exchange are not effective in MMN is extremely scanty, and is discussed in detail later in this chapter. It is difficult, therefore, to place much store on response to therapy in trying to differentiate between MMN and the Lewis-Sumner syndrome. It remains unclear, therefore, whether these two syndromes should be regarded as entirely distinct or as different ends of a spectrum of the same disorder.

3. TREATMENT

3.1. What Is the Evidence for the Efficacy of IVIg in MMN?

There are numerous uncontrolled reports of the efficacy of IVIg in multifocal motor neuropathy (Table 13.6A) as well as data from three randomized controlled trials (Table 13.6B). In the first of these trials, Azulay and colleagues randomized 12 patients to receive either IVIg or placebo in a cross-over study design *(24)*. Not all patients included in this study had MMN because the authors included seven patients with what they described as "lower motor neuron syndrome," which likely refers to the lower motor neuron variant of motor neuron disease (i.e., progressive muscular atrophy). The results for the patients with MMN and those with progressive muscular atrophy were reported separately. Muscle strength score, evaluated using a hand-held dynamometer, was used as the primary outcome measure. The authors reported that there were no differences in baseline muscle strength scores for each patient prior to receipt of IVIg and placebo, but the data they present suggest otherwise in that the baseline differences in muscle strength scores prior to IVIg or placebo treatment are greater than the differences observed between before and after IVIg treatment, casting doubt on the claim that 60% of patients responded to IVIg *(24)*.

The study by Van den Berg and colleagues was not really a randomized controlled trial and the study was susceptible to significant selection bias *(25)*. Patients were first treated with IVIg in an open-label fashion and the efficacy of IVIg was subsequently examined only among those patients who had responded. The authors used what they described as a "single patient double blind placebo controlled ... trial," also known as an "N of 1" trial design. Each patient received IVIg on two occasions and placebo on two occasions, with the treatments administered in a randomized fashion. The basic idea of this study design is that an individual patient's response to treatment can be evaluated in a blinded and placebo-controlled manner. The methodology permits determination that the individual patient responds to a particular therapy but does not permit generalization. It is difficult, therefore, to know how to interpret the finding that five of the six patients studied in this way responded to IVIg.

In the best study to date Federico and colleagues examined the efficacy of IVIg in 16 patients with MMN using a cross-over study design *(26)*. This was a randomized, double-blind and placebo-controlled trial. Patients were randomized to receive either IVIg or placebo first, and were then crossed over to receive the alternate treatment after 28 d or once the patient had returned to their pretreatment baseline condition. The two treatment groups were similar at baseline in terms of neurological disability score (NDS) and grip strength, the two primary outcome measures. The NDS comprises a summed score of strength in 26 muscle groups, sensory function, reflexes, and tremor, with a score of zero indicating no neurological deficit. There was no *a priori* estimation of the magnitude of the treatment effect (i.e., change in NDS or change in grip strength) that would be regarded as indicative of a meaningful clinical improvement. Changes in the degree of conduction block and change in GM1 titers were used as secondary measures of outcome. As shown in Table 13.6C, patients treated with IVIg showed significant improvement in NDS scores and grip strength as well as a reduction in the degree of conduction block. Although mean scores improved, five patients reported no subjective improvement following treatment with IVIg.

The most recent randomized controlled trial of IVIg was also double-blind and placebo-controlled, but employed a parallel treatment design *(27)*. This study included 19 patients with MMN, 10 of whom had not been treated previously with IVIg, and 9 patients who had responded to IVIg in the past. The inclusion of patients who were known to respond to IVIg in the past likely introduced a bias in favor of finding a treatment effect. The primary outcome of this study was the MRC score at 4 months with the patients' subjective evaluation, nerve conduction studies, and anti-GM1 antibody titers used as secondary outcome measures. Among the patients with no prior history of IVIg, four were randomized to receive IVIg (two of whom responded) and five received placebo (two of whom responded). All five of the patients with a history of response to IVIg responded to IVIg during the randomized study, whereas response was seen in none of the placebo treated patients. Although the combined results suggest a small treatment effect, this is clearly due to the inclusion of patients who were known to have responded to IVIg in the past. This study showed no improvement in electrophysiological parameters or in titers of anti-GM1 antibodies.

The weight of evidence, therefore, based primarily on the one high-quality study *(26)*, is that IVIg is effective in patients with MMN, with the expectation that IVIg should lead to improvement in muscle strength and functional status. There are fewer data to answer the question of how quickly the clinical effect becomes apparent and how long the treatment effect lasts, but the available data (mostly from the uncontrolled studies) are summarized in Table 13.6D. These data suggest that improvement is typically seen within a few days and that the effect typically lasts anywhere from 3 to 8 weeks.

3.2. What Is the Evidence for the Efficacy of Cyclophosphamide in Patients With MMN?

There are no controlled trials of the use of cyclophosphamide for the treatment of patients with MMN, although a number of anecdotal reports suggest that it may be effective (Table 13.7A). In their early description of MMN, Pestronk and colleagues reported two patients who had been treated with cyclophosphamide *(3)*. One patient

Table 13.6A
Uncontrolled Reports of the Efficacy of Intravenous Immunoglobulin in Patients With Multifocal Motor Neuropathy

Reference	n	Treatment regimen	Follow-up	Outcome measures	Results
Azulay (24)	18	0.4 g/kg/d × 3–5 d, repeated 6 times over 9–48 mo (mean 25 mo)	25 mo	Maximum voluntary isometric contraction (>30% improvement)	12 improved
Nobile-Orazio (40)	14	2 g/kg over 4–5 d followed by periodic infusions as ~1 g/kg over 2–3d	NR	Rankin Score Rankin score	12 improved 11 improved
Chaudhry (9)	9	Variable dose 1.6–2.4 g/kg over 2–5 d, repeated every 2–4 mo	NR	Hand held dynamometer (at least twofold increase in strength)	9 improved
Jaspert (42)	8	0.4 g/kg/d × 5 d, then regular 1d infusions as required	NR	Functional rating scale Clinical improvement Degree of conduction block	5 improved 8 improved 7 improved
Kermode (43)	5	30 g/d × 3–5 d, repeated monthly	NR	Myometry Nerve conduction studies	2 improved 3 improved
Comi (11)	5	0.4 g/kg/d × 5 d, repeated monthly for at least 2 mo	8 mo	MRC disability score	3 improved
Nobile-Orazio (13)	5	0.4 g/kg/d × 5 d, repeat after 2 mo then further infusions over 1–2 d every 2–4 wk	6–12 mo	Rankin score (1 point improvement)	4 improved
Kaji (29)	2	5 g/d × 3 d every 2 wk	5 mo	Clinical examination Nerve conduction studies	2 improved
Donaghy (30)	2	0.4 g/kg/d × 5 d, repeat for 2 d after 10 wk	20 wk	Clinical examination	2 improved
Charles (44)	1	0.2 g/kg/d × 5 d	NR	Clinical examination	1 improved

NR, not reported; MRC, Medical Research Council.

Table 13.6B
"N of 1" and Randomized Controlled Trials of the Efficacy of Intravenous Immunoglobulin (IVIg) in Multifocal Motor Neuropathy

Reference	n	Methodology	Outcome measures	Results
Azulay (24)	5	Cross-over design (change treatment after 8 wk) Double blind Possibly important differences between treatment groups at baseline No primary outcome specified	Muscle strength score (dynamometer) Norris disability score Nerve conduction studies	2 improved by day 5 and 3 improved by day 28 after IVIg No change in Norris score or electrophysiology
Van den Berg (25)	6	N of 1 trial design among patients who had previously responded to open label IVIg	Myometry (hand-held dynamometer)[a] Rankin score (disability) Nerve conduction studies	5 improved after IVIg
Federico (26)	16	Cross-over design (change treatment after at least 28 d) Placebo and IVIg groups similar at baseline with respect to NDS and grip strength	NDS Maximum grip strength Nerve conduction studies GM$_1$ antibody titers	Significant improvement on NDS and increase in grip strength in the IVIg group
Leger (27)	19	Parallel group design Two groups–those with no prior IVIg use (n = 10) and those with prior response to IVIg (n = 9) Similar baseline characteristics between the two treatment groups	MRC score at 4 mo (primary) Subjective evaluation at 4 mo Nerve conduction studies GM$_1$ antibody titers	Barely significant improvement in MRC score and subjective evaluation in the IVIg group No improvement in electrophysiology and no change in GM$_1$ titers

NDS, neurological disability score; MRC, Medical Research Council.

[a]Improvement defined as ≥ 50% increase in strength of at least 2 muscle groups without ≥ 25% decrease in strength in any other muscle group.

Table 13.6C
Outcome of Patients With Multifocal Motor Neuropathy Treated
With Intravenous Immunoglobulin (IVIg)

	Placebo	IVIg	p value
NDS[a]	↑2.1 points	↓ 6.7 points	<0.05
Grip strength[b]	↓ 1 kg	↑ 6.4kg	<0.005
Conduction block	↑ by 13%	↓13%	0.037

NDS, Neurological Disability Score.
[a]↓ NDS represents an improvement
[b]↑grip strength represents an improvement
Data from ref. 26.

Table 13.6D
Temporal Course of Efficacy of Intravenous Immunoglobulin in Multifocal Motor Neuropathy

Reference	Latency to onset of treatment effect	Latency to peak of treatment effect	Duration of treatment effect
Donaghy (30)	3–14 d	–	42 d
Azulay (32)	–	–	53 d
Chaudhry (9)	4.2 d	14 d	56 d
Comi (11)	–	–	21–56 d
Nobile-Orazio (13)	3–10 d	–	20–30 d
Charles (44)	15 d	–	42–49 d
Jaspert (42)	2–20 d	–	21–28 d
Van den Berg (33)	–		56 d
Van den Berg (25)	–	7–14 d	–

responded to treatment with 3g/m² divided into five doses and administered intravenously over 8 days. She was then placed on oral cyclophosphamide (50 mg 2–3 times per day) for 10 months, after which her response was maintained despite discontinuation of the drug. The second patient also responded to intravenous cyclophosphamide, but relapsed after 3–5 months and required further intravenous and oral therapy (3). In a subsequent report, Pestronk et al. noted that five patients who had been treated with cyclophosphamide had regained motor function when their anti-GM1 antibody titers were reduced by at least 75% (7). This report provided no information regarding the dose and duration of therapy, nor on the criteria by which outcome was judged to be favorable. In their small case series, Krarup and colleagues reported that one of three patients treated with cyclophosphamide showed signs of clinical improvement (4). In the largest case series published to date, Feldman et al. reported their experience with intravenous cyclophosphamide followed by an oral regimen (28). Eight patients were judged to have improved on the basis of an average increase of at least one Medical Research Council (MRC) grade in the strength of weak muscles in at least one extremity. The functional impact of such an "improvement" was not reported. Other authors have similarly reported sporadic cases of clinical improvement in response to cyclophosphamide (9,29,30).

Cyclophosphamide is generally looked upon favorably by neuromuscular specialists as a treatment option for patients with MMN, but it should be apparent from the evidence that the data supporting this view are extremely limited.

3.3. Does the Addition of Cyclophosphamide Reduce the Frequency With Which IVIg is Required?

There is very little published data that informs on this question. In their report of response of MMN patients to IVIg, Nobile-Orazio and colleagues noted that the frequency with which IVIg infusions were required was reduced in the two patients who had been started on oral cyclophosphamide (1.5–3 mg/kg/day) *(13)*. In a subsequent study, the same authors reported a similar finding in a further group of patients with MMN *(31)*. Oral cyclophosphamide was started at a dose of 1.5 to 2 mg/kg/day and subsequently adjusted (0.5–3 mg/kg/day) in order to maintain the white cell count between 3000 and 3500 per μL. After 3–7 months of therapy, they were able to reduce the frequency with which IVIg infusions were required. There are also other anecdotal reports of a reduced requirement for IVIg (frequency and dosage) among patients treated concurrently with cyclophosphamide *(32)*.

3.4. What Is the Evidence That Steroids and Plasmapheresis Have a Detrimental Effect in Patients With MMN?

The efficacy of neither steroids nor plasmapheresis has been examined in a randomized controlled trial. In fact, the evidence for the lack of efficacy and for the claim that they may even be harmful is quite slim. Almost without exception, the literature on the use of steroids in MMN comprises brief remarks in publications of case series of patients with MMN with the authors glibly stating that steroids were of no benefit or resulted in clinical deterioration (Table 13.7B) *(4,7,9,11,13,28–30,32)*. None of these studies used any formal measure of outcome, and most did not even specify the dose and duration for which steroids were used. There is a single case series comprising two patients who were treated with pulses of intravenous dexamethazone for 6 months in which outcome was evaluated using hand-held myometry *(33)*; both patients were reported to deteriorate. Thus, the only evidence supporting the claim that steroids are of no benefit or even harmful, is based on extremely poor-quality data.

As few published data as there are regarding the efficacy of steroids, there are even fewer on the efficacy of plasmapheresis (Table 13.7C) *(2,9,28,34)*. None of these studies set out to formally evaluate plasmapheresis and only one (a case report of a single patient) *(34)* specified the details of the volume and frequency of exchanges. No study used a formal method to evaluate response to therapy.

The only reasonable conclusion that can be drawn would seem to be that there are insufficient data to conclude either way whether steroids and plasmapheresis are beneficial or harmful in patients with MMN.

3.5. Is There a Role for Any Other Immunosuppressive Agents in MMN?

There have been two reports of patients treated with interferon-β1a *(35,36)*. In the first of these reports, Martina and colleagues treated three MMN patients with interferon-β1a

Table 13.7A
Efficacy of Cyclophosphamide in Multifocal Motor Neuropathy

Reference	n	Treatment regimen	Follow-up	Outcome measures	Results
Feldman (28)	9	iv cytoxan 3g/m², & then 2 mg/kg/d PO	2–5 mo	MRC rating scale (≥ 1 point improvement in muscle weakness in at least 1 muscle)	Improvement in 8 patients
Pestronk (7)	5	NR	NR	Clinical evaluation	Improvement in 5 patients
Krarup (4)	3	3 g/m² iv ± 100–150 mg/d PO for 6 mo titrated to clinical response	1 yr	NR	Improvement in 1 patient (the one who received iv cytoxan)
Donaghy (30)	2	100 mg/d PO for 6 mo	6 mo	NR	Disease stabilized in 1 patient
Pestronk (3)	2	3 g/m² iv divided in 5 doses over 8 d ± 100–150 mg/d PO for 10 mo	NR	Clinical evaluation	Improvement in 2 patients
Kaji (29)	1	100 mg/d PO for 1 mo	1 mo	NR	No response

NR, not reported; iv, intravenous; PO, per oral; MRC, Medical Research Council; PE, plasma exchange.

Table 13.7B
Efficacy of Steroids in Multifocal Motor Neuropathy

Reference	n	Treatment regimen	Follow-up	Outcome measures	Results
Feldman (28)	13	High-dose oral prednisone	NR	NR	"No clinical response"
Pestronk (7)	7	High-dose corticosteroids	NR	Clinical examination	1 improved, 6 deteriorated
Chaudhry (9)	6	NR	NR	NR	"No clinical improvement"
Azulay (32)	4	NR	NR	NR	"Four patients were treated previously with steroids without any improvement"
Donaghy (30)	4	60 mg/d	4 wk	NR	"Significant motor deterioration in four patients"
Comi (11)	3	NR	NR	NR	"Three patients were previously treated with steroids but (the response was) considered unsatisfactory"
Kaji (29)	2	50 mg/d for 1 mo ± 100 mg solumedrol iv 2 d/wk for 2 mo	NR	NR	"Further weakening of affected muscles"
Van den Berg (33)	2	Pulse decadron 40 mg/d for 4 d, repeated monthly for 6 mo	6 mo	Hand-held myometry	"Both deteriorated"
Krarup (4)	2	25–60 mg/d PO for 2–9 mo	2–9 mo	NR	"No improvement"
Nobile-Orazio (13)	3	NR	NR	NR	"No effect in two while one had severe and rapid worsening"

NR, not reported; iv, intravenous; PO, per oral; MRC, Medical Research Council; PE, plasma exchange.

Table 13.7C
Efficacy of Plasmapheresis in Multifocal Motor Neuropathy

Reference	n	Treatment Regimen	Follow-up	Outcome measures	Results
Feldman (28)	4	NR	NR	NR	"No clinical response in four patients treated with PE"
Carpo (34)	1	Four PEs on days 1, 3, 8, and 9	NR	Clinical examination	Progressive deterioration during successive exchanges
Chaudhry (9)	2	NR	NR	NR	"No clinical improvement"
Parry (2)	2	NR	NR	NR	"No clinical improvement"

NR, not reported; iv, intravenous; PO, per oral; MRC, Medical Research Council; PE, plasma exchange.

(6 million IU three times per week) for 6 months. Disability status was monitored using the nine hole peg test, 10 m walking test, and the modified Rankin score. Changes in muscle strength, evaluated using the MRC sum score, were used as a secondary outcome measure. Improved disability was seen in all three patients (although only two showed improvement on the Rankin score), as was an increase in muscle strength *(35)*. Van den Berg-Vos and colleagues treated nine MMN patients with the same regimen of interferon-β1a for 6 months *(36)*. The same measures of disability were used to evaluate outcome, and changes in muscle strength were followed using both hand-held dynamometry and the MRC sum score. One important difference was that this study included patients who had previously responded to therapy with IVIg (although the reasons for switching from IVIg to interferon-β1a are not explicitly stated). Only three of the nine patients showed increased muscle strength after 6 months of interferon therapy. In neither study was there any change in the severity of conduction block, and anti-GM1 titers were unchanged in the study by Martina et al. *(35)*.

This limited anecdotal data, therefore, suggest that interferon-β1a may sometimes be effective in MMN patients, although this finding requires validation in a larger controlled trial.

4. PROGNOSIS

4.1. What Is the Long Term Outcome of MMN Patients Treated With Immunosuppressive therapy?

There is very limited data that informs on the long-term prognosis of patients with MMN *(31,37)*. The published studies have reported long-term prognosis following aggressive immunosuppressive therapy either with IVIg alone *(37)* or with IVIg in combination with cyclophosphamide *(31)*. Using the MRC sum score, the authors found statistically significant improvements in muscle strength between the time of initial presentation and final follow-up while the patients were still on therapy *(31,37)*. As shown in Table 13.8A, these benefits appear quite modest, and at least in the one study *(37)* are of questionable clinical significance. Rankin disability scores, however, improved in most patients, suggesting that the benefits were indeed clinical meaningful (Table 13.8B).

Similar results were found in one other study that used the Neuropathy Impairment Score (NIS) to evaluate the progression of disease over time *(38)*. The NIS quantifies and summates the objective weakness of a standard group of muscles, reflexes, and sensory modalities. The scale expresses impairment as a single number ranging from 0 (no impairment) to 244 (total impairment). Based on the 18 patients in this study for whom extended follow-up information was available, it was estimated that muscle weakness declined by 1.3 points per year despite intensive immunosuppressive therapy. Although it is difficult to translate this finding into clinically meaningful terms, these data suggest that MMN is a disorder characterized by slow progression despite treatment. Disability among these patients, however, remains relatively mild *(38)*.

These results seem to suggest that disability from MMN is relatively mild as the majority of patients do not exceed a Rankin score of 2 which implies the presence of only minor disability resulting in some restriction of lifestyle but no interference with the ability to maintain independent existence.

Table 13.8A
Prognosis of Multifocal Motor Neuropathy: Muscle Strength

Reference	Van den Berg (31)	Meucci (37)
Sample size	11	6
Treatment	IVIg	IVIg and cyclophosphamide
Median follow-up (range)	NR (4–8 yr)	46 mo (3–5 yr)
Individual MRC sum score[a]		
Pretreatment	82 77 97 95 98 96 95 96 92 87 94	66 37 81 89 79 65
Last follow-up	86 77 99 99 97 96 97 98 97 91 96	83 83 85 95 86 80
Mean MRC sum score[a]		
Pretreatment	92 (± 7)	69.5
Last follow-up	94 (± 7)	85.3
p value	<0.001	0.0561

NR, not reported; IVIg, intravenous immunoglobulin; MRC, medical research council.
[a]Maximum score of 100.

Table 13.8B
Prognosis of Multifocal Motor Neuropathy: Rankin Disability Score

Reference	Van den Berg (31)	Meucci (37)
Sample size	7	6
Treatment	IVIg	IVIg and cyclophosphamide
Median follow-up (range)	NR (4–8 yr)	46 mo (3–5 yr)
Individual Rankin scores		
Pretreatment	2 2 2 2 2 2 2	2 4 2 2 2 3
Last follow-up	2 2 1 1 1 1 1	1 1 1 1 2 2
Median Rankin score		
Pretreatment	2	2
Last follow-up	1	1
p value	NR	0.0335

NR, not reported; IVIg, intravenous immunoglobulin; MRC, medical research council.

4.2. Are There Any Factors That Predict Outcome in MMN?

There are no data that predict outcome in patients with MMN, but a few studies have tried to determine whether there are any factors that predict a good response to immuno-suppressive therapy. In their randomized controlled trial, for example, Federico and colleagues examined a variety of clinical and laboratory features to determine whether they correlated with clinical improvement after treatment with IVIg (26). They considered age, gender, duration of illness before treatment, anti-GM1 antibody titer, severity of initial weakness, wasting, fasciculations, number of limbs involved clinically and electrophysiologically, number of nerve territories involved clinically and electrophysiologically, temporal dispersion, motor conduction velcotiy, distal motor latency, and F-wave latency. The only variable to correlate with outcome was age with younger patients responding more favorably. The mean age of those who responded was 33 yr, compared to a mean age of 52 yr among those who did not respond (26).

In their retrospective review of 37 patients with lower motor neuron syndromes, all of whom were treated with IVIg, Van den Berg-Vos and colleagues identified younger age of onset, less extensive disease, creatine kinase concentration less than 180 U/L, the presence of elevated anti-GM1 antibody titers, a higher frequency of definite conduction blocks, and preserved distal compound muscle action potential amplitude as predictors of a good response to IVIg *(39)*. Apart from younger age *(26)* and elevated GM1 titers *(32)*, which were also found to predict a better response to IVIg treatment in other studies, these findings have not been validated by other investigators.

The data, therefore, are limited, but younger age and the presence of elevated GM1 antibody titers have each been identified by more than one study as predicting a better response to IVIg.

5. SUMMARY

- MMN is a chronic demyelinating neuropathy closely related to both CIDP and to the Lewis-Sumner syndrome.
- MMN is characterized clinically by asymmetric distal limb weakness, usually beginning in the hand and with minimal or no sensory symptoms; focal atrophy and reflex loss are common.
- The electrophysiological hallmark of MMN is multifocal motor conduction block.
- It is unusual for conduction block to be isolated to proximal nerve segments that are not evaluated by routine nerve conduction studies.
- Conduction block is not the only electrophysiological abnormality in MMN as conduction velocity slowing as well as prolongation of distal latency and F-responses are usually present.
- CSF protein in MMN is typically normal, although it may sometimes be mildly elevated.
- The sensitivity of high titer IgM anti-GM1 ganglioside antibodies is approximately 60–80% whereas the specificity is 90–99%.
- There is evidence from three randomized controlled trials that IVIg is effective in patients with MMN, although repeated infusions are usually required in order to maintain the clinical response.
- There is anecdotal evidence that cyclophosphamide may also be beneficial in patients with MMN, either alone or in conjunction with IVIg.
- The evidence that steroids and plasma exchange are not beneficial in patients with MMN is extremely scant.
- MMN is usually slowly progressive despite immunosuppressive therapy, although disability also accumulates slowly.
- Younger age and the presence of elevated anti-GM1 ganglioside antibody titers may predict a better response to IVIg therapy.

REFERENCES

1. Parry GJ, Clarke S. Pure motor neuropathy with multifocal conduction block masquerading as motor neurone disease. Muscle Nerve 1985;8:617.
2. Parry GJ, Clarke S. Multifocal acquired demyelinating neuropathy masquerading as motor neuron disease. Muscle Nerve 1988;11:103–107.
3. Pestronk A, Cornblath D, Ilyas A, et al. A treatable multifocal motor neuropathy with antibodies to GM1 ganglioside. Ann Neurol 1988;24:73–78.
4. Krarup C, Stewart J, Sumner A, Pestronk A, Lipton S. A syndrome of asymmetric limb weakness with motor conduction block. Neurology 1990;40:118–127.
5. Comi G, Roveri L, Swan A, et al. A randomised controlled trial of intravenous immunoglobulin in IgM paraprotein associated demyelinating neuropathy. J Neurol 2002;249:1370–1377.

6. Bouche P, Moulonguet A, Younes-Chennoufi AB, et al. Multifocal motor neuropathy with conduction block: a study of 24 patients. J Neurol Neurosurg Psychiatry 1995;59:38–44.
7. Pestronk A, Chaudhry V, Feldman E, et al. Lower motor neuron syndromes defined by patterns of weakness, nerve conduction abnormalities, and high titers of antiglycolipid antibodies. Ann Neurol 1990;27:316–326.
8. Katz J, Wolfe G, Bryan W, Jackson C, Amato A, Barohn R. Electrophysiologic findings in multifocal motor neuropathy. Neurology 1997;48:700–707.
9. Chaudhry V, Corse AM, Cornblath DR, et al. Multifocal motor neuropathy: response to human immune globulin. Ann Neurol 1993;33:237–242.
10. Pakiam A, Parry G. Multifocal motor neuropathy without overt conduction block. Muscle Nerve 1998; 21:243–245.
11. Comi G, Amadio S, Galardi G, Fazio R, Nemni R. Clinical and neurophysiological assessment of immunoglobulin therapy in five patients with multifocal motor neuropathy. J Neurol Neurosurg Psychiatry 1994;57(Suppl):35–37.
12. Chaudhry V, Corse AM, Cornblath DR, Kuncl RW, Freimer ML, Griffin JW. Multifocal motor neuropathy: electrodiagnostic features. Muscle Nerve 1994;17:198–205.
13. Nobile-Orazio E, Meucci N, Barbieri S, Carpo M, Scarlato G. High-dose intravenous immunoglobulin therapy in multifocal motor neuropathy. Neurology 1993;43:537–544.
14. Adams D, Kuntzer T, Burger D, et al. Predictive value of anti-GM1 ganglioside antibodies in neuromuscular diseases: a study of 180 sera. J Neuroimmunol 1991;32:223–230.
15. Taylor B, Gross L, Windebank A. The sensitivity and specificity of anti-GM1 antibody testing. Neurology 1996; 47:951–955.
16. Pestronk A, Choksi R. Multifocal motor neuropathy. Serum IgM anti-GM1 ganglioside antibodies in most patients detected using covalent linkage of GM1 to ELISA plates. Neurology 1997; 49:1289–1292.
17. Lewis R, Sumner A, Brown M, Asbury A. Multifocal demyelinating neuropathy with persistent conduction block. Neurology 1982;32:958–964.
18. Saperstein DS, Amato AA, Wolfe GI, et al. Multifocal acquired demyelinating sensory and motor neuropathy: the Lewis-Sumner syndrome. Muscle Nerve 1999;22:560–566.
19. Gorson KC, Ropper AH, Weinberg DH. Upper limb predominant, multifocal chronic inflammatory demyelinating polyneuropathy. Muscle Nerve 1999;22:758–765.
20. Van den Berg-Vos R, Van den Berg L, Franssen H, et al. Multifocal inflammatory demyelinating neuropathy. A distinct clinical entity? Neurology 2000;54:26–32.
21. Oh SJ, Claussen GC, Kim DS. Motor and sensory demyelinating mononeuropathy multiplex (multifocal motor and sensory demyelinating neuropathy): a separate entity or a variant of chronic inflammatory demyelinating polyneuropathy. J Periph Nerv Syst 1997;2:362–369.
22. Viala K, Renie L, Maisonobe T, et al. Follow-up study and response to treatment in 23 patients with Lewis-Sumner syndome. Brain 2004; 127:2010–2017.
23. Verschueren A, Azulay JP, Attarian S, Boucraut J, Pellissier JF, Pouget J. Lewis-Sumner syndrome and multifocal motor neuropathy. Muscle Nerve 2005;31:88–94.
24. Azulay JP, Blin O, Pouget J, et al. Intravenous immunoglobulin treatment in patients with motor neuron syndromes associated with anti-GM1 antibodies: a double-blind, placebo-controlled study. Neurology 1994;44:429–432.
25. Van den Berg L, Kerkhoff H, Oey P, et al. Treatment of multifocal motor neuropathy with high dose intravenous immunoglobulins: a double blind, placebo controlled study. J Neurol Neurosurg Psychiatry 1995; 59:248–252.
26. Federico P, Zochodne D, Hahn A, Brown W, Feasby T. Multifocal motor neuropathy improved by IVIg: randomized, double-blind, placebo-controlled study. Neurology 2000; 55:1256–1262.
27. Leger J, Chassande B, Musset L, Meininger V, Bouche P, Baumann N. Intravenous immunoglobulin therapy in multifocal motor neuropathy: a double-blind, placebo-controlled study. Brain 2001; 124:145–153.
28. Feldman E, Bromberg M, Albers J, Pestronk A. Immunosuppressive treatment in multifocal motor neuropathy. Ann Neurol 1991;30:397–401.
29. Kaji R, Shibasaki H, Kimura J. Multifocal demyelinating motor neuropathy: cranial nerve involvement and immunoglobulin therapy. Neurology 1992;42:506–509.

30. Donaghy M, Mills K, Boniface S, et al. Pure motor demyelinating neuropathy: deterioration after steroid treatment and improvement with intravenous immunoglobulin. J Neurol Neurosurg Psychiatry 1994; 57:778–783.
31. Meucci N, Cappellari A, Barbieri S, Scarlato G, Nobile-Orazio E. Long term effect of intravenous immunoglobulins and oral cyclophosphamide in multifocal motor neuropathy. J Neurol Neurosurg Psychiatry 1997; 63:765–769.
32. Azulay J-P, Rihet P, Pouget J, et al. Long term follow-up of multifocal motor neuropathy with conduction block under treatment. J Neurol Neurosurg Psychiatry 1997; 62:391–394.
33. Van den Berg L, Lokhorst H, Wokke J. Pulsed high-dose dexamethasone is not effective in patients with multifocal motor neuropathy. Neurology 1997; 48:1135.
34. Carpo M, Cappellari A, Mora G, et al. Deterioration of multifocal motor neuropathy after plasma exchange. Neurology 1998; 50:1480–2.
35. Martina I, van Doorn P, Schmitz P, Meulstee J, van der meche F. Chronic motor neuropathies: response to interferon-beta-1a after failure of conventional therapies. J Neurol Neurosurg Psychiatry 1999; 66:917–201.
36. Van den Berg-Vos R, Van den Berg L, Franssen H, van Doorn P, Merkies I, Wokke J. Treatment of multifocal motor neuropathy with interferon-beta-1A. Neurology 2000; 54:1518–1521.
37. Van den Berg L, Franssen H, Wokke J. The long-term effect of intravenous immunoglobulin treatment in multifocal motor neuropathy. Brain 1998; 121 (Pt 3):421–8.
38. Taylor B, Wright R, Harper C, Dyck P. Natural history of 46 patients with multifocal motor neuropathy with conduction block. Muscle Nerve 2000; 23:900–8.
39. Van den Berg-Vos R, Franssen H, Wokke J, Van Es H, Van den Berg L. Multifocal motor neuropathy: diagnostic criteria that predict the response to immunoglobulin treatment. Ann Neurol 2000;48:919–926.
40. Nobile-Orazio E, Cappellari A, Meucci N, et al. Multifocal motor neuropathy: clinical and immunological features and response to IVIg in relation to the presence and degree of motor conduction block. J Neurol Neurosurg Psychiatry 2002;72:761–766.
41. Saperstein DS, Katz JS, Amato AA, Barohn RJ. Clinical spectrum of chronic acquired demyelinating polyneuropathies. Muscle Nerve 2001;24:311–324.
42. Jaspert A, Claus D, Grehl H, Neundorfer B. Multifocal motor neuropathy: clinical and electrophysiological findings. J Neurol 1996;243:684–692.
43. Kermode A, Laing B, Carroll W, Mastaglia F. Intravenous immunoglobulin for multifocal motor neuropathy. Lancet 1992; 340:920–921.
44. Charles N, Benoit P, Vial C, Bierme T, Moreau T, Bady B. Intravenous immunoglobulin treatment in multifocal motor neuropathy. Lancet 1992;340:182.

14 Inherited Neuropathies

1. INTRODUCTION

The inherited neuropathy literature is complex, in part because of the incomplete correlation between genotype and phenotype and in part because of the confusing array of terminology that has been used to describe and classify these disorders. The terms "hereditary motor and sensory neuropathy" (HMSN) and "Charcot-Marie Tooth" (CMT) have both been used to describe the same group of disorders. HMSN-I and HMSN-II are synonymous with CMT-1 and CMT-2 respectively, with the distinction between CMT-1 (HMSN-1) and CMT-2 (HMSN-2) being based on the electrophysiological finding of marked slowing of motor conduction velocities in the former. Recent advances in molecular genetics have shown that mutations in several different genes may underlie the various inherited neuropathies. The expanding array of genetic mutations has further complicated the classification of this group of disorders. The current approach rests on the mode of inheritance and electrophysiological features of the disorder. A simplified classification is presented in Table 14.1. Most of the inherited neuropathy literature has focused on diagnostic issues, with relatively little attention paid to treatment and prognosis. This bias is reflected in this chapter, in which we examine the clinical and electrophysiological features of the hereditary neuropathies and ask whether the various disorders can be differentiated on clinical or electrical grounds. We also consider the electrophysiological differences between acquired and hereditary neuropathies of both the demyelinating and axonal types. Finally, we do consider several treatment and prognosis-related issues.

2. DIAGNOSIS

2.1. What Are the Typical Clinical Manifestations of the Hereditary Neuropathies and Do They Differ Sufficiently to Permit Their Differentiation on Clinical Grounds?

Many of the large series that described the clinical manifestations of patients with inherited neuropathies predate the molecular era and, as a result, almost certainly include genetically heterogeneous groups of patients. For the most part, these early papers defined clinical subgroups based on the electrophysiological and pathological features of these disorders (1–3). There are, however, a number of more recent studies in which the clinical phenotype of genetically homogeneous groups of patients have been described (4–8).

From: *Neuromuscular Disease: Evidence and Analysis in Clinical Neurology*
By: M. Benatar © Humana Press Inc., Totowa, NJ

Table 14.1
Classification of the Inherited Neuropathies

Nomenclature	Inheritance	Physiology	Gene	Chromosome
CMT-1	AD	Demyelinating		
CMT-1A			PMP22	17p11.2
CMT-1B			MPZ	1q22.23
CMT-1C			Unknown	16p13.1–p12.3
CMT-1D			EGR2	10q21.1–q22.1
CMT-2	AD	Axonal	Mitofusin 2	1p36.22
			MPZ, NEFL, KIF1β, GARS, RAB7, HSP22, HSP27	At least 8 loci
CMT-X	X-linked	Intermediate phenotype	GJB1 (Cx32) most common	X
CMT-4	AR	Demyelinating	GDAP1, MTMR2, NDRG1, EGR2, PRX	At least 8 loci
HNPP	AD	–	PMP-22	17p11.2
HNA	AD	–	Unknown	17q25

CMT, Charcot-Marie-Tooth; HNPP, Hereditary neuropathy with liability to pressure palsies; HNA, hereditary neuralgic amyotrophy; AD, autosomal dominant; AR, autosomal recessive; PMP22, peripheral myelin protein-22; MPZ, myelin protein zero; EGR2, early growth response element-2; NEFL, neurofilament light chain; KIF1β, kinesin motor protein-1β; GARS, glycol-tRNA synthetase; RAB7, RAS-associated protein; HSP, heat shock protein; GJB1, gap junction proteinβ1; Cx32, Connexin 32; GDAP-1, ganglioside-induced differentiation associated protein-1; MTMR2, myotubularin-related protein-2 gene; NDRG1, *N*-myc downstream regulated gene-1; PRX, periaxin.

The "generic" phenotype is that of slowly progressive distal muscle weakness and atrophy that primarily affects the intrinsic foot and peroneal-distribution muscles. With time, the intrinsic muscles of the hands and forearm muscles may also become affected. Distal symmetrical sensory deficits are typical and most patients have foot deformities (pes cavus and hammer toes). Distal deep tendon reflexes (notably at the ankle) are typically diminished or absent.

Harding and Thomas provided a detailed description of patients with HMSN-I *(1)*. The 139 patients included in this series were uncomplicated cases of "peroneal muscular atrophy" in whom median motor conduction velocity was less than 38 m/s. Symptom onset was in the first decade in almost two-thirds of patients, and within the first two decades in over 80% (Table 14.2A). Distal weakness in the legs was present in 87% of patients and distal weakness in the arms in 67%. Ankle reflexes were absent in almost 90% of patients and there was complete areflexia in almost 60%. Sensory loss was present in over 50% of patients, with vibration sense most prominently affected and joint position sense more frequently preserved. Foot deformities were common (72%), but not invariable (Table 14.2B).

In their series of 55 patients with peroneal muscular atrophy, Bouche and colleagues used a median motor conduction velocity of less than 30m/s to define patients with CMT-1 *(3)*. The age of onset and clinical manifestations were very similar to those reported by

Table 14.2A
Symptoms in Charcot-Marie-Tooth (CMT)-1A

Sample size	Harding (1) 139	Thomas (6) 61	Nicholson (7) 62	Birouk (4) 119	Bouche (3) 55
Age of onset					
Mean age (range)	NR	NR	NR	19 (2–76)	15
First decade	62%	75%	65%	50%	55%
Second decade	25%	10%	11%	20%	19%
Asymptomatic	NR	NR	18%	NR	NR
Motor symptoms	NR			NR	NR
Difficulty walking/running	NR	34%	45%	NR	NR
Developmental delay	NR	16%	NR	NR	NR
Ankle injury/instability	NR	NR	55%	NR	NR
Foot deformity	NR	33%	NR	NR	NR
Weak grip	NR	NR	26%	NR	NR
Sensory symptoms	NR			NR	NR
Paresthesia	NR	3%	NR	NR	NR
Neuropathic pain	NR	0	NR	NR	NR
Sensory loss	NR	NR	5%	NR	NR
Other					
Muscle cramps	NR	2%	NR	NR	23%

NR, not reported.

Table 14.2B
Physical Signs in Charcot-Marie-Tooth (CMT)-1A

	Harding (1) 139	Thomas (6) 61	Nicholson (7) 62	Birouk (4) 119	Bouche (3) 55
Sample size					
Weakness					NR
None	NR	11%	(19%)[a]	NR	
Legs	87%	NR	81%	78%	
Arms	67%	NR	NR	61%	
Arms and legs	NR	74%	NR	NR	
Diaphragm	NR	5%	NR	NR	
Bulbar	1%	3%	NR	NR	
Foot deformity	72%	72%	77%	95%	70%
Deep tendon reflexes					
Normal reflexes	(11%)[a]	3%	11%	NR	9%
Absent ankle reflexes	89%	NR	69%	NR	NR
Absent ankle & knee reflexes	70%	NR	NR	97%	NR
Areflexia in arms and legs	58%	75%	NR	79%	62%
Extensor plantar responses	2%	5%	NR	0	NR
Sensory loss		43%[b]	NR		64%
Light touch	53%	NR		64%	NR
Pain	53%	NR		64%	NR
Joint position sense	46%	NR		69%	NR
Vibration sense	69%	NR		NR	NR
Tremor/Ataxia			NR		11%
Arms	39%	5%		5%	NR
Legs	23%	NR		NR	NR
Sensorineural hearing loss	NR	NR	NR	5%	NR
Scoliosis	NR	NR	NR	35%	13%

[a]Values in parentheses are extrapolated from figures. NR, not reported.
[b]Said to affect all modalities

252

Harding and Thomas (1) (Tables 14.2A,B). Onset of disease was within the first two decades in 74% of patients. The frequency and distribution of muscle weakness and atrophy were not reported, but foot deformities were present in the majority of patients (70%). All deep tendon reflexes were absent in 62% of patients and sensory loss in 64% (3).

More recently, there have been three studies of genetically confirmed cases of CMT-1A (i.e., presence of the peripheral myelin protein [PMP]-22 duplication) (4,6,7). Age of onset in these studies was also within the first two decades of life in 70–85% of patients (Table 14.2A). The most common symptoms were difficulty walking or running, ankle injury or instability, and foot deformities (7,9). In these studies, distally predominant weakness in the legs was present on examination in approximately 80% of patients and high arched feet and/or hammer toes in 72–95% (4,6,7). Complete areflexia was noted in approximately 80% (4,6) and sensory loss was present in a about 65% (4).

The overall impression from these five studies is that CMT-1A has a fairly consistent clinical phenotype characterized by distal muscle weakness in the legs, complete areflexia, foot deformities, and distal sensory loss. None of these features are invariably present. Age of onset is within the first two decades of life in close to 80% of patients. Although the earlier studies by Harding and Thomas (1) and Bouche and colleagues (3) were undertaken prior to the availability of genetic testing, these case series were likely most representative of CMT-1A given the high frequency of this disorder relative to CMT-1B, 1C, and so on.

The clinical phenotype of patients with CMT-2 was also described in the studies by Harding and Thomas (1), Bouche and colleagues (3), and by Teunissen et al. (9,10). Similar criteria were used to define the phenotype—a median motor conduction velocity greater than 38 m/s (1,10) or greater than 40 m/s (3). Age of onset was within the first two decades in 39–61% of patients (indicating a somewhat older age of onset than CMT-1 patients) with motor symptoms being most common (10) (Table 14.3A). Distal leg weakness with absent ankle reflexes were the most common findings on examination (1), with foot deformities present in approximately 50% of patients and distal sensory loss in only about 35% (1,3,10) (Table 14.3B). The clinical phenotype of CMT-2, therefore, is very similar to that of CMT-1, with the exception that age of onset is relatively less skewed to within the first two decades of life and with a trend towards less frequent finding of foot abnormalities, sensory loss, and complete areflexia. There do not appear, however, to be any clinical features that reliably distinguish the two disorders.

The designation CMT-2, however, encompasses a range of different genetic disorders, and isolated small series suggest that specific forms of CMT-2 do in fact have particular clinical phenotypes. CMT-2B, for example, is reportedly characterized by prominent sensory loss with high prevalence of trophic toe and foot ulcers (11). CMT-2C, on the other hand, is characterized by diaphragmatic and intercostal respiratory muscle weakness as well as vocal cord paresis in addition the more typical clinical manifestations outlined previously (12). Diaphragmatic weakness, however, is not unique to CMT-2C. Hardie and colleagues described 4 CMT-1 patients with diaphragmatic weakness, although the quality of the evidence provided to demonstrate that diaphragmatic weakness was the cause of respiratory insufficiency is variable (13). One other clinical features of CMT-2C patients appears to be the presence of weakness and wasting of the intrinsic hand muscles that occurs in equal frequency to the presence of distal weakness and atrophy in the legs (12).

Table 14.3A. Symptoms in Charcot-Marie-Tooth-(CMT)-2

Sample size	Harding (1) 139	Teunissen (10) 47	Bouche (3) 64
Age of onset		NR	
Mean age (range)	NR		26
First decade	5%		26%
Second decade	34%		35%
Asymptomatic	NR	NR	NR
Motor symptoms	NR	85%	NR
Difficulty walking/running		NR	
Developmental delay		NR	
Ankle injury/instability		NR	
Weak grip		53%	
Sensory symptoms	NR	87%	NR
Paresthesia		NR	
Neuropathic pain		NR	
Sensory loss		NR	
Other			
Muscle cramps	NR	NR	38%

Table 14.3B. Physical Signs in Charcot-Marie-Tooth (CMT)-2

Sample size	Harding (1) 39	Teunissen (10) 47	Bouche (3) 64
Weakness		NR	NR
None	(6%)[a]		
Legs	94%		
Arms	51%		
Arms and legs	NR		
Diaphragm	NR		
Bulbar	2.5%		
Foot deformity	51%	57%	51%
Deep tendon reflexes			
Normal reflexes	NR	NR	13%
Absent ankle reflexes	80%	89%	NR
Absent ankle & knee reflexes	18%	53%	NR
Areflexia in arms and legs	9%	NR	21%
Extensor plantar responses	0	NR	NR
Sensory loss		NR	36%
Light touch	36%		NR
Pain	31%		NR
Joint position sense	25%		NR
Vibration sense	56%		NR
Tremor/Ataxia		28%	16%
Arms	16%	NR	NR
Legs	18%	NR	NR

[a]Values in parentheses are extrapolated from figures.

CMT-X is the X-linked form of Charcot-Marie-Tooth disease. There are several published series of patients with presumed CMT-X based on the pattern of inheritance (no male-to-male transmission) *(2,7)* as well as several series in which affected individuals have demonstrable mutations in the Connexin-32 gene *(5,8)*. In the report by Hahn and colleagues of 42 affected subjects in a large multi-generational family *(2)*, the age of onset was typically earlier in men than in women. Onset was within the first decade of life in all but 2 men and most women first noted symptoms towards the end of the second decade of life *(2)*. The typical clinical manifestations were those of distal muscle weakness in the arms and legs, pes cavus, absent reflexes, and sensory loss. In general, men were more severely affected than women. Similar findings have been reported by other investigators *(5,7,8)* (Table 14.4A). In these studies, age of onset was generally later in women than in men, but the proportion with onset within the first two decades of life varied widely from 47% *(5)* to 95% *(7)* in men and from 30% *(5)* to 35% *(7)* in women. Foot deformities were extremely common, present in the majority of men and women. Weakness is reported in approximately 80% of men and 30-50% of women and sensory loss in 80–90% of men and 60–80% of women (Table 14.4B). The only clinical feature, therefore, that might suggest a diagnosis of CMT-X is that of a family history in which there is no male-to-male transmission and which the men are more severely affected than the women.

For the most part, therefore, there is extensive clinical overlap between the clinical presentations (age of onset, symptoms and abnormalities on physical examination) of patients with CMT-1(A), CMT-2, and CMT-X. Subtle differences include more common onset within the first two decades of life in CMT-1 than CMT-2 and early involvement of respiratory muscles and vocal cords in CMT-2C as well as an X-linked pattern of inheritance (no male-to-male transmission) and a family history in which men are more severely affected than women in CMT-X. Apart from these features, there are few differences between the clinical presentations of the various CMT syndromes.

2.2. What Are the Typical Electrophysiological Features of the Hereditary Neuropathies?

The electrophysiological findings of patients with CMT-1, CMT-2, and CMT-X are summarized in Tables 14.5–14.7. For CMT-1, Birouk and colleagues have provided the most detailed description *(4)*. These data indicate that the neuropathy clearly has demyelinating physiology. Distal latencies are markedly prolonged and conduction velocities are uniformly and markedly slowed, ranging from 7 to 33 m/s for the median nerve and from 5 to 24 m/s for the peroneal nerve *(4)*. The mean motor conduction velocities reported in different studies are quite similar. For example, the mean median motor nerve conduction velocity is approximately 20m/s in all studies *(1,3,4,6)*. There is somewhat more variation in the frequency of sensory nerve conduction abnormalities, with absent median sensory responses reported in 85% *(4)* to 93% *(1)* of patients and absent sural responses in 44% *(3)* to 98% of patients *(4)*.

The available descriptions of the electrophysiology of patients with CMT-2 are in general less detailed, with mean values but not the range of values reported *(1,3,10,11,14)*. This makes it a little more difficult to get a good perspective on the range of abnormalities encountered. As shown in Table 14.6, mean median motor nerve conduction velocity is typically normal (ranging from 48 to 55 m/s), mean tibial motor conduction velocity is mildly slowed (36 m/s) *(10)*, and mean peroneal nerve conduction velocity varies from

Table 14.4A

Symptoms of Charcot-Marie-Tooth (CMT)-X

	Dubourg (8)		Nicholson (7)		Birouk (5)	
	Males	*Females*	*Males*	*Females*	*Males*	*Females*
Sample size	41	52	20	32	21	27
Age of onset						
Mean age (range)	15 (1–40)	19 (1–56)	NR	NR	17 (5–40)	25 (12–56)
First decade	27%	15%	55%	19%	14%	0
Second decade	NR	NR	40%	16%	33%	30%
Asymptomatic	11%	29%	5%	50%	21%	42%
Motor symptoms	NR	NR			NR	NR
Difficulty walking/running			60%	44%		
Ankle injury/instability			95%	75%		
Weak grip			30%	31%		
Sensory symptoms	NR	NR			NR	NR
Paresthesia			NR	NR		
Neuropathic pain			NR	NR		
Sensory loss			15%	22%		

Table 14.4B
Physical Signs in Charcot-Marie Tooth (CMT)-X

	Dubourg (8)		Nicholson (7)		Birouk (5)	
	Males	*Females*	*Males*	*Females*	*Males*	*Females*
Sample size	*41*	*52*	*20*	*32*	*21*	*27*
Weakness	87%	52%		71%	35%	NR
Legs	NR	NR	75%	25%	NR	NR
Arms	NR	NR	15%	12.5%	NR	NR
Foot deformity	97%	79%	90%	78%	90%	85%
Deep tendon reflexes	NR					
Normal		0%	9%	NR	NR	NR
Absent ankle reflexes		100%	72%	NR	NR	NR
Absent ankle & knee reflexes		NR	75%	19%	86%	81%
Sensory loss			90%	75%		
Pain and touch	62%	41%	NR	NR	63%	32%
Proprioception	83%	59%	NR	NR	84%	73%
Tremor	NR	NR	NR	NR	2%[a]	

[a]The gender of the single patient with tremor was not specified

Table 14.5
Electrophysiological Features of Charcot-Marie-Tooth (CMT)-1

	Harding (1)		Bouche (3)		Birouk (4)			Thomas (6)	
	Mean ±SD	Absent	Mean ±SD	Absent	Mean ±SD	Range	Absent	Mean ± SD	Range
Median motor									
DML (ms)					9.8 ± 3	4.6–22.3			
CMAP (mV)					2.42	0.1–9.5			
MCV (m/s)	21.1 ± 7		19.5 ± 5		20.2 ± 5	7–33	3.3%	19.9 ± 1	5–34
Ulnar motor									
DML (ms)					8 ± 3	4.5–16.4			
CMAP (mV)					2.4±2	0.04–8.5			
MCV (m/s)					17.3 ± 5	6–30	0		
Peroneal motor									
DML (ms)					11.9 ± 3	6–19.4			
CMAP (mV)					0.9 ± 1	0.07 – 4			
MCV (m/s)	16.6 ± 8		16.5 ± 5	58%	17 ± 5	5–24	20%	17 ± 1.2	10–22
Sural sensory				44%			98%		
Median sensory		93%					85%		

DML, distal motor latency; CMAP, compound muscle action potential; MCV, motor conduction velocity.

Table 14.6
Electrophysiological Features of Charcot-Marie-Tooth (CMT)-2

	Harding (1)		Bouche (3)		Berciano (14)		Teunissen (10)		Elliot[a] (11)	
	Mean ±SD	Absent	Mean ±SD	Absent	Mean ±SD	Absent	Mean ±SD	Absent	Mean ±SD	Absent
Median motor								0		
DML (ms)					3.6 ± 0.4		4.3 ± 0.7		4 ± 1	
CMAP (mV)					11.9 ± 4		7.4 ± 3		3.7 ± 4	
MCV (m/s)	51.9 ± 9		50.7 ± 6		54 ± 12		55 ± 8		48 9	75%
Ulnar motor								0		
DML (ms)							5.8 ± 1.4			
CMAP (mV)							1.2 ± 1			
MCV (m/s)							36 ± 5			
Peroneal motor										100%
DML (ms)					5 ± 1					
CMAP (mV)					5 ± 3					
MCV (m/s)	44.2 ± 10		37 ± 8		45 ± 9		45. ± 0.4			
Sural sensory		73%		24%	5.5 ± 5	0		50%		100%
Median sensory							6 ± 4	5%		

DML, distal motor latency; CMAP, compound muscle action potential; MCV, motor conduction velocity.

[a]This study included 10 subjects from a single family with CMT-IIB, many of whom had trophic toe and foot ulcers.

259

Table 14.7
Electrophysiological Features of Charcot-Marie-Tooth (CMT)-X

| | Birouk (5) | | | | Dubourg (8) | | | |
| | Males | | Females | | Males | | Females | |
	Mean ± SD	Range	Mean ± SD	Range	Mean ± SD	Range	Mean ± SD	Range
Median motor								
DML (ms)	4.7 ± 1	2.3–7.0	3.8 ± 1	2.7–6.2	4.9 ± 1.2	2.3–8.8	3.8 ± 0.8	2.5–6.2
CMAP (mV)	2.6 ± 2	0.3–6.3	3.9 ± 2	0.8–9.7	2.2 ± 2	0–8.6	4.6 ± 3	0.6–10
MCV (m/s)	36.2 ± 7	31–60	44.± 7	31–55	34.5 ± 7	20–60	44.4 ± 7	28–60
Ulnar motor								
DML (ms)		3.9 ± 1	2.8 ± 6.4	2.9 ± 1	2.3–3.8	3.8–0.5	2.8–5.1	1.9–4.1
CMAP (mV)	3.1 ± 2	0.4–6.0	6.4 ± 3	1.5–11	3.4 ± 2	0–7.8	6.4 ± 3	0.9–12
MCV (m/s)	36.9 ± 6	29–49	46 ± 7	29–59	36.1 ± 5	27–49	44.6 ± 8	29–67
Peroneal motor								
DML (ms)	5.6 ± 2	2.7–8.3	5.5 ± 2	3.3–9.8	6.3 ± 2	2.7–9.9	5 ± 1.5	2.3–9.8
CMAP (mV)	1.9 ± 2	0.05–4.6	2.4 ± 2	0.1–5	0.7–1.6	0–7.4	1.7 ± 2	0–5.4
MCV (m/s)	34.5 ± 11	21–52	37 ± 8	14–52[a]	32 ± 9	17–52	38.6 ± 7	14–52
Median	57%[b]		38%[b]					
Sural	61%[b]		63%[b]					

[a]Manuscript reports range as 14.2 to 7.4, which must be an error. Data presented here is extrapolated from Fig. 3C of the manuscript.
[b]Values represent percentage of patients with absent sensory responses.
DML, distal motor latency; CMAP, compound muscle action potential; MCV, motor conduction velocity.

mildly slowed (37 m/s) *(3)* to normal (45 m/s) *(1,14)*. The narrow standard deviations around these estimates of the mean indicate that the conduction velocity is similarly normal or only mildly slowed in the vast majority of patients. Motor response amplitudes range from mildly reduced *(10,11)* to normal *(1,14)*. The frequency with which sensory responses are absent varies from 5% *(10)* to 73% *(1)* for the median nerve and 25% *(3)* to 100% *(11)* for the sural nerve. These findings, therefore, are clearly different from those described in patients with CMT-1 and indicate a primarily axonal physiology.

The most notable feature of the electrophysiological findings in patients with CMT-X is that they differ substantially between males and females (Table 14.7) *(5,8)*. Estimates of the mean conduction velocity of the median, ulnar, and peroneal nerves are all significantly slower in males compared to females although there is extensive overlap in the range of values reported *(5,8)*. Conduction velocity may vary from normal to markedly slow, indicating that either axonal or demyelinating physiology may be present. Estimates of the mean distal motor latency are similarly more prolonged in men than in women, at least for the median and ulnar nerves *(5,8)*. Motor response amplitudes are also significantly lower in males compared with females although, as with the measurements of conduction velocity, there is substantial overlap in the range of values reported *(5,8)*. CMT-X, therefore, seems to have an intermediate phenotype between the demyelinating physiology of CMT-1 and the axonal physiology of CMT-2.

2.3. Which Are the Most Common Hereditary Neuropathies?

The frequency with which particular mutations are found in patients with the Charcot-Marie Tooth (peroneal muscular atrophy) phenotype is expected to vary depending on the definition used to define the population of interest and may also vary according to the genetic / ethnic background of the subjects studied (Table 14.8). Dubourg and colleagues have reported their experience with 270 patients seen at the Salpêtrière Hospital in Paris *(15)*. This study included patients with a clinical diagnosis of CMT, 63% of whom were classified as CMT-1 on the basis of a median motor conduction velocity less than 40 m/s. The overall frequency of the PMP-22 duplication in the entire study population was 30%, but rose to 48.5% among those with median motor conduction velocity less than 40 m/s and to 67% among those with median motor conduction velocity less than 30 m/s *(15)*. In their study of 75 patients with a clinical diagnosis of CMT in the United States, Wise and colleagues reported an overall frequency of the PMP duplication in 56% of patients *(16)*. The frequency of the PMP duplication was even higher (68%) among those with median motor conduction velocity less than 40 m/s *(16)*. These estimates are somewhat higher than those reported from the French population *(15)*. Interestingly, the frequency of the PMP duplication among patients with median motor conduction velocity less than 40 m/s in a European collaborative study (71%) more closely approximated the estimate from the United States *(17)*.

In the French study the overall frequency of Connexin-32 mutations in the entire study population was 8% and was relatively unchanged (10%) among those with median motor conduction velocity less than 40 m/s *(15)*. The frequency of Connexin-32 mutations was highest among the group of patients with median motor conduction velocity between 30 and 40 m/s (30%) *(15)*.

In a more recent study, Boerkoel and colleagues have reported the relative frequencies of a larger array of mutations in a group of 153 patients in whom the diagnosis of an

Table 14.8
Mutational Frequency in Charcot-Marie-Tooth Disease

	Dubourg (15)	Wise (16)	Nelis (17)	Boerkoel (18)
Sample size	270	75	819	153
Population ethnicity	French	American	European	NR
Proportion of patients with no family history (sporadic)	34%	NR	NR	NR
Proportion of patients with MCV <40 m/s	63%	85%	100%[a]	NR
Proportion of patients with MCV <30 m/s	47%	NR	NR	NR
Overall frequency of PMP duplication	30%	56%	NR	52%
Overall frequency of Cx-32 mutations	8%	NR	NR	7%
Frequency of PMP duplication among those with MCV <40 m/s	48.5%	68%	71%	NR
Frequency of Cx-32 mutations among those with MCV <40 m/s	10%	NR	NR	NR
Frequency of PMP duplication among those with MCV <30 m/s	67%	NR	NR	NR
Frequency of PMP duplication among those with dominant inheritance and MCV <30 m/s	83%	NR	NR	NR
Frequency of PMP duplication among those with dominant inheritance and MCV <40 m/s	63%	NR	85%	NR
Frequency of Cx-32 mutations among those with x-linked inheritance (no male-to-male transmission) and MCV <30 m/s	20%	NR	NR	NR
Frequency of PMP duplication among sporadic cases with MCV <30 m/s	37%	NR	NR	NR
Frequency of PMP duplication among sporadic cases with MCV <40 m/s	33%	NR	53%	NR
Frequency of Cx-32 mutations among sporadic cases with MCV <40 m/s	7%	NR	NR	NR

[a]Patients selected on the basis of motor conduction velocity (MCV) <38 m/s.
PMP, peripheral myelin protein; NR, not reported.

262

hereditary neuropathy was suspected *(18)*. This population of patients was more hetero-geneous than those included in the studies cited above in that they included patients with the CMT phenotype as well as those with Dejerine-Sottas syndrome, congenital hypo-myelinating neuropathy, and hereditary neuropathy with liability to pressure palsies, the effect of which should be to dilute out the relative importance of the PMP duplication (if this mutation is primarily associated with CMT as indicated by prior data). They detected the PMP-22 duplication in 52% of their patients and the Connexin-32 (Gap Junction protein B1) in 7% of patients *(18)*. Other mutations were much less frequent—myelin protein zero (3%), PMP-22 point mutation (3%), early growth response gene 2 (0.65%), periaxin (0.65%), and the neurofilament light change gene (0.65%). No mutation was identified in 33% of subjects *(18)*.

Irrespective of the population studied, the PMP-22 duplication is the most frequently encountered mutation amongst patients with a clinical diagnosis of CMT, accounting for 30% *(15)* to 56% *(16)* of mutations. The frequency with which this mutation is found increases as the study population becomes more focused (e.g., considering only patients with slow median motor conduction velocity and/or dominant inheritance). Mutations in the Connexin-32 (GJB1) gene are the next most commonly encountered, being present in approximately 7–8% of patients *(15,18)*.

2.4. Which Electrophysiological Features Are Most Helpful in Distinguishing Between Hereditary and Acquired Demyelinating Neuropathies?

In their classic paper, Lewis and Sumner compared the electrophysiological features of acquired and hereditary demyelinating neuropathies in 58 patients *(19)*. This was a retrospective study that initially included 75 patients with neuropathy of at least 6 months duration in whom electrophysiological studies indicated demyelinating physiology. Seventeen patients in whom the family history was unclear were excluded, leaving 18 patients with hereditary neuropathy, all of whom had autosomal dominant inheritance, pes cavus, and peroneal muscular atrophy (half of whom also had palpably thickened nerves or onion-bulb formation on nerve biopsy), who were considered to have CMT-1, as well as 40 patients with no family history, all of whom had slowly progressive or relapsing-remitting neuropathy with areflexia, high cerebrospinal fluid (CSF) protein, and segmental demyelination when biopsy was performed (presumed acquired demyeli-nating neuropathy).

They found a number of electrophysiological differences between those with acquired and those with hereditary demyelinating neuropathy. Hereditary neuropathy was charac-terized by uniformity of conduction velocity slowing as well as the absence of conduction block and temporal dispersion *(19)*. The uniformity of conduction velocity slowing was evidenced by two observations. First, the difference in conduction velocity between the median and ulnar nerves never exceeded 5 m/s. Second, the degree of conduction velocity slowing was proportionate to the degree of prolongation of the distal latency in all but one patient, indicating that proximal and distal nerve segments were equally affected *(19)*. Differential slowing of conduction velocity between the median and ulnar nerves was not uniformly present in those with acquired neuropathies. Furthermore, none of the patients with hereditary neuropathy manifested greater than 40% temporal dispersion whereas such dispersion was present in approximately two-thirds of those with acquired neuropathy. Finally, conduction block was never observed among those with hereditary neuropathy, but was present in 30% of those with acquired neuropathy *(19)*. As shown in Table 14.9, the sensitivity of these findings for the diagnosis of an acquired demyelinating neuropathy is relatively low (ranging from as low as 30% to as high as 67%), but the specificity is high (94–100%) *(19)*.

2.5. Are There Any Clinical or Electrophysiological Features That Help to Differentiate Idiopathic Axonal Polyneuropathy From CMT-2?

Teunissen and colleagues compared the clinical and electrophysiological features of patients with chronic idiopathic axonal neuropathy (CIAP) and CMT-2. The diagnosis of CIAP was applied when no cause for the neuropathy could be identified despite extensive clinical and laboratory evaluation including a detailed family history with clinical and neurophysiological evaluation of family members if there was any suspicion of an affected relative *(10)*. Patients with CIAP tended to be older and reported shorter duration of disease. Symptoms were more often sensory in patients with CIAP (60% CIAP vs 15% CMT-2) whereas motor symptoms predominated in patients with CMT-2 (40% CIAP vs 85% CMT-2) *(10)*. Pes cavus and hammer toes were present in 57% and 30% of patients with CMT-2 compared with 13% of patients with CIAP. The major electrophysiological difference between CIAP and CMT-2 was the more frequent finding of ongoing denervation changes (fibrillations and positive sharp waves) as well as chronic reinnervation changes (neurogenic motor unit action potentials) in patients with CMT-2. The sensitivity and specificity of these findings, however, are insufficient to provide a useful means of differentiating the two disorders. For example, the sensitivity and specificity (for the diagnosis of CMT-2) of pes cavus are 0.57 and 0.88, respectively, and the sensitivity and specificity (for the diagnosis of CMT-2) of finding ongoing denervation changes are 0.8 and 0.5, respectively *(10)*. There are, therefore, no reliable clinical or electrophysiological features that permit ready differentiation of CMT-2 from chronic idiopathic acquired axonal neuropathy.

2.6. What Are the Typical Clinical Features of Hereditary Neuropathy With Liability to Pressure Palsies?

The published literature indicates that the clinical presentation of hereditary neuropathy with liability to pressure palsies (HNPP) is heterogeneous (Table 14.10) *(20–22)*. The series by Mouton and colleagues is one of the largest and these authors offered a classification of the different clinical presentations of patients with HNPP harboring the typical 17p11.2 deletion *(20)*. The overwhelming majority of patients (71%) presented with symptoms and signs of acute peripheral nerve palsy. Approximately 14% of patients with the gene deletion were entirely asymptomatic. Other clinical presentations were relatively uncommon and included recurrent short-term positional sensory symptoms (5%), chronic sensorimotor polyneuropathy (4%), chronic sensory polyneuropathy (3%), progressive sensorimotor mononeuropathy of the peroneal nerve (2%) and recurrent episodes of quadraparesis (1%) *(20)*. The smaller series by Amato and colleagues similarly found that the disease manifests as pressure-induced neuropathies in the majority of patients (67%) with other clinical presentations being quite rare *(21)*. In this series, 22% of patients with the gene deletion were asymptomatic and 2 patients (11%) presented with a generalized sensorimotor polyneuropathy *(21)*.

Table 14.9
Diagnostic Accuracy of Electrodiagnostic Findings for Hereditary (vs Acquired) Neuropathy

Electrophysiological finding	Sensitivity	Specificity
Median-Ulnar conduction velocity difference of 5 m/s	54%	100%
Disproportionate slowing of conduction velocity and prolongation of distal latency	37.5%	94%
Temporal dispersion ≥ 40%	67%	100%
Conduction block	30%	100%

Data from ref. *19*

Precise estimates of the frequency with which particular nerves are affected in HNPP vary between studies (Table 14.11), but most suggest that the peroneal and ulnar nerves, as well as the brachial plexus, are most commonly affected. Most studies have emphasized that compression neuropathies are painless *(20,22)*. Generalized areflexia is relatively uncommon (12–21%) amongst those with the gene deletion *(20,22)*, but apparently much more common among those with the less common frame-shift mutation in the PMP-22 gene, being found in 73% of such patients *(22)*.

2.7. What Are the Typical Electrophysiological Features of Hereditary Neuropathy With Liability to Pressure Palsies?

In contrast to the typical clinical presentation with recurrent acute peripheral nerve palsies, the electrophysiological findings in patients with HNPP suggest more diffuse involvement of the peripheral nervous system *(20–24)*. Most *(20,21,23,24)*, but not all *(22)*, studies have emphasized that distal nerve segments are affected more frequently and more severely than the proximal nerve segments. The data in Tables 14.12A and 14.12B are presented in two forms (based on what is available from the literature). For some studies, it has been possible to estimate the degree of distal motor latency prolongation (expressed as a percentage of the upper limit of normal) as well as the degree of slowing of motor conduction velocity (expressed as a percentage of the lower limit of normal), representing the speed of motor nerve conduction along distal and proximal nerve segments, respectively *(20,22,25)*. In the other study, the data for distal motor latency prolongation and conduction velocity slowing are expressed as Z-scores *(21)*. It will be recalled that Z-scores describe the number of standard deviations from the mean for a standard normal population (a population with a mean value of 0 and a standard deviation of 1), with large absolute Z-scores indicating values that are significantly different from the mean. The mean absolute values for distal motor latency, conduction velocity and response amplitude are shown in Table 14.12B. The data shown in Tables 14.12A and 14.12B do suggest that distal motor latency prolongation is more marked and occurs more frequently than slowing of conduction velocity. Another way to appreciate the discrepancy between the degree of distal motor latency prolongation and the severity of proximal conduction velocity is to calculate the terminal latency index (TLI) (terminal distance divided by the product of distal motor latency and conduction velocity). TLIs from two studies are summarized in Table 14.12C. TLI for the median, ulnar, and peroneal nerves are all lower than normal, indicating preferential slowing of distal motor conduction velocity.

Table 14.10
Clinical Features of Hereditary Neuropathy Wth Liability to Pressure Palsies (HNPP)

Reference	n	Genetics	Familial	Sporadic	Clinical syndromes	Clinical features
Mouton (20)	99	17p11.2 deletion	75%	25%	Acute peripheral nerve palsy (n = 70) Recurrent short-term postural sensory symptoms (n = 5) Progressive sensorimotor mononeuropathy (n = 2) Chronic sensory polyneuropathy (n = 3) Chronic sensorimotor polyneuropathy (n = 4) Recurrent episodes of quadraparesis (n = 1) Asymptomatic (n = 14)	Peroneal and ulnar nerves most commonly affected Painless in 100% Pes cavus in 18% Complete areflexia in 12% Absent ankle reflexes in 37% Positional sensory symptoms in 11%
Lenssen (22)	86	17p11.2 deletion (n = 63) PMP22 G-insertion (n = 23)	100%	0	Not reported	Peroneal and ulnar nerves most commonly affected Painless in 100% Pes cavus & complete areflexia in ~73% frame-shift and ~20% deletion patients
Amato (21)	18	17p11.2 deletion (n = 16)	72%	28%	Pressure-induced neuropathies (n = 12) Generalized sensorimotor polyneuropathy (n = 2) Asymptomatic (n = 4)	Peroneal and ulnar nerves most commonly affected
Pareyson (31)	39	17p11.2 deletion	82%	18%[a]	Acute mononeuropathy or brachial plexopathy (n = 25) Chronic symptoms including cramps, paresthesia, myalgia, weakness (n = 13) Asymptomatic (n = 16)	Upper limbs affected more commonly than lower limb nerves; brachial plexopathy also common Painless Pes cavus–38%

[a]May not all have been sporadic, as the parents of apparently sporadically affected siblings could not be examined.

Table 14.11

Frequency of Individual Nerve Involvement in Hereditary Neuropathy With Liability to Pressure Palsies

| | Mouton (20) | Amato (21) | Lenssen (22) | | Hong (23) |
	17p11.2 deletion	17p11.2 deletion	Frame-shift	17p11.2 deletion	17p11.2 deletion
Peroneal	36%	33%	70%	38%	25%
Ulnar	28%	39%	15%	21%	25%
Brachial plexus	20%	22%	10%	25%	–
Radial	13%	–	0	4%	50%
Median	4%	–	5%	11%	12.5%
Tibial	0	–	–	–	–
Facial	2%	–	–	–	–

Focal slowing of conduction velocity at typical sites of nerve compression is commonly encountered at the elbow (80–85%) *(20,22)*, but more variably present at the fibular head (17–64%) *(20,22)*.

There are fewer published sensory electrophysiological data from patients with HNPP, and the available data are quite varied (Table 14.12D). The study by Amato and colleagues suggests that abnormalities of sensory nerve conduction velocity are more prominent than reductions in response amplitudes, as evidenced by the larger Z-scores *(21)*. Data from the other three studies are less clear. All seem to agree, however, that abnormalities of sensory nerve conduction of some sort are fairly diffuse and commonly present.

In summary then, the typical electrophysiological features of HNPP include diffuse abnormalities of both sensory and motor nerves with preferential slowing of conduction velocity in distal nerve segments which manifests as disproportionately prolonged distal motor latencies. Focal slowing of conduction velocity at sites of compression is encountered less frequently that might be expected.

3. TREATMENT

3.1. Does Creatine Supplementation Improve Strength in Patients With Hereditary Neuropathy?

In a small cross-over trial, 39 patients with CMT-1 or CMT-2 were randomized to receive either placebo or supplementation with creatine monohydrate for 1 month, with a 5-week washout period in between each treatment period *(26)*. A variety of outcome measures were used, including a visual analog activities of daily living scale, a 30 m timed walk, maximal grip strength, and maximal voluntary isometric contraction as well as measures of weight and body composition. No significant differences were found between the two treatment groups on any of these outcome measures.

This study has serious methodological shortcomings. No outcome measure was specified as primary, there was no discussion of the changes in outcome measures that would be regarded as clinically meaningful, and there was no power analysis (suggesting that the study was almost certainly underpowered to detect a clinical effect). Furthermore, the method of randomization was not described, allocation concealment was not mentioned, and the methods used to ensure blinding were not reported. The authors' conclusion that creatine supplementation is not beneficial in patients with CMT is, therefore, unjustified, as this study really was inadequate to answer the question. The potential benefit of supplementation with creatine monohydrate remains unknown.

3.2. Is Resistance Training Exercise Beneficial for Patients With Hereditary Neuropathy?

It is has been claimed that patients with CMT respond to resistance training with improved muscle strength and function on the basis of the results of a randomized controlled study *(27)*, but this conclusion is not supported by the data. The study that is cited in support of this conclusion was a trial in which subjects were randomized to receive either resistance exercise training together with creatine supplementation or resistance exercise training with placebo supplementation. The study included 20 patients and

Table 14.12A
Electrophysiological Features of Hereditary Neuropathy With Liability to Pressure Palsies

Reference	Mean DML—%ULN (%nerves DML>ULN)				Mean MCV slowing—% LLN (%nerves MCV<LLN)				Focal slowing at sites of nerve compression	
	Median	Ulnar	Peroneal	Tibial	Median	Ulnar	Peroneal	Tibial	Elbow	Knee
Mouton (20)	164 (99%)	125 (82%)	136 (88%)	125 (77%)	100 (39%)	100 (40%)	88 (78%)	–	80%	17%
Lenssen (22)	–	137 (20%)	176 (64%)	–	–	98 (38%)	86 (82%)	–	–	–
Hong (25)	156	132	121	107	107	96	97	97	–	–
Pareyson (31)	–	154	–	–	–	–	–	–	56%	9%

Reference	DML—mean Z-score				MCV slowing—mean Z-score				Focal slowing at sites of nerve compression	
	Median	Ulnar	Peroneal	Tibial	Median	Ulnar	Peroneal	Tibial	Elbow	Knee
Amato (21)	-5.4	-4.0	-3.9	-1.2	-1.8	-2.8	-3.2	-2.1	85%	64%

DML, distal motor latency; MCV, motor conduction velocity.
ULN, upper limit of normal. LLN, lower limit of normal

Table 14.12B
Electrophysiological Features of Hereditary Neuropathy With Liability to Pressure Palsies

Reference	Mean DML				Mean MCV			
	Median	Ulnar	Peroneal	Tibial	Median	Ulnar	Peroneal	Tibial
Mouton (20)	5.9 ms	3.7 ms	6.8 ms	6.2 ms	48 m/s	50 m/s	37 m/s	–
Lenssen (22)	–	3.7 ms	5.8 ms	–	–	49 m/s	36 m/s	–
Pareyson (31)	5.4 ms	3.7 ms	6.8 ms	–	50 m/s	52 m/s	37 m/s	–
Amato (21)	6.0 ms	3.9 ms	8.1 ms	5.0 ms	50 m/s	50 m/s	40 m/s	40 m/s

Table 14.12C

Terminal Latency Index[a] in Patients With Hereditary Neuropathy With Liability to Pressure Palsies (HNPP)

	Median	Ulnar	Peroneal	Tibial
Hong (23)	0.17	0.32	0.35	0.48
Amato (21)	0.25	0.38	0.27	0.44

[a]Normal values for terminal latency index (TLI) for each nerve are not well established, but the TLIs for the median, ulnar, and peroneal nerves were regarded as significantly smaller for HNPP patients compared with healthy controls in both studies.

Table 14.12D

Sensory Electrophysiology in Hereditary Neuropathy With Liability to Pressure Palsies

Reference	Mean SNAP Amplitude %LLN (% nerves SNAP<LLN)				Mean sensory CV slowing % LLN (% nerves CV<LLN)			
	Median	Ulnar	Peroneal	Tibial	Median	Ulnar	Peroneal	Tibial
Mouton (20)	75 (65%)	75 (66%)	100 (58%)	80 (60%)	–	–	–	–
Lenssen (22)	20 (80%)	–	–	48 (45%)	(90%)	–	–	(63%)
Hong (25)	–	–	–	–	74	78	–	89
	SNAP amplitude—mean Z-score				Sensory CV slowing—mean Z-score			
	Median	Ulnar	Peroneal	Tibial	Medial	Ulnar	Peroneal	Tibial
Amato (21)	–1.3	–1.4	–1.3	–0.9	–9.3	–4.7	–4.0	–6.0

ULN, upper limit normal; LLN, lower limit normal; SNAP, sensory nerve action potential; CV, conduction velocity.

outcome was measured using quantitative muscular assessment and a timed activities of daily living score as well as energy metabolites and muscle biopsy findings. There were no significant differences between the two groups after the 12-week study period *(27)*, supporting the idea that creatine is of no benefit (although there was no discussion of the power of this study to detect a benefit, and so even this conclusion should be treated with caution). Although the study was not designed to examine the effects of resistance exercise training, the authors concluded that such training significantly improved both activities of daily living and strength in patients with CMT *(27)*. The analysis that supports this conclusion is clearly post hoc and uncontrolled (because the randomization and blinding were relevant to the use of creatine/placebo and not exercise). At best, this conclusion may be taken as preliminary data that might be used to justify a new study to examine the effects of resistance training exercise.

4. PROGNOSIS

4.1. What Is the Prognosis for Patients With CMT-1A?

There are limited published data that shed light on the long-term prognosis of patients with CMT-1A *(4,28)*. In their combined cross-sectional and longitudinal study, Dyck and colleagues used the neurological disability score (NDS) to grade the severity of the neuropathy in a group of patients with HMSN type 1 with the phenotype based on the presence of an autosomal dominant demyelinating neuropathy without linkage to the Duffy blood group. It should be recalled that, despite its name, the NDS does not really measure disability. This is a score that quantifies deficits of cranial nerve function, skeletal muscle strength in the arms and legs, deep tendon reflexes, and sensation *(29)*. Linear regression analysis of the data from the cross-sectional part of this study was reported to show that NDS scores increased (i.e., neurological deficits increased) with advancing age, but the slope estimates to describe the strength of this association as well as the R-square values (to quantify how much of the variability in NDS scores could be attributed to the age) are not presented *(28)*. These authors also reported that nerve conduction velocity at the time of initial evaluation was a reliable predictor of final outcome, with slower conduction velocities predicting higher NDS scores (i.e., greater neurological deficit) *(28)*.

In their series of 119 patients with CMT-1A and duplication of 17p11.2, Birouk and colleagues evaluated prognosis using the global neurological disability score (GNDS) *(4)*. Similar to the NDS used by Dyck and colleagues, the GNDS quantifies weakness, sensory loss, and reflex changes in the arms and legs and also does not measure disability. GNDS scores were maximal (worst) in approximately 30% of patients and minimal (scores of 1–5) in approximately 17% of patients. The latter group mostly comprised asymptomatic subjects who had been identified during screening of family members with the disease. These authors also used the Functional Disability Scale (FDS), a scale that ranges from 0 (normal) to 8 (bed bound) to measure disability. They found FDS scores of 0–1 in 35% of patients and scores of 2–3[*] in 60% *(4)*. There was a marked difference in FDS scores between those with age of onset less than 20 and those with older age of

---

[*]A score of 2 indicates inability to run, and a score of 3 indicates some difficulty walking, but still able to ambulate without assistance.

onset. FDS scores of 3 were found in over 40% of those with younger age of onset compared with less than 20% of those with older onset *(4)*.

Although limited in both quality and quantity, these data suggest that neurological deficits and disability increase with advancing age and that those with onset in the first two decades of life are more likely to develop difficulty walking and inability to run as the disease advances. Although it has been suggested that slower nerve conduction velocity predicts subsequent disability, there really is insufficient data to permit reliable prognostication for this disease.

4.2. What Is the Prognosis for Patients With CMT-2?

There are extremely few published data upon which to base any firm conclusions about prognosis for patients with CMT-2. In one small study, 43 of 55 patients with CMT-2 were followed for an average of 5 years *(9)*. In general, there was very gradual progression over time. Approximately 80% of patients reported subjective increase in weakness with supportive findings on examination, and about 50% reported increased sensory loss. At follow-up, the modified Rankin score (mRS) was $\leq 2^{\dagger}$ in most patients (72%), with an mRS of $3^{\S}$ in a further 23% *(9)*. The mRS score increased by one point in one-third of patients over the 5-year duration of the study. Such progression is not insignificant given the relatively short duration of the study. Longer term follow-up data have not been published and there are no reliable data to indicate if any factors are predictive of better or worse outcome.

4.3. What Is the Prognosis for Patients With HNPP?

Very little has been published about the prognosis for recovery in HNPP. In their series of 36 patients with HNPP, Gouider and colleagues reported that recovery was complete within 24 hours in 10% of acute peripheral nerve palsies, delayed for up to 6 months in 62%, and delayed more than 6 months in 28%. Overall, recovery was incomplete in 51% of nerve palsy episodes, but the residual motor deficit was severe in only 9% *(30)*. A similarly low frequency of persistent severe motor deficits was reported by Mouton and colleagues, who found that only 15% of patients had motor weakness worse than Medical Research Council score of 3 at least 3 months after the acute peripheral nerve palsy *(20)*. The prognosis for recovery in HNPP is, therefore, generally good, although a small proportion of patients will have persistent severe weakness.

5. SUMMARY

- The hereditary neuropathies are a clinically and genetically heterogeneous group of disorders.
- CMT type 1, also known as HMSN type 1, is the most common form and is usually due to a duplication on chromosome 17p11.2 that includes the PMP-22 gene.
- PMP-22 duplications account for approximately 30–50% of hereditary neuropathies.

[†]Slight disability; unable to carry out all previous activities, but able to look after own affairs without assistance.

[§]Moderate disability, requiring some help but able to walk without assistance.

- Connexin-32 (also known as the gap junction protein B1 gene) mutations (seen in CMT-X) are the second most common genetic abnormality and account for 7–8% of hereditary neuropathies.
- The typical clinical phenotype of the CMT syndromes is that of progressive distal muscle weakness and wasting, distal symmetric sensory loss, absent distal deep tendon reflexes, and foot deformities (hammer toes and pes cavus).
- There are few clinical differences between CMT-1, CMT-2, and CMT-X. Clues to the underlying genetic abnormality include more frequent onset of symptoms after the second decade of life in CMT-2 and CMT-X (especially in affected females), an X-linked pattern of inheritance (no male-to-male transmission), a family history of a more severe phenotype in men in CMT-X and early involvement of respiratory muscles and vocal cords in CMT-2C.
- There are marked electrophysiological differences between CMT-1, CMT-2, and CMT-X. CMT-1 is a demyelinating neuropathy, CMT-2 has axonal features, and CMT-X has an intermediate phenotype in which either demyelinating or axonal physiology may be present.
- Acquired demyelinating neuropathies may be distinguished from CMT-1 by the presence of differential slowing of conduction velocity across different nerves and across proximal and distal nerve segments, the presence of temporal dispersion and the presence of conduction block. The sensitivity of these findings is relatively low, but their specificity is high.
- There are no reliable electrophysiological features that permit ready differentiation of CMT-2 from acquired idiopathic axonal polyneuropathy.
- The most common clinical presentation of HNPP is that of recurrent acute painless peripheral compression neuropathies, but other clinical phenotypes include recurrent postural sensory symptoms and progressive sensory or sensorimotor polyneuropathy.
- The most common genetic abnormality among patients with HNPP is a deletion on chromosome 17p11.2 that encompasses the PMP-22 gene.
- The typical electrophysiological features of patients with HNPP are diffuse sensory and motor abnormalities, often with more severe involvement of distal nerve segments; focal slowing of conduction velocity at sites of compression is encountered less frequently than might be expected.
- There are no known effective therapies for patients with hereditary neuropathy. Supplementation with creatine monohydrate and resistance training have been examined in small randomized controlled trials, but the results of these studies were inconclusive
- The natural history of CMT-1 is that of gradual progression with increasing motor and sensory deficits. Approximately one-third of patients remain without significant disability and two-thirds develop mild-to-moderate disability (difficulty running and some difficulty walking, but retained ability to ambulate independently). Severe disability may develop, but is uncommon. There is a tendency for more severe disability to develop in those with age of onset before the age of 20 years.
- The natural history of CMT-2 is also one of gradual progression. Worsening of one grade on the mRS scale can be expected in approximately one-third of patients over a 5-year period. Approximately 25% of patients will require assistance with activities of daily living, but retain the ability to ambulate independently.
- The prognosis for recovery of acute peripheral nerve palsies in HNPP is generally good. A small proportion of patients may have permanent motor weakness, but this is rarely severe.

REFERENCES

1. Harding A, Thomas P. The clinical features of hereditary motor and sensory neuropathy types I and II. Brain 1980;103:259–280.

2. Hahn A, Brown W, Koopman W, Feasby T. X-linked dominant hereditary motor and sensory neuropathy. Brain 1990;113:1511–1525.

3. Bouche P, Gherardi R, Cathala H, Lhermitte F, Castaigne P. Peroneal muscular atrophy - Part 1. Clinical and electrophysiological study. J Neurol Sci 1983;61:389–399.

4. Birouk N, Gouider R, LeGuern E, et al. Charcot-Marie-Tooth disease type 1A with 17p11.2 duplication. Clinical and electrophysiological phenotype study and factors influencing disease severity in 119 cases. Brain 1997;120:813–823.

5. Birouk N, LeGuern E, Maisonobe T, et al. X-linked Charcot-Marie-Tooth disease with connexin 32 mutations. Clinical and electrophysiologic study. Neurology 1998;50:1074–1082.

6. Thomas P, Marques W, Davis M, et al. The phenotypic manifestations of chromosome 17p11.2 duplication. Brain 1997;120:465–478.

7. Nicholson G, Nash J. Intermediate nerve conduction velocities define X-linked Charcot-Marie-Tooth neuropathy families. Neurology 1993;43:2558–2564.

8. Dubourg O, Tardieu S, Birouk N, et al. Clinical, electrophysiological and molecular genetic characteristics of 93 patients with X-linked Charcot-Marie-Tooth disease. Brain 2001;124:1958–1967.

9. Teunissen LL, Notermans NC, Franssen H, van Engelen BG, Baas F, Wokke JH. Disease course of Charcot-Marie-Tooth disease type 2. A 5-year follow-up study. Arch Neurol 2003;60:823–828.

10. Teunissen L, Notermans N, Franssen H, et al. Differences between hereditary motor and sensory neuropathy type 2 and chronic idiopathic axonal neuropathy. A clinical and electrophysiological study. Brain 1997;120:955–962.

11. Elliott JL, Kwon JM, Goodfellow PJ, Yee W–C. Hereditary motor and sensory neuropathy IIB: Clinical and electrodiagnostic characteristics. Neurology 1997;48:23–28.

12. Dyck PJ, Litchy WJ, Minnerath S, et al. Hereditary motor and sensory neuropathy with diaphragm and vocal cord paresis. Ann Neurol 1994;35:608–615.

13. Hardie R, Harding A, Hirsch N, Gelder C, Macrae A, Thomas P. Diaphragmatic weakness in hereditary motor and sensory neuropathy. J Neurol Neurosurg Psychiatry 1990;53:348–350.

14. Berciano J, Combarros O, Figols J, et al. Hereditary motor and sensory neuropathy type II. Clinicopathological study of a family. Brain 1986;109:897–914.

15. Dubourg O, Tardieu S, Birouk N, et al. The frequency of 17p11.2 duplication and connexin 32 mutations in 282 Charcot-Marie-Tooth families in relation to the mode of inheritance and motor nerve conduction velocity. Neuromuscul Disord 2001;11:458–463.

16. Wise CA, Garcia CA, Davis SN, et al. Molecular analyses of unrelated Charcot-Marie-Tooth (CMT) disease patients suggest a high frequency of the CMT1A duplication. Am J Hum Genet 1993; 53:853–863.

17. Nelis E, Van Broeckhoven C, De Jonge P, et al. Estimation of the mutation frequencies in Charcot-Marie-Tooth disease type 1 and hereditary neuropathy with liability to pressure palsies: a European collaborative study. Eur J Hum Genet 1996;4:25–33.

18. Boerkoel C, Takashima H, Garcia CA, et al. Charcot-Marie-Tooth disease and related neuropathies: mutation distribution and genotype-phenotype correlation. Ann Neurol 2002;51:190–201.

19. Lewis RA, Sumner AJ. The electrodiagnostic distinctions between chronic familial and acquired demyelinative neuropathies. Neurology 1982;32:592–596.

20. Mouton P, Tardieu S, Gouider R, et al. Spectrum of clinical and electrophysiologic features in HNPP patients with the 17p11.2 deletion. Neurology 1999;52:1440–1446.

21. Amato AA, Gronseth GS, Callerame KJ, Kagan-Hallet KS, Bryan WW, Barohn RJ. Tomaculous neuropathy: a clinical and electrophysiological study in patients with and without 1.5–Mb deletions in chromosome 17p11.2. Muscle Nerve 1996;19:16–22.

22. Lenssen P, Gabreels-Festen A, Valentijn L, et al. Hereditary neuropathy with liability to pressure palsies. Phenotype differences between patients with the common deletion and a PMP22 frame shift mutation. Brain 1998;121:1451–1458.

23. Hong Y, Kim M, Kim H, Sung J, Kim S, Lee K. Clinical and electrophysiologic features of HNPP patients with 17p11.2 deletion. Acta Neurol Scand 2003;108:352–358.

24. Andersson P, Yuen E, Parko K, So YT. Electrodiagnostic features of hereditary neuropathy with liability to pressure palsies. Neurology 2000;54:40–44.
25. Hong CZ, Lee S, Lum P. Cervical radiculopathy. Clinical, radiographic and EMG findings. Orthop Rev 1986;15:433–439.
26. Doherty TJ, Lougheed K, Markez J, Tarnopolsky M. Creatine monohydrate does not increase strength in patients with hereditary neuropathy. Neurology 2001;57:559–560.
27. Chetlin RD, Gutmann L, Tarnopolsky MA, Ullrich IH, Yeater RA. Resistance training exercise and creatine in patients with Charcot-Marie-Tooth disease. Muscle Nerve 2004;30:69–76.
28. Dyck PJ, Karnes JL, Lambert EH. Longitudinal study of neuropathic deficits and nerve conduction abnormalities in hereditary motor and sensory neuropathy type 1. Neurology 1989;39:1302–1308.
29. Dyck P, Sherman W, Hallcher L, et al. Human diabetic endoneurial sorbitol, fructose, and myo-inositol related to sural nerve morphometry. Ann Neurol 1980;8:590–596.
30. Gouider R, LeGuern E, Gugenheim M, et al. Clinical, electrophysiologic, and molecular correlations in 13 families with hereditary neuropathy with liability to pressure palsies and a chromosome 17p11.2 deletion. Neurology 1995;45:2018–2023.
31. Pareyson D, Scaioli V, Taroni F, et al. Phenotype heterogeneity in hereditary neuropathy with liability to pressure palsies associated with chromosome 17p11.2 deletion. Neurology 1996;46:1133–1137.

15 Carpal Tunnel Syndrome

1. INTRODUCTION

Carpal tunnel syndrome (CTS) is a clinical disorder caused by compression of the median nerve at the wrist. The diagnosis can be made with confidence in patients with the typical clinical and electrodiagnostic features. It is the most common entrapment neuropathy with a cumulative lifetime incidence of approximately 8%. As a common cause of pain and functional impairment of the hand, it represents a significant cause of morbidity in the general population.

Because the definition entails the presence of clinical symptoms as well as a specific etiology (i.e., compression of the median nerve within the carpal tunnel), the question arises regarding how best to make the diagnosis. Should the diagnosis be based on clinical symptoms and signs alone or should there be a requirement for electrophysiological evidence for focal compression of the median nerve at the wrist? If clinical criteria are accepted as the gold standard, what are the sensitivity and specificity of the various electrodiagnostic tests for confirming the diagnosis? If neurophysiological evidence for focal compression of the median nerve at the wrist is used as the gold standard, what are the sensitivity and specificity of various clinical features for establishing the diagnosis? Once the diagnosis has been made, how should carpal tunnel syndrome be treated and which factors, if any, predict response to a particular treatment modality? These and other questions are the focus of this chapter.

2. DIAGNOSIS

2.1. What Is the Gold Standard for the Diagnosis of Carpal Tunnel Syndrome?

There is no widespread agreement regarding what constitutes the gold standard for the diagnosis of CTS; some favor clinical parameters and others argue in favor of electrodiagnostic parameters. The problem can be laid out as follows. CTS is a clinical disorder resulting from compression of the median nerve at the wrist. The problem with using clinical criteria alone for the diagnosis of CTS is that a range of other conditions, including polyneuropathy and cervical radiculopathy, may produce identical symptoms. Electrodiagnosis is the only way to prove that the symptoms arise from compression of the median nerve. The problem with relying on electrodiagnostic criteria as the gold standard for the diagnosis of CTS is that sensitivity of these tests is incomplete as evidenced in part by reports of patients with symptoms but normal electrodiagnostic findings, who respond to surgical decompression of the carpal tunnel. Ultimately, then, it is

From: *Neuromuscular Disease: Evidence and Analysis in Clinical Neurology*
By: M. Benatar © Humana Press Inc., Totowa, NJ

necessary to compromise and rely on the combination of clinical and electrophysiological findings, with the caveat that this approach will miss a small number of cases of CTS.

2.2. What Are the Sensitivity and Specificity of Clinical Signs and Symptoms in the Diagnosis of Carpal Tunnel Syndrome?

Attempts to define the sensitivity and specificity of clinical symptoms and signs for the diagnosis of CTS rely on a comparison being made between the diagnostic utility of these clinical features and the gold standard. Because use of a clinico-electrical gold standard would be subject to incorporation bias, attempts to define the diagnostic accuracy of clinical symptoms and signs must rely on the diagnosis being confirmed by electrophysiological tests.

With this in mind, the best source of data to answer the question at hand is the meta-analysis by D'Arcy and McGee (1). These authors included in their review studies in which (a) patients presented with symptoms suggestive of CTS, (b) independent electrophysiological testing was performed, (c) sufficient details were provided regarding how the clinical symptoms and signs were measured, and (d) sufficient data were provided to permit construction of basic 2×2 tables. Twelve articles met these inclusion criteria. A classic or probable hand diagram, diminished pinprick sensation in median nerve distribution, and weakness of thumb abduction were found to be most predictive of the diagnosis of CTS (Table 15.1). Clinical features that were not useful in predicting the diagnosis of CTS based on electrodiagnostic findings included the presence of nocturnal paresthesias, Phalen and Tinel's signs, thenar atrophy, two-point discriminative testing, and monofilament sensory testing.

2.3. What Are the Sensitivity and Specificity of Various Nerve Conduction Studies in the Diagnosis of Carpal Tunnel Syndrome?

The American Association of Electrodiagnostic Medicine has published a meta-analysis of the sensitivity and specificity of the various electrophysiological studies that are used in the diagnosis of carpal tunnel syndrome (2). The pooled summary estimates (with 95% confidence intervals) from this meta-analysis are summarized in Table 15.2.

The specificity for all of the tests is uniformly good. The sensitivity is somewhat variable, being highest for the median and ulnar comparative digit-IV sensory nerve conduction study (NCS) and lowest for the median motor distal latency. Using combinations of these tests, however, can improve the degree of certainty with which the diagnosis of carpal tunnel syndrome can be excluded.

2.4. How Does the Presence of an Underlying Polyneuropathy Affect the Sensitivity and Specificity of Electrophysiological Tests for the Diagnosis of Carpal Tunnel Syndrome?

The value of most electrophysiological tests for the diagnosis of CTS has not been well studied in patients with co-existing polyneuropathy. One study compared the utility of median distal motor latency, median sensory conduction velocity, and the latency difference between median motor study to the second lumbrical with the ulnar motor study to the first palmar interosseous muscle (3).Using a cutoff value of greater than 1 ms, these authors found that the lumbrical-interosseous study provided the greatest specificity

Table 15.1

Accuracy of Symptoms and Signs for the Diagnosis of Carpal Tunnel Syndrome

Clinical feature	No. hands	Sensitivity	Specificity	LR+ (95% CI)	LR− (95% CI)
Classic or probable hand diagram[a]					
Katz (20)	145	0.64	0.73	**2.4** (1.6–3.5)	**0.5** (0.3–0.7)
Impaired pinprick sensation					
Golding (21)	110	0.15	0.93	2.2 (0.7–6.7)	0.9 (0.8–1.1)
Kuhlman (22)	228	0.51	0.85	3.4 (2.0–5.8)	0.6 (0.5–0.7)
Pooled results				**3.1** (2.0–5.1)	**0.7** (0.5–1.1)
Thumb abduction weakness					
Gerr (23)	115	0.62	0.62	1.7 (1.1–2.4)	0.6 (0.4–0.9)
Kuhlman (22)	228	0.66	0.66	2.0 (1.4–2.7)	0.5 (0.4–0.7)
Pooled results				**1.8** (1.4–2.3)	**0.5** (0.4–0.7)

[a]Patients are asked to indicate the distribution of their pain, numbness, and tingling. The following rating scale is used to classify the hand diagrams: Classic: tingling, numbness, or decreased sensation with or without pain in at least two of the digits 1, 2, or 3. Palm and dorsum of the hand excluded; wrist pain or radiation proximal to the wrist allowed: Probable: same as for classic, except palmar symptoms allowed unless confined solely to ulnar aspect. Possible: tingling, numbness, decreased sensation and/or pain in at least one of digits 1, 2, or 3. Unlikely: no symptoms in digits 1, 2, or 3.

LR+, positive likelihood ratio; LR−, negative likelihood ratio; CI, confidence interval.

Table 15.2
Accuracy of Electrophsysiological Studies for the Diagnosis of Carpal Tunnel Syndrome

Electrophysiological study	Sensitivity (95% CI)	Specificity (95% CI)
Median motor distal latency	0.63 (0.61–0.65)	0.98 (0.96–0.99)
Median sensory NCS between wrist and digit	0.65 (0.63–0.67)	0.98 (0.97–0.99)
Median and ulnar mixed palmar sensory NCS	0.71 (0.65–0.77)	0.97 (0.91–0.99)
Median and ulnar digit IV sensory NCS	0.85 (0.80–0.90)	0.97 (0.91–0.99)
Median and radial digit I sensory NCS	0.65 (0.60–0.71)	0.99 (0.96–1.00)

NCS, nerve conduction study.

In order to estimate the posttest probability of carpal tunnel syndrome, the following steps should be taken.

1. Estimate the pretest probability (an estimation based on probability of CTS given the clinical history and findings on examination).
2. Convert pretest probability to pre-test odds, using the equation
Odds = (probability)/(1 – probability).
3. Calculate the positive and negative likelihood ratios; the positive likelihood ratio, which indicates the likelihood of a subject having CTS given a positive test, is defined as sensitivity/(1 – specificity); the negative likelihood ratio, indicating the likelihood that an individual does not have CTS given a negative test result, is defined as (1 – sensitivity)/specificity.
4. Multiply the pretest odds by the relevant likelihood ratio (LR) (LR+ if test is positive and LR– if the test is negative), to yield the posttest odds.
5. If a second (or third) electrodiagnostic test is performed, multiply the posttest odds by the second (or third) likelihood ratio.
6. Convert the posttest odds to the posttest probability using the equation
Probability = (odds)/(1+odds).

This algorithm permits the estimation of the posttest probability that a subject has CTS given an estimated pretest probability and the known sensitivity and specificity of the various electrodiagnostic tests.

(78%) for differentiating CTS plus polyneuropathy from polyneuropathy alone (3). This study did not examine the diagnostic accuracy of other comparative studies (see Table 15.2) and also included patients with both axonal and demyelinating forms of polyneuropathy. This study, however, provides the only empirical data upon which to base the electrodiagnosis of CTS in the face of an underlying polyneuropathy.

3. TREATMENT

3.1. What Is the Evidence Favoring the Efficacy of Splinting in the Treatment of Carpal Tunnel Syndrome?

In an unblinded randomized, controlled study, Celiker and colleagues compared the efficacy of steroid injection with the combination of nonsteroidal anti-inflammatory drugs and splinting *(4)*. They included 23 patients (37 wrists) in whom the diagnosis of CTS was made on the basis of a combination of clinical and electrophysiological parameters. Patients with thenar atrophy were excluded. Outcome was evaluated using a pain visual analog scale (VAS), a symptom severity scale (SSS), and various electrophysiological parameters after 8 weeks. Results were reported in terms of mean changes in VAS and SSS scores as well as changes in motor and sensory distal latencies, rather than the percentage of patients improved in each treatment group. They found significant improvements in both treatment groups compared with baseline in all measures of efficacy, but no significant differences in outcome between the two treatment groups. In a post-hoc analysis, they noted that improvements were only present among patients with symptoms of less than 9 months' duration.

In an effort to refine the use of splinting in CTS, Walker et al. *(5)* randomized 17 patients (24 wrists) to treatment with either full-time or nighttime use of wrist splints. Patients with CTS were identified on the basis of clinical and electrophysiological features and outcome was assessed at 6 weeks using electrodiagnostic parameters as well as a questionnaire incorporating symptoms and function. The found a significant improvement in symptoms, functional measures, and sensory distal latency between baseline and follow-up in both treatment groups; there were no significant differences in outcome measures between the two treatment groups.

The best quality data come from the randomized controlled trial by Gerritsen and colleagues, in which splinting was compared to surgery in patients with electrophysiologically confirmed CTS *(6)*. In this study, patients randomized to receive splinting were instructed to wear the splint during the night for at least 6 weeks. Eighty-nine patients were allocated to splinting. Outcome was evaluated at 1, 3, 6, and 12 months following randomization with improvement scored using a six-point ordinal scale ranging from "much worse" to "completely recovered." Using an intention-to-treat analysis after 1 month of follow-up, 42% of patients in the splinting group had improved. The success rates for the splinting group were somewhat inflated at subsequent follow-up periods because of cross-over from splinting to surgery (7% at 3 months, 31% at 6 months, 39% at 12 months, and 41% at 18 months). If the outcome analysis is repeated using "actual treatment received" rather than an intention-to-treat analysis, then the success rate for splinting alone at 18 months falls to 37% *(6)*.

These data provide evidence that splinting offers some benefit to a minority of patients with carpal tunnel syndrome. In trying to decide whether to offer splinting as a therapeutic measure, however, it is necessary to consider its efficacy in the context of other possible treatments (discussed later).

3.2. Is Local Steroid Injection Effective in the Treatment of the Carpal Tunnel Syndrome?

Controversy has surrounded the use of local steroid injection in the treatment of carpal tunnel syndrome with most studies being either retrospective or prospective, but not randomized. The three studies selected for discussion here all meet the criteria of being prospective, randomized, controlled, and blinded. There are two other studies that also meet these criteria, but have not been included here either because no clinical outcome data were reported (7) or because the actual data on patient outcome were not reported (8). The latter publication only provides the p-values of the statistical tests comparing the treated and control groups. The study by Çeliker et al (discussed in the previous section) was prospective, randomized and controlled, but not blinded (4).

Özdogan et al. (9) randomized 37 patients with CTS diagnosed clinically on the basis of symptoms, to treatment with either local or systemic injection of steroids. The "active treatment" group received 1.5 mg betamethasone (Celestone) injected into the carpal tunnel and a placebo injection into the ipsilateral deltoid muscle. The "control treatment" group received an injection of betamethasone into the deltoid muscle and a placebo injected into the carpal tunnel. Patients classified the severity of their symptoms on a four-point scale (0 – nil, 1 – minimal, 2 – moderate, and 3 – severe) prior to treatment and again 1 week and 1 month after treatment. One month after treatment, significant clinical improvement was present only in the group that received local steroid injection. In the "active treatment" group, nine (50%) patients improved, all of whom reported no symptoms at follow-up. In the "control treatment" group, three (16%) patients reported improvement, only one of whom became symptom free. After a mean of 11 months follow-up, only four (22%) patients remained symptom-free, all of whom were injected with steroid. These results indicate a short-term benefit from local steroid injection.

Dammers et al. (10) randomized 60 patients in a double-blind controlled fashion in order to examine the efficacy of steroid injection proximal to the carpal tunnel. The diagnosis of CTS required the presence of clinical symptoms and signs as well as electrophysiological confirmation. "Active treatment" comprised injection of 40 mg methylprednisolone and 10 mg lignocaine proximal to the carpal tunnel. Controls were injected with lignocaine alone. Treatments were administered in a double-blind fashion. At follow-up, patients were asked whether their symptoms had resolved completely or whether the symptoms were sufficiently mild that they felt no further treatment was required. Those answering affirmatively were classified as "responders." The outcome at 1-month was reported in terms of the relative proportions of "responders" and "nonresponders." The investigators had planned to randomize 80 patients, but the study was stopped prematurely after an interim analysis showed benefit among patients in the steroid-treated group. Twenty-three (77%) of patients in the active treatment group responded, compared with six (20%) in the control treatment group.

Wong et al. (11) randomized 30 patients to steroid injection (1 mg methylprednisolone acetate) and oral placebo, and 30 patients to receive oral steroid (25 mg prednisolone) and saline injection daily for 10 days. Eligible patients had symptoms as well as electrophysiological evidence of CTS. The primary outcome measure of efficacy was the difference in global symptom score (GSS) between the two treatment groups at 2, 8, and 12 weeks after treatment. In a separate analysis, a comparison was made between the pre- and posttreatment GSS scores. Significant improvements in the steroid injection group, but not the oral steroid group, were present at both 8 and 12 weeks ($p = 0.002$ and $p = 0.004$ respectively). A significant improvement in GSS scores at all time points (compared with baseline) was also noted in the steroid-injection group ($p < 0.001$). A significant improvement was also noted in the oral steroid group at 2 weeks ($p = 0.03$) and was attributed by the authors to a placebo effect. The relative proportions of patients in each treatment group whose symptoms improved were not reported.

Apart from the obvious differences between these three studies—eligibility criteria as well as the dose and location of the steroid injections—they also differed significantly in design. In the study by Ozdogan *(9)*, each patient served as his own control with a comparison made between the severity of symptoms before and after treatment. In the study by Dammers *(10)*, the primary analysis involved a comparison between an active treatment and a control group. Both analyses were performed by Wong et al. *(11)*. These first two studies were similar in that the primary outcome measure was a clinical response 1 month after treatment. Wong et al. *(11)* examined clinical outcome after 2 and 3 months. The results, however, are in agreement—that local injection of corticosteroid provides short-term relief from symptoms of CTS.

There have been two systematic reviews of the efficacy of local steroid injection for the treatment of CTS *(12,13)*. Meta-analysis was not performed in either because of the clinical heterogeneity between the various studies. The conclusions from both reviews, in agreement with that based on the data outlined previously, were that there is limited evidence for a short-term (1 month) benefit from injection of the carpal tunnel with steroids.

3.3. What Is the Efficacy of Surgery in the Treatment of Carpal Tunnel Syndrome?

There have been two randomized controlled trials comparing surgery with splinting for the treatment of CTS *(6,14)* and one systematic review *(15)*. There has also been one randomized controlled trial of surgery compared with steroid injection *(16)*. These studies were generally of high quality (Table 15.3A) and showed a benefit of surgery (Table 15.3B) over both a single injection of steroid into the carpal tunnel *(16)* and 6 weeks of splinting *(6)*. The two studies with better methodological quality *(6,16)* are difficult to compare because of the differences in outcome measures used to evaluate treatment efficacy as well as the time period over which treatment efficacy was measured. Hui and colleagues used the GSS, a composite measure of the severity of five symptoms (pain, paresthesia, numbness, nocturnal awakening, and weakness) as the primary outcome measured at 20 weeks after the therapeutic intervention *(16)*. They found a significant improvement in mean score in the surgery group compared to the group treated with a single steroid injection into the carpal tunnel (Table 15.3B) *(16)*. Improvements in the secondary outcome measures of median distal motor latency and median sensory nerve conduction velocity, but not grip strength, were also noted *(16)*. Gerritsen and colleagues measured outcome using a six-point ordinal scale in which responses ranged from "completely recovered" to "much worse" as well as a variety of other measures (Table 15.3B) *(6)*. Patients who reported that symptoms were "completely recovered" or "much improved" were regarded as treatment successes. Outcome was reported at 1, 3, 6, 12, and 18 months. Using an intention-to-treat analysis, the success rates at 3, 6, 12, and 18

Table 15.3A
Methodological Quality of Randomized Controlled Trials of Surgery for Carpal Tunnel Syndrome (CTS)

Reference	Randomization	Allocation concealment	Blinding	Explicit inclusion/ exclusion criteria	Completeness of follow-up
Garland (14)	Inadequate	Inadequate	Not done	Inadequate	Adequate
Gerritsen (6)	Adequate (random number tables)	Adequate (opaque envelopes)	Adequate (observer blinded)	Adequate	Adequate (95% at 1 mo & 84% at 18 mo
Hui (16)	Adequate (computer generated random numbers)	Adequate (opaque envelopes)	Adequate (observer blinded)	Adequate	Adequate (100%)

Table 15.3B
Study Characteristics and Results of Randomized Controlled Trials of Surgery for Carpal Tunnel Syndrome (CTS)

Reference	n	Study population	Comparative treatment	Outcome measure	Interval to end point	Results Surgery	Results Control
Garland (14)	22	Patients with CTS based on DML >4.5 ms	Splinting for 1 mo using plaster-of-paris cast of wrist, hand and arm	Proportion of patients whose symptoms were judged to be improved (no specified criteria used to judge improvement)	Not specified	100%	20%
Gerritsen (6)	176	Patients with CTS of any severity	Splinting × 6 wk	6-point ordinal scale of symptoms ("success rate")	18 mo	90%	75%[a]
				No. nights without awakening with symptoms		3.6 nights	3.2 nights[b]
				Severity of main complaint past week (11-point rating scale)		6.2	5.0[c]
Hui (16)	50	Mild-to-moderate CTS	Single steroid injection	Global symptom score (GSS)	20 wk post intervention	−24.2 points on GSS[d]	−8.7 points on GSS[d]

[a]$p = 0.02$.
[b]$p = 0.44$.
[c]$p = 0.02$.
[d]Reduction in GSS score represents a clinical improvement (difference is significant $p < 0.001$).
DML, distal motor latency.

months favored surgery—80% vs 54% (3 months), 94% vs 68% (6 months), 92% vs 72% (12 months), and 90% vs 75% (18 months) (6).

The results of these studies show that surgery is superior to both a single steroid injection into the carpal tunnel and 6 weeks of splinting. It is relevant to note, however, that successful outcomes were observed in a significant proportion of patients treated conservatively—between 54% and 75% of patients who used a neutral wrist splint—suggesting that surgery should not necessarily be used as first line therapy for patients with CTS. In cautioning against surgery, the authors of the Cochrane systematic review noted the relatively high frequency of adverse effects among the patients treated surgically (15).

4. PROGNOSIS

4.1. Which Factors Predict a Good Clinical Response to Splinting?

This question has been examined using data derived from a randomized controlled study of splinting versus surgery for the treatment of CTS (6). At 12 months following randomization, 60 of 83 patients (72%) randomized to splinting reported that they were "improved" (encompassing the outcomes of completely recovered and much improved). Thirty-four of these patients, however, had actually received additional forms of therapy (largely surgery). If these 34 patients are regarded as treatment failures for splinting, then 28 patients (31%) are left who had improved at the 12-month follow-up visit. Univariate analysis was used to identify features that might be predictive of a good outcome with splinting. The features identified in this way were then examined using multivariate analysis. Only two factors—duration of symptoms (less than 1 year compared with longer than 1 year) and severity of paresthesia at night (a score of 6 or less versus more than 6 on the symptom severity score)—were retained in the final model (17). Using these variables it was possible to reliably predict successful response to splinting at 12 months (Table 15.4).

These data suggest that patients with mild to moderate nocturnal symptoms of less than 1 year's duration are most likely respond to conservative treatment with splinting and that this response is likely to be a durable one, lasting at least 12 months.

4.2. Which Features Predict the Clinical Outcome Following Carpal Tunnel Release?

A number of studies have tried to identify pre-operative features that might predict the response to surgical decompression of the carpal tunnel. There is substantial heterogeneity between these studies with regard to the selection criteria for inclusion of subjects, and the measures used to evaluate outcome as well as the factors that have been examined for their prognostic value. Most studies have employed univariate analysis although a few have used multivariate techniques. The results of these studies are summarized in Table 15.5.

There is conflicting evidence regarding the question of whether increasing duration of symptoms portends a poor prognosis for recovery following carpal tunnel surgery. Similarly controversial is the prognostic value of pre-operative NCSs. This controversy exists in part because of the very different ways in which the prognostic value of NCSs have

Table 15.4
Prognosis for Patients With Carpal Tunnel Syndrome Treated With Splinting

Duration of symptoms	Severity of paresthesia at night[a]	Predicted probability of success at 12 mo	Actual success at 12 mo
>1 yr	>6	5%	13%
>1 yr	6	19%	12%
1 yr	>6	28%	23%
1 yr	6	62%	67%

[a]Severity of symptoms was graded on an 11-point numerical rating scale (with 0 indicating "no symptoms" and 10 indicating "very severe symptoms" used as anchors. Data derived from ref. 17.

Table 15.5
Factors Predicting Outcome Following Surgery for Carpal Tunnel Syndrome

Variable	Predictive value	Reference
Age (increasing)	Poor outcome	19
Gender (male)	Poor outcome	19
Alcohol use	Poor outcome	24
Duration of symptoms (increasing)	Does not predict outcome	18,25–28
	Poor outcome	19,29
Intermittent paresthesias	Good outcome	30
Prominent diurnal pain	Poor outcome	24
Nocturnal symptoms	Good outcome	30
	Does not predict outcome	28
Muscle atrophy	Poor outcome	29
Muscle weakness	Poor outcome	30
Strenuous physical work	Poor outcome	24,28,31
	Does not predict outcome	27
Ongoing legal/insurance claims	Poor outcome	24,28
Results of nerve conduction studies	Does not predict outcome	18,25,28,31,32
	Good outcome	19
Response to carpal tunnel injecion with steroids	Good outcome	33,34

been examined. Many of the studies which concluded that NCSs are of no prognostic value simply compared outcome following carpal tunnel release either in the presence or absence of neurophysiological abnormalities. Those studies that have considered the results of neurophysiological testing in more detail have found that these parameters do have some prognostic value (18,19). Bland recognized seven grades of increasingly severe neurophysiological abnormalities (Table 15.6A) (19) and, using this approach, the outcome following carpal tunnel release was found to vary depending on the severity of pre-operative neurophysiological findings (Table 15.6B).

The results suggest that outcome is best with intermediate grades of neurophysiologic abnormalities. Those with normal nerve conduction studies, those in whom CTS can be diagnosed only using highly sensitive comparative electrodiagnostic studies, and those

Table 15.6A
Grading of Electrophysiological Abnormalities in Carpal Tunnel Syndrome (CTS)

Grade 0 – No neurophysiological abnormality

Grade 1 – CTS detected only with two sensitive (comparative) tests

Grade 2 – Sensory conduction velocity slowed to less than 40 m/s with distal motor latency
            less than 4.5 ms

Grade 3 – Distal motor latency greater than 4.5 ms but less than 6.5 ms with preserved sensory
            response

Grade 4 – Distal motor latency greater than 4.5 ms but less than 6.5 ms with absent sensory
            response

Grade 5 – Distal motor latency greater than 6.5 ms

Grade 6 – Motor amplitude less than 0.2 mV

Grading scheme according to Bland *(19)*.

Table 15.6B
Prognosis for CTS Following Carpal Tunnel Release Based on Pre-Operative
Neurophysiological Grade

Neurophysiological grade	Complete cure/much better	Worse
Grade 0	51%	13%
Grade 1	65%	15%
Grade 2	76%	11%
Grade 3	77%	8%
Grade 4	74%	6%
Grade 5	66%	13%
Grade 6	47%	14%

with markedly reduced motor response amplitudes are least likely to benefit from carpal tunnel release *(19)*.

Choi distinguished three categories of neurophysiological abnormalities based on the severity of distal motor and sensory latencies, sensory amplitude, and the presence or absence of denervation changes on electromyographic examination but failed to find any prognostic value for these neurophysiological changes *(18)*. One explanation may be that the classification employed does not span the full range of electordiagnostic results that may be encountered. The mildest degree of abnormality recognized by Choi, for example, corresponds to Bland's grade 3. Because all of Choi's grades lie within the intermediate grades outlined by Bland, it is perhaps not surprising that Choi found his neurophysiological grades to have no prognostic value.

In conclusion, although some controversy persists, it seems that a reasonable case can be made for arguing that those with very mild neurophysiological abnormalities (detected only with sensitive comparative techniques) and those with very severe abnormalities (evidence by very small or absent motor responses) are least likely to benefit from carpal tunnel release. By contrast, about 75% of those with a wide range of intermediate neurophysiological abnormalities will benefit from release with marked improvement or resolution of symptoms, whereas a small proportion (8–13%) will be worse following surgery *(19)*.

Table 15.7
Summary of the Evidence Supporting Various Treatment Options for Carpal Tunnel Syndrome

Therapeutic modality	Quality of evidence	Treatment efficacy	Reference
Splinting	RCT (unblinded)	6.3-point improvement in mean VAS score at 8 wks	Celiker (4)
	RCT (blinded)	2.2-point improvement in mean symptom severity score at 8 wk[a]	Celiker (4)
		"Completely recovered' or 'much improved" in 42% at 1 mo	Gerritsen (6)
		"Completely recovered' or "much improved" in 72% at 1 yr	
Steroid injection	RCT (unblinded)	5.2-point improvement in mean VAS score at 8 wk	Celiker (4)
		2.3-point improvement in mean symptom severity score at 8 wk[a]	
	RCT (blinded)	Resolution of symptoms in 50% at 1 mo	Ozdogan (9)
		Resolution of symptoms in 22% at 11 mo	
	RCT (blinded)	Resolution of symptoms in 77% at 1 mo	Dammers (10)
	RCT (blinded)	13-point improvement in global symptom score at 2, 8, & 12 wk[b]	Wong (11)
Surgery	RCT (blinded)	"Completely recovered" or "much improved" in 29% at 1 mo	Gerritsen (6)
		"Completely recovered' or "much improved" in 92% at 1 yr	
	RCT (blinded)	24.2-point improvement on global symptom score[b] at 20 wk	Hui (16)

[a]Symptom severity score: a score based on answers to 11 questions including "how severe is the hand or wrist pain that you have at night," "how often do hand or wrist pain wake you up during a typical night in the past two weeks," "do you typically have pain in your hand or wrist during the daytime," "how often do you have hand or wrist pain during the daytime," "how long does an episode of pain last during the daytime," "do you have numbness in your hand," "do you have weakness in your hand or wrist," "do you have tingling sensations in your hand," "how severe is numbness or tingling at night," "how often did hand numbness or tingling wake you up during the last two weeks," "do you have difficulty grasping and using small objects such as keys or pen." Each question has five possible answers with a total possible score of 55 (indicating maximum symptoms).

[b]Global symptom score: this score is based on the severity rating (0 = no symptoms; 10 = severe symptoms) of five symptoms (pain, numbness, paresthesia, weakness/clumsiness and nocturnal awakening). Top score is 50 indicating maximum symptoms.

RCT, randomized controlled trial; VAS, visual analog scale.

288

5. SUMMARY

- CTS is a clinical syndrome caused by compression of the median nerve at the wrist.
- The clinical features that provide the greatest diagnostic accuracy are a classic or probable hand diagram, abnormal pinprick sensation in the distribution of the median nerve, and the presence of weakness of thumb abduction.
- Electrodiagnostic studies provide high specificity, but only intermediate sensitivity for the diagnosis of CTS; the digit-IV and mixed palmar sensory nerve conduction studies provide the highest sensitivity (85% and 71%, respectively).
- In the face of an underlying polyneuropathy, the lumbrical-interosseous motor nerve conduction study provides the greatest specificity for the diagnosis of CTS.
- There is data from several RCTs indicating that a proportion of patients with CTS respond well to splinting. The estimates range from a success rate of 42% at 1 month to 72% at 1 year (Table 15.7).
- Those with symptoms of intermediate severity and duration less than 1 year are most likely to benefit from splinting.
- Data from several RCTs support the short-term efficacy of steroid injection for the treatment of CTS; response rates fall from 50–77% at 1 month to 22% at 1 year (Table 15.7).
- Data from several randomized controlled trials support the role of carpal tunnel release surgery in the management of CTS; response rates rise from 29% 1 month following surgery to 92% at 1 year (Table 15.7).
- Controversy persists regarding which prognostic features predict a good response to carpal tunnel release; those with no or very mild electrophysiologic abnormalities (CTS diagnosed only with sensitive comparative studies) and those with severe abnormalities (markedly reduced or absent motor response) are least likely to benefit from surgery.

REFERENCES

1. D'Arcy CA, McGee S. The rational examination. Does this patient have carpal tunnel syndrome? JAMA 2000;283:3110–3117.
2. Jablecki C. Practice parameter for electrodiagnostic studies in carpal tunnel syndrome: summary statement. Muscle Nerve 2002;25:918–922.
3. Vogt T, Mika A, Thomke F, Hopf HC. Evaluation of carpal tunnel syndrome in patients with polyneuropathy. Muscle Nerve 1997;20:153–157.
4. Çeliker R, Arslan S, Inanici F. Corticosteroid injection vs. nonsteroidal antiinflammatory drug and splinting in carpal tunnel syndrome. Am J Phys Med Rehabil 2002;81:182–186.
5. Walker WC, Metzler M, Cifu DX, Swartz Z. Neutral wrist splinting in carpal tunnel syndrome: a comparison of night-only versus full-time wear instructions. Arch Phys Med Rehabil 2000;81:424–429.
6. Gerritsen AA, de Vet HC, Scholten RJ, Bertelsmann FW, de Krom MC, Bouter LM. Splinting vs surgery in the treatment of carpal tunnel syndrome. A randomized controlled trial. JAMA 2002;288:1245–1251.
7. Wu S, Chan R, Hsu T. Electrodiagnostic evaluation of conservative treatment in carpal tunnel syndrome. Chinese Medical Journal 1991;48:125–130.
8. Girlanda P, Dattola R, Venuto C, Mangiapane R, Nicolosi C, Messina C. Local steroid treatment in idiopathic carpal tunnel syndrome: short- and long-term efficacy. J Neurol 1993;240:187–190.
9. Ozdogan H, Yazici H. The efficacy of local steroid injections in idiopathic carpal tunnel syndrome: a double-blind study. Brit J of Rheumatol 1984;23:272–275.
10. Dammers J, Veering M, Vermeulen M. Injection with methylprednisolone proximal to the carpal tunnel: randomised double blind trial. BMJ 1999;319:884–886.
11. Wong S, Hui A, Tang A, et al. Local vs systemic corticosteroids in the treatment of carpal tunnel syndrome. Neurology 2001;56:1565–1567.
12. Marshall S, Tardif G, Ashworth N. Local corticosteroid injection for carpal tunnel syndrome. Cochrane Database Syst Rev 2002;4:CD001554.

13. Gerritsen AA, de Krom MC, Struijs MA, Scholten RJ, de Vet HC, Bouter LM. Conservative treatment options for carpal tunnel syndrome: a systematic review of randomised controlled trials. J Neurol 2002;249:272–280.

14. Garland J, Langworth E, Taverner D, Clark J. Surgical treatment for the carpal tunnel syndrome. Lancet 1964;13:1129–1130.

15. Verdugo R, Salinas R, Cartillo J, Cea J. Surgical versus non-surgical treatment for carpal tunnel syndrome. Cochrane Database Syst Rev 2003;3:CD001552.

16. Hui A, Wong S, Leung C, et al. A randomized controlled trial of surgery vs steroid injection for carpal tunnel syndrome. Neurology 2005;64:2074–2078.

17. Gerritsen A, Korthals-de Bos I, Laboyrie P, de Vet H, Scholten R, Bouter L. Splinting for carpal tunnel syndrome: prognostic indicators of success. J Neurol Neurosurg Psychiatry 2003;74:1342–1344.

18. Choi SJ, Ahn D-S. Correlation of clinical history and electrodiagnostic abnormalities with outcome after surgery for carpal tunnel syndrome. Plast Reconstr Surg 1998;102:2374–2380.

19. Bland JD. Do nerve conduction studies predict the outcome of carpal tunnel decompression. Muscle Nerve 2001;24:935–940.

20. Katz JN, Larson MG, Sabra A, et al. The carpal tunnel syndrome: diagnostic utility of the history and physical examination findings. Ann Intern Med 1990;112:321–327.

21. Golding D, Rose D, Selvarajah K. Clinical tests for carpal tunnel syndrome: an evaluation. Br J Rheumatol 1986;25:388–390.

22. Kuhlman K, Hennessey W. Sensitivity and specificity of carpal tunnel syndrome signs. Am J Phys Med Rehabi 1997;76:451–457.

23. Gerr F, Letz R, Harris-Abbott D, Hopkins L. Sensitivity and specificity of vibrometry for detection of carpal tunnel syndrome. J Occup Environ Med 1995;37:1108–1115.

24. Katz JN, Losina E, Amick BC, Fossel AH, Bessette L, Keller RB. Predictors of outcome of carpal tunnel release. Arthritis Rheum 2001;44:1184–1193.

25. Cseuz KA, Thomas JE, Lambert EH, Love JG, Lipscomb PR. Long-term results of operation for carpal tunnel syndrome. Mayo Clin Proc 1966;41:232–241.

26. Harris CM, Tanner E, Goldstein MN, Pettee DS. The surgical treatment of the carpal tunnel syndrome correlated with preoperative nerve-conduction studies. J Bone Joint Surg [Am] 1979;61:93–98.

27. Atroshi I, Johnsson R, Ornstein E. Patient satisfaction and return to work after endoscopic carpal tunnel surgery. J Hand Surg [Am] 1998;23:58–65.

28. Al-Qattan M, Bowen V, Manketlow R. Factors associated with poor outcome following primary carpal tunnel release in non-diabetic patients. J Hand Surg [Br] 1994;19:622–625.

29. Muhlau G, Both R, Kunath H. Carpal tunnel syndrome—course and prognosis. J Neurol 1984; 231:83–86.

30. Wintman BI, Winters SC, Gelberman RH, Katz JN. Carpal tunnel release. Correlations with preoperative symptomatology. Clin Orthop Relat Res 1996;326:135–145.

31. Yu G-Z, Firrell J, Tsai T-M. Pre-operative factors and treatment outcome following carpal tunnel release. J Hand Surg [Br] 1992;17:646–650.

32. Clauburgh RH, Beckenbaugh RD, Dobyns JH. Carpal tunnel release in patients with diffuse peripheral neuropathy. J Hand Surg [Am] 1987;12:380–383.

33. Green DP. Diagnostic and therapeutic value of carpal tunnel injection. J Hand Surg [Am] 1984;9:850–854.

34. Edgell SE, McCabe SJ, Breidenbach WC, LaJoie AS, Abell TD. Predicting the outcome of carpal tunnel release. J Hand Surg [Am] 2003;28:255–261.

16 Ulnar Neuropathy at the Elbow

1. INTRODUCTION

Ulnar neuropathy at the elbow (UNE) is the second most commonly encountered entrapment neuropathy after carpal tunnel syndrome. The term "cubital tunnel" syndrome is sometimes used to refer to UNE, but this is misleading as the term accurately describes only compression of the ulnar nerve as it passes beneath the aponeurotic arch of the flexor carpi ulnaris muscle (FCU). Because the ulnar nerve may also be compressed in the ulnar (condylar or retrocondylar) groove behind the medial epicondyle, the term UNE is more encompassing of the range of pathophysiological processes that may lead to ulnar nerve injury in the vicinity of the elbow. Compressive lesions of the ulnar nerve as it passes across the elbow may selectively affect some nerve fascicles more than others, which may cause some difficulty in localizing an ulnar nerve lesion to the elbow. What then are the typical clinical features of ulnar neuropathy at the elbow and how accurate are the various electrophysiologic tests for the diagnosis of UNE? What is the natural history of UNE if left untreated and how do conservative and surgical measures impact this prognosis? These and other questions are the subject of this chapter.

2. DIAGNOSIS

2.1. What Are the Typical Clinical Manifestations of Ulnar Neuropathy at the Elbow?

There are a limited number of studies that have carefully documented the clinical signs that may be encountered in UNE (1,2). In each of these studies, the authors used clearly defined criteria as the gold standard for the diagnosis (Table 16.1). A problem with both studies is that the criteria that were used were largely clinical, thus biasing any estimation of the frequency with which individual clinical signs are encountered. The only way to determine the true frequency of various clinical findings in UNE would be to examine a cohort of patients with UNE defined by nonclinical (e.g., electrophysiological or sonographic) parameters. A further problem with the second study (2) is that the criteria used do not clearly indicate that the ulnar neuropathy is localized to the elbow. The elbow is overwhelmingly the most common site of compression of the ulnar nerve, and so it is not unreasonable to use the data from these studies to estimate the frequency with which the various sensory and motor branches of the ulnar nerve are affected by ulnar neuropathies at the elbow. As shown in Table 16.2, the more distal muscles, abductor digiti minimi (ADM) and first dorsal interosseous (FDI), are more commonly affected than the proximal ulnar-innervated muscles FCU and flexor digitorum profundus-4,5 ($FDP_{4,5}$).

From: *Neuromuscular Disease: Evidence and Analysis in Clinical Neurology*
By: M. Benatar © Humana Press Inc., Totowa, NJ

Table 16.1
Criteria for the Diagnosis of Ulnar Neuropathy at the Elbow (UNE)

Reference	Criteria

Stewart (1)	Numbness and/or weakness in the distribution of one or more of the major branches of the ulnar nerve with no abnormalities of other peripheral nerves in that limb AND at least one of the following three criteria
	• Sensory loss including the palmar and/or dorsal cutaneous branches
	• Definite weakness of FCU or $FDP_{4,5}$ muscles
	• Motor and/or sensory signs restricted to branches at or distal to the wrist together with either
	    (a) conduction block across the elbow segment or
	    (b) EMG abnormalities in FCU or $FDP_{4,5}$

Beekman (2)	Two or more of the following criteria • Symptoms of numbness and paresthesias in the fourth and fifth digits of the hand or subjective weakness or clumsiness of the ulnar innervated muscles • Sensory signs in the ulnar nerve territory • Weakness or wasting of one or more ulnar-innervated muscles
Beekman (13)	Clinical diagnosis based on • Weakness of proximal ulnar muscles accompanied by sensory disturbance in the area of the dorsal cutaneous branch Combined clinical and electrodiagnostic diagnosis based on • Clinical signs that could indicate UNE (weakness of distal ulnar muscles with sensory disturbance only in the palmar cutaneous branch) AND • CMAP reduction across the elbow of >16% OR motor nerve conduction velocity slowing across the elbow to <46 m/s OR >15 m/s slowing of conduction velocity across the elbow compared to forearm conduction velocity OR spontaneous activity on EMG in FCU or $FDP_{4,5}$

FCU, flexor carpi ulnaris; $FDP_{4,5}$, flexor digitorum profundus-4,5; EMG, electromyography; UNE, ulnar neuropathy at the elbow; CMAP, compound muscle action potential.

The one study indicated that FDI was affected more often than ADM (1), but this was not born out by the second study (2). Overall, weakness of ADM and FDI are present in 61–76% and 52%–84% of patients with UNE. The sensory branches supplying the palmar aspect of the hand (palmar cutaneous and terminal digital branches) are affected in 80%–100% of patients with UNE whereas the dorsal cutaneous branch is affected in approximately 90% of patients. These studies, therefore, provide estimates of the sensitivity of the various sensory and motor deficits for the diagnosis of UNE, but do not inform on the specificity of these findings. Studies to evaluate the specificity of these clinical manifestations have not been reported.

Table 16.2
Clinical Abnormalities in Ulnar Neuropathy at the Elbow

	Stewart (1)	*Beekman* (2)
Study sample size	25	109
Weakness/atrophy		
FCU	20%	8%
$FDP_{4,5}$	56%	30%
ADM	76%	61%
FDI	84%	52%
Sensory deficits		
Palmar cutaneous	80%	100%
Digital	92%	NR
Dorsal cutaneous	72%	91%

FCU, flexor carpi ulnaris; $FDP_{4,5}$, flexor digitorum profundus-4,5; ADM, abductor digiti minimi; FDI, first dorsal interosseous; NR, not reported.

2.2. What Is the Accuracy of Provocative Testing for the Diagnosis of UNE?

Based on the recognition that UNE is, at least in part, a compression neuropathy, it has been suggested that the clinical diagnosis may be aided by provocative tests. Such tests are designed to reproduce or exacerbate symptoms by transiently increasing compression of the nerve and include Tinel's sign, the flexion test, and the pressure provocative test (Table 16.3A). The diagnostic accuracy of these tests has been examined in a prospective study of 32 patients with UNE and 33 healthy control subjects *(3)*. The patients with UNE all had symptoms suggestive of an ulnar neuropathy as well as electrophysiological evidence that localized the pathology to the ulnar nerve at the elbow. As shown in Table 16.3B, the sensitivity of these tests range from 70% to 98%, with the specificity uniformly better than 95%. The two major limitations of this study are the failure to blind the investigators to the patient's disease status (i.e., whether they were a case or a control) and the choice of the control group. The authors selected healthy controls rather than patients in whom the diagnosis of UNE had been considered but subsequently established to be due to some other disease process (e.g., cervical radiculopathy). It is this latter group in whom the diagnosis of UNE is more difficult. The inappropriate choice of healthy controls is likely to artificially elevate estimates of sensitivity.

2.3. What Is the Accuracy of Electrophysiological Testing for the Diagnosis of UNE?

Electrophysiological testing plays an important role in the diagnosis of UNE in that it may confirm the presence of an ulnar neuropathy and may demonstrate the location of the lesion. It is also useful in excluding other conditions that may mimic an ulnar neuropathy such as a lower brachial plexopathy or a cervical radiculopathy. Electrophysiological testing typically includes nerve conduction studies of the ulnar sensory and motor nerves as well as electromyographic examination of a selection of muscles. Although infrequently performed, ulnar mixed sensorimotor nerve conduction studies are also an option. The routine motor nerve conduction study records the compound muscle

Table 16.3A
Provocative Tests for Ulnar Neuropathy at the Elbow

Test	Description
Tinel's sign	Examiner applies 4–6 taps to the ulnar nerve just proximal to the cubital tunnel. The presence or absence of a tingling sensation in the distribution of the ulnar nerve is recorded.
Pressure provocative test	The examiner's middle and index fingers are placed over the subject's ulnar nerve immediately proximal to the cubital tunnel with the elbow in 20° flexion and the forearm supinated. Pressure is applied for 60 s and the presence or absence of the patient's subjective symptomatology in the distribution of the ulnar nerve is noted.
Flexion test	The subject's elbow is placed in maximum flexion with full supination and the wrist in neutral. The position is maintained for 60 s. The presence or absence of symptoms in the distribution of the ulnar nerve is noted.

Table 16.3B
Diagnostic Accuracy of Provocative Tests for Ulnar Neuropathy at the Elbow

Test	Sensitivity	Specificity	PPV	NPV
Tinel's sign	0.70	0.98	0.94	0.87
Flexion test	0.75	0.99	0.97	0.98
Pressure test	0.89	0.98	0.95	0.95
Combined flexion and pressure test	0.98	0.95	0.91	0.99

PPV, positive predictive value; NPV, negative predictive value.
Data from ref. 3.

action potential over the ADM muscle, but may also be performed while recording over the FDI muscle. The routine sensory nerve conduction study typically examines the nerve segment between the fifth digit and the ulnar nerve at the wrist, with the nerve impulse recorded either orthodromically (stimulating the fifth digit and recording over the nerve at the wrist) or antidromically (stimulation at the wrist with recording over the fifth digit). At least in theory, the ulnar nerve could also be stimulated (or recorded from) more proximally, both below and above the elbow.

This range of electrophysiological tests may reveal many different abnormalities, only some of which localize the ulnar neuropathy to the elbow. These include the presence of a conduction block between the above-elbow and below-elbow sites of stimulation and the presence of focal slowing of conduction velocity across the elbow segment. The magnitude of the reduction in response amplitude between the above-elbow and below-elbow sites of stimulation that is required for the designation of conduction block has varied between different studies. Most would agree that a fall in response amplitude of less than 16–20% would not constitute a block. Slowing of conduction velocity across the elbow segment may be determined in one of two ways. The velocity may fall below a particular value that defines the absolute lower limit of normal. Alternatively, the difference in conduction velocity between the forearm and elbow segments may be compared and the difference recorded, with differential slowing of velocity across the elbow that exceeds a particular value taken to imply the presence of a focal neuropathy. Finally, the needle electromyographic examination may be used to localize the neuropathy. Although not entirely excluding a proximal forearm ulnar neuropathy, the presence of neurogenic changes (either ongoing denervation or chronic reinnervation changes) in proximal ulnar-innervated muscles such as $FDP_{4,5}$, are usually taken to imply an ulnar neuropathy at the elbow.

There are a number of published studies that have examined various combinations of these electrophysiological tests in order to determine their accuracy for the diagnosis of UNE [1,4–12]. Before evaluating these studies, it is relevant consider two related, but distinct issues — (1) the range of subjects included in the study and (2) the choice of the gold standard for defining the presence of the disease in question (in this case, UNE). It is most appropriate to evaluate the diagnostic accuracy of a test in the framework of the clinical context in which the test will be used. For example, electrophysiological testing will be used to evaluate patients with suspected ulnar neuropathy and not healthy asymptomatic controls or patients with other neurological diseases such as lumbar spondylosis or peroneal neuropathy. Most studies fall prey to this problem in that they report the diagnostic performance of electrophysiological tests among patients with already established ulnar neuropathy and among healthy controls or various disease controls. Failure to evaluate the accuracy of a diagnostic test in a population that mirrors that encountered in clinical practice and includes the full spectrum of subjects with the disease in question will result in falsely elevated estimates of the test's sensitivity and specificity. The second issue relates to the choice of a gold standard for the diagnosis of UNE. It is important that any study that aims to evaluate the diagnostic accuracy of electrophysiological tests should not incorporate the results of these tests in determining the presence or absence of UNE (in order to avoid the error of incorporation bias). Moreover, it seems inadequate to use as a gold standard simply the presence of symptoms and signs suggestive of an ulnar neuropathy. It would be preferable, for example, to categorize patients as having ulnar neuropathy only once greater diagnostic certainty (at a clinical level) has been achieved (e.g., once other relevant diagnoses such as cervical radiculopathy have been excluded).

Finally, note should be made of one technical factor that might affect the diagnostic accuracy of nerve conduction studies—the position of the elbow. Based on cadaver studies, it is apparent that the ulnar nerve lies lax in the epicondylar groove when the elbow is extended and that it become taught once the elbow is flexed. Discordance between the length of nerve over which conduction is being determined and the distance measured over the skin between the two sites of stimulation (above and below the elbow) may result from movement (flexion or extension) of the elbow. Some studies have examined the diagnostic accuracy of nerve conduction studies with the elbow extended, some with the elbow flexed, and yet others have compared the two positions.

As shown in Table 16.4A, the patient populations varied somewhat between the different studies. For the most part, patients were selected on the basis of clinical symptoms and signs suggestive of an ulnar neuropathy, but more specific details were not given. The exception was the study by Stewart, in which definite UNE required the presence of either (1) sensory loss in the palmar and or dorsal cutaneous branches or (2) weakness of the FCU or FDP muscles (*see* Table 16.1) [1]. The gold standard for determining whether UNE was

Table 16.4A
Methodological Characteristics of Studies of Diagnostic Accuracy of Electrodiagnostic Tests
for Ulnar Neuropathy at the Elbow (UNE)

Reference	Patient population	Controls	Elbow position
Bhala (4)	Suspected UNE	Healthy	Flexed 35°
Kimura (6)	Frank clinical signs suggestive of UNE	Healthy	Extended
Pickett (10)	Clinical diagnosis of UNE by referring doctor	Healthy and polyneuroapthy	Extended
Bielawski (5)	Combined clinical, electrical & pathological findings	Healthy and disease[a]	Flexed 90° & extended
Raynor (11)	Referrals for possible UNE (definite and probable based on clinical criteria)	Healthy and disease[a]	Extended
Kothari (7)	Clinical and electrical diagnosis of UNE	Healthy and disease[a]	Flexed and extended
Tackmann (12)	Referrals with diagnosis of UNE	Healthy	Flexed 160°
Odusote (9)	Symptomatic cubital tunnel syndrome	Disease[a]	Extended
Kothari (8)	Clinical symptoms and signs of ulnar neuropathy	Healthy	Flexed 90°
Stewart (1)	Clinical symptoms and signs of ulnar neuropathy (definite and probable based on clinical criteria)	None	Flexed 30°
Gilliatt (43)	UNE "established on clinical grounds"	Healthy and opposite asymptomatic limb in UNE patients	Extended
Payan (44)	"Lesions of the ulnar nerve"	Healthy	Extended

[a]Disease controls included patients with unrelated neurological diseases (e.g., carpal tunnel syndrome, lumbosacral radiculopathy).

in fact the correct diagnosis is rarely described. Many studies for example indicated that patients with suspected UNE or patients referred for evaluation for UNE were studied *(10–12)*, but no further details are given as to how it was determined whether these patients did in fact have UNE. Again, the study by Stewart is exception in providing very explicit clinical criteria by which patients with UNE were selected, but this study did not include a control group. Estimations of specificity, therefore, are either unreliable or cannot be calculated from all of these papers. The discussion that follows, therefore, is focused on the sensitivity of the various electrophysiological tests for the diagnosis of UNE.

As shown in Table 16.4B, the sensitivities of the various tests vary considerably from study to study. Sensitivity of conduction velocity slowing across the elbow (defined either as slowing below a certain threshold or as slowing relative to forearm conduction velocity) ranged from 25 to 100%. All studies reported these sensitivities recording from ADM, and so it is not known whether sensitivity might be improved by recording from the FDI muscle. The presence of conduction block was infrequently mentioned, but the sensitivity ranged from 29% to 48% when recording from ADM, and was as high as 68% when recording from the FDI muscle. The sensitivity of an absent or abnormal ulnar sensory nerve action potential response amplitude varied from 42 to 88%, although it is worth remembering that this finding does not localize the ulnar neuropathy to elbow. Finally, although quite variable, the available data suggest that the sensitivities of the motor nerve conduction tests may be slightly better when the elbow is flexed rather than extended.

Two studies examined the utility of mixed ulnar nerve conduction studies across the elbow *(8,11)*. For this study, mixed nerve potentials are recorded from below the elbow and above the elbow following stimulation at the wrist. Raynor and colleagues reported a sensitivity of approximately 40% for both probable and definite cases of UNE *(11)*, whereas Kothari et al. reported a sensitivity of 57% *(8)*. It would seem, therefore, that the mixed ulnar nerve conduction study does not improve the diagnostic accuracy of the combination of the more routinely used sensory and motor studies.

The results of needle electromyography (EMG) in patients with suspected UNE are summarized in Table 16.4C. Most studies reported the frequency with which ongoing denervation changes (fibrillation potentials and positive sharp waves) were detected in various ulnar-innervated muscles. Fewer studies reported the frequency of chronic reinnervation changes. Sensitivities derived from the examination of FDI and ADM muscles were highest, ranging from 10% to 84% and 10% to 52%, respectively. It is difficult to draw comparisons between the different studies, as most did not report results separately for patients with ulnar neuropathy of differing severity and the frequency with which electromyographic changes are evident varies significantly as a function of the severity of the neuropathy *(9)*. However, when comparisons are drawn between the respective sensitivities of examining the different ulnar-innervated muscles, it is clear that sensitivity is best for ADM and FDI and not very good for $FDP_{4,5}$ and FCU.

The overall impression, therefore, is that the quality of the published data is relatively poor. The available studies do provide some indication of the sensitivity of the various electrodiagnostic tests, but really do not inform on their specificity. The relative utility of recording motor responses from FDI rather than ADM is unknown as is the utility of combining various nerve conduction studies with electromyographic examination.

Table 16.4B
Sensitivity of Electrophysiological Tests for the Diagnosis of Ulnar Neuropathy at the Elbow

Reference	Abnormal sensory response		AE-BE motor CV		Forearm-elbow CV drop-off		AE-BE Conduction Block	
	Sensitivity	Specificity	Sensitivity	Specificity	Sensitivity	Specificity	Sensitivity	Specificity
Bhala (4)	42%[1]	100%	100%[2]	–	81%	–	–	–
Kimura (6)	**100%[2]**	–	**81%**	–	–	–	–	–
Pickett (10)	**49%[3]**	**100%**	**19%[7]**	**100%**	–	–	–	–
Bielawski (5)	–	–	60%[8] 40%[9] **75%[8]** **55%[9]**	100% ?	50%[8] 25%[9] **15%[8]** **15%[9]**	100%[9] ? 100%[9]	–	–
Raynor (11)	–	–	–	– –	37%[9,17] **67%[9,18]**	97%[9]	–	–
Kothari (7)	54%[4]	–	80%[20] **40%[10]**	–	100% **14%**	–	9%[19]	–
Tackmann (12)	57%[2]	–	48%[2,11]	–	48%[2,11]	–	29%	–
Odusote (9)	**54%[1]**	**92%**	28%[12]	96%	–	–	–	–
Kothari (8)	57%[5]	–	71%[13] 81%[14]	–	–	–	–	–
Stewart (1)	88%[1]	–	–	–	–	–	48%[13] 68%[14]	–
Gilliatt (43)	64%[2]	–	86%[15]	–	–	–	–	–
Payan (44)	88%[6]	–	85%[16]	–	–	–	–	–

AE-BE, above elbow-below elbow; CV, conduction velocity.

Boldfaced text represents results when the elbow is extended.

1 - abnormal amplitude defined as <8 μV;
2 - criteria for abnormality not reported;
3 - abnormal amplitude defined as < 6 μV
4 - abnormal amplitude defined as <18 μV
5 - abnormal amplitude defined as <10 μV
6 - age-adjusted (<8.5 μV for 18–65 and <1.5 μV for 70–89)
7 - defined as conduction velocity <42 m/s
8 - abnormal defined as lowest value in control group
9 - defined as 2.5 SD < mean of controls
10 - abnormal defined as velocity <39.6 m/s
11 - results for absolute and relative slowing across the elbow combined
12 - conduction velocity calculated from stimulation of the ulnar nerve above the elbow and at the wrist (i.e., no stimulus below the elbow)
13 - recording abductor digiti minimi
14 - recording first dorsal interosseous
15 - defined as velocity <45 m/s
16 - age-adjusted (<50 m/s for 18–65 <44 m/s for 70–89)
17 - includes only definite cases
18 - definite and probable cases
19 - unclear whether conduction block recorded in the flexed, extended, or both positions
20 - velocity <50 m/s

Table 16.4C
Electromyographic Findings in Patients With Ulnar Neuropathy at the Elbow

Reference	Ongoing denervation changes[a]					Chronic reinnervation changes[b]					Ongoing or chronic changes				
	ADM	FDI	FDP	FCU	Any	ADM	FDI	FDP	FCU	Any	ADM	FDI	FDP	FCU	Any
Bhala (4)	23%	28%	–	28%	–	–	–	–	–	–	–	–	–	–	–
Kimura (6)	50%	53%	20%	6.7%	–	–	–	–	–	–	–	–	–	–	–
Pickett (10)	15%	32%	–	7%	–	55%	58%	–	20%	–	65%	55%	–	22%	–
Kothari (7)	–	–	–	–	–	–	–	–	–	–	–	–	–	–	82%
Stewart (1)	52%	84%	16%	16%	–	100%	–	–	–	–	–	–	–	–	–
Kothari (8)	9.5%	9.5%	4.8%	–	–	–	–	–	–	–	–	–	–	–	–

[a]Fibrillation potentials and/or positive sharp waves.
[b]Large amplitude, long duration and polyphasic motor unit potentials.
ADM, abductor digiti minimi; FDI, first dorsal interosseous; FDP, flexor digitorum profundus-4,5; FCU, flexor carpi radialis.

2.4. What Is the Accuracy of Ultrasound for the Diagnosis of UNE?

In an extremely well designed prospective study, Beekman and colleagues investigated the accuracy of high-resolution sonography for the diagnosis of ulnar neuropathy at the elbow. They included in the study all patients in whom the diagnosis of ulnar neuropathy was considered in the differential diagnosis. The gold standard for the diagnosis of ulnar neuropathy was clearly defined (*see* Table 16.1) *(13)*, and comprised a combination of clinical and electrophysiological features. Importantly, the results of sonography did not feature among these criteria, and the clinical investigators were blinded to the sonographic findings. Similarly, the ultrasonographer was blinded to the results of the clinical evaluation. The study included 136 arms (in 123 patients), in 82 of which the diagnosis of UNE was confirmed and in 45 of which an alternative diagnosis was made. There were nine limbs in which the diagnosis of UNE was suspected clinically, but not confirmed electrophysiologically even though alternate diagnoses were excluded. The authors dealt with this group of patients with probable UNE by performing a sensitivity analysis. With the nine probable-UNE patients included as cases, the sensitivity of sonography for the diagnosis of UNE was 80% and the specificity 91%. With these nine patients excluded, sensitivity remained unchanged, but specificity fell to 75%. Using a receiver operating characteristic curve analysis (plot of sensitivity vs 1-specificity), they determined that sensitivity and specificity were maximized at 81% and 91%, respectively by using an ulnar nerve diameter of 2.5 mm as the cut-off between normal and abnormal. Interestingly, the sensitivity of sonography was highest for patients with slowing across the elbow without conduction block (86%) and for patients in whom electro-diagnostic studies were either nonlocalizing or normal (85%), and lowest for patient with conduction block (71%). Secondary analysis showed that the ulnar nerve was significantly larger on sonography among patients with axonal rather than demyelinating neuropathies.

These results suggest that ultrasonography of the ulnar nerve is likely to prove a useful adjunct in the diagnosis of UNE, particularly given its high sensitivity and specificity amongst symptomatic patients with nonlocalizing or normal electrodiagnostic studies.

3. TREATMENT

3.1. What Is the Efficacy of Splinting in the Treatment of UNE?

In a small uncontrolled study, Seror examined the efficacy of nocturnal splinting with a long elbow splint in the treatment of UNE *(14)*. This study included 22 patients with clinical symptoms and signs of UNE as well as electrophysiological evidence for an ulnar nerve lesion at the elbow. The severity of the ulnar neuropathy prior to treatment was not graded, but 10 patients had muscle weakness (implying a lesion of at least moderate severity) and there was muscle atrophy in only a single patient. Treatment comprised a splint that limited elbow movements to between 15° and 60° flexion, but allowed unrestricted pronation and supination. The patient was instructed to wear the splint all night and every night for 6 months. Follow-up was performed regularly, with the final evaluation performed at 6 months. There was complete resolution of symptoms in 13 patients (59%), with the remainder all reporting improvement in symptoms. Follow-up EMG was available in 17 patients, and although individual patient data are not available, mean motor and sensory nerve conduction velocities as well as sensory response amplitudes were improved for the group as a whole. No attempt was made to correlate outcome with pretreatment severity of the ulnar neuropathy.

Dimond and Lister described (in abstract form) their experience with the treatment of UNE with a long arm splint *(15)*. Improvement was reported in 86% of patients (compared with 58% in a group of patients treated surgically over the same time period). Insufficient details are provided to determine the severity of the ulnar neuropathies in these patients and the criteria for evaluating outcome are not described.

In a small, randomized controlled trial, Hong and colleagues compared the efficacy of splinting alone with the combination of splinting and local steroid injection for the management of UNE *(16)*. They randomized 10 patients (12 nerves) to one of the two treatment groups, but two patients who were noncompliant with use of the splint were not included in the final results (i.e., no intention-to-treat analysis). Patients with ulnar neuropathy of varying severity were included, and the diagnosis was confirmed electrophysiologically in all study subjects. A significant improvement in symptoms (but not clinical signs or electrophysiological features) was found in both treatment groups after both 1 and 6 months' follow-up, with no difference in outcome between the two groups *(16)*.

In a prospective, but uncontrolled, study of conservative management of UNE, Dellon and colleagues employed a treatment regimen that comprised techniques designed to minimize mechanical compression of the ulnar nerve at the elbow *(17)*. These measures included instructions to minimize repetitive elbow flexion, use of an elbow splint at night (to maintain the elbow at less than 30° flexion), and necessary modifications to the work environment to avoid external compression of the nerve. The study population comprised patients with ulnar neuropathy that was "not severe enough to warrant surgery" as well as patients in whom surgery was deemed indicated, but who declined surgical intervention. The presence of muscle wasting, abnormal two-point discrimination, and persistent paresthesiae were regarded as indications for surgery. A 10-point scoring system was used to grade the severity of the ulnar neuropathy at baseline and following 3–6 months of conservative therapy. Those who failed conservative management underwent surgery, with treatment failure defined as the absence of symptomatic improvement, deterioration of symptoms, or a decision by the patient to forgo further conservative management. Twenty-one percent of those with purely sensory symptoms failed conservative therapy whereas 44% were symptom-free at follow-up, suggesting that the prognosis is good for a significant minority of patients with mild ulnar neuropathy. The proportion of patients failing conservative management rose to 33% and 62%, respectively among patients with moderate and severe ulnar neuropathy. Similarly, the proportion of patients with moderate and severe disease who were symptom-free at follow-up fell to 34% and 22%, respectively.

These results seem to suggest that conservative therapy is a reasonable approach for the initial management of UNE irrespective of its severity, as a significant minority (>20%) of patients with severe neuropathy may improve to become asymptomatic in response to conservative measures. It should, however, be recognized that the majority of patients with severe ulnar neuropathy will fail to respond to conservative measures.

3.2. Does Surgery Offer Any Advantage Over Conservative Measures in the Management of UNE?

There have been no prospective controlled studies comparing conservative therapy with surgery in the management of UNE. This makes it extremely difficult, if not impossible, to compare the efficacy of these two treatment modalities. Given the absence of data, the only approach is to compare the outcome of patients treated conservatively (Table 16.5) with the outcome of those treated surgically (Table 16.6A–C) in the different retrospective case series. Apart from being limited by bias and confounding (in that the differences between the patients treated conservatively and those treated surgically, which might be relevant to the outcome, are not controlled), such an approach is also hindered by the relatively small number of patients with moderate or severe ulnar neuropathy whose outcome following conservative therapy has been reported. The available literature, therefore, does not permit any firm conclusions regarding the relative efficacy of surgery and conservative therapy for the treatment of UNE.

3.3. What Are the Relative Advantages of Different Surgical Procedures for the Treatment of UNE?

There are a variety of surgical options for the treatment of UNE. Simple decompression involves freeing the nerve from compressive adhesions and bands throughout its course across the elbow and into the cubital tunnel. An alternative is decompression with anterior transposition of the nerve. Transposition requires more extensive dissection with repositioning of the nerve either within the muscle fascia (submuscular transposition) or within the subcutaneous tissue (subcutaneous transposition). A further option is medial epicondylectomy, but this involves more extensive surgery.

The controversy surrounding the role of surgery for the treatment of UNE exists in large part because of the absence of good quality data. Although there have been many reports of uncontrolled case series of patients with ulnar neuropathy treated with one surgical procedure or another, there have been no prospective controlled trials comparing surgery (of any sort) with conservative measures and only one randomized controlled trial of one surgical procedure against another *(18)*. There have been two systematic reviews of the surgical treatment of UNE *(19,20)*, but each is of limited methodological quality and each reached a different conclusion.

For the purposes of this chapter, the primary literature has been reviewed. A literature search was performed to identify articles relevant to the subject of the surgical treatment of UNE. To be eligible for inclusion in this review, each article had to meet a number of criteria: (1) report the outcome of at least 10 patients treated with a single surgical technique, (2) provide sufficient preoperative clinical information to facilitate assignment of each patient to one of three severity grades—mild, moderate, and severe—with the grading system used based on that proposed by McGowan (*see* Table 16.7), and (3) report the outcome of surgery in sufficient detail to determine overall whether there had been complete alleviation of symptoms, partial improvement, no change, or a deterioration in the clinical state. This search yielded 19 studies, 7 examining simple decompression *(21–28)*, 5 examining anterior subcutaneous transposition *(27–31)*, 3 examining anterior submuscular transposition *(32–34)*, and 6 examining medial epicondylectomy *(26,35–39)* (2 studies reported outcomes of patients treated with decompression and

Table 16.5
Prognosis of Untreated Ulnar Neuropathy of the Elbow (UNE) and UNE Treated Conservatively

Severity of UNE	Full recovery	Treatment	Reference
Mild	20/30 (67%)	None	Eisen (40)
Mild	1/4 (25%)	None	Wadsworth (41)
Mild	53/121 (44%)	Conservative[a]	Dellon (17)
Mild-Moderate	13/22 (59%)	Splinting	Seror (14)
Not specified	63/73 (86%)	Splinting	Dimond (15)
Moderate	41/121 (34%)	Conservative[a]	Dellon (17)
Severe	27/121 (22%)	Conservative[a]	Dellon (17)

Instructions to minimize elbow flexion, elbow splint at night, and avoidance of external compression.

Table 16.6A
Surgical Treatment of Mild Ulnar Neuropathy at the Elbow

	Complete relief	Improvement	No change	Worse
Decompression	36.1 (0–92)	50.9 (0–100)	10.9 (0–15)	1.9 (0–3)
Subcutaneous	17.3 (0–50)	54.7 (0–63)	25.3% (0–100)	2.7 (–25)
Submuscular	81.8 (66–100)	18.2 (0–33)	0	0
Epicondylectomy	84.7 (50–100)	10.6 (7.7–50)	0	0

Results are the proportion of patients with the specified outcome – weighted average (range).

Table 16.6B
Surgical Treatment of Moderate Ulnar Neuropathy at the Elbow

	Complete relief	Improvement	No change	Worse
Decompression	21.9 (0–50)	58.5 (0–67)	19.5 (11–33)	0
Subcutaneous	21.7 (0–36)	56.5 (45–75)	8.7 (0–25)	13.0 (0–25)
Submuscular	53.1 (28–60)	43.8 (20–71)	3.1 (0–20)	0
Epicondylectomy	41.9 (28–67)	27.9 (0–64)	30.1 (0–62)	0

Results are the proportion of patients with the specified outcome – weighted average (range).

Table 16.6C
Surgical Treatment of Severe Ulnar Neuropathy at the Elbow

	Complete relief	Improvement	No change	Worse
Decompression	22.4 (0–50)	62.1 (50–67)	12.1 (0–36)	3.4 (0–8)
Subcutaneous	19.6 (4–3)	50 (27–67)	25 (0–33)	5.4 (0–83)
Submuscular	34.8 (30–67)	60.9 (33–65)	4.3 (0–5)	0
Epicondylectomy	7 (0–14)	52.6 (16–67)	40.4 (0–83)	0

Results are the proportion of patients with the specified outcome – weighted average (range).

patients treated with epicondylectomy). For each surgical procedure and within each severity grade of ulnar neuropathy, the proportions of subjects achieving specific outcomes (complete relief, improvement, no change, or worse) have been calculated. A weighted average of these proportions has also been calculated. The results summarized

Table 16.7
McGowan Classification of the Severity of Ulnar Neuropathy

Grade	Clinical features
I	Exclusively sensory symptoms (paresthesias and numbness)
II	Muscle weakness with mild wasting of the intrinsic hand muscles, with or without accompanying sensory symptoms
III	Severe paralysis with a crippled and often clawed hand

in Tables 16.6A-C include these weighted averages (with larger studies weighted more heavily) as well as the range of values from which these summary values were determined. The most striking feature of these results is the very broad range of values reported for each surgical technique, suggesting that the point estimates (i.e., the weighted averages) do not provide a precise representation of the true efficacy of each surgical technique. Given the poor quality of the available literature as well as the substantial heterogeneity between the different studies, it seems misguided to rely solely on the point estimate of efficacy of each surgical technique. The wide range of reported outcomes is more informative and the conclusion seems to be that no single surgical technique consistently yields more favorable results than the other techniques.

4. PROGNOSIS

4.1. What Is the Natural History of Untreated Ulnar Neuropathy at the Elbow?

There are two published studies that shed light on the natural history of UNE *(40,41)*. The one study only included patients with mild ulnar neuropathy (sensory symptoms only) *(40)*, whereas the other included patients with ulnar neuropathy that ranged in severity from mild to severe *(41)*.

Eisen and Dannon retrospectively reviewed their experience with 30 patients with ulnar neuropathy who were treated conservatively *(40)*. All patients had mild ulnar neuropathy, defined by the presence of sensory symptoms but few or no findings on examination. The diagnosis of ulnar neuropathy was confirmed by electrophysiological testing that showed either slowing of conduction velocity across the elbow, absent ulnar sensory response, or neurogenic motor unit potentials on EMG. It would seem that patients were not treated, thus providing an indication of the natural history of the disorder. Furthermore, the authors did not use any sort of clinical rating scale to grade clinical status prior to treatment and then again at follow up, suggesting that outcome was determined subjectively. Of the 30 patients included in the study, 27 were said to have improved, with 20 of these achieving full recovery (i.e., asymptomatic) and 7 having only intermittent symptoms. The remaining three patients deteriorated, developing weakness, atrophy and/or objective sensory deficits. The authors concluded that the majority of patients with mild ulnar neuropathy recover spontaneously.

Wadsworth reported the outcome of 14 patients with ulnar neuropathy who were not treated surgically *(41)*. He included 3 patients with acute ulnar neuropathy secondary to elbow trauma and 11 patients with more subacute onset of symptoms. The clinical grading scheme proposed by McGowan was used (Table 16.7). The study included four patients with grade-1 ulnar neuropathies, eight patients with grade-2 lesions, and two patients with a grade-3 neuropathy. Improvement at follow-up was seen in 25% of patients in each of grades 1 and 2, and 50% of grade-3 patients *(41)*.

The results of these two studies are somewhat contradictory: the first suggests that the natural history of mild ulnar neuropathy (i.e., ulnar neuropathy manifesting with exclusively sensory symptoms) is quite benign with 90% of patients improving spontaneously *(40)* and 67% recovering completely, whereas the latter suggests that spontaneous improvement is quite unusual, occurring in only 25% of patients *(41)*. The reasons for this disparity are not clear.

4.2. Which Factors, if Any, Predict the Outcome of Surgical Treatment of UNE?

There are no high-quality studies that have examined the impact of various prognostic factors on the outcome of patients with UNE who are treated surgically. However, many of the retrospective surgical case series have included univariate analyses of a few potential prognostic factors. As shown in Table 16.8, there is little agreement between these studies regarding which factors are of prognostic value. The only three factors that emerge as predicting a better outcome in more than one study were shorter duration of symptoms (less than 1 year) *(21,27,42)*, younger age (variably reported as less than 50 or less than 70 years) *(27,42)*, and the absence of muscle atrophy on examination *(21,27)*.

5. SUMMARY

- Estimates of the frequency of various clinical findings in UNE are limited by study methodology, but the available evidence suggests that weakness of abductor digiti minimi and the first dorsal interosseous muscles are present in the majority of patients; sensory deficits are common within territories of the palmar, dorsal cutaneous, and digital branches of the ulnar nerve.
- The diagnostic accuracy of provocative tests for UNE has not been adequately studied, but the available evidence suggests that their sensitivity ranges from 70 to 98%.
- Slowing across the elbow, defined either as a conduction velocity below a certain minimum value or relative to conduction velocity in the forearm, offers the highest sensitivity for the diagnosis of UNE.
- Conduction block across the elbow is encountered less frequently and may be found in the first dorsal interosseous (FDI) muscle more commonly than in abductor digiti minimi (ADM).
- FDI and ADM are affected clinically and electromyographically more commonly than the more proximal ulnar-innervated muscles $FDP_{4,5}$ and FCU.
- Thickening of the ulnar nerve, as determined by ultrasonography, offers high sensitivity and specificity for the diagnosis of UNE, but may be of limited utility as it is a test that is not yet widely available.
- Data on the natural history of untreated UNE are conflicting, but the larger of the two published studies suggests that the outcome is usually good, at least for mild UNE, with the majority of patients improving spontaneously.
- Conservative treatment of UNE may lead to complete resolution of symptoms in almost half of all patients with mild UNE and in a significant minority of patients with moderate-to-severe compressive neuropathy.

Table 16.8
Prognosis for Patients With Ulnar Neuropathy at the Elbow Who Are Treated Surgically

Reference	n	Treatment	Good prognostic factors	Factors not affecting prognosis
Le Roux (21)	51	Decompression	Symptom duration <1 yr Absence of muscle atrophy Mild grade neuropathy	Age Etiology
Davies (42)	128	Decompression or subcutaneous transposition	Symptom duration <1 yr Age <70	–
Novak (45)	100	Subcutaneous transposition	–	Body mass index Preoperative electrodiagnostic findings
Taha (46)	38	Transposition	–	–
Lugnegard (30)	33	Transposition	Age <50 yr No history of alcohol abuse	–
Foster (27)	48	Decompression or subcutaneous transposition	Absence of muscle atrophy Shorter duration of symptoms (trend) Younger age (trend)	–
Nathan (47)	131	Decompression	Male gender Increased height Increased weight	–

- A variety of surgical techniques have been used to treat UNE including simple decompression, anterior transposition (subcutaneous or submuscular) and medial epicondylectomy. There is no good evidence favoring the use of one technique over another for mild or moderately severe UNE. There is no evidence that surgery results in better outcome than conservative management for severe UNE.
- There is conflicting data regarding prognostic factors for outcome of UNE. Limited data suggests that milder disease, younger age and shorter duration of symptoms may portend a better prognosis.

REFERENCES

1. Stewart JD. The variable clinical manifestations of ulnar neuropathies at the elbow. J Neurol Neurosurg Psychiatry 1987;50:252–258.
2. Beekman R, Van Der Plas JP, Uitdehaag BM, Schellens RL, Visser LH. Clinical, electrodiagnostic, and sonographic studies in ulnar neuropathy at the elbow. Muscle Nerve 2004;30:202–208.
3. Novak CB, Lee GW, Mackinnon SE, Lay L. Provocative testing for cubital tunnel syndrome. J Hand Surg [Am] 1994;19A:817–820.
4. Bhala RP. Electrodiagnosis of ulnar nerve lesions at the elbow. Arch Phys Med Rehabil 1976;57:206–212.
5. Bielawski M, Hallett M. Position of the elbow in determination of abnormal motor conduction of the ulnar nerve across the elbow. Muscle Nerve 1989;12:803–809.
6. Kimura I, Ayyar D, Lippmann SM. Early electrodiagnosis of the ulnar entrapment neuropathy at the elbow. Tohoku J Exp Med 1984;142:165–172.
7. Kothari M, Preston D. Comparison of the flexed and extended elbow positions in localizing ulnar neuropathy at the elbow. Muscle Nerve 1995;18:336–340.
8. Kothari MJ, Heistand M, Rutkove SB. Three ulnar nerve conduction studies in patients with ulnar neuropathy at the elbow. Arch Phys Med Rehabil 1998;79:87–89.
9. Odusote K, Eisen A. An electrophysiological quantitation of the cubital tunnel syndrome. Can J Neurol Sci 1979;6:403–410.
10. Pickett JB, Coleman LL. Localizing ulnar nerve lesions to the elbow by motor conduction studies. Electromyogr Clin Neurophysiol 1984;24:343–360.
11. Raynor EM, Shefner JM, Preston DC, Logigian EL. Sensory and mixed nerve conduction studies in the evaluation of ulnar neuropathy at the elbow. Muscle Nerve 1994;17:785–792.
12. Tackmann W, Vogel P, Kaeser H, Ettlin T. Sensitivity and localizing significance of motor and sensory electroneurographic parameters in the diagnosis of ulnar nerve lesions at the elbow. A reappraisal. J Neurol 1984;231:204–211.
13. Beekman R, Schoemaker M, Van Der Plas J, et al. Diagnostic value of high-resolution sonography in ulnar neuropathy at the elbow. Neurology 2004;62:767–773.
14. Seror P. Treatment of ulnar nerve palsy at the elbow with a night splint. J Bone Joint Surg [Br] 1993;75B:322–327.
15. Dimond ML, Lister GD. Cubital tunnel syndrome treated by long-arm splintage. J Hand Surg [Am] 1985;10A:430.
16. Hong CZ, Long A, Kanakamedala RV, Chang Y-M, Yates L. Splinting and local steroid injection for the treatment of ulnar neuropathy at the elbow: clinical and electrophysiological evaluation. Arch Phys Med Rehabil 1996;77:573–577.
17. Dellon AL, Hament W, Gittelshon A. Nonoperative management of cubital tunnel syndrome: an 8-year prospective study. Neurology 1993;43:1673–1677.
18. Geutjens G, Langstaff R, Smith N, Jefferson D, Howell C, Barton N. Medial epicondylectomy or ulnar-nerve transposition for ulnar neuropathy at the elbow? J Bone Joint Surg [Br] 1996;78B:777–779.
19. Mowlavi A, Andrews K, Lille S, Verhulst S, Zook EG, Milner S. The management of cubital tunnel syndrome: a meta-analysis of clinical studies. Plast Reconstr Surg 2000;106:327–334.
20. Bartels RH, Menovsky T, Van Overbeeke JJ, Verhagen WI. Surgical management of ulnar nerve compression at the elbow: an analysis of the literature. J Neurosurg 1998;89:722–727.

21. LeRoux PD, Ensign TD, Burchiel KJ. Surgical decompression without transposition for ulnar neuropathy: factors determining outcome. Neurosurgery 1990;27:709–714.
22. Miller R, Hummel EE. The cubital tunnel syndrome: treatment with simple decompression. Ann Neurol 1980;7:567–569.
23. Wilson DH, Krout R. Surgery of ulnar neuropathy at the elbow: 16 cases treated by decompression without transposition. J Neurosurg 1973;38:780–785.
24. Lavyne MH, Bell WO. Simple decompression and occasional microsurgical epineurolysis under local anesthesia as treatment for ulnar neuropathy at the elbow. Neurosurgery 1982;11:6–11.
25. Manske PR, Johnston R, Pruitt DL, Strecker WB. Ulnar nerve decompression at the cubital tunnel. Clin Orthop Relat Res 1992; 274:231–237.
26. Froimson AI, Anouchi YS, Seitz WH, Winsberg DD. Ulnar nerve decompression with medial epicondylectomy for neuropathy at the elbow. Clin Orthop Relat Res 1991; 265:200–206.
27. Foster RJ, Edshage S. Factors related to the outcome of surgically managed compressive ulnar neuropathy at the elbow level. J Hand Surg [Am]1981;6:181–192.
28. Chan RC, Paine KW, Varughese G. Ulnar neuropathy at the elbow: comparison of simple decompression and anterior transposition. Neurosurgery 1980;7:545–550.
29. Payan J. Anterior transposition of the ulnar nerve: an electrophysiological study. J Neurol Neurosurg Psychiatry 1970;33:157–165.
30. Lugnegard H, Walheim G, Wenneberg A. Operative treatment of ulnar neuropathy in the elbow region. A clinical and electrophysiological study. Acta Orthop Scand 1977;48:168–176.
31. Mooij J. Ulnar nerve pathology at the elbow: the place of anterior transposition today. Acta Neurchirurgica (Wien) 1982;64:75–85.
32. Mass DP, Silverberg B. Cubital tunnel syndrome: anterior transposition with epicondylar osteotomy. Orthopedics 1986;9:711–715.
33. Leffert RD. Anterior submuscular transposition of the ulnar nerves by the Learmonth technique. J Hand Surg [Am] 1982;7:147–155.
34. Nouhan R, Kleinert JM. Ulnar nerve decompression by transposing the nerve and z-lengthening the flexor-pronator mass: clinical outcome. J Hand Surg [Am] 1997;22 A:127–131.
35. Robinson D, Aghasi M, Haperin N. Medial epicondylectomy in cubital tunnel syndrome: an electrodiagnostic study. J Hand Surg [Br] 1992;170B:255–256.
36. Tada H, Hirayama T, Katsuki M, Habaguchi T. Long term results using a modified King's method for cubital tunnel syndrome. Clin Orthop Relat Res 1997;336:107–110.
37. Froimson AI, Zahrawi F. Treatment of compression neuropathy of the ulnar nerve at the elbow by epicondylectomy and neurolysis. J Hand Surg [Am] 1980;5:391–395.
38. Goldberg BJ, Light TR, Blair SJ. Ulnar neuropathy at the elbow: results of medial epicondylectomy. J Hand Surg [Am] 1989;14:182–188.
39. Craven PR, Green DP. Cubital tunnel syndrome. Treatment by medial epicondylectomy. J Bone Joint Surg [Am] 1980;62A:986–989.
40. Eisen A, Danon J. The mild cubital tunnel syndrome. Its natural history and indications for surgical intervention. Neurology 1974;24:608–613.
41. Wadsworth TG. The external compression syndrome of the ulnar nerve at the cubital tunnel. Clin Orthop Relat Res 1977;124:189–204.
42. Davies M, Vonau M, Blum P, Kwok B, Matheson J, Stening W. Results of ulnar neuropathy at the elbow treated by decompression or anterior transposition. Aust NZ J Surg 1991;61:929–934.
43. Gilliatt R, Thomas P. Changes in nerve conduction with ulnar lesions at the elbow. J Neurol Neurosurg Psychiatry 1960;23:312–320.
44. Payan J. Electrophysiological localization of ulnar nerve lesions. J Neurol Neurosurg Psychiatry 1969;32:208–220.
45. Novak CB, Mackinnon SE, Stuebe AM. Patient self-reported outcome after ulnar nerve transposition. Ann Plast Surg 2002;48:274–280.
46. Taha A, Galarza M, Zuccarello M, Taha J. Outcomes of cubital tunnel surgery among patients with absent sensory nerve conduction. Neurosurgery 2004;54:891–895.
47. Nathan P, Keniston R, Meadows K. Outcome study of ulnar nerve compression at the elbow treated with simple decompression and an early programme of physical therapy. J Hand Surg [Br] 1995;20B:628–637.

IV NEUROMUSCULAR JUNCTION DISORDERS

17 Myasthenia Gravis

1. INTRODUCTION

Myasthenia gravis (MG) is an autoimmune disorder in which antibodies are either directed against the muscle nicotinic acetylcholine receptor (nAChR) itself or against other postsynaptic targets such as the muscle specific kinase (MuSK) that indirectly reduce nAChR numbers. The disease may be limited to the extra-ocular muscles and eyelids (ocular myasthenia) or may affect limb, bulbar and respiratory muscles (generalized myasthenia). The relative diagnostic utility of electrophysiological tests and the presence of anti-acetylcholine receptor antibodies vary depending on whether the disease is ocular or generalized. MG is the prototype neurological auto-immune disorder in which both antigen and antibody have been identified, removal of antibody has been shown to lead to clinical improvement, and the disease can be recreated in mice following passive transfer of the auto-antibody. Understandably, therefore, immunosuppressive therapy forms the mainstay of disease-modifying treatment, with acetylcholinesterase inhibitors being reserved for symptomatic management.

What is the accuracy of repetitive nerve stimulation (RNS), single-fiber electromyography (SFEMG), and testing for acetylcholine receptor antibodies for the diagnosis of ocular and generalized myasthenia gravis (MG)? Which immunosuppressive therapies have been shown to be beneficial in myasthenia gravis? Are the beneficial effects of the different treatment strategies comparable? What is the natural history of ocular myasthenia, and is there a role for immunosuppressive therapy in patients who only have ocular disease? What is the prognosis for MG? These and other questions are the focus of this chapter.

2. DIAGNOSIS

2.1. What Is the Diagnostic Accuracy of RNS, SFEMG, and Testing for Anti-Acetylcholine Receptor Antibodies for the Diagnosis of Ocular Myasthenia Gravis?

There are a limited number of studies that have addressed this issue. Useful data can only be obtained from studies that applied the diagnostic test in question both to patients with ocular myasthenia gravis (OMG) and to subjects without OMG. Those studies that have examined the utility of the diagnostic test only among patients with MG have not been included here, as they do not permit estimation of both the sensitivity and specificity

From: *Neuromuscular Disease: Evidence and Analysis in Clinical Neurology*
By: M. Benatar © Humana Press Inc., Totowa, NJ

of the test for the diagnosis of OMG. The relevant features of each of the studies that will be considered here are summarized in Table 17.1.

2.1.2. ANTI-ACETYLCHOLINE RECEPTOR ANTIBODIES

Four studies *(1–4)* evaluated the diagnostic accuracy of anti-nAChR antibodies for OMG. The 2×2 tables below show the data with calculated sensitivities and specificities.

	Padua (1)		*Lefvert* (2)		*Oey* (3)		*Limburg* (4)	
	OMG	no OMG	OMG	no OMG	OMG	no OMG	OMG	no OMG
Antibody +	15	0	7	1	11	0	15	4
Antibody −	19	9	17	225	7	14	15	195
Sensitivity	0.44		0.29		0.61		0.50	
Specificity	1.00		0.99		1.00		0.98	

There are a number of important differences between these studies. Those by Lefvert and Limburg *(2,4)* were case–control studies, with the reference populations including healthy controls and patients with other neurological and autoimmune diseases. The reference populations in the studies by Padua and Oey *(1,3)*, by contrast, included patients referred for evaluation for possible OMG, but who turned out to have another disease. But this difference would be expected to improve the specificity of the test, and because the specificity is equally good in the latter two studies, the difference in choice of reference populations is probably not a cause of significant inter-study heterogeneity.

The pooled sensitivity and specificity may be calculated using a weighted average. The sensitivity or specificity for an individual study is multiplied by the ratio of sample size for the individual study to total number of patients in all four studies combined. Using this method, the pooled sensitivity with 95% confidence interval is 0.59 (0.52–0.66) and the pooled specificity is 0.99 (0.986–0.994). Because the individual study sensitivities do not all fall within the 95% confidence intervals of the pooled estimate, it seems that there is substantial heterogeneity between the individual studies. A pooled estimate is, therefore, inappropriate, and individual study results should be reported. The sensitivity of the assay for anti-acetylcholine receptor antibodies in the diagnosis of OMG, therefore, ranges from 0.29 to 0.61, indicating that this test is relatively insensitive test for the diagnosis of OMG. That is to say, the test will only be positive in 29–61% of subjects who actually have OMG and a negative test result does not help to exclude the diagnosis. By contrast, the specificity is high (99%), indicating that a false-positive test result is extremely rare, occurring in only 1 of 100 cases. A positive test result, therefore, can be taken as reliable evidence for the presence of disease, but a negative test does not help to exclude the diagnosis.

2.1.3. REPETITIVE NERVE STIMULATION

Only two studies have examined the utility of RNS for the diagnosis of OMG *(1,3)*. Although both were follow-up (cohort) studies and the reference population in both was derived from patients referred for evaluation for OMG, Oey and colleagues *(3)* performed RNS of the facial nerve (recording orbicularis oculi), and Padua and colleagues *(1)*

Table 17.1

Characteristics of Studies Examining Diagnostic Accuracy of Various Tests for Ocular Myasthenia Gravis (OMG)

Study	n	Mean age (range)	Gold standard for diagnosis of OMG
Padua (1)	43	45.6 (20–74)	Two of (a) anti-nAChR antibody, (b) response to cholinesterase inhibitors, and (c) abnormal electrophysiology
Rouseev (5)	23	49.6 (19–79)	All of (a) clinical evidence for OMG, (b) no evidence for an alternative diagnosis, (c) clear response to cholinesterase medication
Oey(3)	32	51 (25–74)	History of fluctuating ocular symptoms, together with either (a) good response to cholinesterase inhibitor medication or (b) elevated antibody titers
Limburg (4)	229	Not specified	Typical history and physical signs and response to cholinesterase inhibitors
Lefvert (2)	250	Not specified	Typical history, response to cholinesterase inhibitors, and typical response to repetitive nerve stimulation

stimulated either the ulnar nerve (recording abductor digiti minimi) or the truncus primarius superior (recording from deltoid). The study by Padua and colleagues was also susceptible to incorporation bias in that abnormal electrophysiological tests were used as part of the gold standard for the diagnosis of myasthenia gravis (1). These features suggest that there is substantial heterogeneity between the studies and this is confirmed by the finding that the point estimates for each study do not fall within the 95% confidence intervals of the pooled estimates of sensitivity and specificity. It is, therefore, inappropriate to combine the two studies in a meta-analysis. Instead, each study should be considered independently.

	Padua (1)		Oey (3)	
	OMG	no OMG	OMG	no OMG
RNS+	5	1	8	0
RNS–	29	8	10	14
Sensitivity	0.15		0.44	
Specificity	0.89		1.00	

The varying sensitivities are likely due, in large part, to the different choice of nerve for RNS. The higher sensitivity (0.44) was obtained with stimulation of the facial nerve (3).

As for antibody testing, the sensitivity of RNS for the diagnosis of OMG is low, but the specificity is high. Sensitivity is improved somewhat by stimulating the facial nerve, but remains relatively low. These data suggest that a negative test is not helpful, but a positive test result is extremely useful in confirming the diagnosis of OMG.

Table 17.2

Characteristics of Studies Examining the Accuracy of Single-Fiber Electromyography (SFEMG) for the Diagnosis of Ocular Myasthenia Gravis

Study	Muscle examined	Technique used	Criteria for abnormal jitter
Padua (1)	Orbicularis oculi	Voluntary SFEMG	MCD increased in >15% of pairs OR Abnormal mean jitter with at least 2 of 20 abnormal pairs
Rouseev (5)	Frontalis	Voluntary SFEMG	Mean jitter of 20 fiber pairs >35 μs
Oey (3)	Orbicularis oculi	Stimulated SFEMG	MCD greater than 30 μs in more than 2 of 20 muscle fibers AND mean jitter greater than 20 μs
Milone (6)	Orbicularis oculi	Voluntary SFEMG	Mean MCD >95% of upper limit normal OR MCD of single pair more than 95% upper limit in >10% of fibers

MCD, mean consecutive difference.

2.1.4. SINGLE FIBER ELECTROMYOGRAPHY

For the four studies *(1,3,5,6)* that examined the utility of SFEMG, important methodological considerations are summarized in Tables 17.2 and 17.3.

	Padua (1)		Rouseev (5)		Oey (3)		Milone (6)	
	OMG	no OMG	OMG	no OMG	OMG	no OMG	OMG	no OMG
Abnormal jitter	34	1	5	6	17	1	13	0
Normal jitter	0	8	0	12	1	13	1	8
Sensitivity	1.00		1.00		0.94		0.93	
Specificity	0.89		0.89		0.93		1.00	

In order to decide whether the sensitivities and specificities from these studies can be pooled to yield a summary estimate, it is first necessary to explore the potential sources of heterogeneity between the studies.

Based on the data summarized in Table 17.3, there does appear to be substantial heterogeneity between the various studies. Every study differs from at least one other with respect to at least one important variable. Only one study consecutively recruited all patients referred for evaluation for OMG *(1)*, although this may have been the case in two other studies *(3,5)*; the fourth study compared the diagnostic utility of SFEMG using patients with chronic progressive external ophthalmoplegia as a reference group. Diagnostic threshold was similar across the studies (with the exception of the study by Rouseev *[5]*), but only two of these avoided incorporation bias, the bias that results from the incorporation of the test under investigation (in this case SFEMG) into the gold standard for making the diagnosis of OMG. Incorporation bias tends to inflate the sensitivity of the test.

Table 17.3

Heterogeneity of studies That Examined the Accuracy of Single-Fiber Electromyography
for the Diagnosis of Ocular Myasthenia Gravis (OMG)

	Milone (6)	*Padua* (1)	*Oey* (3)	*Rouseev* (5)
Study design	Case–control	Cohort	Cohort	Cohort
Consecutive series or random sample	No	Consecutive series	Not specified	Not specified
Reference population	CPEO	Patients referred for evaluation for OMG		
Diagnostic threshold	Abnormal mean jitter or jitter of individual fiber pairs abnormal in >10% of fiber pairs			Abnormal mean jitter
Incorporation bias	No	Yes	No	No

CPEO, chronic progressive external opthalmoplegia.

In view of this inter-study heterogeneity, it seems inappropriate to calculate summary measures to describe the diagnostic accuracy of SFEMG. Instead, it is better to rely on the range of values derived from the individual studies. Sensitivity varies from 0.93 to 1.0 and specificity varies from 0.89 to 1.0.

The accuracy of acetylcholine receptor antibodies, RNS, and SFEMG for the diagnosis of OMG are summarized in Table 17.4.

2.2. What Is the Diagnostic Accuracy of RNS, SFEMG, and Testing for Anti-Acetylcholine Receptor Antibodies for the Diagnosis of GMG?

There are even fewer studies that have formally examined the diagnostic utility of these tests in patients with GMG.

2.2.1. ANTI-ACETYLCHOLINE RECEPTOR ANTIBODIES

Two of the studies that examined the diagnostic utility of anti-acetylcholine receptor antibodies in ocular OMG also examined patients with generalized disease (2,4). These were both case–control studies in which the reference populations comprised both healthy controls as well as patients with other neurological and auto-immune diseases. Neither was susceptible to incorporation bias. The homogeneity between these studies suggests that it is appropriate to pool their results. The individual study results are summarized below.

	Lefvert (2)		*Limburg* (4)	
	MG	*no MG*	*MG*	*no MG*
Antibody positive	218	1	213	4
Antibody negative	35	225	37	195
Sensitivity	0.83		0.85	
Specificity	0.996		0.98	

Table 17.4
Summary of Diagnostic Tests in Ocular and Generalized Myasthenia Gravis (MG)

Test	Ocular MG		Generalized MG	
	Sensitivity	Specificity	Sensitivity	Specificity
AChR antibodies[a]	29–61%	99%	84%	99.8%
RNS[b]	15–44%	89–100%	95%[b]	78–100%
SFEMG[c]	93–100%	89–100%	87%	96%

[a]Binding antibodies.
[b]Estimate based on using repetitive nerve stimulation (RNS) in four different nerves.
[c]Using either voluntary or stimulated single-fiber electromyography (SFEMG); muscles tested include frontalis, orbicularis oculi, and extensor digitorum communis.

The pooled sensitivity with 95% confidence intervals is 0.84 (0.83–0.85), and the pooled specificity is 0.998 (0.996–0.999). Anti-acetylchloline receptor antibody testing, therefore, is an excellent test. It is highly specific in that almost everyone with a positive test result will have MG. The sensitivity is also high, with the test being positive in 84% of patients who have the disease.

The foregoing discussion of the utility of anti-acetylcholine receptor antibodies relates to testing for binding antibodies. Two other types of antibodies — *blocking* and *modulating* antibodies—have also been described. Their diagnostic utility has been examined less extensively. Howard and colleagues determined titers of binding, modulating, and blocking antibodies in a large population of patients with MG as well as a large control group with other neurological diseases *(7)*. The results are summarized below.

	Binding		Blocking		Modulating	
	MG	no MG	MG	no MG	MG	no MG
Antibody positive	235	3	142	3	228	4
Antibody negative	27	446	106	446	48	445
Sensitivity	0.90		0.57		0.83	
Specificity	0.99		0.99		0.99	

The sensitivity of modulating antibodies is quite high, but less than that of binding antibodies, and the sensitivity of blocking antibodies is relatively low. The specificity of each type of antibody is high, but is should be noted that there were only four patients with blocking antibodies who did not also have binding antibodies (and all four of these patients also had modulating antibodies), suggesting that the isolated finding of elevated titers of blocking antibodies might represent a false-positive result. There were 27 patients who had only either binding or modulating antibodies.

2.2.2. REPETITIVE NERVE STIMULATION

Ozdemir and Young investigated the utility of RNS, with recordings made from up to four different muscles (abductor digiti minimi, wrist flexors, deltoid and orbicularis oculi) *(8)*. The results of RNS performed in all of these muscles in 80 patients with MG and 40 patients with other neuromuscular diseases are shown in the table.

	MG	*no MG*
RNS +	76	9
RNS −	4	31

The sensitivity of RNS for the diagnosis of MG is 0.95 and the specificity is 0.78. The sensitivity falls to 0.59 if RNS is performed only in abductor digiti minimi, emphasizing the importance of testing multiple sites with RNS. They also noted that the pattern of decremental response differed between the myasthenics and the neuromuscular controls, with an "envelope" pattern in which the response falls initially, but then recovers after more than four to five stimuli, being observed only in MG. Relying on this specific pattern of abnormality, they found that specificity increased to 100%.

2.2.3. SINGLE-FIBER ELECTROMYOGRAPHY

Mercelis examined the diagnostic utility of single fiber SFEMG in 391 consecutive patients referred for evaluation for suspected MG *(9)*. The study designed was susceptible to incorporation bias as the results of SFEMG were used, in part, to determine whether patients were diagnosed with MG. He used stimulated SFEMG in both the extensor digitorum communis (EDC) and orbicularis oculi muscles. Using abnormal mean jitter (>20 µs in orbicularis oculi or >25 µs in EDC) or abnormal jitter in at least 10% of individual muscle fiber pairs (>30 µs in orbicularis oculi or >40 µs in EDC), he obtained the following results:

	MG	*no MG*
SFEMG abnormal	71	20
SFEMG normal	7	293

yielding a sensitivity of 91% and a specificity of 94%. If the stringency of the criteria for defining jitter as abnormal were increased such that more than 10% of individual fibers with abnormal jitter was required, the specificity was improved at the expense of a fall in sensitivity (as shown below).

	MG	*no MG*
SFEMG abnormal	68	12
SFEMG normal	10	301

These more stringent criteria are those that are more widely accepted and commonly used. Stimulated SFEMG, therefore, has a sensitivity of 87% and a specificity of 96% for the diagnosis of MG.

The accuracy of acetylcholine receptor antibodies, RNS, and SFEMG for the diagnosis of GMG are summarized in Table 17.4.

2.3. When Is It Worth Testing for Antibodies Against MuSK?

It has long been recognized that there are a group of patients with myasthenia gravis who do not harbor antibodies directed against the nicotinic acetylcholine receptor despite their clinical similarity to seropositive patients and their responsiveness to immunosuppressive therapy. Antibodies against the tyrosine kinase MuSK have recently been identified in a subset of patients with seronegative MG *(10–12)*. With the identification of a biomarker for these patients, it has emerged that reactivity against MuSK appears to be associated with three somewhat different clinical phenotypes. As previously recognized, some patients are clinically indistinguishable from patients with generalized disease who have antibodies against the acetylcholine receptor. Other patients appear to have prominent oculobulbar symptoms such as ophthalmoparesis, facial weakness, dysarthria, dysphagia, and respiratory muscle weakness *(11)*. Others have little or no ocular involvement but with prominent weakness of the shoulders, of neck extension, and of respiratory muscles *(12)*.

The frequency with which anti-acetylcholine receptor antibodies are identified in patients with purely ocular myasthenia is relatively low. At present, there is no evidence that this group of patients harbor antibodies to MuSK.

3. TREATMENT

3.1. Do Steroids Reduce the Likelihood of Progression From Ocular to Generalized Disease?

A number of retropsective observational studies have addressed the question of whether immunosuppressive therapy has any effect on the natural history of OMG in terms of the risk of progressing to GMG *(13–17)*. Although these studies used different steroid regimens, the methodological quality of these studies (Table 17.5) was otherwise fairly uniform, with reasonably complete follow-up and adquate control for confounding but lack of blinded assessment of outcome. The point estimates of the odds ratios (odds of progression to GMG among those receiving steroids compared with those not receiving steroids) showed a benefit in terms of reducing the risk of progression to generalized MG in four studies *(14–17)*, with the confidence interval spanning unity in the only study that did not show a benefit *(1)* (Table 17.5). Taken together, these data suggest, but do not prove, that patients with OMG may benefit from treatment with steroids. There is, however, no general consensus *(18–20)*.

3.2 What Is the Evidence That Steroids Are of Benefit in Patients With GMG?

The use of corticosteroids in the treatment of MG is an excellent example of a treatment that has become established without ever having been subjected to the rigorous evaluation of a large prospective placebo-controlled trial. Nevertheless, it is useful to reflect on some of the literature that describes the utility of corticosteroids.

The study by Howard et al. *(21)*, published in 1976, was the closest approximation to a placebo-controlled trial. Thirteen patients with mild to moderate generalized myasthenia were randomized to receive either prednisone 100 mg on alternate days or placebo. At two year follow-up, three of six patients in the prednisone group, and three of seven patients who received placebo, were improved. The four patients in the placebo group who were unchanged were then treated with prednisone and an improvement noted in three. Overall, therefore, 70% of patients who were treated responded to prednisone, but this response rate was not significantly different from that in the placebo group. The failure of this study to demonstrate a beneficial effect of alternate-day prednisone was

Table 17.5
Design Characteristics and Outcome of Observational Studies of Steroid Treatment in Ocular Myasthenia

Author (Reference)	n	Study design	Treatment schedule	Control for confounding	Completeness of follow-up	Patient blinding	OR[a] (95% CI)
Papapetropoulos 2003 (13)	28	Case–control	Gradual titration to 60 mg QOD and then tapered to lowest dose required (5–10 mg QOD	Adequate	Adequate 100% ≥8 yr	Not done	4.3 (0.7–25.9)
Mee 2003 (14)	34	Case–control	25 mg QD (mean duration of therapy 33.5 mo)	Adequate	Adequate 100% Mean 4.2 yr	Not done	0.02 (0.001–0.16)
Kupersmith 2003 (15)	147	Cohort	10 mg QD for 2 d, 20 mg QD for 2 d, dose increased to 50–60 mg QD for 4–5 d, 40 mg QD for 1 wk, 30 mg QD for 1 wk, 20 mg QD for 1 wk, 10 mg/20 mg alternating QD for 1 wk, dose further reduced by 2.5 mg QD each week	Adequate	Inadequate 64% Mean 3.6 yr Range 0.5–16 yr	Not done	0.13 (0.04–0.45)
Monsul 2004 (16)	56	Cohort	40–60 mg QD tapered to 2.5.–10 mg QD over 3–6 mo	Adequate	Not done 100% ≥2 yr	Not done	0.24 (0.06–0.99)
Sommer 1997 (17)	78	Cohort	Maximum dose 52 mg QD (mean duration of therapy 32 mo)	Inadequate	Adequate 100%	Not done	0.09 (0.03–0.29)

[a]Odds ratio of progression to generalized myasthenia gravis among those receiving active treatment compared with those receiving control treatment.

likely the consequence of its small sample size. Notwithstanding the results of this study, prednisone continued to be used in the treatment of myasthenia.

Sghirlanzoni and colleagues *(22)* described their experience with 60 patients treated with steroids. They did not use a uniform steroid dosing schedule. Some were treated with a slowly increasing dose, others received high dose therapy on alternate days or every day. Once sustained improvement was achieved and maintained for 3–4 months, the dose was gradually reduced by 10% every 5–7 weeks until the lowest maintenance dose was reached. The response to therapy was described as (1) complete remission (recovery with no requirement for medication), (2) pharmacological remission (clinical recovery, but still requiring pharmacotherapy of some sort), (3) improved, or (4) nonresponsive. Overall, improvement was noted in 72% of patients. Those who received higher dosages achieved a clinical response more rapidly, but by 6 months, the response rates were similar in the two treatment groups provided that a dose of 100 mg prednisone on alternate days had been reached. The only baseline characteristic predictive of a better response to corticosteroid therapy was onset after the age of 40.

Pascuzzi et al. *(23)* studied 116 patients with MG who were treated with the same steroid regimen and followed for between 8 months and 17 years. They designated the response to treatment as satisfactory (remission or marked improvement) or unstatisfactory (unimproved or only moderate improvement). Treatment was initiated with prednisone 60–80 mg for three consecutive days after which the dosage was changed to an equivalent alternate-day schedule. Dose reductions occurred at a rate of approximately 10 mg every 2 months provided that the patient maintained her clinical response. The response was satisfactory in 80% of patients, with marked improvement in 52% and remission in 18%. In those with a satisfactory response, the onset of sustained improvement occurred after a mean of 13 days and the median time to maximal improvement was 5–6 months. Older age was the strongest predictor of a better response to steroid therapy, but the presence of milder disease and symptoms of shorter duration were also important.

Most recently, Evoli and colleagues *(24)* reported their experience with 104 patients with MG who were treated with steroids. The initial prednisone dose varied from 0.8 to 1.5 mg/kg/day, with the higher doses used for patients with more severe disease. This dose was maintained until obvious improvement was apparent (usually about three weeks) and was then gradually changed to an alternate-day regimen. Patients were followed for at least 2 years. The response to treatment was classified as improved (complete remission, pharmacological remission, or marked improvement) or unresponsive (moderate improvement, no improvement, or deterioration). Improvement was noted in 98 patients (94%) and the mean time to onset of objective improvement was 16 days.

The effects of high-dose steroids in MG are summarized in Table 17.6.

3.3. How Problematic Is the Early Clinical Deterioration That May Accompany the Initiation of Steroid Therapy?

The phenomenon of transient worsening of myasthenic symptoms shortly after the initiation of corticosteroid therapy is well recognized. Pascuzzi et al. *(23)*, for example, reported an early deterioration in 48% of patients, in 10 (8.6%) of whom it was severe. The exacerbation occurred between 1 and 17 days after the initiation of therapy (mean onset on day 5). In the retrospective series of Evoli et al. *(25)*, transient early deterioration

Table 17.6
Summary Table of Data Relating to the Use of High-Dose Steroids
in Myasthenia Gravis

Response to treatment with high-dose steroids	
Frequency of improvement	80% *(23)* to 94% *(24)*
Latency to onset of sustained improvement	13 *(23)* to 16 *(24)* d
Median time to maximal improvement	5–6 mo *(23)*
Early deterioration with high-dose steroids	
Frequency	21% *(24)* to 48% *(23)*
Severe	7% *(24)* to 8.6% *(23)*
Mean latency to onset of deterioration	4–5 d *(23,24)*

with initiation of steroid therapy was observed in 22 patients (21%), in approximately one-third of whom it was severe. Typically, the deterioration occurred at a mean of 4 days after the start of therapy. In the study by Sghirlanzoni and colleagues *(22)* a transient deterioration was observed in 38% of patients treated initially with high dose, compared with 19% in those who received a slowly increasing dose. This observation—that the incidence of transient deterioration could be reduced by a gradual initiation of steroid therapy—was not a new one. Seybold and Drachman *(26)* had previously reported their experience with 12 patients in initiating treatment with low-dose steroids. Transient worsening of myasthenic symptoms was not observed in any of their patients.

In these four series, therefore, the incidence of early deterioration varied from 0% to 48%, with there being some indication that early deterioration occurred more frequently in those who were treated with early high-dose steroids.

3.4. What Is the Optimal Dosing Schedule When Steroid Therapy is Initiated?

Broadly speaking, there are two options for the initiation of steroid therapy: high-dose and low-dose. The philosophy behind initiating therapy with high-dose steroids (e.g., prednisone 1 mg/kg day) is that the clinical response is more rapid and that failure to respond to therapy will not be due to underdosage. The competing argument for initiation with low dose steroid (e.g., ~25 mg prednisone every other day) followed by gradual dosage increments) is that the incidence of early deterioration (which may require mechanical ventilation if severe) appears to be less frequent than when therapy is started with high-dose steroids. Other factors that may enter the equation are the severity of the disease (although there is no good evidence indicating whether patients with less severe disease are less likely to experience a marked deterioration) and whether therapy is being initiated in an inpatient or outpatient setting. Although it is difficult to make an evidence-based recommendation, it seems reasonable to begin steroid therapy with a high-dose regimen when patients can be closely monitored and promptly treated if myasthenic symptoms worsen. Low-dose therapy seems more prudent when steroid therapy is initiated in a less controlled or supervised environment.

3.5. Is High-Dose Intravenous Methylprednisolone of Any Benefit?

Arsura and colleagues *(27)* reported rapid improvement in 12 of 15 patients with rapidly progressive severe MG who were treated with high-dose intravenous methyl-prednisolone (IVMP). Patients received an infusion of 2 g over 12 hours, and this was repeated every 5 days if improvement was limited. Those who improved clinically also received 30 mg prednisone followed by a gradual taper. Satisfactory improvement (defined as being asymptomatic or having only minor symptoms which do not interfere with daily activities) occurred in 10 of 15 patients following the second infusion and in 2 more following the third infusion. Improvement began a mean of 3 days after the first infusion, 2 days after the second infusion, and was maximal around 9 days after the last infusion. The latency to clinical improvement, therefore, was substantially shorter than in the studies by Pascuzzi and Evoli, in which the latencies were 13 and 16 days, respectively. At follow-up 15 months later, 10 patients had maintained their level of satisfactory functioning while continuing a prednisone taper.

The efficacy of intravenous methylprednisolone in MG was recently evaluated in a small double-blind placebo controlled trial *(28)*. Twenty patients with moderate to severe GMG with clinical deterioration despite optimal acetylcholinesterase inhibitor therapy were randomized to receive either IVMP (2 g/day for 2 days) or placebo. Apart from two patients in the IVMP group who were taking azathioprine at the time, none of the other patients were receiving any other form of immunosuppressive therapy. A beneficial response to treatment was found in 1 of the 9 patients who received placebo and in 8 of 10 patients treated with IVMP. The duration of clinical response varied from 4 to 14 weeks. In this study, the degree of initial deterioration after IVMP was not systemically evaluated, but one patient did report moderate worsening of myasthenic symptoms.

These studies show that although the degree and duration of response is variable, high-dose IVMP may be of benefit in a significant proportion of patients with worsening MG. The available data do not adequately inform on the frequency or severity of early deterioration.

3.6. How Effective is Azathioprine as a Steroid-Sparing or Adjunctive Agent?

In general, the response to steroids has varied between about 70% and 90%. In many of these studies, however, relapses have occurred with attempts to wean the steroid dose. The long-term toxicity associated with prolonged used of relatively high-dose steroids has led to a search for other treatment strategies.

The use of azathioprine in MG has been the subject of many retrospective uncontrolled studies as well as two prospective controlled studies. The Myasthenia Gravis Clinical Study Group *(29)* randomized patients with severe MG to receive prednisone or azathioprine. Because of the anticipated delayed response to azathioprine, these patients also received prednisone for the first 4 months. Accordingly, the authors felt that the primary outcome of the study should be a measure of long-term outcome which would not be influenced by the early short-term use of prednisone in the azathioprine group. The main endpoint was the time that elapsed prior to the first episode of meaningful clinical deterioration over the 5-year duration of the study. There were 20 patients in the prednisone group and 21 in the azathioprine group. In total, there were 21 events that met the endpoint criterion of a meaningful clinical deterioration, 12 of these occurring in the prednisone group and 9 in the azathioprine group. Although there was no significant difference between the two treatment groups with respect to the time to the first deterioration, the deterioration rate was estimated at 52% and 37% in the prednisone and azathioprine groups, respectively. There are, however, many reasons to be cautious in attributing too much significance to the apparent benefit of azathioprine over prednisone, and the conservative conclusion from this study is that long-term therapy with azathioprine alone is at least as effective as prednisone alone.

In a smaller study of only 10 patients, Bromberg et al. *(30)* randomized patients with MG previously untreated with immunosuppression to receive either prednisone or azathioprine. Two patients randomized to receive azathioprine were crossed-over to receive prednisone because of an idiosyncratic drug response to azathioprine. Only one of the remaining two patients responded to azathioprine. Four patients in the prednisone group responded well to treatment. The two patients who were crossed-over early also responded to prednisone, as did the two patients who failed to respond to azathioprine within the first year of treatment. The authors concluded that prednisone was of greater benefit than azathioprine as a single agent in the treatment of MG.

A related issue is whether the combination of prednisone and azathioprine offers even greater benefit than either treatment alone. The Myasthenia Gravis Study Group performed a randomized double-blind controlled trial comparing prednisolone (100 mg on alternate days) plus placebo to the combination of prednisolone and azathioprine (2.5 mg/kg/day) *(31)*. Patients with myasthenia in whom disabilities interfered with normal activities were eligible for inclusion, and those with restricted ocular disease or those who had received prior immunosuppressive therapy were excluded. The primary outcome measures were the maintenance dose of prednisolone, the number of treatment failures (i.e., failure to achieve remission defined as the absence of symptoms or symptoms that were sufficiently mild that they did not interfere with normal activities) and the duration of the initial remission. Patients were followed for 3 years. After allowance for deaths and withdrawals, there were 10 patients in the prednisolone group and 8 in the combination treatment group. Median prednisolone dose was significantly reduced at 36 months, the difference having first become apparent after 15 months of treatment. There were also significantly more treatment failures among the patients who received prednisolone alone. With respect to the third primary outcome measure, the duration of remission was significantly longer in the group who received prednisolone and azathioprine.

Although the sizes of these studies were limited, the results support the conclusion that the addition of azathioprine to a steroid regimen has the effect of reducing the dose of steroid required, reducing the number of relapses and prolonging the duration of clinical remissions. The efficacy of azathioprine relative to prednisone as a single agent remains unclear.

3.7. Is There a Role for Cyclosporine in the Treatment of MG?

Cyclosporine is an immunosuppressive agent that acts predominantly by inhibiting T-lymphocyte-dependent immune responses. Its efficacy in MG has been evaluated in two randomized double-blind placebo-controlled trials. In the first *(32)*, patients with recent onset moderate to severe GMG who had not undergone thymectomy or received other immunosuppressive therapy were eligible for inclusion if their symptoms were not controlled by anti-acetylcholinesterase medications. Twenty patients were randomized to receive either cyclosporine or placebo and were followed for a period of 12 months. Efficacy was assessed primarily by changes in strength (using a quantitative scoring system). At both 6 and 12 months, the cyclosporine-treated patients fared significantly better than the placebo group with respect to muscle strength score. This improvement was evident as early as 2 weeks after the start of therapy, and the mean time to maximal improvement in the cyclosporine group was 3.6 months. It should be noted, however, that only 4 of 10 patients completed the cyclosporine protocol, that 3 patients in the cyclosporine group received prednisone following a protocol violation or drug failure, and that 6 of 9 patients in the placebo group received some form of immunosuppressive therapy (prednisone, methotrexate, cyclosporine, or plasma exchange) following treatment failure or protocol violation. Significant side effects in the cyclosporine group included nephrotoxicity in 3 of 10 patients that required withdrawal from the study. Risk factors for nephrotoxicity included age over 50 years, preexisting hypertension, or baseline impairment of renal function. In summary, therefore, this study suggested a beneficial effect of cyclosporine, but the number of patients treated was small, the dropout rate was high, and nephrotoxicity was an important side effect.

The second study (33) included patients with generalized myasthenia irrespective of whether they were still receiving corticosteroids or had received azathioprine or undergone thymectomy in the past. Twenty patients were randomized to received cyclosporine and 19 to placebo. The proportion of patients who had received prior immunosuppressive therapy and the concurrent steroid doses were similar between the two groups. The dose of cyclosporine was also reduced from 6 mg/kg/day as a single daily dose in the prior study to 5 mg/kg/day in two divided doses. The primary measures of efficacy were the changes in strength (using a quantitative scoring system) and the percent reduction in steroid dose required. Based on the mean time to maximal benefit of 3.6 months in the prior study, the duration of this study was 6 months. Cyclosporine-treated patients demonstrated significantly greater increase in strength, but there was no difference in the percentage reduction in steroid dose at 6 months. Although not a prespecified endpoint, the percent reduction in steroid dose became more significant between 12 and 24 months. Overall, a sustained improvement was noted in 8 of 20 (40%) cyclosporine-treated patients and only 2 of 19 (11%) who received placebo. Using the lower dose in a divided schedule with trough levels of 300–500 ng/mL, there was no clinically significant nephrotoxicity within the first 6 months, although this subsequently developed in 10% of patients over 12–24 months of follow-up.

These studies demonstrate that cyclosporine is effective in the treatment of MG, and that a meaningful reduction in steroid dose may be achieved by 12 months. However, the utility of cyclosporine compared to azathioprine as steroid-sparing agent remains unclear. Concern has been raised about the potential long-term toxicity of both agents. Prolonged use of azathioprine may be associated with an increased risk of secondary malignancy, but this risk appears small. The risk of nephrotoxicity with prolonged use of cyclosporine appears to be clinically more significant.

3.8. What Is the Evidence for the Efficacy of Mycophenolate Mofetil in MG?

There have been a number of reports of uncontrolled studies of mycophenolate mofetil in MG (34–37) as well as single small randomized controlled trial (38). The randomized controlled trial included patients with chronic, stable myasthenia that had been unrespon-

Table 17.7
Efficacy of Mycophenolate Mofetil in Patients With Myasthenia Gravis

Study	Design	n	Outcome measure	Efficacy	Latency to effect
Ciafaloni (35)	Open-label	12	↓QMG (3 points) ↓MMT (2 point) 50% ↓ steroid dose	50% (QMG, MMT) 17% (steroid dose)	2 mo (improvement in ADLs)
Chaudhry (36)	Retrospective series	32	Improvement ≥1 grade functional status ↓steroid dose (10 mg QOD)	69%	5 mo (2–12)[a]
Meriggioli (37)	Retrospective series	85	MGFA postintervention status	73% (pharmacological remission, minimal manifestation or improved) 37% (↓ steroid dose by 50%) 21% (↓ steroid dose <50%)	Mean latency to initial improvement—8.8. wk (subjective), 10.8 wk (objective) Mean time to maximum improvement 26.7 wk (range 8–104)
Cos (34)	Retrospective series	22	Not specified	68%	Range 2–10 wk

QMG, quantitative Myasthenia Gravis score; MMT, manual muscle testing; ADL, activities of daily living; MGFA, Myasthenia Gravis Fundation of America.
[a]Includes three patients with chronic inflammatory demyelinating polyradiculoneuropathy and three with inflammatory myopathy, because data not reported separately for myasthenia gravis patients.

sive to treatment with prednisone and/or cyclosporine. Fourteen patients were randomized to receive either mycophenolate mofetil (1 g twice per day) or placebo for 5 months with the change in quantitative myasthenia gravis (QMG) score between baseline and follow-up used as the primary outcome measure. The two treatment groups were well balanced for relevant prognostic factors, but there was no power analysis to determine the sample size required to show a beneficial effect. Patients treated with mycophenolate mofetil improved more than patients receiving placebo, but these differences were not significant (attributed to the small study size) (38). The results of one open-label study (35) and three retrospective series (34,36,37) are summarized in Table 17.7. These data suggest that 67–73% of patients with chronic MG respond to treatment with mycopheno- late mofetil with most showing signs of improvement within 2–5 months of initiation of therapy.

3.9. Is There a Role for Plasma Exchange in the Treatment of MG?

As for many of the other treatments used in patients with MG, plasma exchange has become well established as a therapeutic option even though it has not been studied in large prospective controlled trials.

There has been only one randomized controlled trial, and this was published in the French literature (39). The study included 14 patients with either chronic myasthenia (n = 6) or who had presented in myasthenic crisis (n = 8). Patients were randomized to receive either prednisone alone (1 mg/kg/day for 1 month, followed by a slow taper) or the com-bination of prednisone and plasma exchange. Three exchanges were given over 10 days and then continued weekly if needed. There were no significant differences between the two groups at 1 month. Over 12 months of follow-up there were more frequent relapses amongst those patients randomized to receive plasma exchange. It is difficult to draw any firm conclusions from this study given its methodological limitations. As noted in a recent Cochrane systematic review the randomization methodology was not clearly described, there was no placebo in the control group, neither patients nor physicians were blinded to treatment assignment, there were substantive differences at baseline between the two groups and there was no discussion of sample size or the power of the study to detect a difference between the two treatment regimens (40).

In a nonrandomized but controlled trial, Kornfeld and colleagues described their experience with 12 patients who had severe myasthenia unresponsive to other forms of immuno-suppressive therapy (41). Six patients were assigned to the placebo group and six to receive plasma exchange. None of the controls, but all of the plasmapheresed patients responded. Five of the control patients subsequently underwent plasmapheresis, with a good clinical response observed in three. The overall response rate to plasmapher-esis, therefore, was 75%, with clinical remission following plasma exchange typically lasting 3–13 weeks.

In a small randomized study, patients with severe generalized myasthenia unrespon-sive to other forms of therapy were randomized either to receive plasmapheresis (n = 9) or to the control group (n = 7) (41). For varying reasons, six of the control patients, however, were crossed-over to receive plasmapheresis. All of the nine patients initially randomized to plasmapheresis improved and three of the patients initially randomized to the control group also responded to plasmapheresis. The overall response rate, therefore, was 75%. The addition of azathioprine in those receiving plasmapheresis facilitated extension of the interval between exchanges to around 5 weeks. Those who did not also receive azathioprine required exchanges every 2 weeks.

There have also been a number of open studies in which plasma exchange was used in the treatment of MG. The methodological quality of these studies is limited not only by the lack of a control group, but also by the inclusion of heterogeneous patient populations. Some patients had chronic myasthenia refractory to other treatment, some had presented in myasthenic crisis, and others received plasma exchange as a prelude to thymectomy. The frequency with which prednisone and other immunosuppressive treatments were employed also varies greatly between the different studies. The results of these studies and some of their methodological features are summarized in Table 17.8.

The overall impression from the literature is that plasma exchange is of benefit to patients with MG even though this has not been established in high-quality randomized controlled trials. This conclusion is supported by a National Institutes of Health (NIH) consensus statement *(42)*. The precise role of plasma exchange, however, in specific clinical circumstances (chronic myasthenia that is refractory to other therapy, myasthenic crisis, and prethymectomy) is less well defined.

3.10. Is There a Role for Intravenous Immunoglobulin in the Treatment of MG?

There are three randomized controlled trials that have examined the efficacy of intravenous immunoglobulin (IVIg) in patients with MG *(43–45)*. Two of these studies compared IVIg with plasma exchange *(43,44)*, and one compared IVIg with placebo *(42)*. One study examined the efficacy of IVIg for patients presenting with acute exacerbations of myasthenic symptoms *(43)* and the other two examined the efficacy of IVIg in patients with chronic severe (but stable) MG *(44,45)*. Methodological aspects of these studies are summarized in Table 17.9.

Gajdos et al. *(43)* compared plasma exchange and IVIg in a prospective randomized trial. Eighty-seven patients with an exacerbation of MG were randomized to receive plasma exchange for 3 days (41 patients) or IVIg (46 patients), with the latter group randomized to receive IVIg for 3 or 5 days (23 patients each). The primary endpoint was the absolute variation of a myasthenia muscular score ranging from 0 (severe weakness) to 100 (normal) that included assessment of the strength of limb, trunk, and cranial nerve musculature between randomization and day 15. Improvements in the myasthenia muscular score were similar between the two treatment groups. Overall response rates were 66% in the 3-day plasma exchange group, 61% in the 3-day IVIg group, and 39% in the 5-day IVIg group. Median response time was estimated at 9 and 15 days in the plasma exchange and IVIg treatment groups, respectively. The lower incidence of side effects amongst the IVIg-treated patients as well as the absence of a real difference in outcome between the two treatment groups led the authors to suggest IVIg as a safe and effective alternative to plasma exchange.

Rønager et al. performed a randomized cross-over study comparing the clinical efficacy of plasmapheresis and IVIg in patients with stable moderate to severe GMG *(44)*. All patients had received immunosuppressive therapy with azathioprine and/or prednisone in the preceding months. Six patients were randomized to each treatment group and observed for 16 weeks with clinical evaluation performed using the QMG score. Patients who received plasma exchange were improved 1 week after initiation of therapy,

Table 17.8
Uncontrolled Studies of Plasma Exchange in the Treatment of Myasthenia Gravis (MG)

Study	Patient population	n	Plasma exchange	Steroids	Other immune suppressive therapy	Proportion responding	Response duration
Behan (56)	Chronic generalized MG, ocular MG	21	3 per wk for 2–3 wk	21	21	100%	9.9 mo (3–19 mo)
Dau (57)	Chronic generalized MG	60	Weekly for 9–33 exchanges	48	60	73%	≥2 mo in 41/44 responders
Perlo (58)	Poorly controlled MG, Myashenic crisis and preop. for thymectomy	17	3–5 exchanges over 1–2 wk	?	?	65%	?
Olarte (59)	Stable severe MG, recent acute exacerbations	21	2–10 exchanges over 2–14 d	13	12	81%	76 d (7–450 d)
Antozzi (60)	Chronic MG, myasthenic crisis	70	2 exchanges	?	?	70%	<1 mo (4%), 1–4 mo (33%), 4–8mo (35%)
Chiu (61)	Chronic MG, myasthenic crisis, preop. preparation	94	4–5 exchanges over 7–10 d	?	?	85%	?
TOTAL		316				78%	

Table 17.9
Randomized Controlled Trials of Intravenous Immunoglobulin (IVIg) in Myasthenia Gravis (MG)

Study	Study population	n	Treatment	Study quality	Outcome	Immunosuppressive therapy
Gajdos (43)	Acute exacerbation of MG	87	IVIg vs PE	No blinding of patients or physicians	Improvement at day 15	Minority treated with steroids or azathioprine
Ronager (44)	Severe, chronic, stable MG	12	IVIg vs PE	No patient blinding	Change in QMGS at weeks 1, 4, 8, and 16	All treated with steroids or azathioprine
Wolfe (45)	Severe, chronic, stable MG	15	IVIg vs placebo	Inadequate power (premature termination)	Change in QMGS between days 1–42	About half treated with steroids or other immuno-suppression

QMGS, quantitative myasthenia gravis score.

but IVIg-treated patients were not. At 4 weeks follow-up, comparable improvement was noted in both treatment groups. No differences were observed between baseline and 8–16 weeks of follow-up *(44)*.

Wolfe and colleagues reported their results with 15 patients randomized to receive either IVIg or placebo before the study was terminated prematurely (because of insufficient IVIg inventories) *(45)*. Using change in QMG score between day 1 and day 42 as the primary measure of efficacy, they found no significant difference between the two treatment groups. Although the study design was of high methodological quality, the premature termination of the study resulted in limited power to detect a significant clinical improvement *(45)*.

The interpretation of the results of these studies is difficult. The one study that compared IVIg with placebo was underpowered (because it was terminated prematurely), and so limited store can be placed on the conclusion that there was no significant benefit from IVIg. The other two studies compared the efficacy of IVIg with that of plasma exchange, one for acute exacerbation *(43)* and one for chronic severe (but stable) MG *(44)*. The one showed no difference between the two treatment modalities (although an improvement in both from baseline to two weeks following treatment) *(43)*. In the other, patients who received plasma exchange were improved 1 week after treatment, but those treated with IVIg were not *(44)*. No differences were observed at other time points. Notwithstanding the equivocal evidence from these randomized controlled trials, there is a fairly extensive uncontrolled literature that supports the use of IVIg in patients with MG.

The efficacy of plasma exchange and IVIg are summarized in Table 17.10.

3.11. What Is the Role of Thymectomy in Patients With Nonthymomatous MG?

Thymectomy is widely held to be part of the standard care for patients with MG even though this conclusion has not been established in clinical trials. The theoretical rationale for removal of the thymus rests on the recognition that the thymus plays a central role in the pathogenesis of MG as a site of specific auto-antibody production.

A recent evidence-based review by Gronseth and Barohn found that patients who had undergone thymectomy were more likely to achieve medication-free remission and to become asymptomatic or less symptomatic on medication than those who did not undergo thymectomy. They note, however, that this observation must be tempered by the recognition of important confounding differences in baseline characteristics of prognostic significance in all of the available studies. In view of the widespread acceptance of thymectomy their conclusion was remarkably conservative "We cannot determine from the available studies whether the observed association between thymectomy and improved MG outcome was a result of a thymectomy benefit or was merely a result of the multiple differences in baseline characteristics between the surgical and nonsurgical groups. Based on these findings, we conclude that the benefit of thymectomy in nonthymomatous autoimmune MG has not been established conclusively" *(46)*.

In the absence of evidence either way, Lanska *(47)* surveyed 56 neurologists with an interest and expertise in myasthenia. Most advocated thymectomy for patients with thymoma based on the potential for local invasion and the possibility of an improvement in myasthenic symptoms. The most controversy existed regarding patients with generalized myasthenia without evidence of a thymoma. Variables such as age of the patient, severity

Table 17.10
Comparison of the Efficacy of Intravenous Immunoglobulin and Plasma Exchange

	Plasma exchange	*Intravenous immunoglobulin*
Frequency of response	66% *(43)* to 84% *(62)*	52% *(43)*
Median latency to onset of response	9 d *(43)*	>15 d *(43)*
Duration of response	3–13 wk *(63)*	?

of the disease, response to medication, and duration of the disease were used to individualize treatment decisions.

Notwithstanding the absence of evidence regarding the fundamental question of whether thymectomy is beneficial, a number of other controversies surrounding thymectomy have emerged. Which surgical technique—trans-cervical or trans-sternal—is superior? What is the appropriate timing of thymectomy? Are there particular subgroups of patients with MG who are liable to derive greater benefit from thymectomy? Not surprisingly, there are no clear answers to these questions and, in the absence of a carefully designed controlled trial, therapeutic benefit will remain unproven and specific indications and contraindications for thymectomy will be based upon individual preference.

4. PROGNOSIS

4.1. What Is the Natural History of OMG?

The study by Oosterhuis *(48)* provides the most reliable information about the natural history of OMG, as this cohort of patients was essentially untreated. He defined OMG on the basis of symptoms that remained confined to the extra-ocular muscles for 3 months from symptom onset. There are other studies that report the frequency with which symptoms are initially restricted to the extra-ocular muscles as well as the proportion of patients who progress to develop GMG. However, treatment assignments are less clear in these studies, thus limiting the reliability with which they inform on the natural history of the disease. In the study by Grob et al. for example, clinical outcome measures were not stratified or discussed in terms of the different therapies applied *(49)*. And the study by Bever et al. does not report the proportion of patients in each group who were treated and whether any received immunosuppresive therapy *(50)*. The results of these three studies are summarized in Table 17.11.

The proportion of patients in whom the disease remains ocular over prolonged follow-up has varied from 31% *(48)* to 40% *(49,50)* in different studies. GMG, when it does occur, tends to develop within the first year. In one study, for example, the median time to generalization was less than 1 year, with only 9 of 53 patients who generalized doing so after 2 years *(50)*. Similarly, of the 248 patients in another study who developed GMG, the majority (58%) did so within 7 months of the diagnosis *(49)*.

In one Italian study that included 53 patients with OMG at presentation, 32 subsequently developed generalized disease *(51)*. The only significant difference between those who progressed and those who did not was the higher proportion of women among those who developed generalized disease.

Table 17.11
Prognosis of Ocular Myasthenia Gravis (OMG)

Study	Sample size	Ocular at onset	Remaining ocular	Develop GMG
Oosterhuis[a] (48)	73	35	11 (31%)	24 (69%)
Grob (49)	1036	414	166 (40%)	248 (60%)
Bever (50)	108	142	43 (40%)[b]	53 (49%)[b]

[a]The only true natural history study in that essentially none of the patients were treated.
[b]Does not add up to 100% because 11% of patients with initial OMG went into remission.
GMG, generalized myasthenia gravis.

In a summary, therefore, of patients with purely ocular disease at onset, approximately 60–70% will develop generalized disease, and the risk of doing so is greatest within the first year. Progression to generalized disease may be more likely in women than among men.

4.2. What Is the Prognosis for Patients With MG Who Are Treated With Immunosuppressive Therapy?

There are a number of studies that have addressed the question of the prognosis for MG treated with immunosuppressive therapy (51–55), four of which have emerged from Italy (51–54). One difficulty that arises in summarizing this literature is that there appears to be some overlap between the patients described in a number of these studies but without adequate description of the extent of this overlap. The Italian studies all represent a referral-based (hospital) population (51–54) whereas the Danish study is population-based (55). The Danish study was retrospective (55), whereas the most recent Italian study was prospective in design (54). The Italian studies reported outcome in terms of the proportion of patients attaining remission of disease, whereas the Danish study examined survival and mortality rates. Survival rates were 85%, 81%, 69%, and 63% at 3, 5, 10, and 20 years. In multivariate analysis, the only factor predicting increased survival was age less than 60 years (55).

Prognostic factors for remission that were identified in multivariate analysis in the two Italian studies are summarized in the Table 17.12. In both studies, younger age (less than 40 years) and a history of thymectomy were associated with a greater likelihood of attaining remission of disease. The pharmacological remission (asymptomatic with or without medication) rates were 5%, 24%, 33%, and 41% at 1, 3, 5, and 10 years. The completion remission (asymptomatic without medication) rates were 1%, 8%, 13%, and 21% at 1, 3, 5, and 10 years (53).

5. SUMMARY

- The sensitivity of elevated titers of anti-acetylcholine receptor antibodies and RNS is relatively low (less than 60%) for OMG, but much better for GMG (greater than 80%).
- The sensitivity of SFEMG is high (greater than 85%) for both OMG and GMG.
- The specificity of anti-acetylcholine receptor antibodies and SFEMG are excellent (in excess of 95%), that with RNS not quite as good (78%).
- Anti-MuSK antibodies may be present in patients with seronegative MG that is indistinguishable from seropositive GMG, as well as in patients with predominantly oculobulbar

Table 17.12
Prognosis for Remission in Patients With Myasthenia Gravis

Population	n	Mean follow-up	Asymptomatic at follow-up	Favorable prognostic factors			Reference
				Variable	Odds ratio	95% CI	
Rome, Milan, Pavia (1973–1987)	844	5.3 yr	35%	Age less than 40	1.87	1.19–2.93	Beghi (53)
				Disease duration at diagnosis <1 yr	2.51	1.44–4.38	
				Mild disease at time of diagnosis	2.37	1.53–3.67	
				Thymectomy (yes)	1.64	0.93–2.89	
Milan (1981–2001)	756	4.7 yr	53.8%	Age less than 40	2.32	1.47–3.65	Mantegazza (54)
				Thymectomy (yes)	1.63	1.08–2.45	

CI, confidence interval.

333

symptoms and those with weakness of neck extension, shoulders, and respiratory muscles; anti-MuSK antibodies are uncommon in those with exclusively ocular disease.

- Controversy persists as to whether treatment of OMG with steroids reduces the likelihood of progression to GMG, with the available data (albeit of limited quality) suggesting some benefit.
- Steroids, azathioprine, cyclosporine, mycophenolate mofetil, plasmapheresis, IVIg, and thymectomy have each become accepted therapies, notwithstanding the relative lack of data from prospective controlled trials.
- The response rate to corticosteroids (with remission or improvement) varies from 70 to 94%.
- The response rate to plasmapheresis in patients who have failed to respond to other forms of immunosuppressive therapy has varied from 66 to 84%.
- IVIg may be as effective as plasmapheresis, although the effects may take slightly longer to become apparent.
- Azathioprine is an effective adjunctive therapy, facilitating either a reduction in the dose of corticosteroid required or an increase in the interval between plasma exchanges.
- Cyclosporine is probably as effective as azathioprine, but long-term therapy is associated with a significant risk of nephrotoxicity.
- The benefits of thymectomy remain unproven. In particular, there are very few controlled data to guide decisions about the timing of thymectomy or whether to employ the trans-cervical or trans-sternal approach.
- Among patients with OMG, approximately 60–70% will progress to develop generalized disease; this will typically occur within the first year.
- The prognosis for survival with GMG is relatively good (81% at 5 years), with the prognosis for pharmacological remission being 33% at 5 years.
- Age less than 40 and a history of thymectomy are the two factors that predict a better prognosis.

REFERENCES

1. Padua L, Stalberg E, LoMonaco M, Evoli A, Batocchi A, Tonali P. SFEMG in ocular myasthenia gravis diagnosis. Clin Neurophysiol 2000;111:1203–1207.
2. Lefvert A, Bergstrom K, Matell G, Osterman P, Pirskanen R. Determination of acetylcholine receptor antibody in myasthenia gravis: clinical usefulness and pathogenetic implications. J Neurol Neurosurg Psychiatry 1978;41:394–403.
3. Oey PL, Wieneke GH, Hoogenraad TU, van Huffelen AC. Ocular myasthenia gravis: the diagnostic yield of repetitive nerve stimulation and stimulated single fiber EMG of orbicularis oculi muscle and infrared reflection oculography. Muscle Nerve 1993;16:142–149.
4. Limburg P, The T, Hummel-Tappel E, Oosterhuis H. Anti-acetylcholine receptor antibodies in myasthenia gravis. Part 1: relation to clinical parameters in 250 patients. J Neurol Sci 1983;58:357–370.
5. Rouseev R, Ashby P, Basinski A, Sharpe J. Single fiber EMG in the frontalis muscle in ocular myasthenia: specificity and sensitivity. Muscle Nerve 1992;15:399–403.
6. Milone M, Monaco M, Evoli A, Servidei S, Tonali P. Ocular myasthenia: diagnostic value of single fiber EMG in the orbicularis oculi muscle. J Neurol Neurosurg Psychiatry 1993;56:720–721.
7. Howard FM, Lennon VA, Finley J, Matsumoto J, Elveback LR. Clinical correlations of antibodies that bind, block or modulate human acetylcholine receptors in myasthenia gravis. Ann NY Acad Sci 1987;505:526–538.
8. Ozdemir C, Young RR. The results to be expected from electrical testing in the diagnosis of myasthenia gravis. Ann NY Acad Sci 1976;274:203–222.
9. Mercelis R. Abnormal single-fiber electromyography in patients not having myasthenia. Risk for diagnostic confusion. Ann NY Acad Sci 2003;998:509–511.

10. Hoch W, McConville J, Helms S, Newsom-Davis J, Melms A, Vincent A. Auto-antibodies to the receptor tyrosine kinase MuSK in patients with myasthenia gravis without acetylcholine receptor antibodies. Nat Med 2001;7:365–368.

11. Scuderi F, Marino M, Colonna L, et al. Anti-P110 autoantibodies identify a subtype of "seronegative" myasthenia gravis with prominent oculobulbar symptoms. Lab Invest 2002;82:1139–1146.

12. Sanders D, El-Salem K, Massey J, McConville J, Vincent A. Clinical aspects of MuSK antibody positive seronegative MG. Neurology 2003;60:1978–1980.

13. Papapetropoulos TH, Ellul J, Tsibri E. Development of generalized myasthenia gravis in patients with ocular myasthenia gravis. Arch Neurol 2003;60:1491–1492.

14. Mee J, Paine M, Byrne E, King J, Reardon K, O'Day J. Immunotherapy of ocular myasthenia gravis reduces conversion to generalized myasthenia gravis. J Neuroophthalmol 2003;23:251–255.

15. Kupersmith MJ, Latkany R, Homel P. Development of generalized disease at 2 years in patients with ocular myasthenia gravis. Arch Neurol 2003;60:243–248.

16. Monsul NT, Patwa HS, Knorr AM, Lesser RL, Goldstein JM. The effect of prednisone on the progression from ocular to generalized myasthenia gravis. J Neurol Sci 2004;217:131–133.

17. Sommer N, Sigg B, Melms A, Weller M, Schepelmann K, Herzau V, Dichgans J. Ocular myasthenia gravis: response to long-term immunosuppressive treatment. J Neurol Neurosurg Psychiatry 1997;62:156–162.

18. Agius MA. Treatment of ocular myasthenia with corticosteroids: yes. Arch Neurol 2000;57(5):750–751.

19. Kaminski HJ, Daroff RB. Treatment of ocular myasthenia: steroids only when compelled. Arch Neurol 2000;57(5):752–753.

20. Hachinski V. Treatment of ocular myasthenia. Arch Neurol 2000;57(5):753.

21. Howard F, Duane D, Lambert, EH, Daube J. Alternate-day prednisone: preliminary report of a double-blind controlled study. Ann NY Acad Sci 1976;274:596–607.

22. Sghirlanzoni A, Peluchetti D, Mantegazza R, Fiacchino F, Cornelio F. Myasthenia gravis: prolonged treatment with steroids. Neurology 1984;34:170–174.

23. Pascuzzi R, Coslett H, John TR. Long-term corticosteroid treatment of myasthenia gravis: report of 116 patients. Ann Neurol 1984;15:291–298.

24. Evoli A, Batocchi A, Palmisani M, Lon Monaco M, Tonali P. Long-term results of corticosteroid therapy in patients with myasthenia gravis. Eur Neurol 1992;32:37–43.

25. Evoli A, Tonali P, Bartoccioni E, Lo Monaco M. Ocuar myasthenia: diagnostic and therapeutic problems. Acta Neurol Scand 1988;77:31–35.

26. Seybold M, Drachman D. Gradually increasing doses of prednisone in myasthenia gravis. Reducing the hazards of treatment. N Engl J Med 1974;290:81–84.

27. Arsura E, Brunner N, Namba T, Grob D. High-dose intravenous methylprednisolone in myasthenia gravis. Arch Neurol 1985;42:1149–1153.

28. Lindberg C, Andersen O, Lefvert A. Treatment of myasthenia gravis with methylprednisolone pulse: a double-blind study. Acta Neurol Scand 1998;97:370–373.

29. A randomised clinical trial comparing prednisone and azathioprine in myasthenia gravis. Results of the second interim analysis. Myasthenia Gravis Clinical Study Group. J Neurol Neurosurg Psychiatry 1993;56:1157–1163.

30. Bromberg M, Wald J, Forshew D, Feldman E, Alberts J. Randomized trial of azathioprine or prednisone for initial immunosuppressive treatment of myasthenia gravis. J Neurol Sci 1997;150:59–62.

31. Palace J, Newsom-Davis J, Lecky B. A randomized double-blind trial of prednisolone alone or with azathioprine in myasthenia gravis. Myasthenia Gravis Study Group. Neurology 1998;50:1778–1783.

32. Tindall R, Rollins J, Phillips J, Greenlee R, Wells L, Belendiuk G. Preliminary results of a double-blind, randomized, placebo-controlled trial of cyclosporine in myasthenia gravis. N Engl J Med 1987;316:719–724.

33. Tindall R, Phillips J, Rollins J, Wells L, Hall K. A clinical therapeutic trial of cyclosporine in myasthenia gravis. Ann NY Acad Sci 1993;681:539–551.

34. Cos L, Mankodi AK, Tawil R, Thornton CA. Mycophenolate mofetil (MyM) is safe and well-tolerated in myasthenia gravis (MG). Neurology 2000;54:A137.

35. Ciafaloni E, Massey J, Tucker-Lipscomb B, Sanders D. Mycophenolate mofetil for myasthenia gravis: an open-label pilot study. Neurology 2001;56:97–99.

36. Chaudhry V, Cornblath D, Griffin J, O'Brien R, Drachman D. Mycophenolate mofetil: A safe and promising immunosuppressant in neuromuscular diseases. Neurology 2001;56:94–96.

37. Meriggioloi M, Ciafaloni E, Al-Hayk K, et al. Mycophenolate mofetil for myasthenia gravis. An analysis of efficacy, safety and tolerability. Neurology 2003;61:1438–1440.

38. Meriggioloi MN, Rowin J, Richman JG, Leurgans S. Mycophenolate mofetil for myasthenia gravis. A double-blind, placebo-controlled pilot study. Ann NY Acad Sci 2003; 998:494–499.

39. Gajdos P, Simon N, de Rohan-Chabot P, Raphael JC, Goulon M. [Long-term effects of plasma exchanges in myasthenia. Results of a randomized study]. Presse Med 1983;12:939–942.

40. Gajdos P, Chevret S, Toyka K. Plasma exchange for myasthenia gravis. Cochrane Database Syst Rev 2002;4:CD002275.

41. Kornfeld P, Ambinder E, Mittag T, et al. Plasmapheresis in refractory generalized myasthenia gravis. Arch Neurol 1981;38:478–481.

42. The utility of therapeutic plasmapheresis for neurological disorders. NIH Consensus Development. JAMA 1986; 256:1333–1337.

43. Gajdos P, Chevret S, Clair B, Tranchant C, Chastang C. Clinical trial of plasma exchange and high dose immunoglobulin in myasthenia gravis. Myasthenia Gravis Clinical Study Group. Ann Neurol 1997;41:789–796.

44. Ronager J, Ravnborg M, Hermansen I, Vorstrup S. Immunoglobulin treatment versus plasma exchange in patients with chronic moderate to severe myasthenia gravis. Artif Organs 2001;25:967–973.

45. Wolfe GI, Barohn RJ, Foster BM, et al. Randomized, controlled trial of intravenous immunogloublin in myasthenia gravis. Muscle Nerve 2002; 26:549–552.

46. Gronseth G, Baroh R. Practice parameter: thymectomy for autoimmune myasthenia gravis (an evidence-based review). Report of the Quality Standards Subcommittee of the American Academy of Neurology. Neurology 2000; 55:636–643.

47. Lanska D. Indications for thymectomy in myasthenia gravis. Neurology 1990;40:1828–1829.

48. Oosterhuis HJ. The natural course of myasthenia gravis: a long term follow-up study. J Neurol Neurosurg Psychiatry 1989;52:1121–1127.

49. Grob D, Brunner NG, Namba T. The natural course of myasthenia gravis and effect of therapeutic measures. Ann NY Acad Sci 1981;377:652–669.

50. Bever CT, Aquino AV, Penn AS, Lovelace RE, Rowland LP. Prognosis of ocular myasthenia. Ann Neurol 1983;14:516–519.

51. Cosi V, Romani A, Lombardi M, et al. Prognosis of myasthenia gravis: a retrospective study of 380 patients. J Neurol 1997;244:548–555.

52. Mantegazza R, Beghi E, Pareyson D, et al. A multicenter follow-up study of 1152 patients with myasthenia gravis in Italy. J Neurol 1990;237:339–344.

53. Beghi E, Antozzi C, Batocchi AP, et al. Prognosis of myasthenia gravis: a multicenter follow-up study of 844 patients. J Neurol Sci 1991; 106:213–220.

54. Mantegazza R, Baggi F, Antozzi C, et al. Myasthenia gravis (MG): epidemiological data and prognostic factors. Ann NY Acad Sci 2003;998:413–423.

55. Christensen P, Jensen T, Tsiropoulos I, et al. Mortality and survival in myasthenia gravis: a Danish population based study. J Neurol Neurosurg Psychiatry 1998;64:78–83.

56. Behan P, Shakir R, Simpson J, Burnett A, Allan T, Haase G. Plasma-exchange combined with immunosuppressive therapy in myasthenia gravis. Lancet 1979;2:438–440.

57. Dau PC. Response to plasmapheresis and immunosuppressive drug therapy in sixty myasthenia gravis patients. Ann NY Acad Sci 1981;377:700–708.

58. Perlo V, Shahani B, Huggins C, Hunt J, Kosinski K, Potts F. Effect of plasmapheresis in myasthenia gravis. Ann NY Acad Sci 1981;377:709–724.

59. Olarte MR, Schoenfeldt RS, Penn AS, Lovelace RE, Rowland LP. Effect of plasmapheresis in myasthenia gravis 1978–1980. Ann NY Acad Sci 1981;377:725–728.

60. Antozzi C, Gemma M, Regi B, et al. A short plasma exchange protocol is effective in severe myasthenia gravis. J Neurol 1991;238:103–107.

61. Chiu HC, Chen WH, Yeh JH. The six year experience of plasmapheresis in patients with myasthenia gravis. Ther Apher 2000;4:291–295.

62. Yeh J, Chiu H. Double filtration plasmapheresis in myasthenia gravis - analysis of clinical efficacy and prognostic parameters. Acta Neurol Scand 1999;100:305–309.

63. Kornfeld P, Ambinder E, Papatestas A, Bender A, Genkins G. Plasmapheresis in myasthenia gravis: controlled study. Lancet 1979;2:629.

18 Lambert-Eaton Myasthenic Syndrome

1. INTRODUCTION

The Lambert-Eaton myasthenic syndrome (LEMS) is a rare autoimmune presynaptic disorder of neuromuscular transmission in which antibodies are directed against the voltage-gated calcium channel. The classic clinical features include proximal muscle weakness, depressed deep tendon reflexes, and prominent symptoms of autonomic dysfunction. The hallmark electrophysiological finding is a reduction in the size of the compound muscle action potential with facilitation (i.e., increased in amplitude) following brief sustained muscle contraction. In many patients, LEMS may occur in association with an underlying malignancy as a paraneoplastic disorder. How frequently are these clinical and electrophysiological features encountered in patients with LEMS? How specific is the finding of compound muscle action potential facilitation for the diagnosis? Is the presence of antibodies against voltage-gated calcium channels specific for LEMS? Should patients with LEMS be treated with immunosuppressive therapy notwithstanding the frequency with which underlying malignancies are detected? What is the long-term prognosis of LEMS, and does the presence of LEMS affect the prognosis for patients with small cell lung carcinoma? These and other questions are the subject of this chapter.

2. DIAGNOSIS

2.1. What Are the Typical Clinical Features of LEMS?

The clinical features of LEMS have been described in a number of large series of patients (1,2) as well as in a retrospective literature-based review of published cases of LEMS (3). Such case series permit determination of the sensitivity of various symptoms and signs for the diagnosis of LEMS. Apart from one series that compared the distribution of muscle weakness in patients with LEMS and patients with myasthenia gravis, there are no published data on the specificity of these clinical features. The frequencies with which various symptoms and signs are encountered in LEMS are summarized in Tables 18.1A and 18.1B. Weakness is the most common symptom and sign, occurring most often in the legs and typically more prominent proximally (1,2). Distal weakness, involvement of neck flexors or extensors and respiratory muscle involvement may occur, but are unusual (1,3). There is some controversy surrounding the frequency with which oculobulbar symptoms occur. The larger series indicate a prevalence of 20–50% (1,3). Smaller studies have suggested that oculobulbar symptoms and signs occur in as many as 78% of patients, and that they may represent the chief complaint in as many as 30% of patients with LEMS (4). Others have argued that oculobulbar symptoms and signs occur extremely rarely in

From: *Neuromuscular Disease: Evidence and Analysis in Clinical Neurology*
By: M. Benatar © Humana Press Inc., Totowa, NJ

Table 18.1A
Symptoms of Lambert-Eaton Myasthenic Syndrome

Symptom	O'Neill (1) (n = 50)	Wirtz (5)[a] (n = 227)	Nakao (10) (n = 110)	O'Suilleabhain (6) (n = 30)
Muscle weakness	50 (100%)	219 (96%)	–	29 (97%)
Leg weakness	50 (100%)	198 (87%)	–	–
Arm weakness	39 (78%)	126 (55%)	–	–
Fatigability	32 (64%)	75 (33%)	–	–
Autonomic Symptoms	40 (80%)	111 (49%)	–	25 (83%)
Dry mouth	37 (74%)	88 (39%)	34 (31%)	23 (77%)
Sexual dysfunction	13 (26%)	16 (12%)	4 (4%)	6 (20%)
Cranial nerve symptoms	35 (70%)	116 (51%)	–	–
Double vision	25 (50%)	48 (21%)	–	–
Drooping eyelids	21 (42%)	48 (21%)	–	–
Slurred speech	12 (24%)	44 (19%)	–	–
Difficulty swallowing	12 (24%)	54 (24%)	–	–

[a]Data includes the study by O'Neill and colleagues (1).

Table 18.1B
Signs of Lambert-Eaton Myasthenic Syndrome

Signs	O'Neill (1) (n = 50)	Wirtz[a] (5) (n = 227)	Nakao (10) (n = 110)
Muscle weakness	46 (92%)	–	–
Leg weakness	45 (90%)	200 (88%)	107 (97%)
Proximal	45 (90%)	186 (82%)	–
Distal	7 (14%)	60 (26%)	–
Arm weakness	41 (82%)	165 (73%)	88 (80%)
Proximal	41 (82%)	146 (66%)	–
Distal	15 (30%)	47 (21%)	–
Muscle wasting	4 (8%)	33 (14%)	–
Neck weakness	17 (34%)	27 (12%)	–
Respiratory muscle weakness	3 (6%)	13 (6%)	6 (5%)
Cranial nerve signs	31 (62%)	202 (89%)	–
Ptosis	27 (54%)	69 (30%)	31 (28%)
Jaw weakness	2 (4%)	–	–
Facial weakness	8 (16%)	29 (13%)	–
Palatal weakness	4 (8%)	–	–
Tendon Reflexes			
Decreased or absent	46 (92%)	202 (89%)	94 (85%)
Normal	4 (8%)	10 (4%)	–
Posttetanic facilitation	39 (78%)	59 (26%)	–

[a]Data includes the study by O'Neill and colleagues (1).

isolation either at presentation or at the time of maximal disease severity and that the presence of such symptoms or signs is far more suggestive of myasthenia gravis (5). The data from these studies may conflict less than they appear to in that they address different questions - some reporting the mere presence of oculobulbar symptoms and signs and others examining the frequency with which such symptoms and signs occur in the absence of other clinical features of LEMS. Autonomic symptoms are common, reported by 50–80% of patients, with dry mouth being most common (1,3,6).

2.2. What Is the Accuracy of the Voltage-Gated Calcium Channel Antibody Test for the Diagnosis of LEMS?

Patients with LEMS may harbor antibodies against both N and P/Q-type voltage-gated calcium channels, but it is antibodies against the latter which occur with the highest frequency and greatest specificity. The antibody assay involves labeling with radioactive iodine the ω-conotoxin-MVIIC toxin which binds to P/Q-type voltage-gated calcium channels. Labeled channels are mixed with patient serum and then immunoprecipitated by antibodies directed against immunoglobulin. The sensitivity and specificity of this assay have been examined by a number of investigators (7–11) and the results are summarized in Table 18.2. Overall the sensitivity is extremely high, ranging from 82% to 100% (7–11). The specificity varies, depending on the "control" group. For healthy controls, patients with cancer (small cell lung cancer or other cancers) and those with other neurological or autoimmune disorders, the specificity is close to 100%. More variable specificity has been reported for patients with other paraneoplastic disorders of

Table 18.2A
Proportion of Patients With Elevated Titers of Anti-P/Q-Type Voltage-Gated Calcium Channel Antibodies

	LEMS	Cancer	PEM/SN	PCD	ALS	OND	OAID	Healthy
Motomura (7)	56/66	0/10[a]	–	–	0/20	0/10	0/10	
Lennon (9)	62/65	14/90	40/70	0	22/78	5/41	0/28	2/47
Motomura (8)	66/72	0/14[a]	0	0	0	0/10	0/20	0/22
Voltz (11)	11/11	–	8/66	0/27	–	0/9	–	0/22
Nakao (10)	55/67	1/31[a]	–	1/20	0/40	0/92	0/43	0/50

LEMS, Lambert-Eaton myasthenic syndrome; PEM/SN, paraneoplastic encephalomyelitis/sensory neuronopathy; ALS, amyotrophic lateral sclerosis; OND, other neurological diseases; OAID, other autoimmune disorders; PCD, paraneoplastic cerebellar degeneration.

Table 18.2B
Diagnostic Accuracy of Anti-P/Q-type Voltage-Gated Calcium Channel Antibody Assay

	Sensitivity					Specificity		
		Cancer	PEM/SN	PCD	ALS	OND	OAID	Healthy
Motomura (7)	85%	100%[a]	–	–	–	100%	100%	100%
Lennon (9)	95%	85%	43%	–	72%	76%	100%	96%
Motomura (8)	92%	100%[a]	–	–	–	100%	100%	100%
Voltz (11)	100%	–	94%	100%	–	100%	–	100%
Nakao (10)	82%	96.8%[a]	–	95%	100%	100%	100%	100%

[a]Small cell lung cancer.

PEM/SN, paraneoplastic encephalomyelitis/sensory neuronopathy; PCD, paraneoplastic cerebellar degeneration; ALS, amyotrophic lateral sclerosis; OND, other neurological diseases; OAID, other autoimmune disorders.

the central nervous system (ranging from 63% to 94%) and a single study reported relatively low specificity (72%) for amyotrophic lateral sclerosis (9).

2.3. How Useful Is Electrophysiological Testing for the Diagnosis of LEMS?

A number of electrophysiological abnormalities may be seen in patients with LEMS, including a reduced resting compound muscle action potential (CMAP) amplitude, a decrement in CMAP amplitude with slow (2–3 Hz) repetitive stimulation, and an increment in CMAP amplitude in response either to high (20 Hz)-frequency stimulation or to brief (10–15 s) periods of maximal voluntary contraction. It is at least theoretically possible that the sensitivity and specificity of these findings for the diagnosis of LEMS may vary depending on a number of factors, including the specific muscle examined, whether changes in CMAP amplitude or area are measured, and whether "tetanic" stimulation is administered by fast repetitive stimulation or maximal voluntary contraction. For the most part, there are limited data to answer these questions. In this section, we consider only those articles that provide information about both sensitivity and specificity.

2.3.1. What Are the Sensitivity and Specificity of Fast Repetive Nerve Stimulation for the diagnosis of LEMS?

There are two reasonably good-quality studies that shed light on the question of the sensitivity and specificity of fast repetitive nerve stimulation (RNS) for the diagnosis of LEMS (12,13).

In the first study Tim and Sanders examined 25 patients with LEMS, 18 with myasthenia gravis, and 22 healthy controls (12). Among healthy controls, the mean CMAP increment was 5.3%, and so they defined the normal range as 2.5 standard deviations above this (i.e., an increment of 24%). Only one healthy control showed an increment above this threshold (of approximately 26%). All but one of the 25 LEMS patients (96%) showed an increment greater than normal, with an increment of at least 100% present in 18 patients (72%). For differentiating LEMS patients from healthy controls, therefore, the threshold could reasonably be set at 25%, which would provide a sensitivity of 96% and a specificity of 96%. However, 28% of patients with myasthenia gravis also showed an increment above the normal range. The implication is that a threshold increment of 25% would have a specificity of only 72% for differentiating patients with myasthenia from those with LEMS. The maximum increment amongst the patients with myasthenia gravis was 92%, which exceeded the increment observed in three (12%) of the LEMS patients. If a threshold increment of 92% were used, then, based on the available data from this paper, it is possible to estimate the sensitivity and a specificity of RNS for the diagnosis of LEMS as 88% and 100%, respectively (12).

The more recent study by Oh and colleagues reported the results of fast RNS performed in over 500 consecutive patients over a period of 35 years (13). As found in the study by Tim and Sanders (12), the sensitivity and specificity of fast RNS varies depending on the degree of CMAP increment following fast RNS that is used as the threshold for differentiating normal from abnormal (Table 18.3). This point is illustrated by the summary receiver operating characteristic (ROC) curve (Figure 18.1), which shows that diagnostic accuracy (combination of sensitivity and specificity) is maximized when an increment of approximately 90% is used to differentiate patients with LEMS from all others (healthy controls and patients with myasthenia gravis). In an ROC plot, the ideal

Table 18.3

Accuracy of Fast Repetive Nerve Stimulation for the Diagnosis of Lambert-Eaton Myasthenic Syndrome

Percent increment	Sensitivity		Specificity	
	Oh (13)	Tim (12)	Healthy controls	MG
25%	–	96%	96%	72%
43%	97%	–	–	–
50%	94%	–	–	–
60%	94%	–	–	96%
75%	88%	–	–	–
80%	85%	–	–	–
92%	–	88%	–	–
100%	74%	–	100%	100%

MG, myasthenia gravis.

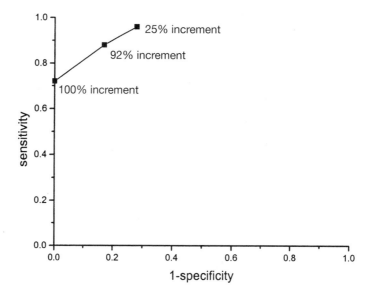

Fig. 18.1. Accuracy of fast repetitive nerve stimulation for the diagnosis of Lambert-Eaton myasthenic syndrome.

curve travels up the vertical axis on the left and then along the horizontal axis on top. Such a curve would be characterized by 100% sensitivity and 100% specificity. Curves that approximate this shape (i.e., that are located in the upper left-hand corner of the ROC plot) indicate that the diagnostic accuracy of a test is extremely good. Based these results, it should be clear that fast RNS is a very good test for diagnosing LEMS.

2.3.2. Does the Choice of Muscle Affect the Accuracy of Fast RNS for the Diagnosis of LEMS?

In an effort to address the question of whether the choice of muscle affects the accuracy of fast RNS, Tim and colleagues examined 73 patients with LEMS and performed fast

RNS in multiple muscles—abductor pollicis brevis (APB), abductor digiti minimi (ADM), extensor digitorum brevis (EDB), and trapezius *(14)*. They observed facilitation (CMAP increment) of at least 100% in similar proportions in the three distal muscles— 62%, 77%, and 59% in APB, ADM, and EDB, respectively. Facilitation was only present in 19% of patients when RNS was performed on the trapezius muscle. Furthermore, facilitation was present in all three muscles in only 41% of patients and in at least two muscles in a further 20%. These findings suggest that the sensitivity of fast RNS for the diagnosis of LEMS is substantially better in distal muscles compared with proximal muscles, and that multiple muscles should be tested before concluding that the test is negative *(14)*.

2.3.3. Is the Diagnostic Accuracy of Fast RNS Affected by Other Technical Factors?

In their study of 25 LEMS patients, 18 patients with myasthenia gravis and 22 healthy controls, Tim and Sanders measured changes in both CMAP amplitude and area before and after 30s of maximal voluntary contraction and in response to 20 Hz RNS. They found that neither 20 Hz RNS (instead of maximal voluntary contraction) nor the use of area instead of amplitude to measure the increment had any impact on the diagnostic performance of RNS.

The available data, therefore, suggest that either amplitude or area may be used to evaluate for the presence of CMAP facilitation. Furthermore, measurement of the change in CMAP following brief maximal voluntary contraction is preferable to fast RNS in view of the discomfort associated with the latter and their equivalent diagnostic accuracy. Finally, an increment of approximately 90% offers the best combination of sensitivity and specificity for the diagnosis of LEMS, particularly when myasthenia gravis forms part of the differential diagnosis.

2.4. What Is the Accuracy of Single-Fiber Electromyography for the Diagnosis of LEMS?

The few reports of single-fiber electromyography (SFEMG) in patients with LEMS suggest a variable relationship between the degree of jitter and frequency of blocking on the one hand and the firing rate (for stimulated SFEMG) on the other *(15–18)*. There are, however, no published studies that provide data on the sensitivity and specificity of SFEMG for the diagnosis of LEMS.

3. TREATMENT

Patients with LEMS may be treated either symptomatically or with immunosuppressive therapy. A third and often complimentary approach is treatment of the underlying malignancy. Symptomatic therapy focuses on drugs such as 3,4-diaminopyridine (DAP)* that increase neurotransmitter release at the neuromuscular junction. DAP is a quaternary ammonium compound that delays closure of voltage-gated potassium channels. The result is prolonged depolarization of the nerve terminal and increased influx

---

*DAP does not yet have US Food and Drug Administration (FDA) approval, and presently is only available in the United States as an investigational drug.

of calcium into the presynaptic terminal resulting in enhanced release of acetylcholine. Immunosuppressive therapy may comprise intravenous immunoglobulin (IVIg), plasma exchange, steroids, or other immunomodulatory agents. Only DAP and IVIg, however, have been the subjects of prospective, randomized placebo-controlled trials.

3.1. What Is the Evidence for the Efficacy of DAP?

In the first of two trials of DAP, 12 patients with LEMS were randomized to receive either the maximal tolerated dose of DAP or placebo for 3 days in a cross-over design [19]. All patients were treated with active drug (i.e., DAP) for the first 8 days of the study, during which time maximal tolerated dose was determined. This run-in phase was followed by a 3-day treatment period in which subjects were randomly assigned to either DAP or placebo, followed by a further 3 days of the alternate therapy. Muscle strength was quantified using isometric testing and the Neurological Disability Scale (NDS)[†]. Other outcome measures included measurement of compound muscle action potential (CMAP) facilitation following exercise as well as quantitative autonomic function testing. The results are presented in terms of mean group changes in outcome measures with the data for individual patients not reported. Average NDS scores were significantly lower (indicating improved strength) among those treated with DAP compared with the placebo group. Improvements in isometric strength and electrophysiological measures (CMAP facilitation) were also noted during treatment with DAP compared to placebo [19].

The second, more recent trial of DAP [20] employed a parallel treatment design rather than the cross-over design of the earlier study [19]. This study included 36 patients with LEMS, 12 of whom were randomized to receive DAP and 14 of whom received placebo. The Quantitative Myasthenia Gravis (QMG)[§] score was used as the primary outcome measure with changes in CMAP amplitude used as a secondary measure of efficacy. After 6 days of study medication, median QMG increased by 0.25 points among those receiving placebo, but decreased by two points (i.e., improved strength) in the DAP group ($p = 0.01$). The QMG improved by at least two points in 7 of 12 patients receiving DAP, with a maximum change of 6.5 points. Although statistically significant, these changes reflect quite modest improvements in muscle strength. CMAP amplitudes were also increased amongst patients receiving DAP, but not in the placebo group ($p < 0.001$) [20].

These two studies (summarized in Table 18.4), therefore, both indicate that DAP produces a functional improvement in muscle strength, the basis for which is the concomitant improvement in CMAP amplitude, a physiological measure of neuromuscular transmission. The degree of functional improvement, however, appears to be relatively small.

3.2. What Is the Evidence for the Efficacy of IVIg?

The efficacy of IVIg in the treatment of LEMS has been examined in a single randomized controlled trial [21]. This was a double-blind, placebo-controlled, cross-over trial in

---

[†]The NDS is derived by testing 25 muscle groups in each arm and leg and assigning a score of 0–4 to each muscle group where 0 - no weakness, 1 - mild weakness, 2 - moderate weakness, 3 - severe weakness, and 4 - no movement.

[§]Scores on the QMG range from 0 to 39. The score is determined by assigning a numeric value from 0 (none) to 3 (severe weakness) to measures of extra-ocular, facial, phargyngeal, respiratory, and limb muscle strength. A final score of 0 indicates no weakness and a score of 39 indicates severe weakness.

Table 18.4
Randomized Controlled Trials in Lambert-Eaton Myasthenic Syndrome

	McEvoy (19)	*Sanders* (20)	*Bain* (21)
Active treatment	3, 4-DAP 20mg tid for 3 d	3, 4-DAP 20mg tid for 6 d	IVIg 1 g/kg d for 2 d
Sample size	12	26	10
No. with cancer	7	10	0
Study design	Cross-over	Parallel group	Cross-over
Outcome measures	NDS, myometric limb strength, CMAP amplitude, & autonomic function	QMG, CMAP amplitude	Myometric limb strength, respiratory & bulbar measures calcium channel antibody titers
Methodological problems	Inadequate patient & observer blinding Outcome criteria not clearly specified	–	It is difficult to discern the clinical relevance of the outcome measures

DAP, 3, 4-diaminopyridine; NDS, neurological disability score; CMAP, compound muscle action potential; QMG, Quantitative Myasthenia Gravis Score.

which IVIg was administered at a dose of 2 g/kg divided over 2 days and outcome measured after 8 weeks, just prior to cross-over to the alternate treatment. The study included 10 patients, although one subject did not complete the study because of a severe adverse reaction (meningitis) and was excluded from the analysis. The primary outcome measure was a change in limb muscle strength measured by myometry, but the results are presented in such a way that it is difficult to appreciate their clinical relevance. The strength of five muscles was measured with myometry at baseline and at various time points over the 8-week duration of the study. The myometry measurements were expressed as a percentage of the lower limits of normal and were analyzed using the area-under-the-curve approach. The results, as presented in the original manuscript, are shown in Table 18.5. Statistically significant improvement in strength measures was first observed at 2 weeks, was at its best at 2–4 weeks, and had begun to decline by 8 weeks. The authors describe these results as showing a statistically significant improvement in limb, respiratory, and bulbar muscle strength, but the clinical significance of these findings is not at all clear.

In summary, therefore, IVIg is generally regarded as being beneficial in patients with LEMS based on the results of this single randomized controlled trial (summarized in Table 18.4). However, the magnitude of the clinical response that may be anticipated is not clear.

3.3. Is there Any Evidence for the Efficacy of Prednisone, Azathioprine, or Plasma Exchange in Patients With LEMS?

None of these therapeutic modalities have been examined in randomized controlled trials. There is, however, some retrospective uncontrolled data suggesting that each might be beneficial. Newsom-Davis and Murray reported their experience treating nine LEMS patients with prednisone, azathioprine and plasma exchange (22). Eight of the nine patients were reported to show a short-term clinical response to a course of plasma

Table 18.5
Effects of Intravenous Immunoglobulin (IVIg) in Lambert-Eaton Myasthenic Syndrome

	Mean[a] ± SD	n	Median[a]	p value
Limb strength				
IVIg	118.2 ± 33.4	9	124.3	0.038
Placebo	101.8 ± 43.9		101.8	
Vital capacity				
IVIg	69.5 ±14.6	9	69.3	0.028
Placebo	46.8 ±15.3		67.0	

[a]Results are expressed as a percentage of the lower limit of normal (see text for details).

exchange (although the criteria for defining "response" are not specified). Of the six patients without an associated malignancy, three who were treated with prednisone and azathioprine developed almost complete remission of symptoms, and three (including two who were treated with alternate day prednisone only) responded but less completely. Of the three patients with an associated malignancy, two had responded initially to the combination of prednisone and azathioprine, but relapsed when the cancer presented and failed to respond to further immunosuppressive therapy.

There are, therefore, anectodal data suggesting that patients with LEMS respond to treatment with prednisone with or without azathioprine and that short-term benefit may be derived from plasma exchange. The real efficacy of these therapeutic measures, however, has not been demonstrated in randomized controlled trials.

3.4. How Effective is Treatment of the Underlying Malignancy With Regard to Symptoms of LEMS?

Data from retrospective studies suggest that remission of LEMS may be facilitated by treatment of the underlying neoplasm. Chalk and colleagues reported their experienced with 16 patients with LEMS and SCLC (23). Eleven of these patients received anti-neoplastic treatment (some combination of chemotherapy, radiotherapy, and surgery). There was complete and sustained remission of the cancer in four patients, in three of whom this was accompanied by sustained improvement in LEMS. Sustained improvement in LEMS was observed in four of six patients with temporary remission of the cancer. LEMS was temporarily improved in two further patients (one with sustained cancer remission and one with temporary remission of the cancer). The cancer did not respond to anti-neoplastic therapy in the last patient, but the LEMS did improve temporarily. In summary, therefore, among the 10 patients whose cancer responded (albeit temporarily in some) to anti-neoplastic therapy, LEMS was improved in 8. It should be noted that all patients also received immunosuppressive therapy (prednisone, azathioprine, and/or plasma exchange), and so it is not entirely clear that the LEMS responded to treatment of the underlying cancer rather than to the immune suppressive therapy or to a synergistic effect of the two.

The presence of an underlying cancer obviously warrants treatment in its own right. Whether treatment of the underlying cancer without additional immunosuppressive therapy is sufficient, however, remains unclear.

4. PROGNOSIS

4.1. What Is the Long-Term Prognosis for LEMS Patients Without Cancer?

Maddison and colleagues reported their experience of 47 consecutive patients with LEMS without cancer who were seen in Oxford *(24)*. The median duration of follow-up was 10.5 years (range 2.3 to 36 years). Most patients (*n* = 44) had been treated with alternate-day prednisone (94%), which was combined with azathioprine in 37 cases (84%). Plasma exchange had been used in 26 of 44 patients (59%) in conjunction with other immunosuppressive therapy in order to induce a rapid clinical response.

At follow-up, 37 of the 44 patients who had received immunosuppressive therapy of some sort were still alive, and 31 (84%) of these still required prednisone with or without a steroid-sparing agent (azathioprine, methotrexate or cyclosporine). Two patients were taking DAP alone. Sustained clinical remission was achieved by 20 of 44 patients (45%), of whom all but four required ongoing immunosuppressive therapy. Survival analysis showed that most patients who achieved clinical remission did so within the first 3 years.

The overall impression from these data, therefore, is that most patients with LEMS require long-term immunosuppressive therapy (usually with some combination of alternate-day prednisone and a steroid-sparing agent) and that approximately one-half will achieve clinical remission. The vast majority of those who do go into remission will do so within the first 3 years of therapy, and maintenance of remission will usually require ongoing immunosuppressive therapy.

4.2. Does the Presence of LEMS Improve the Prognosis for Patients With Small Cell Lung Carcinoma?

In an effort to address this question, Maddison and colleagues compared the survival of 15 LEMS patients with small cell lung carcinoma (SCLC) with 81 patients with SCLC but not LEMS. Patients were matched on the variables sex, age at diagnosis of cancer, extent of the tumor and treatment received (chemotherapy or radiotherapy). Kaplan-Meier analysis showed a significantly shorter median survival time from diagnosis of SCLC amongst patients without LEMS (10 months vs 17.3 months, $p = 0.048$). It has been suggested that the improved survival of SCLC patients who also have LEMS may be due to the autoimmune response in LEMS that retards tumor growth. It is also possible that the diagnosis of LEMS (which typically precedes the diagnosis of the cancer) results in greater vigilance and hence earlier diagnosis of the cancer.

5. SUMMARY

- Weakness is the most common presenting symptom in patients with LEMS, but autonomic symptoms such as dry mouth are also present in approximately 50–80% of patients.
- The sensitivity of finding anti-P/Q type voltage-gated calcium channel antibodies in the serum is generally high, with estimates ranging from 82%–100%; the specificity of these antibodies is extremely good and approaches 100% in most series.
- The sensitivity and specificity of an incremental CMAP response following repetitive nerve stimulation (using an increment of greater than 92% as the threshold) are 88% and 100%, respectively; in general, the sensitivity of repetitive nerve stimulation is best in distal muscles.

- There are no published studies that inform on the sensitivity and specificity of SFEMG for the diagnosis of LEMS.
- There is data from two randomized controlled trials supporting the use of DAP in patients with LEMS.
- The efficacy of IVIg in the treatment of LEMS has been demonstrated in a single randomized controlled trial, but the magnitude of the clinical benefit that may be expected is not entirely clear.
- The efficacy of steroids, azathioprine, and plasma exchange have not been formally evaluated in randomized controlled trials, but uncontrolled retrospective data support their use.
- It remains unclear whether LEMS may be expected to improve following treatment of the underlying malignancy.
- Most patients with LEMS require long-term immunosuppressive therapy, and approximately one-half will achieve clinical remission.
- There is some suggestion that the prognosis for patients with small cell lung cancer may be improved by the presence of LEMS.

REFERENCES

1. O'Neill J, Murray N, Newsom-Davis J. The Lambert-Eaton myasthenic syndrome. Brain 1988; 111:577–596.
2. Nakao Y, Motomura M, Fukudome T, et al. Seronegative Lambert-Eaton myasthenic syndrome. Study of 110 Japanese patients. Neurology 2002;59:1773–1775.
3. Wirtz PW, Smallegange TM, Wintzen AR, Verschuuren JJ. Differences in clinical features between the Lambert-Eaton myasthenic syndrome with and without cancer: an analysis of 227 published cases. Clin Neurol Neurosurg 2002;104:359–363.
4. Burns TM, Russell JA, LaChance DH, Jones HR. Oculobulbar involvement is typical with Lambert-Eaton myasthenic syndrome. Ann Neurol 2003;53:270–273.
5. Wirtz P, Sotodeh M, Nijnuis M, et al. Difference in distribution of muscle weakness between myasthenia gravis and the Lambert-Eaton myasthenic syndrome. J Neurol Neurosurg Psychiatry 2002;73:766–768.
6. O'Suilleabhain P, Low PA, Lennon VA. Autonomic dysfunction in the Lambert-Eaton myasthenic syndrome. Serologic and clinical correlates. Neurology 1998;50:88–93.
7. Motomura M, Johnston I, Lang B, Vincent A, Newsom-Davis J. An improved diagnostic assay for Lambert-Eaton myasthenic syndrome. J Neurol Neurosurg Psychiatry 1995;58:85–87.
8. Motomura M, Lang B, Johnston I, Palace J, Vincent A, Newsom-Davis J. Incidence of serum anti-P/Q and anti-N-type calcium channel autoantibodies in the Lambert-Eaton myasthenic syndrome. J Neurolog Sci 1997;147:35–42.
9. Lennon VA, Kryzer TJ, Griesmann GE, et al. Calcium-channel antibodies in the Lambert-Eaton syndrome and other paraneoplastic syndromes. N Engl J Med 1995;332:1467–1474.
10. Nakao YK, Motomura M, Suenaga A, et al. Specificity of omega-conotoxin MVIIC-binding and – blocking calcium channel antibodies in Lambert-Eaton myasthenic syndrome. J Neurol 1999;246:38–44.
11. Voltz R, Carpentier AF, Rosenfeld MR, Posner JB, Dalmau J. P/Q-Type voltage gated calcium channel antibodies in paraneoplastic disorders of the central nervous system. Muscle Nerve 1999;22:119–122.
12. Tim RW, Sanders DB. Repetitive nerve stimulation studies in the Lambert-Eaton myasthenic syndrome. Muscle Nerve 1994;17:995–1001.
13. Oh SJ, Kurokawa K, Classen GC, Ryan HF. Electrophysiological diagnostic criteria of Lambert-Eaton myasthenic syndrome. Muscle Nerve 2005;32:515–520.
14. Tim RW, Massey JM, Sanders DB. Lambert-Eaton myasthenic syndrome: Electrodiagnostic findings and response to treatment. Neurology 2000;54:2176–2178.
15. Lambert EH, Rooke D. Myasthenic state and lung cancer. In: Brain W, Norris F, eds. The remote effects of cancer on the nervous system. Grune and Stratton, New York:1965;pp.67–79.

16. Trontelj J, Stalberg E. Single motor end-plates in myasthenia gravis and LEMS at different firing rates. Muscle Nerve 1991;14:226–232.

17. Sanders DB. The effect of firing rate on neuromuscular jitter in Lambert-Eaton myasthenic syndrome. Muscle Nerve 1992;15:256–258.

18. Trontelj JV, Stalberg E. The effect of firing rate on neuromuscular jitter in Lambert-Eaton myasthenic syndrome. A reply. Muscle Nerve 1992;15:258.

19. McEvoy K, Windebank AJ, Daube JR, Low PA. 3,4-Diaminopyridine in the treatment of Lambert-Eaton myasthenic syndrome. N Engl J Med 1989;321:1567–1571.

20. Sanders DB, Massey JM, Sanders LL, Edwards LJ. A randomized trial of 3,4-diaminopyridine in Lambert-Eaton myasthenic syndrome. Neurology 2000;54:603–607.

21. Bain P, Motomura M, Newsom-Davis J, et al. Effects of intravenous immunoglobulin on muscle weakness and calcium-channel autoantibodies in the Lambert-Eaton myasthenic syndrome. Neurology 1996; 47:678–683.

22. Newsom-Davis J, Murray NM. Plasma exchange and immunosuppressive drug treatment in the Lambert-Eaton myasthenic syndrome. Neurology 1984;34:480–485.

23. Chalk C, Murray N, Newsom-Davis J, O'Neill J, Spiro S. Response of the Lambert-Eaton myasthenic syndrome to treatment of associated small cell lung carcinoma. Neurology 1990;40:1552–1556.

24. Maddison P, Lang B, Mills K, Newsom-Davis J. Long term outcome in Lambert-Eaton myasthenic syndrome without lung cancer. J Neurol Neurosurg Psychiatry 2001;70:212–217.

V   MUSCLE DISEASE

19 Inflammatory Myopathy

1. INTRODUCTION

The idiopathic inflammatory myopathies include polymyositis (PM), dermatomyositis (DM), and sporadic inclusion body myositis (s-IBM). Although the clinical presentation of PM and DM may be very similar apart from the presence of a skin rash in the latter, it is important to note that DM is not simply "PM with a rash." Similarly, although there are histolopathological similarities between PM and s-IBM at the light-microscopic level, inclusion body myositis is not merely "PM that is unresponsive to steroids." PM, DM, and s-IBM are, in fact, three immunopathologically distinct entities. In PM, the immune attack is directed primarily at the muscle fiber. There is increased major histocompatibility (MHC)-I antigen expression on muscle fibers and there is cytotoxic (CD_8) T-cell mediated destruction of otherwise healthy muscle fibers. In DM, by contrast, the immune-attack is primarily directed against intra-muscular blood vessels, i.e., it is a microvascular angiopathy with muscle fiber destruction being a secondary phenomenon. The pathophysiology of s-IBM is less clear. Although it is typically characterized by an endomysial cytotoxic T-cell inflammatory infilatrate, as seen in PM, it is unclear whether the inflammatory infiltrate is the primary event. The presence of vacuoles containing a variety of proteins including amyloid and ubiquitin suggests a primary degenerative disorder of muscle.

The literature relating to the diagnosis, treatment, and prognosis of the idiopathic inflammatory myopathies, however, is difficult to read in part because the distinction between PM, DM, and s-IBM has not always been made as clearly as it should. For example, the Bohan and Peter criteria (*see* "Diagnosis") make no distinction between PM and s-IBM and many studies investigating the sensitivity of various diagnostic tests or reporting the treatment and prognosis of PM have relied upon these diagnostic criteria. For this reason, interpretation of the literature is particularly difficult.

2. DIAGNOSIS

2.1. What Are the Diagnostic Criteria for the Inflammatory Myopathies?

There is ongoing controversy regarding the appropriate diagnostic criteria for the inflammatory myopathies. In a paper published in 1975, Bohan and Peter offered a set of criteria (Table 19.1A) that have continued to be used until very recently despite their limitations (*1*). They suggested that PM be classified as "definite" if four criteria were present, "probable" with three criteria, and "possible" with two; whereas DM would be classified as "definite" with three or four criteria, "probable" with two, and "possible" with one; all cases of DM required the presence of the characteristic rash. A notable

From: *Neuromuscular Disease: Evidence and Analysis in Clinical Neurology*
By: M. Benatar © Humana Press Inc., Totowa, NJ

Table 19.1A
Bohan and Peter Diagnostic Criteria for Inflammatory Myopathy

1. Symmetrical proximal muscle weakness with or without dysphagia and respiratory muscle weakness
2. Elevation of the serum enzymes, especially the CPK, but also the transaminases, the LDH and the aldolase
3. The electromyographic triad of
   a. small amplitude, short-duration, polyphasic motor unit potentials
   b. fibrillations, positive sharp waves, increased insertional irritability, or
   c. spontaneous bizarre high frequency discharges
4. Muscle biopsy abnormalities of degeneration, regeneration, necrosis, phagocytosis, and an interstitial mononuclear infiltrate
5. The typical skin rash of dematomyositis

CPK, creatine phosphokinase; LDH, lactic dehydrogenase.

354

Table 19.1B
Proposed Diagnostic Criteria for the Inflammatory Myopathies

Criterion	Polymyositis		Dermatomyositis		Inclusion body myositis
	Definite	Probable	Definite	Probable	Definite
Muscle strength	Myapthic muscle weakness[a]	Myopathic muscle weakness[a]	Myopathic muscle weakness[a]	Apparently normal strength[b]	Myopathic muscle weakness with early involvement of distal muscles[a]
Electromyographic findings	Myopathic	Myopathic	Myopathic	Myopathic or nonspecific	Myopathic with mixed potentials
Creatine kinase	Increased (up to 50-fold)	Increased (up to 50-fold)	Normal or increased (up to 50-fold)	Normal or increased (up to 10-fold)	Normal or increased (up to 10-fold)
Muscle biopsy	Diagnostic for this type of inflammatory myopathy[c]	Nonspecific myopathy without signs of primary inflammation	Diagnostic[d]	Nonspecific or diagnostic	Diagnostic[e]
Rash or calcinosis	Absent	Absent	Present	Present	Absent

[a]Myopathic muscle weakness, affecting proximal muscles more than distal ones and sparing eye and facial muscles, is characterized by a subacute onset (weeks to months) and rapid progression in patients who have no family history of neuromuscular disease, no endocrinopathy, no exposure to myotoxic drugs or toxins, and no biochemical muscle disease (excluded on the basis of muscle-biopsy findings).

[b]Although strength is apparently normal, patients often report new onset of fatigue, myalgia, and reduced endurance. Careful muscle testing may reveal mild muscle weakness.

[c]Endomysial inflammatory infiltrate with scattered invasion of nonnecrotic muscle fibers that are not necessarily near areas of inflammation.

[d]Inflammatory infiltrate perivascular and perifascicular; endothelial hyperplasia with capillary obliteration of intramuscular blood vessels; necrotic, degeneration, and regenerating fibers are mostly in groups involving a portion of a muscle fasciculus and are often the result of micro-infarction; perifascicular atrophy.

[e]Endomysial inflammatory infiltrate with invasion of nonnecrotic muscle fibers; basophilic granular inclusions distributed around the edge of slit-like vacuoles (rimmed vacuoles), eosinophilic inclusions, and angulated fibers; cytoplasmic filamentous inclusions on electron microscopy.

Data from ref. 2.

355

feature of these criteria is that only skin features are used to differentiate DM from polymyositis PM. Furthermore, these criteria did not recognize the entity of s-IBM, which has since been characterized and included among the idiopathic inflammatory myopathies.

Dalakas has proposed alternative criteria *(2,3)* with the pathological findings on muscle biopsy being most important for the diagnosis (Table 19.1B). In both PM and s-IBM, there is primary endomysial inflammation. The term primary is used to indicate that lymphocytes (CD_8) invade histologically healthy (nonnecrotic) muscle fibers that express MHC-I antigens. In s-IBM, however, there are also slit-like vacuoles surrounded by basophilic granular inclusions, producing the so-called "rimmed vacuoles." Cytoplasmic eosinophilic inclusions and angulated fibers may also be seen. Cytoplasmic filamentous inclusions are visible on electron-microscopy. In DM, the inflammatory infiltrate is perivascular and perifascicular. There is endothelial hyperplasia with obliteration of intramuscular capillaries. Necrotic, degenerating, and regenerating fibers are found in groups involving a portion of a muscle fasciculus and are often the result of microinfarction. Perifascicular atrophy, the presence of layers of atrophic fibers at the periphery of a fascicle, is pathognomonic of DM, although not always present.

It is important to emphasize that these criteria have been proposed but never evaluated (either retrospectively or prospectively) to determine their sensitivity and specificity. These criteria have also been criticized *(4)* because they require specialized immunopathological testing for CD_8 staining and MHC-I expression, which are not widely available. Although these are indeed valid concerns, the criteria do at least represent a conceptual improvement over the Bohan and Peter criteria which clearly do lack specificity.

2.2. Is There a Distinctive Distribution of Muscle Weakness in PM, DM, and s-IBM That Permits their Clinical Differentiation?

In the early case series by Bohan and colleagues, proximal muscle weakness was regarded as the sine qua non for the diagnosis of PM. It was the presenting symptom in 105 of 153 (69%) patients and developed subsequently in all but two of the remaining patients *(5)*. Dysphagia was encountered in 12% of cases. DeVere and Bradley *(6)* noted proximal upper and lower limb weakness in 86% and 92% of their series of 118 patients. Distal upper and lower limb weakness was noted in one-third of patients. More specific details are not provided. It should be recalled, however, that s-IBM was not a recognized diagnostic entity at the time of these studies and so a peculiar pattern of weakness in a subset of patients with s-IBM would have been overlooked.

Textbooks commonly note that early involvement of forearm finger and wrist flexor muscles, as well as quadriceps femoris and tibialis anterior, is common in s-IBM, in contrast to the proximal shoulder and hip girdle weakness that is typically encountered in patients with PM and DM. What is the evidential basis for this claim?

A number of studies have suggested that the pattern of weakness in s-IBM is distinctive. In their retrospective review of 40 histopathologically confirmed cases of s-IBM, Lotz and colleagues *(7)* noted that the biceps, triceps, iliopsoas, quadriceps, and tibialis anterior muscles were the most severely affected, with deltoid, forearm, and intrinsic hand muscles affected to a lesser degree. Facial muscles were occasionally affected, and extra-ocular muscles were spared in every case. Overall, some distal weakness was detected in 50% of cases, but in only 35% was the weakness more prominent distally than proximally *(7)*. More prominent distal weakness was similarly noted in approximately 50% of patients in two other series *(8,9)*, but in a much smaller proportion of patients in yet another *(10)*. Phillips and colleagues similarly observed a propensity for involvement of quadriceps femoris (seen in 17 of their 18 cases) as well as the long finger extensors and the wrist flexors and extensors *(11)*. The authors commented, however, on the variability of the pattern of weakness between different patients. Asymmetry of muscle weakness is also said to be typical of s-IBM. This was noted in approximately one-half of the patients in one study *(11)*, but only about 30% in another *(10)*.

Dysphagia was present in 40% of the patients described in the series by Lotz and colleagues *(7)* at the time of diagnosis and was reported to be present in 30% of cases in Ringel's series *(10)*. Facial weakness may occur in two-third of patients *(10)*, and neck flexor weakness may be found in around 50% of patients *(11)*.

Amato and colleagues retrospectively reviewed the records of their patients with newly diagnosed inflammatory myopathy to determine whether patterns of weakness were helpful in distinguishing s-IBM from DM and PM *(12)*. Their study included 15 patients with s-IBM, 22 with PM, and 9 with DM, with all diagnoses being confirmed with muscle biopsy and typical histopathological findings. They found that the finger flexors, wrist flexors, ankle dorsiflexors, and quadriceps muscles were significantly weaker in patients with s-IBM than in patients with DM and PM *(12)*. Asymmetric weakness was also noted in s-IBM more frequently (12 of 15 patients) than in DM (0 of 9 patients) or PM (7 of 22 patients).

These data, therefore, suggest that the pattern of clinical weakness, in terms of the specific muscle groups affected as well as the symmetry of muscle weakness, is useful in the clinical differentiation of s-IBM from DM/PM.

2.3. How Useful Is Measurement of Serum Creatine Kinase in the Diagnosis of Inflammatory Myopathy?

There are no studies that have reported serum creatine kinase (CK) concentrations among all patients in whom the diagnosis of inflammatory myopathy was considered clinically. There have been a number of studies, however, in which pretreatment serum CK concentrations in patients with idiopathic inflammatory myopathy, have been reported. The data from these studies are summarized in Table 19.2, and are presented in terms of the number (percentage) of patients in each study in whom the serum CK concentration was normal, as well as the mean (± standard deviation) CK concentration. In most of these studies, the diagnosis of inflammatory myopathy was based on histopathological evidence. In the others, diagnosis was made on the basis of the Bohan and Peter criteria, which may variably have involved muscle biopsy. In large part because of the diagnostic criteria employed, these studies have not reliably distinguished PM/DM on the one hand from s-IBM on the other. Some studies have focused exclusively on s-IBM. It should be evident from Table 19.2 that these data are extremely heterogeneous. If the data from all of these studies are pooled (a dubious analysis in itself), the serum CK was found to be normal in 54 of the 316 (15%) patients, with (for the most part) biopsy proven inflammatory myopathy.

Based on these data, it is possible to only partially complete a 2×2 table.

	Inflammatory myopathy	No inflammatory myopathy	TOTAL
Increased CK	316	?	?
Normal CK	54	?	?
TOTAL	370	?	?

It is possible, therefore, to estimate the sensitivity of estimation of CK concentration for the diagnosis of inflammatory myopathy. Sensitivity describes the proportion of patients with the disease in question in whom a positive test result is found. (i.e., sensitivity = true positive/[true positive + false negative]). Based on the data in Table 19.2 (and summarized above), therefore, sensitivity = 316/370 = 85%. Although there are insufficient data to calculate the specificity of the test, an intuitive approximation can be made. Because there are many known causes of elevated serum CK concentration other than inflammatory myopathy, the specificity of this test is likely to be quite low.

Serum CK, therefore, performs reasonably well as a screening test in that it will be elevated in 85% of patients with inflammatory myopathy. Clearly, however, a normal serum CK does not exclude the diagnosis. Similarly, an elevated serum CK, although consistent with the diagnosis of inflammatory myoapthy, is not diagnostic and further investigations are required.

2.4. Does Serum CK Concentration Help to Differentiate s-IBM From DM/PM?

The data summarized in Table 19.2 also suggest that the serum CK concentration is lower in patients with s-IBM compared with those with PM/DM. One reason for being cautious in drawing this conclusion from the data is that the diagnosis of PM/DM in these series was frequently based on the Bohan and Peter criteria, which do not reliably distinguish between PM and s-IBM. The study by Amato et al., however, lends support to the notion that serum CK tends to be lower in patients with s-IBM *(12)*. In this retrospective review, which included 15 patients with s-IBM, 22 with PM, and 9 with DM, they found mean (±SD) CK concentrations to be 5758 (±6929) for DM, 5097 (±7706) for PM, and 698 (±430) for s-IBM. The available data, therefore, suggest that serum CK tends to be lower in patients with s-IBM. Whether serum CK is more often normal in this group of patients is not clear from the available data.

2.5. Which Muscles Should be Examined During Electromyography to Offer the Highest Diagnostic Yield?

There are relatively few studies that provide adequate data to answer this question *(13, 14)*. Needle electromyographic examination in patients with inflammatory myopathy may show "myopathic" features, characterized by the early recruitment of short-duration polyphasic motor unit action potentials (MUAPs) and/or fibrillation potentials (and positive sharp waves).

Streib and colleagues *(13)* retrospectively reviewed their experience with 40 patients diagnosed with inflammatory myopathy on the basis of the Bohan and Peter criteria. At

Table 19.2
Serum Creatine Kinase (CK) Concentrations in Patients With Inflammatory Myopathy

Myopathy	Basis for Dx	No. (%) with normal CK	Sample size	Mean (±SD)	Reference
DM, PM, & s-IBM	B&P criteria	7 (4.6%)	153	Insufficient data	5
PM & s-IBM	B&P criteria	21 (36%)	58	Insufficient data	6
DM, PM, & s-IBM	Histopathology	4 (33%)[a]	12	2039 ± 4767	15
PM, DM	Histopathology	3 (11%)	28	Insufficient data	59
s-IBM	Histopathology	8 (20%)	40	Insufficient data	7
s-IBM	Histopathology	2 (25%)[a]	8	385 ± 275	41
s-IBM	Histopathology	3 (50%)	6	Insufficient data	8
s-IBM	Histopathology	0[b]	7	374 ± 245	9
PM	Histopathology	2 (12.5%)[a]	16	1637 ± 1587	21
s-IBM	Histopathology	1 (6%)	17	553 ± 250	11
DM, PM, & s-IBM	B&P criteria	2 (10%)[c]	20	1178 ± 1320	34
DM, PM, & s-IBM	B&P criteria	0	11	1587 ± 1789	32
DM, PM, & s-IBM	B&P criteria	2 (18%)	11	1932 ± 1740	30

Dx, diagnosis; B&P, Bohan and Peter criteria; DM, dermatomyosis; PM, polymyositis; s-IBM, sporadic inclusion body myositis.

[a]Normal CK not defined by authors. A value of <200 IU was defined as normal for the purposes of this analysis.

[b]Serum CK was less than twice normal in 3 of these 7 cases.

[c]Serum CK was less than twice normal in 2 additional patients.

359

Table 19.3A
Distribution of Fibrillation Potentials in Upper Limb Muscles in Inflammatory Myopathy

Muscle examined	No. of muscles examined	No. of muscles with fibrillation potentials
Paraspinal	40	37 (93%)
Infraspinatus	36	27 (75%)
Deltoid	36	26 (72%)
Biceps	38	29 (76%)
Triceps	24	16 (67%)
Brachioradialis	33	26 (79%)
First dorsal interosseous	34	16 (47%)

Data from ref. *13*.

Table 19.3B
Distribution of Fibrillation Potentials in Lower Limb Muscles in Inflammatory Myopathy

Muscle examined	No. of muscles examined	No. of muscles with fibrillation potentials
Paraspinal	40	37 (93%)
Gluteus	30	22 (73%)
Iliacus	33	25 (76%)
Vastus lateralis	39	25 (64%)
Gastrocnemius	24	13 (54%)
Tibialis anterior	40	28 (70%)

Data from ref. *13*.

least eight limb muscles as well as the paraspinal muscles were examined in each patient. In this study, fibrillation potentials were identified in all muscles examined in 35% of patients, in more than one-half of the muscles examined in further 35%, in less than one-half of the muscles examined in 20%, and in only one to two muscles in 10%. These authors also provided a breakdown of the specific muscle distribution of fibrillation potentials (Tables 19.3A and 19.3B). These data show that fibrillation potentials are most often identified (93% of patients) in the paraspinal muscles and more frequently in other proximal rather than in distal muscles. Other estimates of the frequency with which fibrillation potentials are identified in parapsinal muscles are not quite as high. Bohan et al. *(5)*, for example, noted them in only 90 of 122 (74%) patients.

Fredericks reported his experience with needle electromyographic examination in 53 patients with PM or DM *(14)*. The data for myopathic MUAPs and fibrillation potentials were not reported separately (summarized in Table 19.4).

The predominant involvement of paraspinal muscles in the inflammatory myopathies raises the question of how frequently the abnormal findings on needle electromyography are confined to this muscle group. Data from a number of studies indicate that this does occur but in a minority of cases, with estimates ranging from a low of 1.6% *(5)* to a high of 8% *(15)* to 37.5% *(16)*. The latter estimates may be inaccurate, as they are based on the study of a small number of patients (*n* = 8 *[15]* and *n* = 12 *[16]*). The lower estimate

Table 19.4
Distribution of Fibrillations and Myopathic MUAPs in Inflammatory Myopathy

Muscle examined	No. of muscles examined	No. of muscles with fibrillations or myopathic MUAPs
Parapsinal	45	41 (91%)
Iliopsoas	48	42 (86%)
Deltoid	53	44 (83%)
Biceps brachii	50	33 (66%)
Infraspinatus	47	30 (64%)
Latissimus dorsi	42	27 (64%)
Glueus medius	44	24 (55%)
Triceps	48	20 (42%)
Rectus femoris	42	16 (38%)
Tibialis anterior	50	15 (30%)
Vastus medialis	41	8 (20%)
First dorsal interosseous	43	3 (7%)

Data from ref. *14*.
MUAP, motor unit action potential.

may be more reliable, as it is based on a larger sample size ($n = 122$) and is in closer agreement with the estimate of 2.5% *(13)* from an intermediately sized sample ($n = 40$).

Overall, therefore, the paraspinal muscles are the most important muscle group to examine, in part because they offer the highest diagnostic yield and, in part because they may occasionally be the only muscles affected. Outside of the paraspinal muscles, it is important also to examine other proximal muscles. How many muscles should be sampled, remains an unanswered question, but in the studies cited here *(13,14)* that demonstrate the importance of paraspinal muscle examination, at least 6-8 muscles were examined.

2.6. What Are the Characteristic Histopathological Changes Seen in PM, DM, and s-IBM?

In DM, the immune attack is primarily directed against the intra-muscular capillaries. The inflammatory infiltrate is predominantly perivascular and perimysial and is composed predominantly of CD_4^+ T-cells. There is deposition of immunoglobulin and membrane attack complex on blood vessels; the intramuscular blood vessels show endothelial hyperplasia with tubuloreticular inclusions in endothelial cells. There is myofiber necrosis with regeneration, micro-infarcts, and perifascicular atrophy.

Myofiber necrosis and regeneration are also seen in PM, although the pattern of involvement of muscle fibers differs from that seen in DM (single-fiber pattern in PM, compared with groups of fibers in DM). The mononuclear infiltrate primarily comprises CD_8^+ T-cells and is most pronounced in the endomysial space. There is increased MHC-I antigen expression and invasion of nonnecrotic muscle fibers.

The histopathology of s-IBM bears many resemblances to that of PM. The inflammatory infiltrate is predominantly composed of CD_8^+ T-cells, and this mononuclear cell infiltrate is predominantly endomysial with infiltration of nonnecrotic muscle fibers. MHC-I antigen is upregulated on the surface of muscle fibers, although MHC staining

Table 19.5A
Pathology of Polymyositis

Pathological features	Reference
Myofiber necrosis and regeneration	60[a]
Primarily CD8 mononuclear cell infiltrate (endomysial)	61,62
Mononuclear cell invasion of nonnecrotic muscle fibers	60[a]
MHC-I expression on muscle fibers	60[a]

[a]Ref. 60 is to a chapter in the text Myology edited by Engel and Franzi-Armstrong. Efforts to find original data to support the claim that these pathological features are characteristic of polymyositis or dermatomyositis were unsuccessful.

Table 19.5B
Pathology of Dermatomyositis

Pathological features	Reference
Myofiber necrosis and regeneration	60[a]
Micro-infarcts	60[a]
Perifascicular atrophy	60[a]
Predominantly CD4 mononuclear cell infiltrate (perivascular, perimysial)	63
Vascular membrane attack complex and Ig deposition	64–66
Endothelial cell tubuloreticular inclusions	64

[a]Ref. 60 is to a chapter in the text Myology edited by Engel and Franzi-Armstrong. Efforts to find original data to support the claim that these pathological features are characteristic of polymyositis or dermatomyositis were unsuccessful.

Table 19.5C
Pathology of Inclusion Body Myositis

Pathological features	Reference
Rimmed vacuoles	7–9
Mononuclear infiltrates	7–9
Endomysial infiltrate	7,8
Myofiber necrosis	3–5
Regenerating fibers	8,9
Tubulofilamentous inclusions (nuclear or cytoplasmic)	7–9
Amyloid deposits in muscle fibers	67,68
Ubiquitin positive inclusions in muscle fibers	69,70

is not typically part of the routine diagnostic evaluation. The characteristic pathological feature of s-IBM at the light microscopic level is the presence of subsarcolemmal or centrally placed vacuoles that are lined by granular material. The vacuoles are most easily identified on the modified Gomori-Trichrome stain. The characteristic feature on electron microscopy is the presence of cytoplasmic tubulofilamentous inclusions. More recently, immunohistochemical techniques have been used to demonstrate the presence of β-amyloid, ubiquitin and β-crystalin.

The range of histopathological changes that occur in patients with PM, DM, and s-IBM, together with the relevant supporting references, are summarized in Tables 19.5A–19.5C.

3. TREATMENT

3.1 What Is the Evidence for the Efficacy of Prednisone in DM/PM?

Steroid treatment in patients with PM/DM has never been evaluated in either a prospective study or in a randomized controlled trial. The available data are all retrospective and uncontrolled.

In the study by Bohan et al., 40 patients treated with prednisone had been examined carefully both before and after the initiation of treatment (5). The proportion of patients with strength graded as ≥4/5 increased from 25% before treatment to 63% following steroid treatment (5). In a retrospective series of 118 patients with inflammatory myopathy treated with prednisone 30–100 mg per day, it was reported that 104 (88%) were "adequately" treated, although no details are provided regarding what constituted an "adequate" response (6). In another retrospective series of 107 patients in which 102 were treated with prednisolone in varying doses (17), approximately 60% showed improvement on a four-point disability scale. In yet another retrospective series of 113 patients with infammatory myositis (including PM/DM and s-IBM) who were treated with at least 0.75 mg/kd/day of prednisone for 8 weeks, Joffe et al. found an overall complete clinical response (i.e., full clinical recovery) rate of 25%, with 61% of patients responding only partially (with the term "partial response" covering a spectrum from minimal to almost complete response) (18). When they considered the subgroups of inflammatory myopathy separately, they observed a complete response in 11% and 30% of patients with PM and DM respectively. Partial response rates in PM and DM were 73% and 60%, respectively (18).

Cook and colleagues, in a retrospective review of 35 children with DM/PM, compared the efficacy of daily and alternate-day steroids as initial treatment (19). Twenty-six children were treated with 1–2 mg/kg/day, and 9 received 2–3 mg/kg every other day. They reported no difference in efficacy between the two groups (without specifying the outcome measure used), although they noted a higher frequency of adverse effects in the daily prednisone group (19).

There is, therefore, an abundance of anecdotal data showing a beneficial effect of steroids in patients with DM/PM and, notwithstanding the absence of any quality data from a randomized controlled trial, steroids are regarded as the mainstay of the pharmacotherapy for patients with PM/DM (2,3,20).

3.2. What Is the Evidence for the Efficacy of Azathoprine in DM/PM?

There has been one small randomized, double-blind, placebo-controlled trial of azathioprine among patients with PM (21). Azathioprine was used at a dose of 2 mg/kg/day for a period of 3 months. All patients were also treated with prednisone 60 mg per day. Manual muscle testing of 18 pairs of muscles was used to estimate an average muscle strength score, which was used as the clinical outcome measure. Although the improvement in strength was greater in the azathioprine group than in the control group, the difference was not significant at the end of the 3-month treatment period (21). One

Table 19.6.
Efficacy of Various Immunosuppressive Regimens in Polymyositis/Dermatomyositis

	Sample size	*Complete response*	*Partial response*	*Reference*
Azathioprine	44	5 (11%)	23 (52%)	Joffe *(18)*
Methotrexate	55	9 (16%)	31 (56%)	Joffe *(18)*
	22	4 (18%)	13 (59%)	Metzger *(24)*
Cyclosporine A	6	3 (50%)	3 (50%)	Qushmaq *(26)*
	19	6 (32%)	13 (68%)	Danieli *(27)*
Cyclophosphamide	7	–	4 (57%)	Haga *(29)*
	11	–	1 (9%)	Cronin *(30)*

potential problem with this study was its relatively short duration in terms of the expectation that azathioprine might not exert its maximal effect for up to 6–9 months.

In their retrospective series of 113 patients who were initially treated with prednisone, Joffe and colleagues also included 44 patients who had a trial of azathioprine (75 mg/day for 8 weeks) that was given concurrently with prednisone *(18)*. Only 5 of these 44 patients (11%) had a complete clinical response, with a further 23 (52%) responding partially *(18)*. One difficulty in interpreting these results is that the term "partial response" was used to describe any response from minimal to almost complete. As in the study by Bunch et al. *(21)*, the duration of the trial of azathioprine was relatively brief. Furthermore, the dose of 75 mg/day is relatively low (with current practice in other clinical contexts being to use a dose of around 2.5–3 mg/kg/day).

The remaining data on the efficacy of azathioprine in PM is very scant, comprising a few small case series *(22,23)*. Benson and colleagues, for example, reported their experience with four patients with polymyositis in whom the addition of azathioprine led to clinical improvement and permitted a reduction in the dose of concurrently administered steroid *(22)*.

In conclusion, therefore, there really are no good quality data to support the use of azathioprine in the treatment of PM, but in truth, this practice has not yet been adequately put to the test (Table 19.6).

3.3. What Is the Evidence for the Efficacy of Methotrexate in DM/PM?

In their retrospective series of 113 patients who were initially treated with prednisone, Joffe and colleagues also included 55 patients who had a trial of methotrexate (5 mg/week for 8 weeks) that was given concurrently with prednisone *(18)*. Nine (16%) responded completely and 31 (56%) had a partial response. Although the authors explain that none of the patients with s-IBM responded completely, they do not indicate how many of the complete and partial responders had PM or DM. As noted before in reference to this study, the term "partial response" was taken to include a spectrum spanning minimal to almost complete response, and this impacts the ease with which these results can be interpreted.

Metzger and colleagues retrospectively reported their experience with 22 patients with PM/DM who were treated with a combination of prednisone and intravenous methotrexate *(24)*. All (except for two) patients had failed to show significant improvement in muscle strength despite 2 months of treatment with prednisone at a dose of 40 mg/day. The methotrexate dosing regimen was somewhat complex, starting at 10–15mg initially and then titrating up to 0.5–0.8 mg/kg (30–50 mg) every 5–7 days; once a response was achieved, the frequency with which the methotrexate was administered was decreased to every other week, every third week, or every month. The response to methotrexate was assessed in terms of an improvement in muscle strength and/or improvement in the skin rash (in cases of DM); the results are not reported separately for these two outcome measures. Seventeen (77%) showed a definite response in terms of muscle strength, cutaneous manifestations or both *(24)*. Four patients (18%) had a complete response and 13 (59%) had a partial response; these results are very similar to those reported by Joffe and colleagues *(18)*. The improvement in muscle strength occurred, on average, after 13 weeks of therapy and after a mean cumulative dose of 500 mg (range 120–1200 mg).

The available data, therefore, albeit of limited quality, suggest that a significant proportion of patients with PM/DM may derive at least some benefit from methotrexate (Table 19.6).

3.4. Is There Any Evidence for a Benefit of the Combination of Azathioprine and Methotrexate?

The efficacy of a combination of azathioprine and oral methotrexate in patients with treatment-resistant myositis was examined in a small randomized open-label study that employed a cross-over design *(25)*. Thirty patients with either DM or PM that had been resistant to prior immunosuppressive therapy were randomized to receive 6 months of therapy with one of two treatment regimens. The first regimen comprised methotrexate 7.5 mg/week and azathioprine 50 mg/day for 1 month, methotrexate 15 mg/week and azathioprine 100 mg/day for 1 month, and methotrexate 22.5–25 mg/week and azathioprine 150 mg/week for 4 months. The second regimen comprised intravenous methotrexate (500 mg/m^2) with leucovorin resecue (50 mg/m^2 every 6 hours for four doses, beginning 24 hours after methotrexate infusion) every 2 weeks. Efficacy was measured using a combination of muscle strength and functional assessment of activities of daily living (ADL). Response to therapy was defined in advance (increment of at least one grade of strength in at least two affected muscle groups as well as improvement of at least one functional level on the Convery Assessment scale). Baseline characteristics of the two groups were similar, and there was no interaction between treatment and the sequence in which treatments were received (initial period vs cross-over period). In total, 13 of 28 patients treated with azathioprine and oral methotrexate were classified as improved compared with 5 of 26 patients treated with intravenous methotrexate *(25)*. A response rate of 46% with the combined oral regimen was considered favorable given the nature of the study population—patients with myositis that had been resistant to prior immunosuppressive therapy.

3.5. What Is the Evidence for the Efficacy of Cyclosporine in DM/PM?

Qushmaq and colleagues retrospectively reported their experience with six PM/DM patients who were treated with cyclosporine A (average dose 3.5 mg/kg/day). All had been treated with prednisone (1 mg/kg/day) and had been refractory to other immunosuppressive therapies. Recovery was complete in three patients and partial in the other three *(26)*. These authors also reviewed the literature and identified 59 other patients who had been treated with cyclosporine A (average dose of 5.3 mg/kg/day). Thirty-eight of these 59 patients (64%) improved clinically *(26)*.

In the study by Danieli and colleagues of 19 patients with PM/DM, patients all received prednisone and cyclosporine, but some also received either plasmapheresis or intravenous immunoglobulin (IVIg), making it difficult to disentangle and isolate the efficacy of the cyclosporine 27. In general, cyclosporine was used initially at a dose of 3 mg/kg/day and subsequently tapered to 2 mg/kg/day. Outcome was evaluated using manual muscle testing, and 6 patients (32%) showed a complete response and 13 (68%) showed a partial response *(27)*.

There is, therefore, some retrospective and uncontrolled data that suggests a beneficial effect of cyclosporine in conjunction with other immunosuppressive therapies (Table 19.6).

The efficacy of cyclosporine was compared with that of methotrexate in small randomized trial *(28)*. Thirty six patients with PM or DM were randomized to receive either 7.5–15 mg methotrexate per week or 3–3.5 mg/kg/day cyclosporine for 6 months. All patients also received 0.5–1 mg/kg prednisone each day. Treatment efficacy was examined using a variety of outcome measures including the "muscle endurance together with functional test" (MEFT), a semiquantitative clinical assessment (CA) (in which the presence of various symptoms and signs contributed to an overall score), and a global patient assessment (GPA) of disability. Improvements in the methotrexate and cyclosporine groups were noted in 33% and 47% of patients using the MEFT, 73% and 58% using the CA, and 67% and 68% using the GPA (28). The differences in response rates between the two treatment groups were not significant, arguing in favor of a comparable effect of cyclosporine and methotrexate, each in combination with prednisone, for the treatment of PM and DM. Important limitations of this study include the lack of any discussion about the power of the study to detect differences in the efficacy of these two agents as well as the absence of any attempt to blind patients or observers to the treatment received.

3.6. What Is the Evidence for the Efficacy of Cyclophosphamide in DM/PM?

One study of the effects of intravenous cyclophosphamide in a variety of connective tissue diseases included seven patients with PM/DM *(29)*. They were treated with a mean of 3.6 pulses and a mean cumulative dose of 1.6 g. Four patients (57%) showed some improvement in muscle strength. A second study of monthly (for 6 months) pulses of intravenous cyclophosphamide (0.75 g/m^2) in 11 patients with refractory inflammatory myopathy (including patients with PM, DM, and s-IBM) showed poor results with 1 patient improving, 1 deteriorating, and the others remaining unchanged *(30)*.

There really has been very little investigation of the efficacy of cyclophosphamide (intravenous) in patients with PM/DM, but the little evidence available suggests that it is of limited value (Table 19.6).

3.7. Is There Any Evidence for the Use of Rituximab in DM?

In a small open-label and uncontrolled study, Levine examined the efficacy of Rituximab in seven patients with DM *(31)*. Study patients had failed to respond to prior immunosuppressive therapy and were treated with four intravenous infusions of

Rituximab (dose varied from 100 mg/m^2 to 375 mg/m^2) at weekly intervals. Outcome was examined using manual muscle testing and quantitative myometry with the prespecified criterion for success defined as improvement in muscle strength by >12% at 24 and 52 weeks following therapy. Treatment was successful in all six patients (one patient was lost to follow-up), with improvement seen as early as 4 weeks after the initial infusion and maximum benefit between 12 and 24 weeks *(31)*. The results of this study are difficult to interpret given the small sample size, absence of a control group, and lack of blinding of the patients and investigators. Nevertheless, the data do suggest that Rituximab warrants further investigation in a randomized controlled fashion.

3.8. What Is the Evidence Supporting the Use of IVIg in the Treatment of DM and PM?

Most of the literature relevant to the use of IVIg in the treatment of inflammatory myopathy comprises uncontrolled case series. This limitation of the literature is further compounded by the failure of most studies to make a clear distinction between PM and inclusion body myositis. This shortcoming is due, in large part, to reliance on the outdated Bohan and Peter criteria, which were suggested before inclusion body myositis was a recognized entity. If s-IBM is genuinely unresponsive to immunotherapy (as seems to be the case), then inclusion of such patients together with subjects with PM has the effect of reducing the power of the study in question to show any benefit of the immunosuppressive therapy being studied in patients with PM. Finally, IVIg has been used to treat patients with inflammatory myopathy in two different contexts. Most studies have focused on the use of IVIg in subjects who had been resistant to all forms of prior immunosuppressive therapy. There is, however, also a small (uncontrolled) literature on the use of IVIg as initial (and sole) therapy *(32)*.

There is a single prospective randomized placebo-controlled trial of IVIg in patients with DM who had been resistant to previous immunosuppressive therapy *(33)*. The study population comprised 15 subjects with active disease resistant to treatment with steroids or other immunosuppressive agents. Active treatment comprised two doses of IVIg (1 g/kg per dose), administered monthly for 3 months. This was followed by a 1-month wash-out period, after which patients were offered the opportunity to cross-over to the alternate treatment arm. Outcome was measured using a neuromuscular-symptoms scale, an ADL scale (based on the Barthel Index), and a modified Medical Research Council (MRC) scale to measure muscle strength as well as photographs of the skin rash. Eight patients were randomized to receive IVIg and seven were randomized to the placebo group. The majority of patients in both groups were taking other immunosuppressant drugs during the study. After 3 months, all eight patients randomized to receive IVIg had improved. Of the seven patients who received placebo, three worsened, two remained the same, and two showed mild improvement. Mean improvements in the MRC and neuromuscular symptom scores (NSS) are shown in Table 19.7. Four of the eight patients who initially received placebo were subsequently crossed-over and were treated with IVIg. All four improved (Table 19.7). In open long-term follow-up of six patients treated with IVIg, all continued to require an infusion approximately every 6 weeks in order to maintain their response.

Table 19.7
Response to Intravenous Immunoglobulin (IVIg) in Patients With Dermatomyositis

Therapy	No. of patients	MRC Score[a]		Neuromuscular symptom score[b]	
		Pre-Rx	Post-Rx	Pre-Rx	Post-Rx
IVIg	8	77 ± 6	85 ± 5	44 ± 8	51 ± 6
Placebo	7	79 ± 6	77 ± 8	46 ± 9	46 ± 11
Placebo-then IVIg	4	74 ± 6	83 ± 6	38 ± 9	49 ± 11

Data from ref. 33.
[a]Maximum score (normal) = 90. Increased score represents improvement.
[b]Maximum score (normal) = 60. Increased score represents improvement.

The remaining literature on the use of IVIg in the treatment of patients with inflammatory myopathy is uncontrolled (34,35). In an open study of 20 patients with refractory PM and DM, Cherin and colleagues examined the efficacy of IVIg as "add-on" immunosuppressive therapy (34). The diagnosis was based on the Bohan and Peter criteria, and 19 of 20 patients had not responded or had been intolerant of previous immunosuppressive therapy. Response to therapy was evaluated using the MRC grading system of muscle strength. Out of a theoretically maximum score of 88 points, a clinical improvement was defined as ≥ 18-point improvement. Fifteen patients improved, four remained unchanged and one deteriorated. Because the scoring system was very similar to that used by Dalakas et al. in their randomized controlled trial, it is possible to compare the outcome data in this uncontrolled trial (Table 19.7). The mean MRC score after three IVIg infusions (for all 20 patients combined) improved from 44 ±13 to 66 ± 18 (34). In an even smaller uncontrolled trial of IVIg in 11 patients with PM or DM (four in association with systemic sclerosis), 9 patients responded with partial or complete remission of disease (35).

The evidence, therefore, supports the use of IVIg in patients with DM or PM who have not responded to other forms of immunosuppressive therapy. The one caveat is that, for the most part, the efficacy of IVIg has been demonstrated in patients who were also taking other immunosuppressive agents. It may be, therefore, that it is the combination therapy that is effective. Relevant to this concern is the single open study by Cherin and colleagues of IVIg as initial therapy in patients with DM or PM (i.e., in the absence of other immunosuppressive therapy), in which clinical improvement was observed in only 3 of 11 patients (32).

3.9. Is Plasmapheresis Effective in the Treatment of PM/DM?

The efficacy of plasmapheresis in patients with PM/DM has been the subject of a number of uncontrolled studies (36,37) as well as of a single double-blind, randomized, placebo-controlled trial (38). Although the uncontrolled studies (36,37) suggested a beneficial effect of plasma exchange, this was not borne out by the randomized controlled trial (38). The randomized controlled study included 42 patients randomized to receive plasmapheresis, leukapheresis, or sham pheresis (three times per week for 4 weeks). All patients had previously been treated with high-dose prednisone; some had also received other immunosuppressive therapy, but not during the study period. Outcome was evaluated using both manual muscle testing and a functional assessment of ADL *(38)*. The authors of the more recent uncontrolled series of PM/DM patients treated with plasmapheresis *(37)* attributed their finding a beneficial effect of plasmapheresis (while the randomized controlled trial did not) to the fact that the randomized controlled trial had included small patient numbers and had focused on patients with chronic disease. With regard to the former criticism, the randomized controlled trial appears to have been adequately powered (80%) to detect a 16% improvement in muscle strength *(38)*.

The available evidence, therefore, does not support the use of plasmapheresis in patients with DM/PM.

3.10. Are Steroids Effective in the Treatment of s-IBM?

Traditional wisdom is that s-IBM is resistant to treatment with corticosteroids and, although this is probably true, the data supporting this contention are actually quite poor. There have been no formal studies of the efficacy of prednisone in the treatment of s-IBM. In describing the histopathology in six patients with s-IBM, Carpenter et al. noted that there had been no clinical response to treatment with corticosteroids in varying doses for variable periods of time *(8)*. In their larger case series of 40 patients, Lotz and colleagues noted that 29 had been treated with at least 40 mg of prednisone per day for 3 months. Twenty-five subjects had been followed for more than 2 years, and there had been progression of the disease in all despite treatment *(7)*.

Some data about the potential efficacy of prednisone can also be gleaned from one of the double-blind controlled trials of IVIg, in which 22 patients were randomized to monthly infusions of placebo or IVIg for 6 months; all subjects also received prednisone 60 mg per day for 1 month with subsequent gradual taper to 60 mg every other day *(39)*. Outcome at 3 months was examined using the MRC and quantitative muscle testing (QMT) scores. Relevant to the potential effects of prednisone are not the differences between the two groups, but rather the differences between baseline and follow-up. There were small (but insignificant) losses in muscle strength between baseline and follow-up in both treatment groups. One might be inclined to interpret these data as demonstrating a stabilizing effect of prednisone on the course of the disease (because the natural history of s-IBM is thought to be one of slow relentless progression). Caveats, however, include the relatively short duration of follow-up and the fact that this study did not include a control group for prednisone treatment because it was not designed to examine the efficacy of steroids.

In the retrospective series by Joffe and colleagues that included 14 patients with s-IBM, the authors commented on the relatively poor response of this group of patients to steroids *(18)*. Interestingly, more than one-half of these patients were described as having a partial response to prednisone. As noted elsewhere, however, the term "partial response" in this study spanned a broad spectrum from minimal to almost complete. Without further data, it is impossible to know whether any of these patients with s-IBM really showed any signs of improvement.

In summary, therefore, although steroids are widely regarded as ineffective in the treatment of s-IBM, this conclusion is based entirely on anecdotal (although consistent) observations.

3.11. Is There Evidence to Support the Use of IVIg in Patients With s-IBM?

The use of IVIg in patients with s-IBM has been the subject of a number of investigations *(39–43)*. Soueidan and Dalakas suggested that IVIg might be effective after they treated four patients with IVIg for 2 months and followed them over a period of 9–12 months. Using cumulative MRC scores, they noted an improvement in three of the four patients *(40)*. Amato and colleagues reported their experience with 9 patients who were treated with monthly IVIg for 3 months, noting no improvement in any patients and deterioration in six *(41)*.

In their first controlled trial of IVIg in patients with s-IBM, Dalakas and colleagues randomized 22 patients to treatment with monthly infusions of either IVIg or placebo for 3 months *(42)*. Overall, they noted no significant treatment effect of IVIg, but did report that six of the nine patients treated with IVIg showed a ≥10-point improvement on the cumulative MRC score, and they also described a regional effect in which there was improvement in certain muscle groups but deterioration in others, producing no net change. They suggested that dysphagia might be improved by IVIg *(42)*. In their second, slightly larger controlled trial, Dalakas and colleagues randomized patients to treatment with prednisone plus IVIg or prednisone plus placebo *(39)*. The IVIg (or placebo) infusions were administered monthly for 3 months and all patients received adequate doses of steroids (60 mg per day initially, subsequently tapered to 60 mg every other day). Nineteen patients received IVIg and 17 were treated with placebo. They found no significant difference between the two treatment groups in the cumulative MRC scores of muscle strength over the 3-month duration of the study. Although some subjects reported a subjective improvement in strength, this likely reflected an expression of improved endurance rather than strength; overall, there was a minor deterioration in strength in both treatment groups. The regional effect and improvement in dysphagia noted in their previous study were not confirmed in the second study.

In one other controlled trial, patients were randomized to received either IVIg or placebo for 6 months in a cross-over design study *(43)*. Patients received one of the two treatments for 6 months and were then crossed over to receive the alternate treatment for 6 months. The cumulative MRC muscle strength score and the neuromuscular symptoms scale were used to evaluate outcome. These investigators noted a significant improvement in muscle strength in both groups (IVIg → placebo and placebo → IVIg) over the entire 12-month duration of the study. They also reported a significant improvement in the NSS in the IVIg group compared with the placebo group over the first 6 months of the study (although this effect may have been confounded by the baseline differences in the NSS between the two groups).

The results of these studies generally paint a picture of poor responsiveness to treatment with IVIg, but they also raise the possibility that a select few patients may benefit in terms of slowed progression of the disease. Although there have been no formal studies of whether IVIg slows progression of the disease, the therapeutic dilemma that remains is whether individual patients with s-IBM warrant a careful trial of IVIg, especially given the absence of any other effective therapy. This remains an unanswered question, and individual decisions will need to be made on a case-by-case basis.

4. PROGNOSIS

4.1. What Is the Risk of Malignancy in Patients with Inflammatory Myopathy?

There are a number of studies that have addressed the relationship between the inflammatory myopathies, notably DM and PM, and malignancy. Four population-based studies provide the most reliable estimates of this risk (44–47). These four studies were similar in that they were all retrospective cohort studies. In each study, subjects with the diagnosis of inflammatory myopathy were identified and then matched to a national cancer registry to determine which patients with inflammatory myopathy had also been diagnosed with a malignancy (other than skin cancer). This provided data on the "observed" number of cases of malignancy in the population of patients with inflammatory myopathy. The "expected" number of cases of cancer were then estimated using age- and gender-specific cancer rates from the cancer registry. The expected number of cancers was calculated by multiplying the age- and gender-specific rates from the standard population (the cancer registry) by the size of the population under investigation (those with inflammatory myopathy). The standardized incidence ratio (SIR) was then calculated as the ratio of the number of observed cases divided by the expected number of cases. The studies differed primarily in the certainty with which the diagnosis of inflammatory myopathy was established. In the Danish study, for example, cases were identified based on International Classification of Diseases (ICD) codes from hospital discharge with no effort made to verify the diagnosis (46). In the Swedish study, approximately 10% of the medical records were reviewed and the diagnosis of inflammatory myoapthy confirmed in over 90% of cases (44). The Finnish investigators reviewed all of the medical records and only included those in which the diagnosis was confirmed (45). The Australian investigators, on the other hand, identified cases from a central diagnostic neuropathology service that reviewed all muscle biopsies performed in the state of Victoria (47). All of these investigators were primarily interested in malignancies that developed at, or after, the time of diagnosis of the inflammatory myopathy. As show in Table 19.8, these studies yielded SIRs for malignancy in association with DM that ranged from 2.4 to 8.3, indicating that the incidence of malignancy among patients with DM varied from 2.4 to 8.3 times the incidence among the general population. The SIR for malignancy in PM ranged from 1.7 to 2.0, indicating a more modest increase in the risk of malignancy.

A meta-analysis of the Swedish, Danish, and Finnish studies provided more reliable estimates of (1) the cancer-specific incidence rates and (2) the timing of the increased risk of malignancy (48). These pooled data indicate an increased risk for ovarian, lung, pancreatic, gastric, and colorectal cancer among subjects with DM and an increased risk of lung cancer, non-Hodgkin's lymphoma, and bladder cancer in patients with PM (Table 19.9). Finally, these data indicate that the risk of malignancy is greatest within the first

Table 19.8
Risk of Malignancy in Polymyositis (PM) and Dermatomyositis (DM)

Study	Population	Study design	Sample size DM	Sample size PM	No. cancers DM	No. cancers PM	SIR[a] DM	SIR[a] PM
Sigurgeirsson (44)	Sweden—population-based	Cases identified by ICD codes from hospital discharges. Reviewed 10% of records (93% diagnostic accuracy of ICD codes)	392	396	61	42	M **2.4** (1.6–3.6) F **3.4** (2.4.–4.7)	M **1.8** (1.1–2.7) F **1.7** (1.0–2.5)
Airio (45)	Finland—population-based	Cases identified by ICD codes from hospital discharges. Reviewed all medical records to confirm diagnosis	311		34		M **8.3** (3.0–18)[b] F **6.0** (3.2–10)[b]	
Chow (46)	Denmark—population-based	Cases identified from hospital discharge records. No comment regarding medical record review—presumably none	203	336	31	26	**3.8** (2.5–5.4)[c]	**1.7** (1.1–2.4)[c]
Buchbinder (47)	Australia (state of Victoria—population-based	Cases identified based on diagnoses made at the centralized Victorian neuropathology service. Review of all biopsies to confirm the diagnosis	321	85	58	36	**6.2** (3.9–10)	**2.0** (1.4–2.7)

[a]SIR, standardized incidence ratio, i.e., the number of cancer cases that arose among dermatomyositis or polymyositis patients divided by the expected number of cancer cases according to nation age-specific, gender-specific, and period-specific cancer rates.

[b]Excess risk of cancer observed only in patients over the age of 50 at the time of diagnosis of DM.

[c]Estimates are based primarily on patients older than 45 (only 4 of the 57 cases of cancer occurred in subjects less than 45 years). ICD, international classification of diseases.

Table 19.9
Standardized Incidence Ratios for Cancer After the Diagnosis
of Dermatomyositis/Polymyositis

Cancer type	Dermatomyositis (n = 618)		Polymyositis (n = 914)	
	No.	SIR (95% CI)	No.	SIR (95% CI)
All	115	**3** (2.5–3.6)	95	**1.3** (1.0–1.6)
Lung, trachea, bronchus	19	**5.9** (3.7–9.2)	20	**2.8** (1.8–4.4)
Ovary	13	**10.5** (6.1–18.1)	2	–
Pancreas	5	**3.8** (1.6–9.0)	1	–
Stomach	7	**3.5** (1.7–7.3)	1	–
Colorectal	12	**2.5** (1.4–4.4)	10	–
Non-Hodgkin's lymphoma	3	–	6	**3.7** (1.7–8.2)
Bladder	3	–	9	**2.4** (1.3–4.7)

CI, confidence interval; SIR, standardized incidence ratio.
Data from ref. *48*.

year following the diagnosis of inflammatory myopathy. The risk of malignancy falls with time, returning to normal amongst those with PM by 5 years but remaining marginally increased among those with DM.

The argument has been made that the increased risk of malignancy shortly after the diagnosis of DM/PM may be related to increased cancer surveillance, and that the increased risk of cancer many years after the diagnosis may be due to the side effects of prolonged immunosuppressive therapy used in the treatment of DM/PM. The evidence against the increased risk being due to heightened surveillance comes from a number of sources. First, in the Swedish study, Sigurgeirsson and colleagues also examined cancer mortality rates and found these to be increased among both men and women with DM and, to a lesser extent, among men with PM *(44)*. Second, although not described in detail, these population-based studies also found an increased risk of malignancy in the years preceding the diagnosis of DM/PM. Finally, in the Finnish study, the risk of malignancy was approximately 30% lower among the patients with DM/PM who had received immunosuppressive therapy compared with those who did not (45), and the declining risk of malignancy with increased duration of immunosuppressive therapy would be surprising if such therapy was important in the pathogenesis of these malignancies.

In summary, therefore, there is an overall increased risk of malignancy among patients with inflammatory myopathy. This risk is greatest for those with DM, especially (but not exclusively) for those older than 50 years of age. The risk is also greatest in the first year following the diagnosis and declines with time, although remains elevated even up to 5 years after diagnosis. The risk is greatest for ovarian and lung cancers, although is also increased for a broad spectrum of other malignancies. The data regarding the relationship between cancer and PM are less robust. The small overall magnitude of the risk, as well as the observation that the risk is only increased in the first year following diagnosis, suggest that case ascertainment bias could account for a significant component of the documented association between cancer and PM.

Table 19.10
Mortality Rates in Polymyositis and Dermatomyositis

Study	Cumulative mortality rates			
	1 yr	2 yr	5 yr	8–9 yr
Hochberg (1986) (71)	5.5%	~12%	19.6%	27.2%
Marie (2001) (51)	17%	18%	23%	
Maugars (1996) (50)	17.5%	26.1%	35.3%	44.6%
Basset-Seguin (1990) (72)	28%			
Medsger (1971) (52)	28%	28%	35%	
Sigurgeirsson (1992) (44)	22%		48%	
Benbassat (1985) (49)			48%	

4.2. What Is the Prognosis of Patients With PM/DM?

Because it has long been recognized that PM and DM are responsive to immunosuppressive therapy, all published series of the long-term outcome of patients with PM/DM represent the outcome given the best available treatment at the time rather than the true natural history of the disease.

In considering the prognosis of patients with PM/DM, it is worth making a distinction between the mortality rates and causes of death, the functional outcome among survivors, and risk of recurrence among the survivors as well as the factors that are predictive of a poor outcome. For the sake of clarity, each of these will be considered separately.

Varying mortality rates have been reported in different studies (Table 19.10), but the trend is the same, with an early increase in mortality within the first year followed by a more gradual increase in mortality thereafter. Based on the data in the table, mean cumulative survival is approximately 80% at 1 year, 79% at 2 years, and 65% at 5 years.

The most common causes of death among patients with PM/DM are cardiac (myocarditis, arrhythmia), pulmonary (interstitial lung disease, aspiration pneumonia), and carcinomatous (49–51). Cardiac deaths are most prominent among patients with PM, whereas pulmonary and carcinomatous deaths are more common in patients with DM (50).

A number of studies have tried to determine which factors are predictive of a poor outcome. One study from 1971 identified advancing age, the presence of pulmonary infiltrates on chest X-ray, the presence of dysphagia, and the presence of more severe proximal muscle weakness as predictive of mortality (52). Another study, published in 1985, suggested that older age, dysphagia, shorter duration of disease, and failure to respond to treatment represented the most important adverse prognostic factors (49). Using more sophisticated modeling techniques and a multivariate analysis, Maugars and colleagues identified old age, the presence of dysphonia, pulmonary interstitial fibrosis, the absence of myalgia, the absence of dysphagia, and the presence of asthenia-anorexia as being the most important prognostic factors for death in their retrospective review of 69 patients with PM or DM (50). Although there is some disagreement, most studies have concurred in identifying older age and the presence of interstitial pulmonary disease as being predictive of worse outcome and increased mortality.

What about the prognosis of those who survive? Some studies have reported outcome in terms of the proportion of patients who enter remission (i.e., have no persistent muscle weakness). Because clinical remission is typically defined in terms of recovery of full strength, such an outcome measure does not shed light on overall functional outcome. Other investigators, therefore, have evaluated outcome using more global measures such as the Medical Outcomes Study Short Form Healthy Survey (SF-36) or the Health Assessment Questionnaire (HAQ) to evaluate patients' subjective assessments of muscle strength, disease-related complications, and treatment-related complications.

Varying remission rates have been described, with one study reporting that approximately 85% of surviving patients had either insignificant or no muscle weakness at follow-up *(50)*, whereas others have suggested that the rate of remission is much lower, of the order of 31% *(53)* to 40% *(51)*.

The prospective study by Clark and colleagues provides some information about the change in disability over time. They found that among patients less than 60 years of age, disability remained fairly stable over time but with a tendency to gradually increase. Disability increased more rapidly among patients over the age of 60, especially those who developed avascular necrosis of the femoral head or compression fractures as a result of long-term corticosteroid use *(54)*. Information about the degree of disability can be gleaned from the retrospective cohort study by Marie and colleagues. In this study, 10 of 16 subjects (62.5%) with complete remission reported persistent fatigue with moderately decreased activities (HAQ score <0.75). By comparison, among those with nonremitting disease, 17 (55%) reported persistent muscle effort fatigue (HAQ <0.75) and 12 (39%) described marked muscle weakness with severe reduction of activities (0.75 < HAQ < 1.5). In their review of 105 patients with inflammatory myositis, Ponyi and colleagues also used the HAQ to evaluate functional outcome *(55)*. They found that 17.5% of patients reported no disability, 39% were mildly disabled, 31% moderately disabled, and 12.5% severely disabled *(55)*. These and other investigators have similarly found that the subjective sense of well-being among patients with inflammatory myositis was significantly worse than the general population, irrespective of whether the disease remained active or was in remission *(55,56)*. These studies, therefore, indicate that inflammatory myositis is a disease associated with chronic disability, irrespective of the use and success of treatment. Immunosuppressive therapy has the potential to impact on the disease and to improve muscle strength, but may also be associated with significant morbidity.

Finally, there is the matter of recurrence. If remission of disease, either partial or complete, is achieved, is the disease likely to remain in abeyance? If not, what is the likelihood of relapse and what is the latency to relapse? Again, there are limited data to reliably answer these questions, but some information can be gleaned from the literature. Marie and colleagues, for example, noted clinical recurrence of PM/DM in nine patients (12%) in their study. The latency to recurrence after discontinuation of therapy ranged from 3 months to 9 years *(51)*.

In conclusion, therefore, mortality is increased in patients with PM/DM as compared with the general population, particularly in the first year following diagnosis. Factors that have consistently been identified as predictive of a poor outcome include older age of onset and the presence of interstitial lung disease. Amongst the survivors, approximately 40% can be expected to achieve clinical remission. Irrespective of whether remission is achieved, significant disability often persists in this group of patients, with ongoing complaints of fatigue and limitation of daily activities. Finally, there is a small risk of recurrence of disease after discontinuation of therapy among those who achieve remission, with the latency to recurrence ranging anywhere from 3 months to 9 years.

4.3. What Is the Natural History of s-IBM?

There are very limited published data about the natural history of s-IBM. In one study, Rose and colleagues followed 11 patients over a 6-month period, using lean body mass, muscle mass, and strength to evaluate progression of the disease *(57)*. Maximal voluntary isometric contraction (MVIC) was used to quantify muscle strength. They found an overall decline in composite strength score of 4% between baseline and the time of follow-up, but noted significant variability, with four patients showing no decline. No significant changes were noted in the measurements of lean body and muscle mass *(57)*. Two obvious limitations of this study are the small sample size and limited duration of follow-up. In a retrospective review, Felice and colleagues reported the 4-year outcome of eight patients with s-IBM *(58)*. Overall MRC scores declined by 3.5% per year (0.3% per month), with mean grip strength falling by 10.7% per year (0.9% per month) *(58)*.

These data suggest that s-IBM is characterized by progressive muscle weakness, but the rate of progression has not been reliably established. Neither are there good data to indicate the proportion of patients who deteriorate, the final degree of disability attained, or whether there are any factors that are predictive of a particularly poor outcome.

5. SUMMARY

- Consensus has not yet been reached on the criteria that should be used for the diagnosis of the inflammatory myopathies. The Bohan and Peter criteria from the 1970s are the most widely accepted, but these are limited by failing to make a distinction between PM and s-IBM and by the sole reliance on the presence or absence of a skin rash to distinguish PM from DM. Dalakas has proposed a set of revised criteria that place much greater weight on histropathological findings, but these criteria have not yet been validated either prospectively or retrospectively.
- The pattern of muscle weakness may help to distinguish s-IBM on the one hand from PM/ DM on the other. Most case series of patients with s-IBM have emphasized the involvement of select muscle groups including forearm, wrist and finger flexors, and extensors as well as the quadriceps femoris and tibialis anterior muscles. Asymmetric muscle weakness is also characteristic of s-IBM.
- The sensitivity of elevated CK in the diagnosis of inflammatory myoapthy is approximately 85%. The degree of CK elevation in s-IBM tends to be less than that found in patients with PM/DM.
- Electromyographic examination of the paraspinal muscles offers the greatest yield in the diagnosis of the inflammatory myopathies. At least six to eight muscles should be examined.
- PM, DM, and s-IBM have characteristic histopathological findings, but specialized immunohistochemical techniques may be required to identify these specific changes.

- Steroids remain the mainstay of treatment of PM and DM, even though they have never been studied in a prospective or controlled fashion.
- Steroids are thought to be ineffective in s-IBM even though there have never been any prospective or controlled trials.
- There have been five controlled studies of immunosuppressive therapy in PM/DM:
  - The combination of azathioprine and placebo showed no benefit over prednisone alone, but the negative results may at least in part be due to the short duration of the study.
  - The trial of plasmapheresis and leukapheresis failed to show any benefit.
  - A placebo-controlled trial showed the efficacy of IVIg in patients with DM.
  - A randomized open-label study showed a benefit of combined azathioprine and oral methotrexate over intravenous methotrexate with leucovorin rescue over a 6-month period in patients with treatment-resistant myositis.
  - A randomized open-label study indicated equivalency of methotrexate and cyclosporine, each in combination with oral prednisone.
- The efficacy of IVIg in PM is based on uncontrolled data.
- There are conflicting data regarding whether IVIg may offer some limited benefit to patients with s-IBM.
- The risk of malignancy is increased among patients with DM, particularly in the first year following diagnosis. The greatest risk is for ovarian and lung cancers. The risk of malignancy falls with time following diagnosis, but remains marginally elevated at 5 years.
- Mortality is increased among patients with PM/DM, with cumulative survival rates of 80% at 1 year and 65% at 5 years.
- Older age and the presence of interstitial lung disease portend a worse prognosis (in terms of increased mortality) among patients with PM/DM.
- Approximately 30–40% of patients with PM/DM will achieve complete clinical remission with appropriate treatment; the risk of subsequent recurrence of disease is approximately 10%
- The natural history of s-IBM is poorly characterized. The temporal course of clinical deterioration is unclear.

REFERENCES

1. Bohan A, Peter J. Polymyositis and dematomyositis. N Engl J Med 1975;292:344–347 and 403–407.
2. Dalakas MC. Polymyositis, dermatomyositis, and inclusion-body myositis. N Engl J Med 1991; 325:1487–1498.
3. Dalakas MC, Hohlfeld R. Polymyositis and dermatomyositis. Lancet 2003;362:971–982.
4. Miller FW, Rider LG, Plotz PH, Isenberg DA, Oddis CV. Diagnostic criteria for polymyositis and dermatomyositis. Lancet 2003;362:1762–1763.
5. Bohan A, Peter JB, Bowman RL, Pearson CM. A computer-assisted analysis of 153 patients with polymyositis and dermatomyositis. Medicine (Baltimore) 1977;56:255–286.
6. DeVere R, Bradley W. Polymyositis: its presentation, morbidity and mortality. Brain 1975; 98:637–666.
7. Lotz B, Engel A, Nishino H, Stevens J, Litchy W. Inclusion body myositis. Observations in 40 patients. Brain 1989;112:727–747.
8. Carpenter S, Karpati G, Heller I, Eisen A. Inclusion body myositis: a distinct variety of idiopathic inflammatory myopathy. Neurology 1978;28:8–17.
9. Danon MJ, Reyes MG, Perurena OH, Masdeu JC, Manaligod JR. Inclusion body myositis. A corticosteroids-resistant idiopathic inflammatory myopathy. Arch Neurol 1982;39:760–764.

10. Ringel SP, Kenny CE, Neville HE, Giorno R, Carry MR. Spectrum of inclusion body myositis. Arch Neurol 1987;44:1154–1157.

11. Phillips BA, Cala LA, Thickbroom GW, Melsom A, Zilko PJ, Mastaglia FL. Patterns of muscle involvement in inclusion body myositis: clinical and magnetic resonance imaging study. Muscle Nerve 2001;24:1526–1534.

12. Amato AA, Gronseth GS, Jackson CE, et al. Inclusion body myositis: clinical and pathological boundaries. Ann Neurol 1996;40:581–586.

13. Streib EW, Wilbourn AJ, Mitsumoto H. Spontaneous electrical muscle fiber activity in polymyositis and dermatomyositis. Muscle Nerve 1979; 2:14–18.

14. Fredericks EJ. Electromyography in polymyositis and dermatomyositis. Muscle Nerve 1994,17:1235–1236.

15. Mitz M, Chang G, Albers J, Sulaiman A. Electromyographic and histologic paraspinal abnormalities in polymyositis/dermatomyositis. Arch Phys Med Rehabil 1981;62:118–121.

16. Streib E, Daube J. Electromyography of paraspinal muscles. Neurology 1975; 25:386.

17. Henriksson K, Sandstedt P. Polymyositis - treatment and prognosis. A study of 107 patients. Acta Neurol Scand 1982;65:280–300.

18. Joffe MM, Love LA, Leff RL, et al. Drug therapy of the idiopathic inflammatory myopathies: predictors of response to prednisone, azathioprine and methotrexate and a comparison of their efficacy. Am J Med 1993;94:379–387.

19. Cook JD, Fink CW, Henderson-Tilton AC. Comparison of the initial response of childhood dermatopolymyositis to daily versus alternate-day corticosteroid administration: a retrospective study. Ann Neurol 1984;16:400–401.

20. Mastaglia FL, Phillips BA, Zilko P. Treatment of inflammatory myopathies. Muscle Nerve 1997; 20:651–664.

21. Bunch TW, Worthington JW, Combs JJ, Ilstrup DM, Engel AG. Azathioprine with prednisone for polymyositis. A controlled clinical trial. Ann Int Med 1980;92:365–369.

22. Benson MD, Aldo MA, Azathioprine therapy in polymyositis. Arch Int Med 1973; 132:447–451.

23. McFarlin DE, Griggs RC. Treatment of inflammatory myopathies with azathioprine. Trans Am Neurol Assoc 1968;93:244–6.

24. Metzger AL, Bohan A, Goldberg LS, Bluestone R, Pearson CM. Polymyositis and dermatomyositis: combined methotrexate and corticosteroid therpay. Ann Int Med 1974; 81:182–189.

25. Villalba L, Hick JE, Adams EM, et al. Treatment of refractory myositis. A randomized crossover study of two new cytotoxic regimens. Arthritis Rheum 1998;41:392–399.

26. Qushmaq KA, Chalmers A, Esdaile JM. Cyclosporin A in the treatment of refractory adult polymyositis/dermatomyositis: population based experience in 6 patients and literature review. J Rheumatol 2000;27:2855–2859.

27. Danieli M, Malcangi G, Palmieri C, et al. Cyclosporin A and intravenous immunoglobulin treatment in polymyositis/dermatomyositis. Ann Rheum Dis 2002; 261:37–41.

28. Vencovsky J, Karsova K, Machacek S, et al. Cyclosporin A versus methotrexate in the treatment of polymyositis and dermatomyositis. Scan J Rheumatol 2000; 29:95–102.

29. Haga H-J, D'Cruz D, Asherson R, Hughes GR. Short term effects of intravenous pulses of cyclophosphamide in the treatment of connective tissue disease crisis. Ann Rheum Dis 1992;51:885–888.

30. Cronin ME, Miller FW, Hicks JE, Dalakas M, Plotz PH. The failure of intravenous cyclophosphamide therapy in refractory idiopathic inflammatory myopathy. J Rheumatol 1989;16:1225–1228.

31. Levine TD. Rituximab in the treatment of dermatomyositis: an open label pilot study. Arthritis Rheum 2005;52:601–607.

32. Cherin P, Piette J-C, Wechsler B, et al. Intravenous gamma globulin as first line therapy in polymyositis and dematomyositis: an open study with 11 adult patients. J Rheumatol 1994;21:1092–1097.

33. Dalakas MC. Controlled studies with high-dose intravenous immunoglobulin in the treatment of dermatomyositis, inclusion body myositis and polymyositis. Neurology 1998;51(Suppl 5):S37–S45.

34. Cherin P, Herson S, Wechsler B, et al. Efficacy of intravenous gammaglobulin therapy in chronic refractory polymyositis and dermatomyositis: an open study with 20 adult patients. Am J Med 1991; 91:162–168.

35. Mastaglia F, Phillips B, Ziko P. Immunoglobulin therapy in inflammatory myopathies. J Neurol Neurosurg Psychiatry 1998;65:107–110.

36. Dau PC. Plasmapheresis in idiopathic inflammatory myopathy. Arch Neurol 1981; 38:544–552.

37. Cherin P, Auperin L, Bussel A, Pourrat J, Herson S. Plasma exchange in polymyositis and dermatomyositis: a multicenter study of 57 cases. Clin Exp Rheumatol 1995;13:270–271.

38. Miller FW, Leitman S, F, Cronin ME, et al. Controlled trial of plasma exchange and leukapheresis in polymyositis and dermatomyositis. N Engl J Med 1992; 326:1380–1384.

39. Dalakas M, Koffman B, Fujii M, Spector S, Sivakumar K, Cupler E. A controlled study of intravenous immunoglobulin combined with prednisone in the treatment of IBM. Neurology 2001;56:323–327.

40. Soueidan SA, Dalakas MC. Treatment of inclusion-body myositis with high-dose intravenous immunoglobulin. Neurology 1993; 43:876–879.

41. Amato A, Barohn R, Jackson C, Pappert E, Sahenk Z, Kissel J. Inclusion body myositis: Treatment with intravenous immunoglobulin. Neurology 1994; 44:1516–1518.

42. Dalakas M, Sonies B, Dambrosia J, Sekul E, Cupler E, Sivakumar K. Treatment of inclusion-body myositis with IVIg: a double-blind, placebo-controlled trial. Neurology 1997;48:712–716.

43. Walter MC, Lochmüller H, Toepfer M, et al. High-dose immunoglobulin therapy in sporadic inclusion body myositis: a double-blind, placebo-controlled study. J Neurol 2000;247:22–28.

44. Sigurgeirsson B, Lindelöf B, Edhag O, Allander E. Risk of cancer in patients with dermatomyositis or polymyositis: A population–based study. N Engl J Med 1992;326:363–367.

45. Airio A, Pukkala E, Isomäki H. Elevated cancer incidence in patients with dermatomyositis: a population based study. J Rheumatol 1995; 22:1300–1303.

46. Chow WH, Gridley G, Mellemkjær L, McLaughlin JK, Olsen JH, Fraumeni JF. Cancer risk following polymyositis and dermatomyositis: a nationwide cohort study in Denmark. Cancer Causes Control 1995;6:9–13.

47. Buchbinder R, Forbes A, Hall S, Dennett X, Giles G. Incidence of malignant disease in biopsy-proven inflammatory myopathy. A population-based cohort study. Ann Intern Med 2001;134:1087–1095.

48. Hill CL, Zhang Y, Sigurgeirsson B, et al. Frequency of specific cancer types in dermatomyositis and polymyositis: a population-based study. Lancet 2001;357:96–100.

49. Benbassat J, Gefel D, Larholt K, Sukenik S, Morgenstern V, Zlotnick A. Prognostic factors in polymyositis/dermatomyositis. Arthritis Rheum 1985; 28:249–255.

50. Maugars Y, Berthelot JM, Abbas A, Mussini JM, Nguyen JM, Prost A. Long-term prognosis of 69 patients with dermatomyositis or polymyositis. Clin Exp Rheumatol 1996;14:263–274.

51. Marie I, Hachulla E, Hatron PY, et al. Polymyositis and dermatomyositis: short term and longterm outcome, and predictive factors of prognosis. J Rheumatol 2001;28:2230–2237.

52. Medsger TA, Robinson H, Masi A. Factors affecting survivorship in polymyositis. A life–table study of 124 patients. Arthritis Rheum 1971;14:249–258.

53. Lilley H, Dennet X, Byrne E. Biopsy proven polymyositis in Victoria 1982–1987: analysis of prognostic factors. J R Soc Med 1994;87:323–326.

54. Clarke AE, Bloch DA, Medsger TA, Oddis CV. A longitudinal study of functional disability in a national cohort of patients with polymyositis/dermatomyositis. Arthritis Rheum 1995;38:1218–1224.

55. Ponyi A, Borgulya G, Constantin T, Vancsa A, Gergely L, Danko K. Functional outcome and quality of life in adult patients with idiopathic inflammatory myositis. Rheumatology (Oxford) 2005;44:83–88.

56. Sultan S, Ioannou Y, Moss K, Isenberg D. Outcome in patients with idiopathic inflammatory myositis: morbidity and mortality. Rheumatology 2002;41:22–26.

57. Rose M, McDermott M, Thornton C, Palenski C, Martens W, Griggs R. A prospective natural history study of inclusion body myositis: implications for clinical trials. Neurology 2001;57:548–550.

58. Felice KJ, North WA. Inclusion body myositis in Connecticut. Observations in 35 patients during an 8-year period. Medicine (Baltimore) 2001;80:320–327.

59. Lacomis D, Chad DA, Smith TW. Myopathy in the elderly: evaluation of the histopathologic spectrum and the accuracy of clinical diagnosis. Neurology 1993;43:825–828.

60. Engel AG, Hohlfeld R, Banker BQ. Inflammatory myopathies. The polymyositis and dermatomyositis syndromes. In: Franzini-Armstrong C, ed. Myology. Vol. 2. McGraw-Hill, New York: 1994; pp.1335–1383.

61. Arahata K, Engel AG. Monoclonal antibody analysis of mononuclear cells in myopathies. I: Quantitation of subsets according to diagnosis and sites of accumulation and demonstration and counts of muscle fibers invaded by T-cells. Ann Neurol 1984;16:193–208.

62. Engel AG, Arahata K. Monoclonal antibody analysis of mononuclear cells in myopathies. II: phenotypes of autoinvasive cells in polymyositis and inclusion body myositis. Ann Neurol 1984;16:209–215.

63. Carpenter S, Karpati G, Rothman S, Watters G. The childhood type of dermatomyositis. Neurology 1976;26:952–962.

64. De Visser M, Emslie-Smith A, Engel A. Early ultrastructural alterations in adult dermatomyositis. Capillary abnormalities precede other structural changes in muscle. J Neurol Sci 1989;94:181–192.

65. Emslie-Smith AM, Engel AG. Microvascular changes in early and advanced dermatomyositis: a quantitative study. Ann Neurol 1990;27:343–356.

66. Kissel JT, Mendell JR, Rammohan KW. Microvascular deposition of complement membrane attack complex in dermatomyositis. N Engl J Med 1986;314:329–334.

67. Mendell JR, Sahenk Z, Gales T, Paul L. Amyloid filaments in inclusion body myositis. Novel findings provide insight into nature of filaments. Arch Neurol 1991;48:1229–1234.

68. Askanas V, Engel WK, Alvarez RB. Light and electron microscopic localization of ß-amyloid protein in muscle biopsies of patients with inclusion-body myositis. Am J Pathol 1992;141:31–36.

69. Askanas V, Serdaroglu P, Engel WK, Alvarez RB. Immunocytochemical localization of ubiquitin in inclusion body myositis allows its light mircroscopic distinction from polymyositis. Neurology 1992;42:460–461.

70. Prayson RA, Cohen ML. Ubiquitin immunostaining and inclusion body myositis: study of 30 patients with inclusion body myositis. Hum Pathol 1997;28:887–892.

71. Hochberg MC, Feldman D, Stevens MB. Adult onset polymyositis/dermatomyositis: an analysis of clinical and laboratory features and survival in 76 patients with a review of the literature. Semin Arthritis Rheum 1986;15:168–178.

72. Basset-Seguin N, Roujeau J-C, Gherardi R, Guillaume J-C, Revuz J, Touraine R. Prognostic factors and predictive signs of malignancy in adult dermatomyo111sitis. A study of 32 cases. Arch Dermatol 1990;126:633-637.

20 Idiopathic Hyper-CK-emia

1. INTRODUCTION

Idiopathic hyper-CK-emia is a term used to describe the finding of an elevated serum creatine kinase (CK) concentration in the absence of symptoms (or only minimal symptoms) that can be attributed to an underlying neuromuscular disease. The discovery of a high serum CK, even when asymptomatic or pauci-symptomatic, raises the prospect of an underlying neuromuscular disorder and typically prompts referral for further evaluation. The next diagnostic steps are likely to involve electromyography (EMG) and muscle biopsy. Questions arise, however, regarding the diagnostic yield of these investigations and the frequency with which a definitive diagnosis can be made and, more importantly, the frequency with which a disorder which warrants (and is likely to respond to) therapy can be identified. This chapter focuses on the diagnostic yield of EMG and muscle biopsy and the relationship between idiopathic hyper-CK-emia and the risk of malignant hyperthermia.

2. DIAGNOSIS

2.1. What Is the Utility of EMG in the Evaluation of Patients With Unexplained Hyper-CK-emia?

Because EMG is less invasive than muscle biopsy, there is a natural tendency to perform EMG in advance of deciding whether muscle biopsy should be performed. This approach raises the question of how well abnormalities on EMG predict the presence of pathological abnormalities on muscle biopsy. Unfortunately, there is a paucity of data in the literature that are helpful in trying to answer this question. The study by Prelle et al. *(1)* provides some useful information. This was a retrospective review of 114 patients with asymptomatic or minimally symptomatic hyper-CK-emia, 100 of whom underwent both electromyography and muscle biopsy. The data presented in this study (Table 20.1A) permit estimation of the accuracy of EMG for detecting pathological abnormalities on muscle biopsy. Sensitivity was 0.73 and specificity 0.53. EMG, therefore, is reasonably useful for excluding pathological abnormalities on muscle biopsy, as the rate of false negative (normal) EMG is only 27%. EMG, however, is not very useful for predicting which patients are likely to have pathological findings on muscle biopsy as an abnormal EMG is accompanied by a normal muscle biopsy in 47% of patients. EMG, therefore, is a reasonably good screening tool in that it will "pick up" the majority (73%) of patients who will have abnormalities on muscle biopsy. High specificity is not necessarily required for a good screening test.

From: *Neuromuscular Disease: Evidence and Analysis in Clinical Neurology*
By: M. Benatar © Humana Press Inc., Totowa, NJ

Table 20.1A

Predictive Value of Electromyography (EMG) for Abnormalities on Muscle Biopsy
in People With Unexplained Hyper-CK-emia

	Normal biopsy	Pathological biopsy	Totals
Normal EMG	32	11	43
Pathological EMG	28	29	57
Totals	60	40	100

Data from ref. *1*.

Table 20.1B

Predictive Value of Electromyography (EMG) for Abnormalities on Muscle Biopsy
in People With Unexplained Hyper-CK-emia

	Normal biopsy	Pathological biopsy	Totals
Normal EMG	4	1	5
Pathological EMG	0	14	14
Totals	4	15	19

Data from ref. *2*.

The problem with these data is that the goal is not to identify pathological features on
muscle biopsy, but rather to make a definitive diagnosis. In the study by Prelle et al., the
term "pathologic biopsy" was used to refer to the results of routine histological and
histochemical analysis, but such abnormalities appeared to have limited value in predicting those patients in whom a definitive diagnosis will be made following the application
of more specialized testing such as immunohistochemistry and biochemical analysis. Of
the 21 definitive diagnoses established in the study by Prelle and colleagues *(1)*, 8 were
made in patients with normal muscle biopsy based on routine testing and a further 5 were
made in patients with mild nonspecific findings on routine histology and histochemistry.
The minority of definitive diagnoses, therefore, were made in samples that were felt to
be abnormal based on routine testing. Based on these results, the sensitivity of abnormalities on routine pathology for the establishment of a definitive diagnosis was only 62%.

In their study of 19 patients, Joy and Oh *(2)* also provided the results of both EMG and
muscle biopsy in each patient, permitting calculation of the sensitivity and specificity of
EMG for predicting which muscle biopsies are likely to be abnormal. The available data
also permit calculation of the sensitivity and specificity of EMG for predicting those
patients in whom a definitive diagnosis will eventually be made. Based on these data
(Tables 20.1B), the sensitivity of EMG for the finding of abnormal muscle biopsy is 93%
and the specificity is 100%. The sensitivity of EMG for a definitive diagnosis based on
muscle biopsy is 92% and the specificity is 57% (Table 20.2).

The available data, therefore, are conflicting. The data from the larger (*n* = 114) of the
two retrospective studies *(1)* suggest that EMG is not particularly helpful in predicting
which patients are likely to have an abnormal muscle biopsy, whereas the smaller study (*n*
= 19) suggests otherwise. Apart from the difference in sample size between the two studies,
it may be relevant to note that, compared with other studies *(1,3,4)*, the report by Joy and

Table 20.2
Predictive Value of Electromyography (EMG) for Definitive Diagnosis Following Muscle
Biopsy

	No definitive diagnosis	Definitive diagnosis	Totals
Normal EMG	4	1	5
Pathological EMG	3	11	14
Totals	7	12	19

Data from ref. 2.

Oh (2) stands out as an exception in the high frequency with which a definitive diagnosis
was made. Notwithstanding these differences, the two studies are in agreement that EMG
is a useful screening test to determine which patients should undergo muscle biopsy.

2.2. What Is the Diagnostic Yield of Muscle Biopsy in Patients With Pauci- or Asymptomatic Hyper-CK-emia?

It is not surprising that the diagnostic yield of muscle biopsy depends on the extent of the
testing that is performed on the pathological sample. Such testing may include (1) routine
histological and histochemical study (hematoxilin and eosin, modified Gomori trichrome,
cytochrome c oxidase, succinate dehydrogenase, NADH dehydrogenase, adenosine triph-
osphatase at acid and alkaline pH, acid phosphatase, period-acid Schiff, and oil red O), (2)
immunohistochemistry (with antibodies directed against dystrophin, the sarcoglycans,
merosin, dysferlin, desmin, and caveolin) and (3) biochemical analysis (phosphorylase,
phosphorylase b kinase, phosphofructokinase, phosphoglycerate kinase, phosphorglycerate
mutase, lactate dehydrogenase, and carnitine palmitoyltransferase). It might also be expected
that the diagnostic yield should increase together with our understanding of the pathobiology
of muscle disease and the development of an increasing number of diagnostic tests.

There have been a number of studies over the last 15 years that have reported the
diagnostic yield of muscle biopsy in series of patients with asymptomatic or minimally
symptomatic elevations of serum CK. The results have varied quite widely, with some
studies describing a high frequency (5,6) and others a low frequency (1,3,4) of specific
diagnoses. The explanation for these discrepancies lies, in part, in the details of how these
studies were performed.

Brewster and de Visser (5) retrospectively reviewed their records to identify 14 patients
with persistently elevated CK levels with normal neurological examination and no identifiable etiology based on the exclusion of thyroid disease, the lack of a family history of
neuromuscular disease, the absence of medications that might cause an elevation of CK
as well as nondiagnostic EMG and muscle biopsy studied by light microscopy. Upon
review, they were able to identify the cause of the increased CK level in 10 patients. In
eight patients, the elevated CK was attributed to strenuous physical activity, one patient
was found to have subclinical hypothyroidism, and two (including one in the physical
activity group) had myoadenylate deminase deficiency. The high diagnostic yield in this
study, therefore, was a function of the way in which the cases were initially defined. In
truth, none of the 14 patients was found unequivocally to have an underlying muscle

disease of any significance.* In their series of 19 patients with incidentally discovered persistent elevation of CK, Joy and Oh *(2)* found diagnostic abnormalities on muscle biopsy in 12 patients (63%) (Table 20.3).

The diagnostic yield of muscle biopsy has been much lower in most other studies. In the largest, albeit retrospective, series to date, Prelle et al. *(1)* examined 114 asymptomatic or minimally symptomatic subjects with persistent hyper-CK-emia. The muscle biopsy specimens were examined with all of the routine histological and histochemical methods as well as the immunohistochemical and biochemical studies listed at the beginning of this section. Despite this extensive array of tests, a definitive diagnosis was possible in only 21 patients (18.4%) (Table 20.3)

Simmons and colleagues reported the results of a similar (although not quite as extensive) array of diagnostic tests in 20 patients with unexplained hyper-CK-emia *(4)*. They were able to make a definitive diagnosis in six patients (30%) (Table 20.3).

In their retrospective review, Reijneveld and colleagues*(7)* reported the results of muscle biopsy in 31 patients with persistently elevated serum CK despite a normal neurological examination. In addition to routine studies, they obtained immunohistochemistry for dystrophin and sarcoglycan as well as measurement of lymphocyte α-glucosidase activity in most patients and ischemic exercise testing in about a third of patients. Muscle biopsy showed nondiagnostic abnormalities in 77% and was normal in the remainder. No definitive diagnoses were made, and patients remained clinically stable over a mean follow-up period of 7 years. Their conclusion was that idiopathic hyper-CK-emia is not a prelude to a neuromuscular disorder if adequate initial ancillary investigations have been performed. This conclusion, however, should be tempered by the fact that the array of diagnostic tests performed on each muscle biopsy specimen was somewhat limited.

This review of the available literature shows that widely varying rates of definitive diagnosis have been reported following muscle biopsy (Table 20.3). The variation cannot be attributed to differences in the specific immunohistochemical and biochemical tests that were performed, because two of the studies with low diagnostic yields *(1,4)* included the widest array of diagnostic tests. With the exception of the study by Joy and Oh *(2)*, in which muscle biopsy led to the diagnosis of polymyositis in a number of patients, the remaining studies did not yield diagnoses for which there are currently any recognized forms of treatment. If muscle biopsy is to be undertaken in patients with persistently elevated asymptomatic or minimally symptomatic hyper-CK-emia, it is important for the patient and physician to recognize that the diagnostic yield is relatively low (probably around 18–30%) and that the likelihood of making a definitive diagnosis is highly dependent on the availability of advanced immunohistochemical and biochemical testing. Finally, it is extremely unlikely that a treatable myopathy will be discovered.

3. TREATMENT

There are no published data to suggest that idiopathic hyper-CK-emia requires treatment.

---

* The entity of myoadenylate deminase (MADA) deficiency remains controversial, with most authorities not recognizing it as a real diagnostic entity of any significance.

Table 20.3
Frequency of Definitive Diagnoses in Idiopathic Hyper-CK-emia

Reference	n	Definitive diagnosis	Diagnoses
Joy *(2)*	19	12 (63%)	Polymyositis ($n = 5$)
			Mitochondrial myopathy ($n = 2$)
			Central core disease ($n = 1$)
			Multicore myopathy ($n = 1$)
			Sarcoid myopathy ($n = 1$)
			Inclusion body myositis ($n = 1$)
			McArdle's disease ($n = 1$)
Prelle *(1)*	114	21 (18%)	Dystrophinopathy ($n = 5$)
			Carnitine palmitoyl transferase deficiency ($n = 4$)
			Malignant hyperthermia ($n = 3$)
			Mitochondrial myopathy ($n = 2$)
			Desminopathy ($n = 1$)
			Tubular aggregate myopathy ($n = 1$)
			Central core myopathy ($n = 1$)
			Myoadenylate deaminase deficiency ($n = 1$)
			Dysferlinopathy ($n = 1$)
			Myotonia fluctuans ($n = 1$)
			Limb girdle muscular dystrophy ($n = 1$)
Simmons *(4)*	20	6 (30%)	Phosphorylase b kinase deficiency ($n = 3$)
			Carnitine palmitoyl transferase deficiency ($n = 2$)
			Myoadenylate deaminase deficiency ($n = 1$)
Reijnveld *(7)*	31	0	–

4. PROGNOSIS

4.1. Is the Presence of Idiopathic Hyper-CK-emia a Risk Factor for Malignant Hyperthermia?

In order to answer this question, it is necessary to distinguish it from two related questions. The first is whether serum CK levels can be used as a screening test to identify patients at risk for developing malignant hyperthermia during general anesthesia. The second is whether there is a correlation between the malignant hyperthermia genetic trait and the presence of raised levels of CK in certain families. The latter two questions are relevant insofar as they should not be confused with the question of whether patients with idiopathic hyper-CK-emia are at an increased risk for developing malignant hyperthermia, and hence whether any special precautions are required when these patients undergo general anesthesia.

Any attempt to answer this question is complicated by the criteria used to identify patients with malignant hyperthermia. The syndrome is characterized by a rapid rise in body temperature, acidosis, hyperkalemia, and muscle rigidity following exposure to "triggering" anesthetic agents such as halothane and enflurane, commonly used inhalational anesthetics. The trait is inherited in an autosomal dominant fashion. One difficulty is that a susceptible individual may have a history of prior uncomplicated anesthesia,

Table 20.4
Association Between Increased Creatine Kinase (CK) Concentration and Malignant
Hyperthermia

Diagnosis	Elevated CK	Normal CK	Totals
Malignant hyperthermia	1	1	2
No malignant hyperthermia	108	1690	1798
Totals	109	1691	1800

which complicates identification of which individuals carry the susceptibility trait. The
in vitro muscle contraction test has been developed in an effort to identify muscle biopsy
specimens that show abnormal reactivity to halothane and caffeine, as a means of predicting who is at risk for the development of malignant hyperthermia in response to these
"triggering" agents. But the sensitivity and specificity of this test are unknown because
a gold standard for the diagnosis of malignant hyperthermia is lacking.

The prospective population-based study by Amaranath and colleagues (8) provides the
best evidence that serum CK lacks both sensitivity and specificity as a screening tool for
the diagnosis of malignant hyperthermia. This study included 1800 consecutive healthy
subjects undergoing outpatient surgery. Serum CK was measured as part of their routine
pre-anesthetic evaluation. Patients with malignant hyperthermia were identified on the
basis of a prior documented history of the syndrome or the development of the classic
signs during the actual anesthetic. Only two patients with malignant hyperthermia were
identified, and CK was elevated in 109 subjects, including one of the malignant hyperthermia patients. As shown in Table 20.4, the sensitivity and specificity of serum CK for
the diagnosis of malignant hyperthermia are 50% and 94%, respectively. The positive
predictive value (defined as the number of true positives divided by all positive test
results) is less than 1%. Expressed another way, for every true positive result, there are
100 false-positive results. Elevated serum CK concentration, therefore, is a poor screening test for identifying those at risk for malignant hyperthermia.

The sensitivity and positive predictive value of any diagnostic test are dependent on
the frequency of the disease in question. It might be asked, therefore, whether elevated
CK is a more useful marker of predisposition to malignant hyperthermia in a group of
high-risk patients. The studies by Paasuke and Bronwell (9) and Ellis and colleagues (10)
were designed to answer this question. Paasuke and Bronwell performed muscle biopsy
and in vitro caffeine contracture studies in patients selected either because of a suspected
malignant hyperthermia reaction under anesthesia or because they were relatives of
patients known to have malignant hyperthermia. Although the mean CK level was slightly
higher in the group of 34 patients with malignant hyperthermia, the levels were all within
the normal range, as were those in the 87 patients without malignant hyperthermia. They
appropriately concluded that CK levels are not useful in the identification of patients with
malignant hyperthermia. Ellis and colleagues (10) performed in vitro halothane contracture testing in 52 patients selected for being at risk for malignant hyperthermia based on
personal or family history. They found significant overlap in the CK concentrations
between patients with and without malignant hyperthermia, and similarly concluded that

serum CK level was unhelpful in predicting which patients were susceptible to malignant hyperthermia.

These studies, therefore, establish that elevation of serum CK is not helpful in predicting subjects at risk of malignant hyperthermia, irrespective of the prevalence of the syndrome in the population under investigation.

A related, but slightly different, question is whether in vitro contracture testing should be performed in patients with elevated serum CK concentration in order to determine which patients are at risk of developing malignant hyperthermia. This question has been the subject of two studies. In a small retrospective study, Lingaraju and Rosenberg performed in vitro halothane contracture testing in seven patients with persistently elevated CK levels *(11)* and found that three patients were susceptible to the development of malignant hyperthermia. In a larger study, Weglinski and colleagues *(12)* performed in vitro contracture testing in 49 patients with persistently elevated CK levels. On the basis of a positive response either to halothane of caffeine, they found that 24 patients were susceptible to the development of malignant hyperthermia. The results of these two studies suggest that the frequency of malignant hyperthermia is substantially higher in a population of patients with unexplained elevation of CK concentration compared to the general population in whom the prevalence is estimated to be approximately 1 in 50,000.

The final word, therefore, has not yet been said on the subject of whether patients with persistently elevated CK levels should undergo in vitro contracture testing. On the basis of the results presented here, some authors have recommended that contracture testing be considered as part of the work-up of these patients, especially once a decision has been made to undertake muscle biopsy for general diagnostic purposes *(12)*.

5. SUMMARY

- On the basis of the available data it ,might reasonably be argued that EMG is a useful screening test (in advance of muscle biopsy) in the evaluation of patients with pauci- or asymptomatic hyper-CK-emia.
- Most of the available literature supports the conclusion that the diagnostic yield of muscle biopsy is relatively low (18–30%) in asymptomatic patients with elevated serum CK concentrations.
- The likelihood of making a definitive diagnosis is highly dependent on the availability of advanced immunohistochemical and biochemical testing.
- It is extremely unlikely that muscle biopsy in patients with asymptomatic elevation in serum CK will lead to a the diagnosis of a treatable myopathy.
- There is no consensus as to whether subjects with persistently elevated serum CK should undergo muscle biopsy and in vitro muscle contracting testing to determine their risk for malignant hyperthermia.

REFERENCES

1. Prelle A, Tancredi L, Sciacco M, et al. Retrospective study of a large population of patients with asymptomatic or minimally symptomatic raised serum creatine kinase levels. J Neurol 2002;249:305–311.
2. Joy JL, Oh SJ. Asymptomatic hyper-CK-emia: an electrophysiologic and histopathologic study. Muscle Nerve 1989;12:206–209.

3. Kleppe B, Reimers CD, Altmann C, Pongratz DE. [Findings in 100 patients with unexplained hyperCKemia]. Med Klinik (Munich) 1995;90:623–627.

4. Simmons Z, Peterlin BL, Boyer PJ, Towfighi J. Muscle biopsy in the evaluation of patients with modestly elevated creatine kinase levels. Muscle Nerve 2003;27:242–244.

5. Brewster L, de Visser M. Persistent hyperCKemia: fourteen patients studied in retrospect. Acta Neurologica Scandinavica 1988;77:60–63.

6. Galassi G, Rowland LP, Hays AP, Hopkins LC, DiMauro S. High serum levels of creatine kinase: asymptomatic prelude to distal myopathy. Muscle Nerve 1987;10:346–350.

7. Reijneveld JC, Notermans NC, Linssen WH, Wokke JH. Bengin prognosis in idiopathic hyper-CK-emia. Muscle Nerve 2000;23:575–579.

8. Amaranath L, Lavin TJ, Trusso RA, Boutros AR. Evaluation of creatine phosphokinase screening as a predictor of malignant hyperthemia. A prospective study. Br J Anaesth 1983;55:531–533.

9. Paasuke RT, Brownell AK. Serum creatine kinase level as a screening test for susceptibility to malignant hyperthermia. JAMA 1986;255:769–771.

10. Ellis FR, Clarke I, Modgill M, Currie S, Harriman D. Evaluation of creatine phosphokinase in screening patients for malignant hyperpyrexia. Br Med J 1975;3:511–513.

11. Lingaraju N, Rosenberg H. Unexplained increases in serum creatine kinase levels: its relation to malignant hyperthermia susceptibility. Anesth Analg 1991;72:702–705.

12. Weglinski MR, Wedel DJ, Engel AG. Malignant hyperthermia testing in patients with persistently increased serum creatine kinase levels. Anesthe Analg 1997;84:1038–1041.

21 Statin-Induced Myopathy

1. INTRODUCTION

Statins (3-hydroxy-3-methylglutaryl-coezyme A [HMG-CoA] reductase inhibitors) are a highly effective group of cholesterol-lowering drugs. Although generally well tolerated, they may exert a toxic effect on skeletal muscle. In considering the myotoxicity of the statins, it is helpful to make a distinction between minimally or asymptomatic elevations in serum creatine kinase (CK) concentrations on the one hand, and the presentation with myositis or rhabdomyolysis on the other. In the relevant literature, significant elevations of serum CK concentration are taken to be those that are at least 9–10 times the upper limit of normal. Asymptomatic or minimally symptomatic patients with such elevations of CK have been distinguished from those with myositis (muscle pain and/or weakness) that is accompanied by a marked (greater than 10 times the upper limit of normal) elevation of serum CK concentration. The term "rhabdomyolysis" has variably been used to describe this latter syndrome, especially when accompanied by renal failure. In some studies, the term rhabdomyolysis is reserved for those in whom the CK concentration is at least 40 times the upper limit of normal. The potential for such severe statin-induced myotoxicity achieved particular prominence following the voluntary withdrawal of cerivastatin from the US market in 2001 because of the apparently high risk of rhabdomyolysis. Notwithstanding this adverse publicity, the statins remain a frequently prescribed class of dugs given their efficacy in reducing the risk of coronary heart disease.

The frequent use of statins together with the increased recognition of their potential for myotoxicity had led to the use of serum CK measurement as a screening tool to identify patients with drug-induced muscle injury. But this practice raises a number of important questions. What is the significance of the finding of an elevated serum CK concentration in patients taking a statin? Does it matter whether the raised CK occurs in the context of symptoms attributable to muscle disease or whether the patient is entirely asymptomatic? Is the magnitude of the CK elevation helpful in deciding whether it is safe to continue statin therapy or whether the medication should be discontinued? Is the statin-induced increase in CK concentration simply due to the toxic effect of the drug or has the statin somehow unmasked an underlying (previously undetected) muscle disease? For how long does the CK elevation persist following discontinuation of the statin?

In order to think rationally about these issues, however, it is helpful to have an idea of the frequency with which statins cause a rise in serum CK and the extent to which this finding is attributable solely to the use of the statin rather than to the use of a statin in combination with other drugs.

From: *Neuromuscular Disease: Evidence and Analysis in Clinical Neurology*
By: M. Benatar © Humana Press Inc., Totowa, NJ

2. DIAGNOSIS

2.1. What Is the Frequency With Which Statins Cause Asymptomatic Hyper-CK-emia?

The diagnosis of statin-induced myotoxicity is usually considered when a patient who has been taking a statin either reports symptoms such as myalgias and weakness or is found to have an elevated serum CK concentration on routine blood work. There has been almost nothing published on the subject of the accuracy of various tests (serum CK, electromyography [EMG], and muscle biopsy) for the diagnosis of myopathy. This may reflect the lack of consensus regarding the gold standard for the diagnosis of statin-induced myotoxicity. Is the presence of myopathic symptoms sufficient to make the diagnosis, or is an elevation in serum CK required? Are the EMG and findings on muscle biopsy always abnormal? In the absence of answers to these questions, the presumption that the statin is responsible for the symptoms and/or elevation in serum CK is typically based on (1) the recognition that statins may cause myotoxicity and (2) the temporal sequence between the initiation of the drug (or change in dose) and the onset of symptoms. It is relevant, therefore, to consider the frequency with which statins are associated with an increase in serum CK concentration. In an effort to address this question, it is helpful to begin with a review of what is known about the incidence of hyper-CK-emia in patients receiving statin therapy.

The safety and efficacy of the first-generation statins (lovastatin, pravastatin, and simvastatin) have been evaluated in a series of large clinical trials involving more than 50,000 patients. The myotoxicity data from these studies in summarized in Table 21.1.

In their systematic review of all of the randomized controlled statin trials, Thompson and colleagues (1) reported similar results. Among 42,323 patients who were treated with statins, they identified 49 (~0.1%) with CK elevations greater than 10 times the upper limit of normal. CK elevations of a similar magnitude were found in a comparable number (44 of 41,535) of patients in the placebo group.

In summary, therefore, the combined data from these studies suggest that the first-generation statins are associated with a low risk of myotoxicity, and that this risk appears to be no greater than that observed in patients treated with placebo. The observed frequency of mild elevations of CK has varied from 0.1% to 11% in different studies. The frequency of more marked increases in serum CK (to greater than 10 times the upper limit of normal) is more constant, varying between 0.1% and 0.6%. These data seem to conflict with the clinical impression that statin use is indeed associated with symptoms of myotoxicity and elevations in serum CK concentration. This discrepancy is partially addressed by postmarketing surveillance data (discussed in the following section), but may only be resolved with further studies.

2.2. What Is the Risk of Statin-Induced Myositis and/or Rhabdomyolysis?

The risk of myositis and rhabdomyolysis are considered together, in part because both represent examples of symptomatic myotoxicity, and in part because of the variable definitions used to distinguish the two. In the Heart Protection Study (4) and the Prospective Pravastatin Pooling Project (5), for example, myopathy was defined as the presence

Table 21.1
Statin-Induced Hyper-CK-emia in Randomized Controlled Trials

Study	Asymptomatic mild ↑ CK		Asymptomatic moderate ↑ CK	
	Active drug	Placebo	Active drug	Placebo
PPP (5)[a]	578/5245 (11%)	561/5233 (11%)	9/5245 (0.2%)	2/5233 (<0.1%)
4S (2)	Not reported	Not reported	6/2221 (0.2%)	1/2223 (<0.1%)
AFCAPS (3)	Not reported	Not reported	21/3242 (0.6%)	21/3248 (0.6%)
HPS (4)[b]	19/10269 (0.2%)	13/10267 (0.1%)	11/10269 (0.1%)	6/10267 (<0.1%)

CK, creatine kinase; PPP, Prospective Pravastatin Pooling; 4S, Scandinavian Simvastatin Survival Study; AFCAPS, Air Force/Texas Coronary Atherosclerosis Prevention Study; HPS, Heart Protection Study.

[a]Mild increase defined as 1.5–9 times the upper limit of normal; moderate increase defined as >9 times the upper limit of normal.
[b]Mild increase defined as 4–10 times the upper limit of normal; moderate increase defined as >10 times the upper limit of normal.

of muscle symptoms in association with a CK elevation to greater than 10 times the upper limit of normal. The term "rhabdomyolysis" was used when the CK rose to greater than 40 times the upper limit of normal *(4)*. Based on these definitions, the combined incidence of myopathy and rhabdomylolysis are summarized in Table 21.2.

Postmarketing surveillance data indicate that rhabdomyolysis may occur more frequently than was initially suggested by these randomized controlled trials. Thompson and colleagues *(1)* reviewed the Food and Drug Administration (FDA) Adverse Event Reporting System database and identified 3339 cases of statin-associated rhabdomyolysis during the 12-year period 1990–2002. Fifty-seven percent of these cases were associated with the use of cerivastatin (that has since been withdrawn from the market), with each of the other statins associated with a smaller number of cases—simvastatin (18%), atorvastatin (11.5%), pravastatin (7.3%), lovastatin (4.4%), and fluvastatin (1.6%). These data should be interpreted with caution, as they rely on voluntary physician reporting and do not employ a uniform definition of rhabdomyolysis. Based on these data and estimates of the number of statin prescriptions, the reported rates of fatal rhabdomyolysis for the various statins are estimated as follows: lovastatin 0.19, pravastatin 0.04, simvastatin 0.12, fluvastatin 0, atrovastatin 0.04, and cerivastatin 3.16 *(6)*. These rates are not true incidence rates and are likely to be underestimates given that they are based on voluntary physician reporting, and that the number of prescriptions was used as the denominator rather than the number of patients actually using the relevant drug.

2.3. Is Statin-Induced Myotoxicity Simply Due to the Toxic Effect of the Drug, or has the Statin Unmasked an Underlying (Previously Undetected) Muscle Disease?

The observation that the majority of patients with only mildly symptomatic or asymptomatic elevations in serum CK may recover spontaneously despite continuation of the medication argues against the presence of an underlying, previously undetected muscle disease. The time course with which serum CK can be expected to return to normal is unclear. Whether the persistent elevation of serum CK despite discontinuation of the offending drug is more suggestive of an underlying myopathy is unclear. Similarly, whether instances of rhabdomyolysis represent the unmasking of an underlying myopathy is a question that is not readily answered based on the available data.

3. TREATMENT

That statin-induced symptomatic muscle disease with marked elevation of CK, together with potential or actual renal damage, mandates discontinuation of the drug is little debated. More controversial, perhaps, is the appropriate response to mildly or asymptomatic elevations in serum CK concentrations in patients using statins.

Discontinuation of the offending agent is often recommended on intuitive grounds, but there are no published studies that indicate whether such measures are always required. Furthermore, there are no published studies that support the use of any particular treatment for statin-induced myopathy.

Table 21.2
Statin-Induced Rhabdomyolysis in Randomized Controlled Trials

	Myopathy/rhabdomyolysis	
Study	Active drug	Placebo
PPP (5)	0/5245	0/5233
4S (2)	1/2221 (< 0.1%)	0/2223
AFCAPS/TexCAPS (3)	1/3242 (< 0.1%)	2/3248 (< 0.1%)
HPS (4)	10/10269 (<0.1%)	4/10267 (< 0.1%)

PPP, Prospective Pravastatin Pooling; 4S, Scandinavian Simvastatin Survival Study; AFCAPS/TexCAPS, Air Force/Texas Coronary Atherosclerosis Prevention Study; HPS, Heart Protection Study.

4. PROGNOSIS

4.1. What Is the Natural History of Statin-Induced Asymptomatic Hyper-CK-emia?

There is relatively little data to inform on this question. In the Scandinavian Simvastatin Survival Study (2), six patients treated with active drug developed an asymptomatic rise in serum CK to greater than 10 times the upper limit of normal. The study reports that this degree of elevation was not maintained in repeated samples, but no further information is provided. Similarly, in the Air Force/Texas Coronary Atherosclerosis Prevention Study (AFCAPS/TexCAPS) study (3), there were 21 patients with CK elevations to greater than 10 times the upper limit of normal. Twenty of these patients recovered while on treatment and the remaining patient, after a brief interruption of therapy, resumed statin treatment without a subsequent rise in serum CK. Neither the Heart Protection Study (4) nor the Prospective Pravastatin Pooling Project (5) reported the outcome of patients with asymptomatic elevations in serum CK. The available data, therefore, although limited, suggest that the natural history of asymptomatic statin-induced hyper-CK-emia is relatively benign. It is perhaps relevant to note that no differences in outcome were observed between those with mild and more marked asymptomatic elevations in CK.

4.2. What Are the Risk Factors for Statin-Induced Myositis/ Rhabdomyolysis?

The risk of statin-induced rhabdomyolysis increases with serum concentration of these drugs. Serum concentration is increased by factors that affect the volume of distribution (such as body size and gender) as well as factors that reduce drug metabolism (impaired renal and hepatic function, advancing age, hypothyroidism, diabetes, and concomitant use of medications that inhibit the cytochrome P-450 system).

Lovastatin, simvastatin, and atorvastatin are primarily metabolized by the cytochrome P450 3A4 system. Fluvastatin is metabolized by cytochrome P450 2C9 and pravastatin is primarily excreted by the kidneys with minimal metabolism by the cytochrome P450 system. Cerivastatin is metabolized by both the P450 3A4, and 2C8 systems, a feature of the drug design that was thought would, but did not, reduce the risk of rhabdomyolysis. Medications that inhibit CytP450 3A4 such as the macrolide antibiotics, azole antifungals, and cyclosporine, increase serum concentrations of selected statins and hence the risk of rhabdomyolysis. Glucuronidation is probably also important in the excretion of statins and relevant to the effect of gemfibrozil in increasing the risk of statin-induced rhabdomyolysis. Fifty-eight percent of the 1339 cases reported to the FDA over the 12-year period from 1990 to 2002 were associated with the use of drugs that are known to affect the metabolism of statins (1). Based on these data, concomitant use of certain medications has the effect of approximately doubling the risk of statin-induced myositis/rhabdomyolysis.

5. SUMMARY

- The evidence that informs on the questions about statin-induced myotoxicity that are addressed in this chapter is extremely limited. The result is that conclusions are based more on "expert" opinion than on evidence.
- Broadly speaking, there are three grades of severity of statin-induced myotoxicity: (1) asymptomatic, mild-to-moderate elevation in serum CK (up to nine times the upper limit of normal), (2) asymptomatic, marked increase in serum CK (greater than 10 times the upper limit of normal), and (3) symptomatic elevation in serum CK concentration.
- Mild, asymptomatic elevations of CK may occur in an many as 11% of patients treated with a statin.
- Moderate-to-marked increases in serum CK occur in approximately 0.1% to 0.6% of patients treated with a statin.
- Myositis and/or rhabdomyolysis occurs in approximately 0.1% of statin-treated patients.
- Symptoms matter. The available data suggest that the natural history of asymptomatic statin-induced hyper-CK-emia is relatively benign.
- Size matters. The greater the rise in serum CK, the greater the likelihood of symptoms and progression to rhabdomyolysis.
- Based on these data and the guidelines issued by the ACA/AHA/NHLBI clinical advisory on statins (7), the following recommendations can be made:
  1. Obtain baseline CK measurement prior to the initiation of statin therapy. This recommendation is based on the reasoning that asymptomatic CK elevations are common and knowledge of the pretreatment CK concentration will prove useful in subsequent evaluation and management.
  2. Routine measurement of CK concentration in asymptomatic individuals is not necessary, but it is reasonable to measure the CK concentration in response to the report of muscle symptoms.
  3. Statin therapy should be discontinued if the CK is elevated to greater than 10 times the upper limit of normal in symptomatic patients.
  4. Statin therapy may be continued if the CK is elevated to less than 10 times the upper limit of normal, but close monitoring of symptoms and CK concentration is prudent.
  5. Caution should be exercised when prescribing statin therapy for those at increased risk for myotoxicity. Risk factors for myotoxicity are summarized as follows:
     – Advancing age (especially over the age of 80 years)
     – Female gender

- Small body frame and frailty
- Multisystem disease (diabetes, renal failure, hepatic failure)
- Concurrent drug therapy (Fibric acid derivatives, especially gemfibrozil, Macrolide antibiotics, Azole anti-fungals, Cyclosporine, HIV protease inhibitors, Nefazodone, Amiodarone, Verapamil)
- Perioperative period

REFERENCES

1. Thompson PD, Clarkson P, Karas RH. Statin-association myopathy. JAMA 2003;289:1681–1690.
2. Randomised trial of cholesterol lowering in 4444 patients with coronary heart disease: the Scandinavian Simvastatin Survival Study (4S). Lancet 1994; 344:1383–1389.
3. Downs JR, Clearfield M, Tyroler A, et al. Air Force/Texas Coronary Atherosclerosis Prevention Study (AFCAPS/TexCAPS): additional perspectives on tolerability of long-term treatment with lovastatin. Am J Cardiol 2001;87:1074–1079.
4. MRC/BHF Heart Protection Study of cholesterol lowering with simvastatin in 20,536 high-risk individuals: a randomised placebo-controlled trial. Lancet 2002; 360:7–22.
5. Pfeffer MA, Keech A, Sacks FM, et al. Safety and tolerability of pravastatin in long-term clinical trials. Prospective Pravastatin Pooling (PPP) Project. Circulation 2002;105:2341–2346.
6. Staffa JA, Chang J, Green L. Cerivastatin and reports of fatal rhabdomyolysis. N Engl J Med 2003;346:539–540.
7. Pasternak RC, Smith SC, Bairey-Merez CN, Grundy SM, Cleeman JI, Lenfant C. ACC/AHA/NHLBI clinical advisory on the use and safety of statins. J Am Coll Cardiol 2002;40:567–572.

22 Metabolic Myopathy

1. INTRODUCTION

1.1. Background

The metabolic myopathies are a group of disorders characterized by impaired energy production in muscle that results from inherited defects in glycogen, lipid, or mitochondrial metabolism. Although onset in the neonatal period and during infancy is typical of many of these disorders, others may present for the first time during adolescence of adulthood. The typical presentation in adolescence or adulthood is with either (1) dynamic (i.e., fluctuating) symptoms like myoglobinuria and muscle weakness related to exercise that resolve completely, or (2) static (present all the time) symptoms such as slowly progressive muscle weakness. The gold standard for the diagnosis of these disorders usually relies on biochemical analysis of a muscle biopsy specimen with demonstration of the specific enzymatic defect. Such testing, however, is not part of the routine evaluation of every muscle biopsy, and because biochemical evaluation of muscle requires special preparation of the tissue sample at the time of biopsy, it cannot be requested post hoc. The diagnosis of a metabolic myopathy, therefore, requires a high index of clinical suspicion so that the appropriate testing can be arranged at the time of muscle biopsy. What are the typical presentations of the adult-onset metabolic myopathies? And what is the utility of more readily available investigations such as serum creatine kinase (CK), electromyography (EMG), and the forearm exercise test in ranking the likelihood of the presence or absence of a metabolic myopathy? Questions such as these, relating to the diagnosis of metabolic myopathy, form the bulk of this chapter, although some attention is also paid to the role of therapeutic interventions such as dietary modifications (e.g., low-carbohydrate or low-fat diets) as well as supplements like creatine and coenzyme Q10.

1.2. Muscle Energy Metabolism

In order to understand this group of disorders, it is helpful to have some insight into normal muscle energy metabolism. Glycogen, glucose, and free fatty acids are the main energy substrates for muscle. Their metabolism produces adenosine triphosphate (ATP), the hydrolysis of which is required for muscle contraction and relaxation. Fatty acids (metabolized via β-oxidation) are the major substrate for energy at rest and during prolonged low-intensity exercise. Omega-oxidation of fatty acids in liver microsomes occurs during prolonged fasting with production of dicarboxylic acids that are transported to the mitochondria for β-oxidation. Aerobic glycolysis is the main energy source during

From: *Neuromuscular Disease: Evidence and Analysis in Clinical Neurology*
By: M. Benatar © Humana Press Inc., Totowa, NJ

dynamic forms of exercise such as walking or jogging. Anaerobic glycolysis is primarily responsible for the supply of energy under conditions of sustained high-intensity isometric muscle activity (e.g., lifting heavy objects), during which there is limited blood flow and oxygen supply to muscles. A detailed review of the relevant biochemical pathways is beyond the scope of this text.

Muscle metabolism of lipids occurs by way of β-oxidation of free fatty acids that are derived either from circulating very low density lipoproteins or from muscle stores of triglyceride. Once in the cytoplasm, short and medium chain fatty acids (up to 10 carbon atoms in length) can diffuse across the mitochondrial membrane where they undergo β-oxidation. The mitochondrial membrane is impermeable to long-chain fatty acids. Their entry into the mitochondrial matrix requires first that they be converted to their coenzyme-A thioesters (via long chain acyl-CoA synthetase). These long-chain acyl-CoA-thioesters then enter the mitochondrial matrix by way of the carnitine transport system. Using carnitine (that enters the cytosol via the plasma membrane carnitine transporter), carnitine palmitoyl-transferase (CPT)-I catalyzes the formation of long-chain-acylcarnitine esters at the outer mitochondrial membrane. Carnitine-acylcarnitine translocase (CACT) transports these acylcarnitine esters across the inner mitochondrial membrane in exchange for carnitine. CPT-II then catalyzes the reverse reaction of CPT-I, regenerating the long-chain acylcarnitine esters and free carnitine within the mitochondrial matrix. These long-chain acylcarnitine esters then undergo β-oxidation via a sequence of four enzymatic reactions (a dehydrogenase, a hydratase, a second dehydrogenase and finally a thioketolase) to produce long-chain acylcarnitines two carbon atoms shorter as well as an acetyl-CoA molecule that then enters the Krebs cycle. This intra-mitochondrial β-oxidation of fatty acids requires fatty acid carbon chain length-specific enzymes—short-chain, medium-chain, long-chain and very-long-chain acyl-CoA dehydrogenase (SCAD, MCAD, LCAD, and VLCAD). Unlike SCAD, MCAD and LCAD that are found within the mitochondrial matrix, VLCAD is located in the inner mitochondrial membrane. The last three enzymatic reactions of β-oxidation for very-long chain (VLC) fatty acids are accomplished by the trifunctional protein that is also located in the inner mitochondrial membrane.

Glycogen stores in muscle provide a substrate for energy production under both aerobic and anaerobic conditions via glycogenolysis and glycolysis. (Myo)phosphorylase is responsible for the conversion of glycogen to glucose-1-phosphate (which may then be converted to glucose-6-phosphate for glycolytic metabolism). Phosphorylase exists in a less active "b" form and a more active "a" form. Phosphorylase b kinase (PbK) catalyzes the conversion of phosphorylase from the less active to the more active form. Glycolysis proceeds via a series of enzymatic reactions catalyzed by phosphofructokinase (PFK), phosphoglycerate kinase (PGK), phosphoglycerate mutase (PGAM), and lactate dehydrogenase (LDH). Under anaerobic conditions, pyruvate, the end product of glycolysis, is converted to lactate. Under aerobic conditions, pyruvate undergoes oxidative decarboxylation via the pyruvate dehydrogenase complex to produce acetyl-coenzyme-A, which then enters the Krebs (citric acid) cycle.

Thus, both oxidation of pyruvate through the pyruvate dehydrogenase complex, and metabolism of fatty acyl-CoAs through β-oxidation, result in the production of acetyl-CoA which is then metabolized through the Krebs cycle. β-oxidation and metabolism through the Krebs cycle produce reducing equivalents that are passed along the electron transport chain. The electron transport chain comprises four multimeric protein complexes (I through IV) as well as two electron carriers, coenzyme Q (ubiquinone) and cytochrome c. The energy that is generated is used to create an electrochemical gradient across the mitochondrial membrane. A fifth multimeric protein complex (complex V) then converts the energy of this electrochemical gradient into ATP in a process known as oxidation-phosphorylation coupling.

2. DIAGNOSIS

2.1. What Are the Clinical Manifestations of Adult-Onset Metabolic Muscle Disease?

Metabolic muscle disease may manifest with either dynamic or static symptoms, or a combination of the two. Dynamic symptoms include exercise-induced muscle pain, stiffness, cramps, and weakness and, when severe, muscle breakdown (rhabdomyolysis) with attendant myoglobinuria (1). The term "exercise intolerance" describes the limitation of physical activity that results from some or all of these symptoms. Static symptoms comprise fixed (permanent) muscle weakness that may be slowly progressive over time (2–10). Because the differential diagnosis of each of these presentations differs (see Tables 22.1 and 22.2), each clinical syndrome will be considered separately. Certain disorders may have accompanying systemic manifestations such as hemolytic anemia in phosphofructokinase deficiency.

2.2. What Are the Most Common Inherited Metabolic Causes of Recurrent Myoglobinuria?

Only a few studies have addressed this question, with somewhat differing results depending on the population under study (1,11). In an effort to determine the relative frequency of the different hereditary enzyme defects that cause recurrent myoglobinuria, Tonin and colleagues retrospectively reviewed the biochemical results of 77 patients studied in New York over a 4-year period (1). They divided these subjects into two groups, those with at least one attack of confirmed myoglobinuria (CK > 20,000 or detection of myoglobin in the urine) and those with suspected myoglobinuria (based on exercise-induced myalgia and weakness with accompanying gross discoloration of urine). Biochemical studies for eight enzyme defects were routinely performed, including phosphorylase, PbK, PFK, PGK, PGAM, LDH, CPT, and myoadenylate deaminase (MAD). Overall, a specific enzyme defect was identified in 36 of 77 (46%) patients, with a greater proportion amongst those with confirmed myoglobinuria. CPT deficiency was most common (17 patients; 22%), followed by phosphorylase deficiency (10 patients; 13%) and PbK deficiency (4 patients; 5%) (1). In a study of similar design conducted in Finland, Löfberg and colleagues examined 22 patients with recurrent myoglobinuria (11). Tests for phosphorylase, PbK, PFK, CPT, and MAD were routinely performed. Overall, a specific enzymatic defect was identified in six patients (27%). Phosphorylase deficiency was found in four patients (18%), PbK deficiency in one patient, and PFK deficiency in one other (11). The differences in the frequency with which a definitive diagnosis was made (46% vs 27%) as well as the relative frequencies of the specific enzymatic defects (22% versus 0% with CPT deficiency) are likely the result of to the ethnic differences between the two study populations. Taken together, however, these data suggest that CPT

Table 22.1
Differential Diagnosis of Adult-Onset Hereditary Recurrent Myoglobinuria

Glycogen-storage diseases
    Myophosphorylase deficiency (McArdle's disease) *(99–101)*
    Phosphorylase b kinase deficiency *(25–27,29)*
    Phosphofructokinase deficiency (Tarui's disease) *(22,23)*
    Phosphoglycerate kinase deficiency *(102)*
    Phosphoglycerate mutase deficiency *(103–105)*
    Lactate dehydrogenase deficiency

Lipid storage diseases
    Carnitine palmitoyltransferase-II deficiency *(41–620)*
    Trifunctional protein deficiency *(106,107)*
    Very long-chain acyl-coenzyme A dehydrogenase deficiency *(108–111)*
    Medium chain acyl-coenzyme A dehydrogenase deficiency *(112)*

Mitochondrial disease
    Complex II *(113)*

and (myo)phosphorylase deficiency are, respectively, the most common lipid and glycogen storage diseases that cause recurrent myoglobinuria.

2.3. What Are the Most Common Inherited Metabolic Causes of Adult-Onset Fixed Muscle Weakness?

There are no published series of patients with suspected inherited metabolic myopathies manifesting as fixed muscle weakness in which extensive investigation has been performed. Furthermore, because most (if not all) of the literature on the subject comprises case reports and small case series, there are no reliable estimates of the relative frequencies with which the various metabolic myopathies are responsible for causing fixed muscle weakness. As shown in Table 22.2, the range of metabolic myopathies that cause fixed muscle weakness is quite narrow. Of these diseases, acid maltase deficiency would appear to be the most common, based simply on the number of published case reports. Debrancher disease, defective carnitine transport, acyl-CoA dehydrogenase deficiency and trifunctional protein deficiency appear to be quite uncommon, again based on the number of published case reports.

2.4. What Is the Clinical Phenotype of Adult-Onset McArdle's Disease, and How Useful Are Paraclinical Investigations for Confirming the Diagnosis?

McArdle's disease is the eponymous term used to describe (myo)phosphorylase deficiency, also known as glycogenosis type V. The overwhelming majority of patients describe symptoms of exercise intolerance, with only about one-half of the patients having episodes of myoglobinuria *(12,13)* (Table 22.3). It is said that symptoms are typically precipitated either by brief intense isometric muscle contraction (e.g. weight lifting) or less intense more sustained exercise dynamic exercise (e.g., climbing stairs) *(12)*, but the reliability with which such a specific exercise history can be obtained, is not clear. Around one-third of patients develop fixed muscle weakness *(12,13)*. How often

Table 22.2
Differential Diagnosis of Adult-Onset Progressive Muscle Weakness

Glycogen storage diseases
      Acid maltase deficiency *(7–10)*
      Debrancher deficiency *(4–6,30)*
      Phosphofructokinase deficiency (less common) *(22,23)*
      Phosphorylase b kinase deficiency (less common) *(27)*

Lipid storage diseases
      Muscle carnitine deficiency *(65–77)*

Mitochondrial diseases
      Complex I deficiency *(114–121)*
      Complex II deficiency *(113,122)*
      Complex III deficiency *(117,123–126)*
      Complex IV deficiency

Table 22.3
Myophosphorylase Deficiency (McArdle's Disease)

	No. of cases/all cases	*Percentage*
Exercise intolerance	146/166	87
Myoglobinuria	88 /166	53
+ renal failure	15/56	27
Fixed weakness	46/166	28
Muscle cramps[a]	50/54	93
Myalgia[a]	46/54	74
Wasting	13/112	12
Positive family history	51/97	53
Increased serum creatine kinase at rest	62/67	93
Abnormal forearm exercise test	55/55	100
Abnormal electromyography at rest	29/59	49
Undetectable phosphorylase activity (histochemistry)	56/74	76

    Denominator varies depending on the number of cases for which data is available for the clinical feature in question.

    [a]Muscle cramps and myalgia might have occurred alone or as part of a constellation of symptoms causing "exercise intolerance."

    Data from refs. *12,13*.

patients report only symptoms such as tiredness and poor stamina is not clear, but a number of investigators have described such patients. The series by Martin and colleagues, for example, included two children aged 6 and 8 years who only reported such nonspecific symptoms; in these cases, the diagnosis was suspected because of an affected older sibling *(13)*.

    Although the onset of symptoms is usually within the first decade of life, diagnosis is typically not made until well into adulthood *(12,13)*. Based on the few published case reports, it seems to be very uncommon for symptoms to begin only in adulthood *(14)*. A family history is present in only around one-half of all patients *(12)*.

Serum CK concentration (in between episodes of myoglobinuria) is increased in more than 90% of patients *(12,13)*. The forearm ischemic exercise test shows either an abnormally low or absent rise in venous lactate concentration in almost all patients *(12,13)*. Electromyographic examination (in between episodes of myoglobinuria) is abnormal in approximately 50% of patients *(12)*. Routine muscle biopsy may show sub-sarcolemmal glycogen deposits (stained with periodic acid-Schiff) or vacuolar changes within muscle fibers. Electron microscopy may similarly show the accumulations of glycogen. The frequency with which routine muscle biopsy shows such changes (either on light or electron microscopy), however, is unclear. A histochemical reaction for myosphosphorylase may be useful with staining of intramuscular blood vessels but not of normal muscle fibers. Using this technique, there is undetectable myophosphorylase activity in 75% of patients *(12,13)*; false-positive histochemical reactions may result from expression of a different isoenzyme in regenerating muscle fibers.

Although McArdle's disease is genetically heterogeneous, a nonsense point mutation (C-to-T) at codon 49 in exon 1 that changes an arginine (CGA) to a stop codone (TGA), is the most commonly encountered genetic defect in American *(15,16)* and British *(17)* subjects. In the American population this mutation was identified in 92 of 144 alleles (89%) *(15,16)*. These findings suggest that McArdle's disease may be diagnosed using genomic DNA isolated from peripheral blood lymphocytes in approximately 90% of patients, thus avoiding the need for a muscle biopsy.

2.5. What Is the Clinical Phenotype of Phosphofructokinase Deficiency, and How Useful Are Paraclinical Investigations for Confirming the Diagnosis?

The usual presentation of phosphofructokinase deficiency, also known as Tarui's disease or glycogenosis type VII, is clinically indistinguishable from myophosphorylase deficiency. Most (if not all) patients describe exercise intolerance, with around 60% also reporting episodes of myoglobinuria *(12,18–20)* (Table 22.4). There are three case reports of patients whose presentation was dominated by fixed (slowly progressive) muscle weakness rather than exercise intolerance, none of whom reported episodes of myoglobinuria *(21–23)*. A family history of similar affected individuals is present in one-third of cases *(24)*. Serum CK concentration is increased, and the forearm exercise test shows an abnormally small rise in venous lactate concentration in the majority (80–90%) of patients *(12,18–20,22–24)*. Evidence of compensated hemolysis (high bilirubin, increased lactate dehydrogenase, or mild reticulocytosis) may be present in as many as 80% of patients *(12,18–20,22,23)*, as a result of concomitant partial phosphofructokinase deficiency in red blood cells. Although abnormal insertional activity (fibrillations and positive sharp waves) is found in around one-half of patients with PFK deficiency *(18,20, 23)*, myopathic motor unit potentials (short duration, low-amplitude polyphasic units) have been reported only in patients with fixed muscle weakness *(22,23)*.

Routine muscle biopsy shows subsarcolemmal glycogen deposits (stained with periodic acid-Schiff) or vacuolar changes within muscle fibers, and electron microscopy similarly shows the accumulations of glycogen in most patients *(18,20,22,23)*. A specific stain for PFK permits histochemical diagnosis, but the sensitivity of this assay has not

Table 22.4
Phosphofructokinase Deficiency

	No. of cases/all cases	Percentage
Exercise Intolerance	25/25	100
Myoglobinuria	10/16	63
Renal failure	1/13	8
Fixed weakness	3/25	12
Muscle cramps	3/6	50
Nausea and vomiting with exercise	3/6	50
Positive family history	3/9	33
High serum creatine kinase	14/17	82
Abnormal forearm exercise test	13/14	93
Electromyography		
Myopathic	1/6	17
Mixed (neurogenic + myopathic)	1/6	17
Increased insertional activity	3/6	50
Hemolytic anemia	5/6	83
Subsarcolemmal glycogen accumulation	5/5	100

Data from refs. *12,18–20,22–24.*
Denominator varies depending on the number of cases for which data are available for the
clinical feature in question.

been determined. The gold standard for confirmation of the diagnosis is biochemical
testing of a muscle biopsy specimen, demonstrating PFK deficiency.

Tarui's disease is genetically heterogeneous. Unlike MrArdle's disease, in which a
single mutation accounts for most cases of the disease within British and American
populations, there is no predominant mutation in the PFK gene that would permit molecular diagnosis.

2.6. What Is the Clinical Phenotype of PbK Deficiency, and How Useful Are Paraclinical investigations for Confirming the Diagnosis?

PbK deficiency, as a cause of myopathy in adults, is probably quite uncommon, as
there are only 15 cases described in the literature *(25–29).* The gold standard for the
diagnosis is biochemical evidence of PbK deficiency in a muscle biopsy specimen.

The clinical profile of these patients is summarized in Table 22.5. Most (~87%) report
symptoms of exercise intolerance with cramps (40%) and myalgias (47%). Almost one-
half of the patients reported had episodes of recurrent myoglobinuria *(25–29).* Examination of strength is normal in most patients, but approximately one-third may have some
degree of weakness on examination, which may be either proximal *(26,29)* or distal *(27).*
All but two patients with weakness also had a history of recurrent myoglobinuria *(27,29)*
and there is only a single report of a patient with clinically detectable weakness, but no
history of exercise intolerance *(27).* Symptoms may begin either in childhood *(26–29)* or
as in adulthood *(25,27,29).* Among the 15 patients reported in the literature, the mean age
of onset was 23 years, with a range from 5 to 35 years. A family history of similarly
affected individuals is present in only a minority (21%) of patients.

Table 22.5
Phosphorylase b Kinase Deficiency

	No. of cases/all cases	Percentage
Exercise intolerance	13/15	87
Myoglobinuria	7/15	47
Fixed weakness	5/15	33
Muscle cramps	6/15	40
Myalgia	7/15	47
Positive family history	3/14	21
Increased serum creatine kinase	9/15	60
Abnormal forearm exercise test	4/11	36
Myopathic electromyography	4/10	40
Abnormal muscle biopsy	9/14	64

Data from refs. *25–29.*

Denominator varies depending on the number of cases for which data are available for the clinical feature in question.

CK is elevated in 60% of patients, with the increase varying from "slight" *(28)* to 1500 IU/liter *(26)*. Forearm exercise testing showed a blunted or absent venous lactate response in 4 of the 11 patients (36%) examined *(25–27,29)*, and EMG showed "myopathic" features in 4 of the 10 patients in whom it was performed *(25–27,29)*. Muscle biopsy was abnormal in 9 of the 14 patients, evidenced by increased staining with periodic acid-Schiff reaction as well as subsarcolemmal glycogen accumulation visible on electron microscopy *(25–27,29)*.

2.7. What Is the Clinical Phenotype of Debrancher Deficiency, and How Useful are Paraclinical Investigations for Confirming the Diagnosis?

Debrancher (amylo-1,6-glucosidase) deficiency, also known as type III glycogenosis, is usually a benign disease of childhood characterized by hepatomegaly and fasting hypoglycemia. It may, however, also present in adulthood as a syndrome of muscle weakness and wasting *(4–6,30)*. The extent to which the adult-onset myopathy represents the very first manifestation of the disease is difficult to determine from the literature, as the available case reports suggest that there may be a childhood history of hepatomegaly, fasting intolerance, or vague nonspecific symptoms such as difficulty keeping up physically with other children. For the purposes of this discussion, adult-onset is taken to mean that medical evaluation is first sought during adulthood for new symptoms related to muscle dysfunction.

The literature on debrancher deficiency comprises a few cases reports and small case series *(4–6,30,31)*. Patients typically present with static rather than dynamic symptoms (Table 22.6). Weakness is usually symmetric and may be either proximal *(5)* or distal *(4, 6)*. Wasting of distal muscles, especially the intrinsic muscles of the hand *(6)*, is characteristic occurring in approximately 63% of patients. The degree of weakness is usually mild (MRC grade 4 or better) *(30)*. There may be associated hepatomegaly *(5)* and cardiac dysfunction *(4,5,30)*. Family history of a similarly affected relative is present in only 40%

Table 22.6
Debrancher Deficiency

	No. of cases/all cases	Percentage
Fixed weakness	11/11	100
Proximal > distal	3/11	27
Proximal = distal	3/11	27
Proximal < distal	2/11	18
Unspecified	3/11	27
Muscle wasting	5/8	63
Cardiac involvement	8/10	80
Hepatomegaly	3/8	38
Positive family history	2/8	25
Increased serum creatine kinase	8/8	100
Abnormal forearm exercise test	9/9	100
Abnormal nerve conduction studies	3/8	38
Electromyography		
Myopathic	6/8	75
Neurogenic	2/8	25
Fibrillations, positive sharp waves	6/8	75
Abnormal glucose tolerance test	7/7	100
Abnormal muscle biopsy	10/10	100

Data from refs. *4–6,30,31*.

Denominator varies depending on the number of cases for which data are available for the clinical feature in question.

of cases *(4,6,30)*. Serum creatine kinase concentration is increased and the forearm exercise test shows a blunted or absent rise in venous lactate concentration in all patients *(4–6,30)*. Nerve conduction studies are abnormal, showing slowing of conduction velocity and prolongation of distal latency, in a small proportion of cases *(4,5)*. EMG may show either myopathic *(5,6)* or neurogenic *(5)* changes, with fibrillations and positive sharp waves identified in the majority of cases *(5,6,30)*. A "diabetic" response to glucose tolerance testing is seen in all patients *(4–6)* as is an abnormally low glucose response to the infusion of glucagon or epinephrine *(4–6,31)*. Muscle biopsy shows abnormal subsarcolemmal and intermyobrillary accumulations of glycogen on both light and electron microscopy in all patients *(4–6,30)*. The clinical and laboratory features of patients with debhrancher deficiency are summarized in Table 22.6.

In summary, therefore, adult-onset debrancher deficiency is a syndrome characterized by relatively mild muscle weakness, often with marked wasting of distal musculature. CK is invariably increased, and there is an abnormal glucose response to infusion of glucose, glucagon, or epinephrine. There may be an associated peripheral neuropathy and the EMG may show either myopathic or neurogenic changes (or a combination of the two), often in conjunction with fibrillations and positive sharp waves. Abnormal accumulations of glycogen are apparent on muscle biopsy with both light and electron microscopy.

Table 22.7
Acid Maltase Deficiency

	No. of cases/all cases	Percentage
Weakness	50/50	100
Proximal > distal	49/50	98
Pelvic > shoulder girdle	38/50	76
Respiratory	27/50	52
Respiratory > limb	10/50	20
Exercise intolerance	10/50	20
Family history	6/30	20
Increased creatine kinase[a]	48/50	96
Electromyography		
Myopathic	32/46	70
Fibrillations & positive sharps	15/46	33
Myotonic discharges	14/46	30
Muscle biopsy		
Vacuolar changes	37/49	76
Acid phosphatase staining	22/25	88

[a]CK increase was quite variable, but often only mildly elevated.
Data from refs. *7–10,32–40,127,128.*

2.8. What Is the Clinical Phenotype of Acid Maltase Deficiency, and How Useful Are Paraclinical Investigations for Confirming the Diagnosis?

Acid maltase (α-1,4-glucosidase) deficiency may present during infancy, during childhood, or in adulthood, with the clinical manifestations varying depending on the age of onset. The adult form of the disease typically presents as slowly progressive proximal muscle weakness *(7–10,32–35)*, with more severe involvement of the pelvic rather than the shoulder girdle *(7–10,33,34)* (Table 22.7). Respiratory muscle involvement is common, occurring in approximately 50% of cases *(7–10,32,33,35–38)*. Respiratory muscle weakness may occasionally be the presenting manifestation of the disease *(35–38)* and there may be a poor correlation between the severity of limb and respiratory muscle weakness *(7)*. Only around 20% of patients report a family history of a similarly affected relative *(8,9)*. Serum CK concentration is increased in 96% of patients, although the extent of the increase is quite variable and often only mildly elevated *(33–35)*. The EMG is usually, but not invariably, abnormal, showing myopathic motor units in around 70% of patients *(7,8,10,34,36–40)*. Myotonic discharges (in the absence of clinical myotonia) and fibrillations/positive sharp waves are seen in approximately 30% *(7,8,34)*. Routine muscle biopsy shows vacuolar changes in the majority of patients (~76%), and an even greater proportion (~88%) show positive histochemical staining with acid phosphatase *(7–10,32–36)* (Table 22.7).

In summary, adult-onset acid maltase deficiency is a disorder characterized by proximal muscle weakness (with or without wasting) that affects the pelvic girdle more severely than the shoulder girdle. Respiratory muscle involvement is common, and this may be the initial manifestation of the disease. There is no good correlation between the severity of

Table 22.8
Carnitine Palmitoyltransferase II Deficiency

	No. of cases/all cases	Percentage
Recurrent myoglobinuria	25/28	89
Precipitated by		
Prolonged exercise	22/28	79
Fasting (± exercise)	9/28	32
Infection	2/28	7
Exposure to cold (+ exercise)	1/28	4
No apparent cause	4/28	14
Renal failure	7/28	25
Fixed weakness	1/23	4
Positive family history	12/22	56
Increased serum creatine kinase at rest	7/19	37
Abnormal electromyography at rest	4/18	22
Increased lipid in muscle biopsy	7/27	26

Data from refs. *41–62*.

involvement of limb and respiratory muscles. A positive family history is uncommon. Serum CK is almost always increased, and EMG usually shows myopathic motor unit potentials. The diagnosis can usually be made with routine muscle biopsy showing vacuolar changes and positive histochemical staining for acid phosphatase.

2.9. What Is the Clinical Phenotype of CPT-II Deficiency, and How Useful Are Paraclinical Investigations for Confirming the Diagnosis?

CPT-II deficiency is a syndrome characterized by recurrent episodes of myoglobinuria *(41–60)*, occasionally accompanied by renal failure *(41,43,44,48,50,53,61)*. Attacks are typically, but not always, precipitated by prolonged exercise *(41–59)*, fasting, or a combination of the two *(43,46,55,57)* (Table 22.8). The age of onset of symptoms varies. Although onset is in the first two decades of life in about two-thirds of patients, symptoms may not begin until as late as the fifth decade. Unlike patients with recurrent myoglobinuria due to glycogen storage disease, those with CPT-II deficiency typically do not report exercise intolerance. Symptoms of muscle pain (myalgia), cramps, and weakness typically begin several hours after the period of sustained exercise, especially if undertaken while fasting. Because symptoms develop only after (rather than during) exercise, the onset of symptoms cannot serve as a warning signal to stop the exercise and thus perhaps abort the attack of myoglobinuria. When symptoms do develop, the symptoms may either be generalized or affect only the exercised muscles. In between attacks, there is typically no permanent weakness *(41–43,46–60)* and serum CK *(41,43,48,51,53,54, 57,58,60,61)* and EMG examination *(42,43,46,48,50,53–55,57–60,62)* are usually normal. Muscle biopsy may show lipid accumulation, but such findings are present in only about one-quarter of patients *(41,43,47,54,57,62)* and electron microscopy may be required to demonstrate this abnormality. A family history of similarly affected individuals is present in about one-half of all patients *(41–43,49–51,55,56,61)*.

The gold standard for the diagnosis of CPT-II deficiency remains biochemical evaluation of a fresh muscle biopsy specimen. Genetic mutational analysis, however, has become increasingly useful with the recognition that a C-to-T transition at nucleotide 439 that leads to a serine-to-leucine substitution at codon 113 (9S113L) is the mutation most commonly responsible for the disease in patients of European *(63)* and American *(64)* descent.

2.10. What Is the Clinical Phenotype of Carnitine Deficiency, and How Useful Are Paraclinical Investigations for Confirming the Diagnosis?

The term "carnitine deficiency" is used to describe a number of different clinical entities including primary muscle carnitine deficiency, primary systemic carnitine deficiency, and secondary carnitine deficiency.

Primary muscle carnitine deficiency is a rare disorder, with only a handful of cases described in the literature. Onset is usually, but not exclusively, in childhood *(65–77)*. The syndrome is characterized by progressive weakness. Serum CK is typically increased and electromyographic examination shows myopathic motor unit potentials with increased insertional activity. Lipid accumulation is apparent on muscle biopsy. Serum carnitine levels are normal (or only slightly decreased) whereas muscle carnitine levels are low. Some patient may respond to treatment with oral carnitine or prednisone (Table 22.9).

Primary systemic carnitine deficiency is a disorder of childhood and, although most patients have permanent muscle weakness, they also have recurrent episodes of hepatic encephalopathy (summarized in ref. *78)*. Given the age of onset and accompanying history of recurrent encephalopathy, this syndrome will not be considered further.

As might be expected from the diversity of causes, secondary carnitine deficiency is a clinically more heterogeneous disorder. Secondary (acquired) carnitine deficiency may occur in primary defects of β-oxidation with organic aciduria and in association with mitochondrial respiratory chain disorders as well as with treatment with a variety of drugs (most notably valproate).

In summary, therefore, it is only really primary muscle carnitine deficiency that may occasionally produce an adult-onset slowly progressive myopathy. Measurement of serum carnitine is not helpful diagnostically, but serum CK is typically elevated, the EMG shows myopathic features, and evidence of abnormal lipid accumulation should be apparent on muscle biopsy (Table 22.9).

2.11. What Is the Clinical Phenotype of Mitochondrial Respiratory Chain Defects, and How Useful Are Paraclinical Investigations for Confirming the Diagnosis?

Disorders of the mitochondrial respiratory chain are frequently characterized by a progressive encephalopmyopathy that comprises varying combinations of dementia, seizures, stroke, short stature, deafness, ataxia, cardiomyopathy, pigmentary retinopathy, involuntary movements, progressive external ophthalmoplegia, and neuropathy. It is this multi-systemic nature of the syndrome that often points to the diagnosis of a mitochondrial respiratory chain defect. Myopathy may occur as part of this multi-system presentation, but may also occasionally be the only (or most prominent) manifestation of the disease. It is this group of mitochondrial disorders that is the focus of the present discussion.

Table 22.9
Primary Muscle Carnitine Deficiency

	No. of cases /total no. of cases	Percentage
Age of onset		
Infancy/childhood/adolescence	7/11	64
Adulthood	4/11	36
Progressive weakness	10/11	91
Myoglobinuria	1/11	9
Family history	1/4	25
Increased serum creatine kinase	10/10	100
Electromyography		
Myopathic	4/6	67
Fibrillations, positive sharp waves	3/6	50
Myotonic discharges	1/6	17
Abnormal muscle biopsy[a]	11/11	100
Normal serum carnitine	11/11	100
Responsive to carnitine replacement	4/6	67
Responsive to corticosteroids	3/5	60

[a]Vacuolar changes with excess lipid accumulation.
Data from refs. 65–77.

The literature describing the clinical presentation and diagnosis of myopathy due mitochondrial respiratory chain disorders is scanty and comprises a collection of case reports and small case series. Approximately 13 cases of complex-I, 2 cases of complex-II, 4 cases of complex-III, and a single case of complex-IV deficiency have been described. The clinical features and results of paraclinical investigations described in these reports are summarized in Table 22.10.

2.12. Are There Any Clinical Features that Help Discern the Cause of Recurrent Myoglobinuria?

Whether there are clinical features that help one discern the cause of recurrent myoglobinuria is a difficult question to answer, because there have been no studies, either prospective or retrospective, that have addressed this matter. It is not possible, therefore, to estimate the sensitivity and specificity of the various clinical features for any particular diagnosis. It is said that the occurrence of a "second-wind" phenomenon occurs in McArdle's disease and that episodes of myoglobinuria are precipitated by short bursts of strenuous activity in the glycogen storage diseases. Conversely, it is sustained, lower- intensity exercise, especially in the context of fasting, that is said to more commonly precipitate myobloginuria in CPT-II deficiency. In distinguishing between McArdle's and CPT-II deficiency, the two most common metabolic causes of recurrent myoglobinuria, it is useful to consider the serum CK (which is elevated in the majority of patients with McArdle's and in the minority of patients with CPT-II deficiency) and the results of forearm exercise testing. A blunted rise in serum lactate following forearm exercise is expected in all patients with McArdle's (and in the majority of patients with other glycogen storage diseases), whereas this is not a feature of CPT-II deficiency (Table 22.11). The presence of a hemolytic anemia should

Table 22.10
Mitochondrial Respiratory Chain Disorders

	Complex I (114–121) No./total cases (%)	Complex II (113,122) No./total cases (%)	Complex III (117,123–126) No./total cases (%)	Complex IV (129) No./total cases (%)
Age of onset	Infancy → 18 yr[a]	Childhood → 14 yr	Infancy → 24 yr	Childhood
Weakness	11/11 (100%)	1/2 (50%)	2/3 (67%)	1/1 (100%)
Exercise intolerance	12 / 12 (100%)	2 / 2 (100%)	4 / 4 (100%)	1 / 1 (100%)
Muscle pain	9/10 (90%)	1/1 (100%)	2/2 (100%)	0/1
Metabolic acidosis	4/6 (67%)	Not specified	1/1 (100%)	1/1 (100%)
Increased serum lactate	6/6 (100%)	1/2 (50%)	1/2 (50%)	1/1 (100%)
Positive family history	6/10 (60%)	0/1	1/3 (33%)	0/1
Increased serum creatine kinase	2/5 (40%)	0/1	0/3	0/1
Myopathic electromyography	3/5 (60%)	Not specified	1/3 (33%)	0/1
Abnormal muscle biopsy	8/9 (89%)[b]	2/2 (100%)[b]	3/3 (100%)	1/1 (100%)

Denominator varies depending on the frequency with which the particular feature is described in each case report.

[a] With the exception of a single patient who first developed symptoms at the age of 47.

[b] Abnormalities include excess lipid accumulation, ragged red fibers, abnormalities of cytochrome c or succinate dehydrogenase staining.

Table 22.11
Comparison of the Clinical Features of the Metabolic Myopathies

	Weakness	Exercise intolerance	Myoglobinuria	↑CK	Myopathic EMG	Abnormal FET	Abnormal biopsy	Comments
McArdle's	28	87	53	93	49	100	76	2nd most common cause of myoglobinuria
PFK	12	100	63	82	17	93	100	Hemolytic anemia
PbK	33	87	47	60	40	36	40	–
CPT-II	4	79	89	37	22	–	26	Most common cause of myoglobinuria
Debrancher	100	–	–	100	75	100	100	Distal muscle weakness and wasting; cardiac & liver involvement
Acid maltase	100	20	–	90	70	–	76	Respiratory muscles commonly affected
Carnitine	91	–	9	100	67	–	100	Rare; onset usually in childhood
Mitochondrial	88	100	5	20	44	–	93	Metabolic acidosis with ↑ serum lactate in the majority

Values in the table represent the percentage of patients with particular clinical features.

CK, creatine kinase; EMG, electromyography; FET, forearm exercise test; PFK, phosphofructokinase; PbK, phorphorylase b kinase, CPT-II, carnitine palmitoyl-transferase II.

411

suggest Tarui's disease (phosphofructokinase deficiency) as the cause of recurrent myogloinuria.

Among those disorders that present with progressive weakness rather than exercise intolerance and recurrent myoglobinuria, acid maltase deficiency is probably the most common (although reliable epidemiological data are not available). The early or prominent involvement of respiratory muscles strongly suggests this diagnosis. Debrancher deficiency should be suspected if there is prominent distal muscle weakness and wasting or if there are neurogenic changes on the EMG. The presence of a lactic acidosis should point toward mitochondrial disease. These and other differences between the clinical characteristics of the various metabolic myopathies are summarized in Table 22.11.

3. TREATMENT

3.1. Is There a Role for Dietary Modification in the Treatment of the Metabolic Myopathies?

Historically, therapy directed at improving exercise tolerance in patients with McArdle's disease has been chosen based on the understanding that it is the failure to provide muscle with a source of fuel during exercise that is responsible for the symptoms. Because the problem lies with utilization of glycogen stores, it has been suggested that raising serum free fatty acid concentrations might enable muscle to metabolize fatty acids instead of carbohydrate. The suggestion, however, that dietary modification might improve exercise tolerance in patients with McArdle's disease is based entirely on anecdotal case reports. For example, some reports have suggested that raising plasma free fatty acids by infusion of emulsified fat (79) or fasting (80) may improve exercise tolerance, but the more practical application of a low-carbohydrate, high-fat diet was unsuccessful in another patient (81).

With the similar goal of providing fuel downstream of the metabolic block, others have suggested that work capacity may be increased by the intravenous infusion or oral administration of glucose or fructose (79,81–85), but a beneficial effect has not always been observed (86). Similarly inconsistent results have been observed following administration of glucagon (86,87). There are two case reports suggesting that exercise tolerance may be improved with a high-protein diet (88,89). Finally, a recent single-blind, randomized, placebo-controlled crossover trial of oral sucrose ingestion prior to exercise showed a marked improvement in exercise tolerance in all 12 patients with McArdle's disease (90). Although effective, such therapy may not be practical on a daily basis.

Dietary modification has also been recommended for patients with CPT-II deficiency. A number of authors have suggested the use of a high-carbohydrate, low-fat diet with frequent meals and extra carbohydrate intake before and during sustained exercise (91, 92). These recommendations, however, are based on an understanding of the metabolic defect rather than on evidence for their efficacy. One author suggested that a low-fat diet supplemented with medium-chain triglycerides might be beneficial (in terms of lowering serum triglyceride levels rather than in improving exercise capacity) (93), but others have suggested that caution should be exercised, as the capacity of other enzyme systems to handle medium chain triglycerides may easily be exceeded in patients with CPT-II deficiency (94).

3.2. Is There a Role for Physical Exercise in the Treatment of the Metabolic Myopathies?

A small case series (comprising four patients) suggests that aerobic training may improve exercise capacity among subjects with McArdle's disease *(95)*. Patients with McArdle's disease may utilize the "second wind" phenomenon to prolong the duration of the period that they are able to exercise. One important difference between those with McArdle's disease and those with CPT-II deficiency is that those with McArdle's tend to develop painful muscle cramps (really contractures) that limit exercise tolerance. Those with CPT-II deficiency, on the other hand, typically do not develop these exercise-limiting symptoms. It is more common, therefore, for those with CPT-II deficiency to present with symptoms of rhabdomyolysis and myoglobinuria some hours after strenuous exercise. Because those with CPT-II deficiency do not develop these "warning" signs during exercise, they should perhaps be more cautious in engaging in prolonged physical activity. This recommendation, however, is again based on an understanding of the metabolic defect rather than on the presence of any evidence.

3.3. Is There a Role for Creatine Therapy in the Treatment of Metabolic Myopathies?

A small placebo-controlled crossover study of creatine therapy for 5 weeks was performed in nine patients with McArdle's disease. No difference was found in overall exercise tolerance (using the fatigue severity scale) between those treated with creatine and those who received placebo *(96)*.

A small randomized trial of creatine supplementation for 3 weeks was also performed in patients with mitochondrial myopathy. This found minor improvements among those treated with carnitine. The outcome measures for which an effect was demonstrated included the nonischemic dorsiflexion torque and ischemic isometric grip strength *(97)*. It is not clear whether these findings have any clinical significance.

3.4. Is There a Role for Steroids in the Treatment of Metabolic Myopathies?

There are a number of case reports of patients with primary muscle carnitine deficiency being successfully treated with prednisone *(65,72,73,98)*. There is, however, no controlled data to support of refute this possibility. The use of steroids has not been suggested for the treatment of any of the other metabolic myopathies.

4. PROGNOSIS

There really are no good prognostic data that can be used reliably to predict the natural history of the metabolic myopathies.

5. SUMMARY

- The typical presentation of the adult-onset metabolic myopathies is either with exercise intolerance and recurrent myoglobinuria or with fixed and progressive muscle weakness.
- The most common causes of recurrent episodes of myoglobinuria include CPT-II deficiency, McArdle's disease, and phosphofructokinase deficiency.

- Mitochondrial disease appears to be an uncommon cause of isolated myopathic symptoms, although neuromuscular symptoms may be just one of manifestation of a multi-system presentation including cognitive impairment, seizures and sensorineural hearing loss.
- Short periods of high-intensity exercise are the usual precipitant for myoglobinuria in patients with glycogen-storage diseases; prolonged submaximal exercise, especially in the context of an overnight fast, is the more common precipitant for myoglobinuria in patients with lipid-storage myopathies including CPT-II deficiency.
- Acid maltase deficiency is the metabolic myopathy that most commonly causes fixed and progressive muscle weakness; other, less common causes include debrancher, phosphofructokinase and phosphorylase b kinase deficiency as well as mitochondrial disease, and primary muscle carnitine deficiency.
- CPT-II deficiency and McArdle's disease are the two most commonly encountered metabolic myopathies that cause recurrent myoglobinuria.
- Almost all patients with McArdle's disease report exercise intolerance, and about one-half will have recurrent episodes of myoglobinuria; serum CK is increased (in between attacks) in the majority and EMG is abnormal in about one-half; the forearm exercise test almost invariably shows a blunted rise in serum lactate.
- The diagnosis of McArdle's disease may be confirmed by mutational analysis using peripheral blood leukocytes, by histochemical analysis of a muscle biopsy (staining for phosphorylase), or by biochemical analysis on a muscle biopsy specimen.
- Most patients with CPT-II deficiency will experience recurrent episodes of recurrent myoglobinuria; in between attacks, the neurological examination, serum CK, EMG, and muscle biopsy are usually normal.
- The diagnosis of CPT-II may be confirmed by mutational analysis using peripheral blood leukocytes or by biochemical analysis performed on a fresh muscle biopsy specimen.
- Acid maltase defieicncy typically presents as fixed and progressive muscle weakness with early or prominent involvement of respiratory muscles.
- There are no proven treatments for any of the metabolic myopathies, although patients should be instructed to avoid obvious precipitating factors
- There is no firm basis to recommend specific dietary modifications for patients with metabolic myopathies despite the intuitive appeal of a low-fat diet for patients with CPT-II deficiency and a low-carbohydrate diet for those with glycogen-storage disease.

REFERENCES

1. Tonin P, Lewis P, Servidei S, DiMauro S. Metabolic causes of myoglobinuria. Ann Neurol 1990; 27:181–185.
2. Engel AG, Siekert RG. Lipid storage myopathy responsive to prednisone. Arch Neurol 1972;27:174–181.
3. Engel AG, Angelini C. Carnitine deficiency of human skeletal muscle with associated lipid storage myopathy: a new syndrome. Science 1973;179:899–902.
4. Cornelio F, Bresolin N, Singer PA, DiMauro S, Rowland LP. Clinical varieties of neuromuscular disease in Debrancher deficiency. Arch Neurol 1984;41:1027–1032.
5. DiMauro S, Hartwig GB, Hays A, et al. Debrancher Deficiency: Neuromuscular disorder in 5 adults. Ann Neurol 1979;5:422–436.
6. Brunberg JA, McCormick WF, Schochet SS. Type 3 Glycogenosis: An adult with diffuse weakness and muscle wasting. Arch Neurol 1971;25:171–178.
7. Engel AG, Gomez MR, Seybold M, Lambert EH. The spectrum and diagnosis of acid maltase deficiency. Neurology 1973;23:95–106.

8. Trend PS, Wiles C, Spencer G, Morgan-Hughes J, Lake B, Patrick A. Acid maltase deficiency in adults. Diagnosis and management in five cases. Brain 1985;108:845–860.

9. Swash M, Schwartz M, Apps M. Adult onset acid maltase deficiency. Distribution and progression of clinical and pathological abnormality in a family. J Neurol Sci 1985;68:61–74.

10. Laforet P, Nicolino M, Eymard PB, et al. Juvenile and adult-onset acid maltase deficiency in France. Genotype-phenotype correlation. Neurology 2000;55:1122–1128.

11. Lofberg M, Jankala H, Paetau A, Harkonen M, Somer H. Metabolic causes of recurrent rhabdomyolysis. Acta Neurol Scand 1998;98:268–275.

12. DiMauro S, Tsujino S. Nonlysosomal glycogenoses. In: Engel AG, Franzini-Armstrong C, eds. Myology. Vol. 2. McGraw-Hill, New York:1994;pp.1554–1576.

13. Martin MA, Rubio JC, Buchbinder J, et al. Molecular heterogeneity of myophosphorylase deficiency (McArdle's disease): a genotype-phenotype correlation study. Ann Neurol 2001;50:574–581.

14. Wolfe GI, Baker NS, Haller RG, Burns DK, Barohn RJ. McArdle's disease presenting with asymmetric, late–onset arm weakness. Muscle Nerve 2000;23:641–645.

15. Tsujino S, Shanske S, DiMauro S. Molecular genetic heterogeneity of myopshophorylase deficiency (McArdle's disease). N Engl J Med 1993;329:241–245.

16. el-Schahawi M, Tsujino S, Shanske S, DiMauro S. Diagnosis of McArdle's disease by molecular genetic analysis of blood. Neurology 1996;47:579–580.

17. Bartram C, Edwards RH, Clague J, Beynon RJ. McArdle's disease: a nonsense mutation in exon 1 of the muscle glycogen phosphorylase gene explains some but not all cases. Hum Mol Genet 1993; 2:1291–1293.

18. Agamanolis DP, Askari AD, DiMauro S, et al. Muscle phosphofructokinase deficiency: two cases with unusual polysaccharide accumulation and immunologically active enzyme protein. Muscle Nerve 1980;3:456–467.

19. Layzer RB, Rowland LP, Ranney HM. Muscle phosphofructokinase deficiency. Arch Neurol 1967; 17:512–523.

20. Tobin WE, Huijing F, Porro RS, Salzman RT. Muscle phosphofructokinase deficiency. Arch Neurol 1973;28:128–130.

21. Serratrice G, Monges A, Roux H, Aquaron R, Gambarelli D. Forme myopathique du deficit en phosphofructokinase. Rev Neurol (Paris) 1969;120:271–277.

22. Hays AP, Hallett M, Delfs J, et al. Muscle phosphofructokinase deficiency: abnormal polysaccharide in a case of late-onset myopathy. Neurology 1981;31:1077–1086.

23. Danon MJ, Servidei S, DiMauro S, Vora S. Late-onset muscle phosphofructokinase deficiency. Neurology 1988;38:956–960.

24. Tarui S, Okuno G, Ikura Y, Tanaka T, Suda M, Nishikawa M. Phosphofructokinase deficiency in skeletal muscle. A new type of glycogenosis. Biochem Biophys Res Commun 1965;19:517–523.

25. Abarbanel J, Bashan N, Potashnik R, Osimani A, Moses S, Herishanu Y. Adult muscle phosphorylase "b" kinase deficiency. Neurology 1986;36:560–562.

26. Carrier H, Maire I, Vial C, Rambaud G, Flocard F, Flechaire A. Myopathic evolution of an exertional muscle pain syndrome with phosphorylase b kinase deficiency. Acta Neuropathol (Berlin) 1990;81:84–88.

27. Clemens PR, Yamamoto M, Engel AG. Adult phosphorylase b kinase deficiency. Ann Neurol 1990; 28:529–538.

28. Iwamasa T, Fukuda S, Tokumitsu S, Ninomiya N, Matsuda I, Osame M. Myopathy due to glycogen storage disease: pathological and biochemical studies in relation to glycogenosome formation. Exp Mol Pathol 1983;38:405–420.

29. Wilkinson D, Tonin P, Shanske S, Lombes A, Carlson G, DiMauro S. Clinical and biochemical features of 10 adult patients with muslce phosphorylase kinase deficiency. Neurology 1994;44:461–466.

30. Moses S, Gadoth N, Bashan N, Ben-David E, Slonim A, Wanderman K. Neuromuscular involvement in glycogen storage disease type III. Acta Paediatr Scand 1986;75:289–296.

31. Oliner L, Schulman M, Larner J. Myopathy associated with glycogen deposition resulting from generalized lack of amylo-1,6-glucosidase. Clin Res 1961;9:243.

32. Engel AG. Acid maltase deficiency in adults: studies in four cases of a syndrome which may mimic muscular dystrophy or other myopathies. Brain 1970;93:599–616.

33. Karpati G, Carpenter S, Eisen A, Aube M, DiMauro S. The adult from of acid maltase (alpha-1,4-Glucosidase) deficiency. Ann Neurol 1977;1:276–280.

34. Bertagnolio B, Di Donato S, Peluchetti D, Rimoldi M, Storchi G, Cornelio F. Acid maltase deficiency in adults: clinical, morphological and biochemical study of three patients. Eur Neurol 1978;17:193–204.

35. Sivak ED, Salanga V, D, Wilbourn AJ, Mitsumoto H, Golish J. Adult-onset acid maltase deficiency presenting as diaphragmatic paralysis. Ann Neurol 1981;9:613–615.

36. Rosenow EC, Engel AG. Acid maltase deficiency in adults presenting as respiratory failure. Am J Med 1978; 64:485–491.

37. Keunen R, Lambregts P, Op De Coul A, Joosten E. Respiratory failure as initial manifestation of acid maltase deficiency. J Neurol, Neurosurg Psychiatry 1984;47:549–552.

38. Bellamy D, Newsom-Davis J, Hicky B, Benatar S, Clark T. A case of primary alveolar hypoventilation associated with mild proximal myopathy. Am Rev Respir Dis 1975;112:867–873.

39. Schlenska G, Heene R, Spalke G, Seiler D. The symptomatology, morphology and biochemistry of glycogenosis type II (Pompe) in the adult. J Neurol 1976;212:237–252.

40. Hudgson P, Gardner-Medwin D, Worsfold M, Pennington R, Walton JN. Adult myopathy from glycogen storage disease due to acid maltase deficiency. Brain 1968;91:435–462.

41. Angelini C, Freddo L, Battistella P, et al. Carnitine palmityl transferase deficiency: clinical variability, carrier detection, and autosomal recessive inheritance. Neurology 1981;31:883–886.

42. Argov Z, DiMauro S. Recurrent exertional myalgia and myoglobinuria due to carnitine palmityltransferase deficiency. Isr J Med Sci 1983;19:552–554.

43. Bank WJ, DiMauro S, Bonilla E, Capuzzi DM, Rowland LP. A disorder of muscle metabolism and myoglobinuria. Absence of carnitine palmityl transferase. N Engl J Med 1975;292:443–449.

44. Brownell A, Selverson D, Thompson C, Fletcher T. Cold induced rhabdomyolysis in carnitine palmityl transferase deficiency. Can J Neurol Sci 1979;6:367–370.

45. Carey M, Poulton K, Hawkins C, Murphy R. Carnitine palmitoyl transfase deficiency with an atypical presentation and ultrastructual mitochondrial abnormalities. J Neurol, Neurosurg Psychiatry 1987;50:1060–1062.

46. Carroll JE, Brooke MH, DeVivo DC, Kaiser KK, Hagberg JM. Biochemical and physiologic consequences of carnitine palmityltransferase deficiency. Muscle Nerve 1978;1:103–110.

47. Cumming W, Hardy M, Hudgson P, Walls J. Carnitine-palmityl-transferase deficiency. J Neurol Sci 1976;30:247–258.

48. Di Donato S, Castiglione A, Rimoldi M, Vendemia F, Cardace G, Bertagnolio B. Heterogeneity of carnitine-palmitoyltransfase deficiency. J Neurol Sci 1981;50:207–215.

49. DiMauro S, DiMauro PM. Muscle carnitine palmityltransferase deficiency and myoglobinuria. Science 1973;182:929–931.

50. Skard HM, Dietrichson P, Landaas S. Familial combined deficiency of muscle carnitine and carnitine palmityl transferase (CPT). Acta Neurol Scand 1986;74:479–485.

51. Ionasescu V, Hug G, Hoppel C. Combined partial deficiency of muscle carnitine palmitoyltransferase and carnitine with autosomal dominant inheritance. J Neurol Neurosurg Psychiatry 1980;43:679–682.

52. Layzer RB, Havel RJ, McIlroy MB. Partial deficiency of carnitine palmityltransferase: physiologic and biochemical consequences. Neurology 1980;30:627–633.

53. Meola G, Bresolin N, Rimoldi M, Velicogna M, Furtunato F, Scarlato G. Recessive carnitine palmityl transferase deficiency: biochemical studies in tissue cultures and platelets. J Neurol 1987;235:74–79.

54. Mongini T, Doriguzzi C, Palmucci L, Chado-Piat L, Maniscalco M, Schiffer D. Myoglobinuria and carnitine palmityl transferase deficiency in father and son. J Neurol 1991;238:323–324.

55. Patten BM, Wood JM, Harati Y, Heffernan P, Howell RR. Familial recurrent rhabdomyolysis due to carnitine palmityl transferase deficiency. Am J Med 1979;67:167–171.

56. Pula T, Max S, Zielke H, et al. Selective carnitine palmitoyltransferase deficiency in fibroblasts from a patient with muscle CPT deficiency. Ann Neurol 1981;10:196–198.

57. Reza MJ, Kar NC, Pearson CM, Kark RA. Recurrent myoglobinuria due to muscle carnitine palmityl transferase deficiency. Ann Intern Med 1978;88:610–615.

58. Scholte H, Jennekens F, Bouvy J. Carnitine palmitoyltransferase II deficiency with normal carnitine palmitoyltransferase I in skeletal muscle and leucocytes. Journal of the Neurological Sciences 1979; 40:39–51.

59. Trevisan CP, Angelini C, Freddo L, Isaya G, Martinuzzi A. Myoglobinuria and carnitine palmityltrans-fease (CPT) deficiency: studies with malonyl-CoA suggest absence of only CPT-II. Neurology 1984;34:353–356.

60. Herman J, Nadler HL. Recurrent myoglobinuria and muscle carnitine palmityltransferase deficiency. J Pediatr 1977;91:247–250.

61. Ross NS, Hoppel CL. Partial muscle carnitine palmitoyltransferase-A deficiency. Rhabdomyolysis associated with transiently decreased muscle carnitine content after ibuprofen therapy. JAMA 1987;257:62–65.

62. Bertorini T, Yeh YY, Trevisan CP, Stadlan E, Sabesin S, DiMauro S. Carnitine palmityl transferase deficiency: myoglobinuria and respiratory failure. Neurology 1980;30:263–271.

63. Taroni F, Verderio E, Dworzak F, Willems PJ, Cavadini P, DiDonato S. Identification of a common mutation in the carnitine palmitoyltransferase II gene in familial recurrent myoglobinuria patients. Nat Genet 1993;4:314–320.

64. Kaufmann P, el-Schahawi M, DiMauro S. Carnitine palmitoyltransferase II deficiency: diagnosis by molecular analysis of blood. Mol Cell Biochem 1997;174:237–239.

65. Engel A, Siekert R. Lipid storage myopathy responsive to prednisone. Arch Neurol 1972;27:174-181.

66. Engel A, Angelini C. Carnitine deficiency of human skeletal muscle with associated lipid storage myopathy: a new syndrome. Science 1973;179:899–902.

67. Markesbery W, McQuillen M, Procopis P, Harrison A, Engel A. Muscle carnitine deficiency: association with lipid myopathy, vaculoar neuropathy and vacuolated leukocytes. Arch Neurol 1974;31:320–324.

68. Smyth D, Lake B, Mac Dermot J, Wilson J. Inborn errors of carnitine metabolism ('carnitine deficiency') in man. Lancet 1975;1:1198–1199.

69. Van Dyke D, Griggs R, Markesbery W, DiMauro S. Hereditary carnitine deficiency of muscle. Neurology 1975;25:154–159.

70. Hart Z, Chang C, DiMauro S, Farooki Q, Ayyar R. Muscle carnitine deficiency and fatal cardiomyopathy. Neurology 1978;28:147–151.

71. Willner J, DiMauro S, Eastwood A, Hays A, Roohi F, Lovelace R. Muscle carnitine deficiency: genetic heterogeneity. J Neurol Sci 1979;41:235–246.

72. Bradley W, Hudgson P, Gardner-Medwin D, Walton J. Myopathy associated with abnormal lipid metabolism in skeletal muscle. Lancet 1969;1:495–498.

73. Bradley W, Jenkison M, Park D, et al. A myopathy associated with lipid storage. J Neurol Sci 1972;16:137–154.

74. Bradley W, Tomlinson B, Hardy M. Further studies of mitochondrial and lipid storage myopathies. J Neurol Sci 1978;35:201–210.

75. Angelini C, Govoni E, Bragaglia M, Vergani L. Carnitine deficiency: acute post-partum crisis. Ann Neurol 1978;4:558–561.

76. Prockop LD, Engel WK, Shug AL. Nearly fatal muscle carnitine deficiency with full recovery after replacement therapy. Neurology 1983;33:1629–1633.

77. Koller H, Stoll G, Neuen-Jacob E. Postpartum manifestation of a necrotizing lipid storage myopathy associated with muscle carnitine deficiency. J Neurol, Neurosurg Psychiatry 1998;64:407–408.

78. DiMauro S, Trevisan C, Hays A. Disorders of lipid metabolism in muscle. Muscle Nerve 1980;3:369-388.

79. Pearson CM, Rimer DC, Mommaerts F. A metabolic myopathy due to absence of muscle phosphorylase. Am J Med 1961;30:502–517.

80. Carroll HE, DeVivo DC, Brooke MH, Planer GJ, Hagberg JH. Fasting as a provocative test in neuromuscular diseases. Metabolism 1979;28:683–687.

81. Hockaday T, Downey J, Mottram R. A case of McArdle's syndrome with a positive family history. J Neurol, Neurosurg Psychiatry 1964;27:186–197.

82. Schmid R, Mahler R. Chronic progressive myopathy with myoglobinuria: demonstration of a glycogenolytic defect in the muscle. J Clin Invest 1959;38:2044–2058.

83. Mellick R, Mahler R, Hughes B. McArdle's syndrome: phosphorylase–deficiency myopathy. Lancet 1962;1:1045–1048.

84. Porte D, Crawford DW, Jennings DB, Aber C, McIlrov MB. Cardiovascular and metabolic responses to exercise in a patient with McArdle's syndrome. N Engl J Med 1966;275:406–412.

85. Cochrane P, Hughes R, Buxton P, Yorke R. Myophosphorylase deficiency (McArdle's disease) in two interrelated families. J Neurol, Neurosurg Psychiatry 1973;36:217-224.

86. Rowland LP, Lovelace RE, Schotland DL, Araki S, Carmel P. The clinical diagnosis of McArdle's disease. Identification of another family with deficiency of muscle phosphorylase. Neurology 1966;16:93–100.

87. Rowland LP, Fahn S, Schotland DL. McArdle's disease: Hereditary myopathy due to absence of muscle phosphorylase. Arch Neurol 1963;9:325–342.

88. Slonim A, Goans PJ. Myopathy in McArdle's syndrome. Improvement with a high-protein diet. N Engl J Med 1985;312:355–359.

89. Jensen K, Jakobsen J, Thomsen C, Henriksen O. Improved energy kinetics following high protein diet in McArdle's syndrome. A 31P magnetic resonance spectroscopy study. Acta Neurol Scand 1990;81:499–503.

90. Vissing J, Haller RG. The effect of oral sucrose on exercise tolerance in patients with McArdle's disease. N Engl J Med 2003;349:2503–2509.

91. Bonnefont JP, Demaugre F, Prip-Buus C, et al. Carnitine palmitoyltransferase deficiencies. Mol Genet Metab 1999;68:424–440.

92. Zierz S. Carnitine palmitoyltransferase deficiency. In: Engel A, Franzini-Armstrong C, eds. Myology. Vol. 2. McGraw Hill, New York:1994;pp.1577–1586.

93. Scott TF, Virella-Lopes M, Malone MJ. Hypertriglyceridemia in carnitine palmityl transferase deficiency: lipid profile and treatment with medium chain trigylcerides. Muscle Nerve 1991;14:676–677.

94. Schaefer J, Jackson S, Taroni F, Swift P, Turnbull DM. Characterization of carnitine palmitoyltransferases in patients with a carnitine palmitoyltransferase deficiency: implications for diagnosis and therapy. J Neurol Neurosurg Psychiatry 1997;62:169–176.

95. Haller RG, Wyrick P, Cavender D, Wall A, Vissing J. Aerobic conditioning: an effective therapy in McArdle's disease. Neurology 1998;50:A369.

96. Vorgerd M, Grehl T, Jager M, et al. Creatine therapy in myophosphorylase deficiency (McArdle's disease). A placebo-controlled crossover trial. Arch Neurol 2000;57:956–963.

97. Tarnopolsky M, Roy B, MacDonald J. A randomized, controlled trial of creatine monohydrate in patients with mitochondrial cytopathies. Muscle Nerve 1997;20:1502–1509.

98. Johnson MA, Fulthorpe J, Hudgson P. Lipid storage myopathy: a recognizable clinicopathological entity? Acta Neuropathol (Berlin) 1973;24:97–106.

99. Mastaglia F, McCollum J, Larson P, Hudgson P. Steroid myopathy complicating McArdle's disease. J Neurol Neurosurg Psychiatry 1970;33:111–120.

100. Hewlett R, Gardner-Thorpe. McArdle's disease—what limit to the age of onset? S Afr Med J 1978;53:60–63.

101. Pourmand R, Sanders DB, Corwin HM. Late-onset McArdle's disease with unusual electromyographic findings. Arch Neurol 1983;40:374–377.

102. Tonin P, Shanske S, Miranda A, et al. Phosphoglycerate kinase deficiency: Biochemical and molecular genetic studies in a new myopathic variant (PGK Alberta). Neurology 1993;43:387–391.

103. DiMauro S, Miranda AF, Olarte M, Friedman R, Hays AP. Muscle phosphoglycerate mutase deficiency. Neurology 1982;32:584–591.

104. Bresolin N, Ro YI, Reyes M, Miranda AF, DiMauro S. Muscle phosphoglycerate mutase (PGAM) deficiency: a second cause. Neurology 1983;33:1049–1053.

105. Vita G, Toscano A, Bresolin N, et al. Muscle phosphoglycerate mutase (PGAM) deficiency in the 1st Caucasian patient. Neurology 1990;40:296.

106. Schaefer H, Jackson S, Dick DJ, Turnbull DM. Trifunctional enzyme deficiency: adult presentation of a usually fatal β-oxidation defect. Ann Neurol 1996;40:597–602.

107. Miyajima H, Orii K, Shindo Y, et al. Mitochondrial trifunctional protein deficiency associated with recurrent myoglobinuria in adolescence. Neurology 1997;49:833–837.

108. Ogilvie I, Pourfarzam M, Jackson S, Stockdale C, Bartlet K, Turnbull D. Very long-chain acyl coenzyme A dehydrogenase deficiency presenting with exercise-induced myoglobinuria. Neurology 1994;44:467–473.

109. Straussberg R, Harel L, Versano I, Elpeleg ON, Shamir R, Amir J. Recurrent myoglobinuria as a presenting manifestation of very long chain acyl coenzyme A dehydrogenase deficiency. Pediatrics 1997;99:894–896.

110. Smelt A, Poorthuis J, Onkenhout W, et al. Very long chain acyl-coenzyme A dehydrogenase deficiency with adult onset. Ann Neurol 1998;43:540–544.

111. Pons R, Cavadini P, Baratta S, et al. Clinical and molecular heterogeneity in very-long chain acyl-coenzyme A dehydrogenase deficiency. Pediatr Neurol 2000;22:98–105.

112. Ruitenbeek W, Poels P, Turnbull D, et al. Rhabdomyolysis and acute encephalopathy in late onset medium chain acyl-CoA dehydrogenase deficiency. J Neurol Neurosurg Psychiatry 1995;58:209–214.

113. Haller RG, Henriksson K, Jorfeldt L, et al. Deficiency of skeletal muscle succinate dehydrogenase and aconitase. Pathophysiology of exercise in a novel human muscle oxidative defect. J Clin Invest 1991;88:1197–1206.

114. Morgan-Hughes J, Darveniza P, Landon D, Land J, Clark J. A mitochondrial myopathy with a deficiency of respiratory chain NADH-CoQ reductase activity. J Neurol Sci 1979;43:27–46.

115. Land JM, Morgan-Hughes JA, Clark JB. Mitochondrial myopathy. Biochemical studies revealing a deficiency of NADH-cytochrome b reductase activity. J Neurolog Sci 1981;50:1–13.

116. Clark J, Hayes D, Morgan-Hughes J. Byrne E. Mitochondrial myopathies: disorders of the respiratory chain and oxidative phosphorylation. J Inherit Metab Dis 1984;7:62–68.

117. Morgan-Hughes JA, Hayes DJ, Cooper M, Clark JB. Mitochondrial myopathies: deficiencies localized to complex I and complex III of the mitochondrial respiratory chain. Biochem Soci Trans 1985;13:648–650.

118. Arts W, Scholte H, Bogaard J, Kerrebijn K, Luyt-Houwen I. NADH-CoQ reductase deficient myopathy: successful treatment with riboflavin. Lancet 1983;2:581–582.

119. Koga Y, Nonaka I, Kobayashi M, Tojyo M, Nihei K. Findings in muscle in complex I (NADH Coenzyme Q reductase) deficiency. Ann Neurol 1988;24:749–756.

120. Watmough N, Birch-Machin M, Bindoff L, et al. Tissue specific defect of complex I of the mitochondrial respiratory chain. Biochem Biophys Res Commun 1989;160:623–627.

121. Watmough NJ, Bindoff LA, Birch-Machin MA, et al. Impaired mitochondrial ß-oxidation in a patient with an abnormality of the respiratory chain. Studies in skeletal muscle mitochondria. J Clin Invest 1990;85:177–184.

122. Garavaglia B, Antozzi C, Girotti F, et al. A mitochondrial myopathy with complex II deficiency. Neurology 1990;40:294.

123. Morgan-Hughes JA, Darveniza P, Kahn S, et al. A mitochondrial myopathy characterized by a deficiency in reducible cytochome b. Brain 1977;100:617–640.

124. Hayes D, Lecky B, Landon DN, Morgan-Hughes JA, Clark JB. A new mitochondrial myopathy: biochemical studies revealing a deficiency in the cytochrome b-c1 complex (complex III) of the respiratory chain. Brain 1984;107:1165–1177.

125. Reichmann H, Rohkamm R, Zeviani M, Servidei S, Ricker K, DiMauro S. Mitochondrial myopathy due to complex III deficiency with normal reducible cytochrome b concentration. Arch Neurol 1986;43:957–961.

126. Schapira AH, Cooper JM, Morgan-Hughes JA, Landon DN, Clark JB. Mitochondrial myopathy with a defect of mitochondrial-protein transport. N Engl J Med 1990;323:37–42.

127. Martin J, de Barsy T, den Tandt W. Acid maltase deficiency in non-identical adult twins: a morphological and biochemical study. J Neurol 1976;213:105–118.

128. Wokke JH, Ausems MG, van den Boogaard MJ, et al. Genotype-phenotype correlation in adult-onset acid maltase deficiency. Ann Neurol 1995;38:450–454.

129. Haller RG, Lewis SF, Estabrook RW, DiMauro S, Servidei S, Foster DW. Exercise intolerance, lactic acidosis, and abnormal cardiopulmonary regulation in exercise associated with adult skeletal muscle cytochrome c oxidase deficiency. J Clin Invest 1989;84:155–161.

23 Critical Illness Weakness

1. INTRODUCTION

Weakness may complicate the course of a significant number of intensive care unit (ICU) patients. This weakness may affect the respiratory musculature, in which case it is usually recognized as a failure to wean from the ventilator. It may also commonly affect limb muscles, and more rarely, both facial and extra-ocular muscles. Critical illness polyneuropathy (CIP) and critical illness myopathy (CIM) are two of the better recognized causes of such weakness that arise during the course of the ICU stay.

Much has been made of the distinction between the two and indeed, in their classic presentation, the two are easily differentiated. The initial reports of CIM described patients who were intubated and ventilated for severe asthma exacerbations and who had received a combination of high-dose intravenous glucorcorticoids as well as prolonged paralysis with neuromuscular blocking agents (NMBAs). By contrast, CIP was originally described in the context of systemic sepsis and multi-organ failure. There are also said to be clear electrophysiological differences between the two disorders, which facilitates their distinction. Although compound muscle action potential (CMAP) amplitudes are reduced in both CIP and CIM, sensory nerve action potential (SNAP) responses are abnormally low in CIP and relatively preserved in CIM. The pattern of voluntary motor unit potential (MUP) recruitment also differs, with low amplitude, short duration, and polyphasic units recruited early in CIM. In contrast, MUP recruitment is reduced in CIP, and MUP morphology is neurogenic (large amplitude, polyhasic, and long duration). The reality of electrodiagnostic testing in critically ill patients in the ICU, however, is such that superimposed encephalopathy or simply the presence of severe weakness may preclude the recording of voluntary MUPs. Similarly, SNAP amplitudes may be reduced because of tissue edema that increases the distance between the nerve and recording electrode. It may, therefore, sometimes be difficult to distinguish CIP from CIM. As it turns out, both disorders may occur in the context of systemic sepsis and multi-organ failure, in which case the clinical context may be less helpful for differentiating the two than anticipated.

A number of questions emerge when one is faced with the clinical problem of critical illness weakness. What is the spectrum of neuromuscular disease encountered in the ICU that may be responsible for respiratory muscle and limb weakness? How useful are the clinical context and a history of corticosteroid and neuromuscular blocking agent (NMBA) use in suggesting myopathy rather than polyneuropathy as the cause of acquired weakness in the ICU? Are there clinical or electrodiagnostic variables that permit reliable distinction between CIP and CIM? If not, how important is it to distinguish the two

From: *Neuromuscular Disease: Evidence and Analysis in Clinical Neurology*
By: M. Benatar © Humana Press Inc., Totowa, NJ

entities? Does the prognosis for neuromuscular recovery, for example, differ for the two diagnostic entities? These and other questions are the focus of this chapter.

2. DIAGNOSIS

2.1. What Is the Spectrum of Neuromuscular Complications Encountered in the ICU?

The range of neuromuscular diseases that may be encountered in the ICU is quite broad. A useful way to consider these disorders is to make a distinction between those conditions that cause sufficient weakness to warrant admission to the ICU (e.g., severe myasthenia gravis or the Guillain-Barré syndrome) and those diseases that develop during, and often because of, the ICU stay. The focus in this chapter is on those neuromuscular disorders that arise as a consequence of the critical illness or treatment modalities employed in the management of these critically ill patients. CIP and CIM are the two primary considerations, although a syndrome of prolonged neuromuscular junction blockade is also recognized. Whether CIP and CIM represent distinct entities or whether there is overlap in their pathophysiology, or at least their clinical occurrence, is part of an ongoing controversy.

2.2. What Are the Clinical and Electrophysiological Manifestations of Critical Illness Polyneuropathy?

The syndrome of CIP was first described by Bolton and colleagues in a series of publications (1–3). These successive papers do not seem to describe different cohorts of patients, but rather represent these authors' cumulative experience over a period of a number of years. For the delineation of this syndrome, polyneuropathy was defined electrophysiologically by the presence of reduced compound muscle and sensory nerve action potentials as well as fibrillation potentials in the muscles of at least two limbs. The designation of the polyneuropathy as being etiologically linked to critical illness relied on (1) the presence of septicemia or a septic focus with systemic effects and (2) the presence of critical illness, defined as involvement of at least two major organs. Using these criteria, they identified 15 patients with CIP, who formed the basis for the description of the syndrome. The use of steroids and NMBAs was not reported. Limb weakness was present in all of the patients, with the legs more affected than the arms and the distal limb muscles more severely affected than proximal muscles. Facial weakness was present in three patients. Deep tendon reflexes were depressed or absent. Sensory symptoms were mild, and varying degrees of a distal glove and stocking pattern of sensory loss might be present when examination is possible. Autonomic dysfunction was not evident clinically. Electrodiagnostic testing showed clearly reduced CMAP and SNAP amplitudes with only mild abnormalities of conduction velocities, distal latencies, and F-responses. The absent or reduced SNAP responses were confirmed in a majority of patients with near nerve recordings in order to circumvent the technical difficulty that might result from prominent tissue edema. Repetitive nerve stimulation in 10 patients showed no evidence of a defect in neuromuscular transmission. Needle electromyography showed abundant acute denervation changes (fibrillation potentials and positive sharp waves) with a relatively high incidence of myotonic and complex repetitive discharges. MUP morphology and recruitment pattern were not described, although follow-up neuropathology, available in six patients, confirmed the presence of an axonal polyneuropathy affecting both motor and sensory fibers with predominant distal involvement. A superimposed myopathy was noted in one patient.

2.3. What Are the Clinical and Electrophysiological Manifestations of Critical Illness Myopathy?

Increasingly, a syndrome of critical illness weakness due to primary muscle disease has also been recognized as an important cause of respiratory and limb muscle weakness in ICU patients. This syndrome has gone by a variety of names, including myopathy with thick filament (myosin) loss, acute quadriplegic myopathy, and acute necrotizing myopathy of the ICU. Although muscle necrosis or selective myosin loss is not present in every case, these entities all likely represent part of the same spectrum of disease, and so the term "critical illness myopathy" has been used to encompass them all.

Much of the literature on CIM comprises case reports and small case series *(4–6)*, which makes it difficult to adequately characterize the typical medical context, clinical semiology, and electrodiagnostic findings. Although the early reports of CIM were of patients with status asthmaticus treated with steroids and NMBAs *(7–9)*, in the largest series of 14 patients with CIM *(6)*, only five had severe chronic obstructive pulmonary disease (COPD) and the others were post-liver transplantation. Similarly, in Zochodne and colleagues' series of seven patients *(5)*, only two were admitted with status asthmaticus, with the remaining patients in the ICU having sepsis and multi-organ failure.

In the study by Lacomis and colleagues *(6)* all 14 patients received high-dose corticosteroids, and NMBAs were administered in all but one patient. Weakness was generalized and always affected the neck flexors. Distal weakness predominated in nine patients, and five patients showed similar weakness in proximal and distal muscles. Five patients had facial weakness and extra-ocular muscle weakness was noted in one. The pattern of weakness is not described in the series by Zochodne and Ramsay *(4,5)*, but in each series, two patients were noted to have involvement of the extra-ocular muscles.

In general, the CMAPs were reduced in amplitude and the SNAP amplitudes were relatively preserved. In the study by Ramsay et al., in which electrodiagnostic testing was only performed in three of the five patients *(4)*, the sural SNAPs were absent in two patients and showed reduced amplitude in the third. The relevance of tissue edema to the findings of low SNAP amplitudes is not clear, as near nerve recordings were not obtained. Repetitive nerve stimulation (RNS) was performed on three patients in one study, and an abnormal decrement was noted in each case *(5)*. In each of these patients, vecuronium had been discontinued less than 7 days prior.

By and large, needle examination showed fibrillation potentials and positive sharp wave activity (21 of the 24 patients examined in these three case series) in some (but not all) muscles evaluated. No particular pattern of denervation changes was noted, with fibrillations and positive sharp waves noted in both proximal and distal muscles in both the arms and the legs *(5,6)*. Myopathic MUPs were recorded in 7 of 14 patients in one study *(6)* and 4 of 7 patients in another *(5)*. In some patients, no voluntary MUPs were recorded.

In summary, therefore, these reports suggest that although the clinical context of high-dose steroid and NMBA use might suggest CIM as the neuromuscular cause of weakness in a given patient, the absence of such a history is not helpful in differentiating CIP from CIM. Limb weakness is most common, with a small proportion of patients also showing facial and extra-ocular muscle weakness. There is no particular predilection for proximal limb muscles to be affected. The electrodiagnostic findings are typically those of reduced CMAP response amplitude, although SNAP response amplitudes may also be reduced in ICU patients for technical reasons. Ongoing muscle denervation on needle examination is usually seen, although again without predilection for particular muscles. When voluntary MUPs are recruited, they tend to be polyphasic and of low amplitude and short duration. Not infrequently, however, weakness may be sufficiently severe (or movement may be impossible for other reasons such as a septic encephalopathy) that MUP morphology cannot be reliably ascertained.

2.4. Can CIP and CIM be Differentiated on Clinical and Electrophysiological Grounds?

To appreciate the similarities and differences between the polyneuropathy and myopathy of the ICU, it is helpful to consider the data outlined in Table 23.1, which are more noticeable for the similarities between CIP and CIM than for the differences. Both CIP and CIM may occur in the context of sepsis and multi-organ failure. The available data simply do not inform on the issue as to whether high-dose steroids and NMBAs predispose more to CIM than CIP, in that the use of these agents was not reported in the largest series of CIP patients published to date. Similarly, the pattern of weakness is not obviously helpful, in that both proximal and distal weakness may be encountered in both CIP and CIM. One noticeable difference is the occurrence of extra-ocular muscle weakness only in patients with CIM. The electrodiagnostic examination is, unfortunately, similarly disappointing. CMAP amplitudes, as expected, are reduced in both disorders. A substantial proportion of patients with CIM were also found to have either reduced SNAP amplitudes or absent responses. Even though this finding may have been due to technical factors related to tissue edema, it does not detract from the observation that abnormal SNAP responses are less useful than might be expected in differentiating CIP from CIM. Finally, consider the electromyographical examination. The MUPs were generally small and polyphasic, a morphology consistent with both a myopathic and a severe neurogenic process. The differentiation between these two processes, at least in theory, hinges upon the MUP recruitment pattern, being reduced in a neurogenic process and occurring early in a myopathic process. Regrettably, the severity of weakness so often encountered in neuromuscular weakness in the ICU, together with a superimposed encephalopathy, means that there is often very little if any voluntary activity. It should be apparent, therefore, that it may be extremely difficult at times to differentiate CIP from CIM (Table 23.1).

Rich and colleagues have suggested that direct muscle stimulation might provide a reliable means to differentiate the polyneuropathy and myopathy of critical illness *(10, 11)*. They hypothesized that the decrease in CMAP amplitude in patients with CIM is due to a loss of muscle membrane excitability. If this were true, then direct stimulation of muscle should evoke a small or no CMAP, similar to that elicited by motor nerve stimulation. By contrast, normal CMAP amplitude would be expected from direct muscle stimulation in the face of a polyneuropathy even though the nerve-evoked CMAP is

Table 23.1
Clinical Features of Critical Illness Polyneuropathy (CIP) and Critical Ilness Myopathy (CIM)

	Zochodne (3)	Lacomis (6)	Zochodne (5)	Ramsay (4)
Critical illness syndrome	CIP	CIM	CIM	CIM
Sample size	$n = 19$	$n = 14$	$n = 7$	$n = 5$
Clinical Context				
Sepsis/multi-organ failure	19	1	7	5
Status asthmaticus	–	5	–	–
Other	–	8	–	–
Medications				
High-dose steroids	NS	14	4	5
NMBAs	NS	13	7	5
Pattern of weakness				
Limb proximal > distal	–	0	"Severe"	"Severe"
Limb distal > proximal	"Usually"	9	flaccid	flaccid
Limb distal = proximal	–	5	paralysis"	paralysis"
Facial	3	5	0	0
Extra-ocular muscles	0	1	2	2
Electrophysiology				
Decreased CMAP amplitude	17/17	13/14	6/7	3/3
Decreased SNAP amplitude	17/17	3/3	3/7	2/3
Fibrillations/positive sharps	17/17	11/14	7/7	3/3
Decrement on RNS	0/2	–	3/3	–
MUP morphology	Normal or small and polyphasisc	Small, short, polyphasic in 12/14	Small, short polyphasic in 4/7	Small, short polyphasic in 1/3
MUP recruitment pattern	Reduced	NS	NS	NS

NS, not stated; NMBA, neuromuscular blocking agent; CMAP, compound muscle action potential; SNAP, sensory nerve action potential; RNS, repetitive nerve stimulation; MUP, motor unit potential.

markedly reduced. Using the ratio of nerve-evoked to direct muscle stimulated CMAP amplitude, they were able to show that muscle membrane is relatively unexcitable in 11 of 14 patients suspected of having CIM (11). The utility of this test is greatest when weakness is profound or when voluntary activity is limited by concurrent pathology, such as a septic encephalopathy. The pattern of motor unit recruitment can be used to differentiate myopathy from polyneuropathy when adequate voluntary motor activity is possible. The use of direct muscle stimulation has not gained widespread usage, probably in large part because, as described, it requires the use of intramuscular recording and stimulating electrodes.

3. TREATMENT

3.1. Are There Any Treatment Modalities That Impact Outcome in Patients With CIP or CIM?

There are no studies that have directly addressed the impact of any sort of treatment modality in patients with critical illness polyneuropathy and myopathy. The only clue, perhaps, derives from the observation that the administration of even a single dose of corticosteroid *(12)* represents a risk factor for the development of ICU acquired paresis. On the basis of this finding, these authors cautioned that physicians should "... carefully weigh the indications [for] corticosteroids in critically ill patients and restrict their use to conditions such as septic shock, unresolved adult respiratory distress syndrome, and status asthmaticus in which corticosteroids have been shown to have a significant impact on morbidity and mortality" *(12)*. Finally, the observation by the same authors that the duration of multiple organ dysfunction represents an important risk factor for ICU-acquired paresis (ICUAP) suggests that preventative or therapeutic strategies to reduce the risk of multi-organ dysfunction might also reduce the risk of ICUAP.

4. PROGNOSIS

4.1. What Are the Risk Factors for the Development of Neuromuscular Weakness in the ICU?

Most of the retrospective studies of risk factors for the occurrence of critical illness neuromuscular weakness have not included data from control groups that would enable legitimate determination of risk factors for the development of critical illness neuromuscular weakness. There has been one retrospective study that did provide such data *(13)*, as well as two prospective studies *(12,14)*, the results of which are discussed here.

In the retrospective study, 50 consecutive patients with acute respiratory distress syndrome were divided into two groups—those with critical illness neuropathy/myopathy and those without neuromuscular weakness *(13)*. The characteristics of the patients in these two groups were compared. Those with neuromuscular weakness were found to be older, to have been in the ICU and have required mechanical ventilation for significantly longer periods of time, and to have higher mean daily blood glucose concentrations *(13)*. Duration of sepsis, severity of illness, and the use of nondepolarizing muscle NMBAs were no different between the two groups.

One prospective study of 98 critically ill patients included 31 patients with CIP or CIM and 67 patients without neuromuscular weakness *(14)*. Multivariate Cox-Proportional Hazards regression analysis showed that the presence of the systemic inflammatory response syndrome (SIRS) and the Acute Physiology and Chronic Health Evaluation (APACHE) III score (severity of critical illness) were the only significant risk factors for the occurrence of ICU neuromuscular weakness. The use of nondepolarizing neuromuscular blocking agents, steroids, and aminoglycoside antibiotics were considered in the model, but found not to have meaningful predictive value.

The second prospective study included consecutive patients admitted to an ICU who required mechanical ventilation for more than 7 days *(12)*. Patients were screened daily for level of arousal and, once sufficient arousal and comprehension were established, they were evaluated both clinically and electrophysiologically for evidence of neuromuscular weakness. Twenty-four patients were identified with intensive care unit acquired paresis (ICUAP), a syndromic diagnosis encompassing both critical illness myopathy and polyneuropathy. The study also included 71 patients without ICUAP. They examined a number of baseline patient characteristics and a variety of metabolic variables as well as a range of organ dysfunction-related variables in an effort to identify risk factors for the development of ICUAP.

Table 23.2
Risk Factors for Critical Illness Neuromuscular Weakness

	de Letter (14)	Bercker (13)	De Jonghe (12)
Study design	Prospective	Retrospective	Prospective
Study population	ICU patients requiring ventilation for >4 d	ARDS	ICU patients requiring ventilation for >7 d
Sample size	98	50	24
Analysis	Multivariate	Univariate	Multivariate
Risk factors for neuromuscular weakness	1. SIRS 2. APACHE III score	1. Older age 2. Longer duration of ICU stay 3. Longer duration of mechanical ventilation 4. Higher mean daily blood glucose concentration	1. Female gender 2. Longer duration of multi-organ failure 3. Longer duration of ventilation prior to awakening 4. Administration of corticosteroids

ARDS, Acute Respiratory Distress Syndrome; SIRS, Systemic Inflammatory Response Syndrome; APACHE Score, Acute Physiology and Chronic Health Evaluation Score.

The results of these studies are summarized in Table 23.2. Each study examined a different range of potential risk factors with the result that there is little agreement between these studies regarding the risk factors for critical illness neuromuscular weakness.

4.2. Does the Presence of CIP or CIM Impact on Morbidity and Mortality in the ICU?

There are a few prospective studies that have examined the impact of critical illness neuromuscular weakness on the clinical course in the ICU. Berek et al. (15) recruited all patients with SIRS over a 1-year period, excluding those with a pre-existing neurological disorder. They identified 22 patients whom they investigated clinically and electrophysiologically. Although their criteria for the diagnosis of polyneuropathy are a little unclear, they identified 16 patients with evidence of an axonal polyneuropathy and an additional 2 patients with a mixed axonal and demyelinating polyneuropathy (not typically recognized as being part of the spectrum of CIP). There were seven deaths among these patients in the ICU as a result of multiple organ failure. There are no data reported from a control group (i.e., ICU patients without evidence of critical illness polyneuropathy), however, which makes it difficult to know the prognostic significance of the presence of CIP.

Similar results were reported by Douglass and colleagues in their prospective study of 25 consecutive patients who required mechanical ventilation for severe asthma (16). Myopathy developed in nine of these patients, and the need for mechanical ventilation was significantly longer in these patients compared with controls (12.9 days vs 3.1 days, $p < 0.02$). There were three deaths in this study, only one of which occurred among the patients with myopathy.

Leijten et al. (17) prospectively studied all patients in the ICU who required mechanical ventilation for more than 7 days. They excluded those with pre-existing neurological conditions and screened the remainder for electrophysiological evidence of a polyneuropathy. They defined CIP on the basis of the electrodiagnostic findings of abnormal spontaneous activity in combination with reduced response amplitude in at least two muscles or nerves. (Note that these criteria could include patients with CIM as well as CIP.) Their sample included 38 patients, 18 of whom developed CIP. They provided comparative data from both groups of patients—those with and those without evidence of CIP. They found that the CIP patients required longer periods of ventilation (34 vs 20 days [$p = 0.02$]) and had a higher mortality than the non-CIP group (44% vs 20% [$p = 0.11$] despite similar APACHE II scores at the time of admission to the ICU. The median number of different organs affected, as well as the mean maximal multiple organ dysfunction scale (MODS) scores, were also significantly higher in the CIP patients. It is unclear, therefore, whether the CIP is the cause or the consequence of more severe illness in the ICU. At the very least, the presence of CIP seems to be associated with a poorer prognosis while in the ICU.

The prospective cohort study of De Jonghe et al. (12) showed similar results. This study included 24 patients with ICUAP, a combination of CIP and CIM, as well as 71 controls. The mean total duration of mechanical ventilation was significantly longer in the ICUAP group (35 days vs 18 days), $p < 0.01$), and there was a trend toward a longer ICU stay in the ICUAP patients (28 vs 15 days, $p = 0.06$).

4.3. What Is the Long-Term Outcome of Patients With CIM or CIP?

Although there have been a number of prospective studies of patients with critical illness neuromuscular weakness *(12,15–19)*, the long-term outcome has, in general, been poorly documented. In their study of myopathy in patients with severe asthma, Douglass and colleagues *(16)* reported that "... the mean duration of myopathy ... was 27 ± 12 days," although it is not entirely clear what is meant by this statement. In the 18 patients with CIP in the study by Berek et al. *(15)*, 11 subjects survived and were discharged from the ICU. Follow-up 3 months later revealed clinical evidence of polyneuropathy in seven, mostly comprising reduced deep tendon reflexes and mild motor and sensory loss. There was electrophysiological evidence of polyneuropathy in all 11 patients. Nevertheless, all patients were improved, even the patient with the most severe neuropathy initially. Finally, in the most recent study of ICU acquired paresis by De Jonghe et al. *(12)*, the mean duration of paresis in survivors after regaining wakefulness was 45 days (with a median of 21 days). At follow-up 9 months later, of the 19 ICUAP patients who survived the ICU, 3 subsequently died, 1 was lost to follow-up, and the remaining 15 all achieved an Medical Research Council (MRC) score of at least 48 (i.e., at least MRC grade 4/5 in each of the three muscles tested in each limb).

It would seem, therefore, that most patients with ICU-acquired neuromuscular weakness who are discharged from the ICU do survive, and eventually show signs of improvement.

4.4. Are There Prognostic Implications to the Differentiation Between CIP and CIM?

Whether there are prognostic implications to the differentiation between CIP and CIM is an extremely difficult question to answer based on the available data. The statement by Douglass et al. *(16)* that "... the mean duration of myopathy ... was 27 ± 12 days" seems to suggest that recovery from myopathy may occur over a relatively short time period. In contrast, the limited follow-up data from studies of patients with polyneuropathy *(12,15)* indicate that there is usually residual disease (both clinically and electrophysiologically) even after many months of follow-up. These data create the impression that patients with CIM tend to recover more quickly than those with CIP, although the quality of data supporting this conclusion is quite limited.

5. SUMMARY

- CIP is characterized clinically by limb weakness that affects the legs more severely than the arms and distal muscles more severely than proximal muscles; facial weakness is uncommon; deep tendon reflexes are usually absent and distal loss of sensation can be demonstrated in patients who are sufficiently awake to cooperate with the sensory examination.
- CIP is characterized electrophysiologically by reduced CMAPs, reduced sensory nerve action potential amplitudes, and abundant fibrillations and positive sharp waves on needle electromyography.
- The pattern of weakness in critical illness myopathy is diverse, and either proximal or distal muscle weakness may predominate; facial and extra-ocular muscle weakness may occasionally be present.

- CMAP amplitudes are reduced in CIM, but SNAP amplitudes are relatively preserved (unless obscured by technical difficulties encountered in recording sensory responses in the ICU); needle electromyography reveals fibrillations and positive sharp waves in both proximal and distal muscles.
- There is extensive overlap in the clinical manifestations of CIP and CIM; notable differentiating features are the presence of extra-ocular muscle weakness only in patients with myopathy and the more commonly absent SNAP responses in patients with neuropathy; although the morphology of motor units and their recruitment should, in theory, help to differentiate these disorders, weakness in these patients in frequently sufficiently severe that no voluntarily motor units are recorded.
- Female gender, the use of corticosteroids, and the duration of multi-organ dysfunction appear to be important risk factors for the development of critical illness neuromuscular weakness.
- Data from two prospective studies have shown that patients with critical illness polyneuropathy require longer periods of ventilation and have a higher mortality than patients without CIP.
- The long-term outcome of patients with critical illness neuromuscular weakness has not been well characterized; the available data suggest that most who survive their ICU stay eventually shows signs of improvement.
- There are limited data suggesting that the prognosis for patients with CIM is somewhat better than that for patients with CIP.

REFERENCES

1. Bolton CF, Gilbert JJ, Hahn AF, Sibbald WJ. Polyneuropathy in critically ill patients. J Neurol, Neurosurg Psychiatry 1984;47:1223–1231.
2. Bolton CF, Laverty DH, Brown JD, Witt NJ, Hahn AF, Sibbald WJ. Critically ill polyneuropathy: electrophysiological studies and differentiation from Guillain-Barre syndrome. J Neurol, Neurosurg Psychiatry 1986; 49:563–573.
3. Zochodne DW, Bolton CF, Wells GA, et al. Critical illness polyneuropathy. A complication of sepsis and multiple organ failure. Brain 1987;110:819–842.
4. Ramsay D, Zochodne D, Robertson D, Nag S, Ludwin S. A syndrome of acute severe muscle necrosis in intensive care unit patients. J Neuropathol Exp Neurol 1993;52:387–398.
5. Zochodne DW, Ramsay DA, Saly V, Shelley S, Moffatt S. Acute necrotizing myopathy of intensive care: electrophysiological studies. Muscle Nerve 1994;17:285–292.
6. Lacomis D, Giuliani MJ, Van Cott A, Kramer DJ. Acute myopathy of intensive care: clinical, electromyographic and pathological aspects. Ann Neurol 1996;40:645–654.
7. MacFarlane I, Rosenthal F. Severe myopathy after status asthmaticus. Lancet 1977;2:615.
8. Van Marle W, Woods K. Acute hydrocortisone myopathy. Br Med J 1980;2:271–272.
9. Williams TJ, O'Hehir RE, Czarny D, Horne M, Bowes G. Acute myopathy in severe acute asthma treated with intravenously administered corticosteroids. Am Rev Respir Dis 1988;137:460–463.
10. Rich M, Teener J, Raps E, Schotland D, Bird S. Muscle is electrically inexcitable in acute quadriplegic myopathy. Neurology 1996;46:731–736.
11. Rich MM, Bird SJ, Raps EC, McCluskey LF, Teener JW. Direct muscle stimulation in acute quadriplegia myopathy. Muscle Nerve 1997;20:665–673.
12. De Jonghe B, Sharshar T, Lefaucheur JP, et al. Paresis acquired in the intensive care unit. A prospective multicenter study. JAMA 2002;288:2859–2867.
13. Bercker S, Weber–Carstens S, Deja M, et al. Critical illness polyneuropathy and myopathy in patients with acute respiratory distress syndrome. Criti Care Med 2005;33:711–715.
14. de Letter M, Schmitz PI, Visser LH, et al. Risk factors for the development of polyneuropathy and myopathy in critically ill patients. Criti Care Med 2001;29:2281–2286.

15. Berek K, Margreiter J, Willeit J, Berek A, Schmutzhard E, Mutz N. Polyneuropathies in critically in patients: a prospective evaluation. Intensive Care Med 1996;22:849–855.
16. Douglass JA, Tuxen DV, Horne M, et al. Myopathy in severe asthma. Am Rev Respir Dis 1992; 146:517–519.
17. Leijten F, De Weerd A, Poortvliet D, De Ridder V, Ulrich C, Harinck–De Weerd J. Critical illness polyneuropathy in multiple organ dysfunction syndrome and weaning from the ventilator. Intensive Care Medicine 1996;22:856–861.
18. Spitzer AR, Giancarlo T, Maher L, Awerbuch G, Bowles A. Neuromuscular causes of prolonged ventilator dependency. Muscle Nerve 1992;15:682–686.
19. Witt NJ, Zochodne DW, Bolton CF, et al. Peripheral nerve function in sepsis and multiple organ failure. Chest 1991; 99:176–184.

24 Myotonic Dystrophy

1. INTRODUCTION

Myotonic dystrophy (MD) is the most common adult-onset muscular dystrophy with a prevalence reported as approximately 2.5 to 5.5 per 100,000. Inheritance is autosomal-dominant. Early linkage studies assigned the MD gene to chromosome 19, and the mutation underlying the most common form of MD, dystrophia myotonica type 1 (DM1) was subsequently identified as a CTG triplet repeat expansion in the 3' untranslated region of the dystrophia myotonica protein kinase (DMPK) gene. Subsequent studies have revealed a second genetic locus on chromosome 3, with the responsible mutation being an expansion of a CCTG tetranucleotide repeat in an apparently unrelated gene, the zinc finger transcription factor 9 gene; this genotype is referred to as dystrophia myotonica type 2 (DM2). MD is characterized by tremendous variability in the phenotypic expression and severity of the disease. In the congenital form of the disease, infants are born with severe generalized weakness and hypotonia and death ensues from respiratory failure. In the noncongenital forms of the disease, age of onset may vary from the teenage years to the sixth decade of life. The phenotype may be sufficiently mild that the affected individual is entirely asymptomatic.

MD is a multi-system disease in which skeletal muscle, the central nervous system, the heart, eyes, endocrine system, and gastrointestinal tract may all be affected. The focus on this chapter is on the neuromuscular, cardiac, and central nervous system manifestations of the disease. What is the typical pattern of weakness and myotonia in the noncongenital forms of the disease? How common are cardiac abnormalities, and how are they best diagnosed? Why do MD patients have excessive daytime somnolence, and how should this problem be managed? How severe is the muscle weakness in MD, how rapidly does skeletal muscle weakness progress, and what sort of disability can patients with MD expect to develop over the course of their lives? These and other questions are the focus of this chapter.

2. DIAGNOSIS

2.1. What Is the Typical Clinical Phenotype of Myotonic Dystrophy?

Review of the literature has not disclosed any large series of patients with MD that shed light on the typical clinical phenotype. Most texts reference the monograph by Peter Harper *(1)*. The description of the clinical phenotype described in this monograph is, no doubt, based on the experience of the author, but the text does not disclose the number of patients studied or the gold standard that was used for the diagnosis and does not provide numeric data to indicate the relative frequencies of the different clinical symp-

From: *Neuromuscular Disease: Evidence and Analysis in Clinical Neurology*
By: M. Benatar © Humana Press Inc., Totowa, NJ

toms and signs. As such, an evidence-based description of the clinical phenotype is difficult. Nevertheless, because no better source has been identified, this monograph has been referenced here.

The distinction between DM1 and DM2 had not been made at the time that Harper's monograph was published (1), but because DM1 is by far the most common, it is likely that the clinical phenotype that he describes is mostly relevant to DM1.

The muscles most frequently affected in myotonic dystrophy are the facial muscles, levator palpebrae superficialis, temporalis, sternomastoids, the distal muscles of the forearm, and the ankle dorsiflexors. Less commonly, the quadriceps, respiratory muscles, intrinsic muscles of the hands and feet, palatal and pharyngeal muscles, tongue, and extra-ocular muscles may be involved. Muscles of the pelvic girdle, the hamstrings and ankle plantarflexors are typically spared (1).

Myotonia is the hallmark of myotonic dystrophy and "... can be elicited in almost every symptomatic patient with the disease, and also is probably the single most valuable sign of the disorder in presymptomatic individuals bearing the abnormal gene" (1). Myotonia is most easily demonstrated in the hands—there is delayed relaxation following a forceful grip (grip myotonia) and a firm tap on the thenar eminence with the patellar hammer will elicit a stereotyped abnormal movement of the thumb (percussion myotonia). Although almost invariably present, myotonia typically does not lead to prominent clinical symptoms.

In a small study, Avaria and Patterson reported the frequency of weakness of specific muscles in 20 patients with MD (2). The study implies that these patients all had DM1, but the evidence to support this conclusion is not provided. Facial muscles, neck flexors, and external rotators of the shoulder were weak in all patients (2). Hip flexion weakness was present in only approximately 40% of patients, and proximal arm weakness was only slightly more frequent. Apart from the frequent finding of weakness of shoulder external rotation and involvement of hip flexors in a significant minority of patients, these findings are consistent with those described by Harper (1).

In an effort to define the symptoms and signs of patients with DM2, Day and colleagues have described the clinical features that were present in 234 patients with genetically confirmed DM2 (3). Neck flexor weakness, present in 75% of patients, was the most common clinical finding, with hip flexion weakness present in 64% and thumb/finger deep flexor weakness detected in 55%. Facial muscles and ankle dorsiflexors were weak in 12% and 16% of patients, respectively. The differences in the pattern of weakness seen in patients with DM1 and DM2 are summarized in Table 24.1 (with the data from DM1 derived from Harper's monograph). These data suggest a few notable clinical differences between DM1 and DM2. The frequent involvement of hip flexors and the relatively infrequent facial weakness in DM2 are the two most striking features that set this disorder apart from DM1 (3).

2.2. Which Muscles Are Most Likely to Show Myotonia on Electromyography?

Streib and Sun examined 25 newly diagnosed patients with MD using a fairly standardized approach (4). All but two patients had clinical evidence of myotonia. The distal muscles of the upper extremity and the facial muscles were most frequently abnormal. The first dorsal interosseous, the abductor pollicis previs, and the flexor pollicis longus

Table 24.1
Clinical Phenotype of Dystrophia Myotonica Type 1 (DM1) and Type 2 (DM2)

Clinical feature	DM1[a]	DM2
Weakness of neck flexion	+++	75%
Facial weakness	++	12%
Weakness of hip flexion	+	64%
Weakness of thumb/finger deep flexors	+++	55%
Weakness of ankle dorsiflexion	++	16%
Weakness of shoulder abductors	++	20%
Weakness of elbow extension	++	31%
Myotonia on examination	+++	75%
Cataracts	++	60%

[a]Actual percentages are not provided, as these are not available.
Data from refs. *1,3*.

showed myotonic discharges in 92%, 96%, and 96% of patients, respectively. Orbicularis oris was similarly abnormal in 95% of patients. Only 3 of the 25 patients had myotonia in every muscle examined *(4)*. Although the distal arm and facial muscles provide high diagnostic yield, no muscle was abnormal in every patient examined, underlying the importance of sampling a number of muscles before concluding that myotonia is absent.

2.3. What Is the Nature of the Cardiac Involvement in MD?

There are relatively few studies that have described the frequency and nature of cardiac symptoms in patients with myotonic dystrophy. Church described the cardiac symptoms and electrocardiogram (ECG) findings of 17 patients with myotonic dystrophy and reviewed the pertinent literature on 252 other cases *(5)*. She found that 23% of her 17 patients and only 16% of those reported in the literature had symptoms referable to the cardiovascular system *(5)*. Symptoms among her series of 17 patients included palpitations, dyspnea, orthopnea, and pedal edema, but the specific symptoms amongst the larger number of patients from the literature review were not reported.

In contrast to the relatively few descriptions of cardiac symptoms among patients with MD, there have been numerous reports of the electrocardiographic abnormalities in these patients (Table 24.2) *(6–14)*. These studies show that atrioventricular and intraventricular conduction disturbances are the most common abnormalities, indicating that the His–Purkinje system bears the brunt of the disease, with consequent prolongation of the PR interval and QRS complex. The studies by Olofsson *(6)*, Fragola *(7)* and Florek *(8)* likely provide the most reliable estimates of the frequency of various ECG abnormalities as these three series included consecutive patients. The studies summarized in Table 24.2 did not provide a clear description of the selection criteria that were used to include patients, and so it is likely that selection bias exists in these studies, although the nature and extent of this bias cannot be determined. The study by Griggs and colleagues provides a good example in that one-half of the patients included in the study warranted investigation with invasive electrophysiological studies, suggesting that the study population may have been biased toward those with more prominent cardiac involvement *(14)*.

Table 24.2
Cardiac Conduction Abnormalities in Myotonic Dystrophy

Reference	n	Study population	1st degree AVB	LBB	RBB	LAFB	ST/T-wave abnormalities
Olofsson (6)	65	Consecutive series	20%	5%	5%	17%	16%
Fragola (7)	56	Consecutive series	29%	9%	16%	16%	–
Florek (8)	45	Consecutive series	20%	7%	2%	7%	–
Hawley (9)	31	Case series (selection criteria not specified)	61%	10%	6%	19%	–
Melacini (10)	42	Case series (selection criteria not specified)	29%	14%	17%	19%	–
Nguyen (11)	12	Case series of patients undergoing autopsy for whom heart tissue available	50%	25%	17%	25%	–
Hiromasa (12)	10	Case series (3 patients referred for palpitations)	80%	10%	0	60%	–
Motta (13)	8	Case series (2 patients referred for palpitations)	25%	12.5%	12.5%	–	–
Griggs (14)	26	Case series (selection criteria not specified—13 patients underwent EPS)	65%	8%	19%	8%	–

AVB, atrioventricular block; LBBB, left bundle branch block; RBBB, right bundle branch block; LAFB, left anterior fascicular block; EPS, electrophysiological studies.

These data, therefore, indicate that there is a discrepancy between the frequency with which patients complain of cardiovascular symptoms and the frequency with which abnormalities may be found on the ECG. The most common ECG findings are atrioventricular and intraventricular conduction disturbances. First-degree atrioventricular block is present in 20–30% of patients and bundle branch block in 10–15%.

2.4. Which Arrhythmias Occur Most Frequently in Patients With MD?

A number of studies present data from routine surface ECG and 24-hour ambulatory ECG monitoring that provide information about the occurrence of various arrhythmias (Table 24.3A,B) *(6,7,9–13,15,16)*. These data indicate that atrial flutter and atrial fibrillation occur most frequently, with a smaller number of patients experiencing ventricular and supraventricular tachycardia. Only two of these studies included consecutive patients *(6,7)*. Most studies either did not report the criteria used to select patients for inclusion in the study or selected patients at high risk for cardiac involvement (either referral for electrophysiological evaluation *(15)* or autopsy with heart tissue available for study *[11]*), indicating the likely presence of significant selection bias. It is, therefore, difficult to obtain a reliable estimate of either the incidence or prevalence of these arrhythmias.

2.5. How useful is 24-Hour Ambulatory ECG Monitoring for the Diagnosis of Myotonic Heart Disease?

There are a limited number of studies that shed light on this question (Table 24.3B) *(10, 12,13,16)* and those studies that have reported the results of 24-hour ambulatory ECG monitoring in patients with MD have frequently not provided information regarding the correlation between the electrocardiographic findings and the presence of symptoms or signs of cardiac disease. Furthermore, to reliably answer the question of the utility of 24-hour ambulatory ECG recording, it is necessary to know the frequency with which the results of the study have some clinical impact (either in terms of prompting further investigation or altering management). None of the published studies provide data that help to answer this question.

From the available literature, it seems that ambulatory ECG monitoring may detect cardiac arrhythmias in patients in whom these were not evidenct on routine 12-lead ECG *(10,12,13,16)*. A proportion of those patients in whom ambulatory monitoring has shown abnormalities might be considered at high risk because of the presence of conduction disturbances on routine 12-lead ECG (*see* Table 24.3B), but this is not invariably the case. In seems reasonable to investigate all patients who have symptoms with 24-hour ambulatory ECG. It might even be argued that all patients with abnormalities on 12-lead ECG should undergo 24-hour ambulatory monitoring, but there is little evidence to support this conclusion. It remains unclear whether asymptomatic MD patients without abnormalities on 12-lead ECG should also undergo such monitoring.

2.6. How Common Is Excessive Daytime Sleepiness Among Patients With MD?

Excessive daytime sleepiness (EDS) is said to be a common feature of MD, but there are relatively few studies that provide a reliable estimate of the frequency of this symp-

Table 24.3A
Cardiac Arrhythmias in Myotonic Dystrophy (12-Lead Surface Electrocardiogram)

Reference	Study population	n	Atrial fibrillation/ flutter	Ventricular tachycardia	Premature ventricular complexes
Motta (13)	Case series (selection criteria not specified)	8	1	0	0
Komajda (15)	Series of patients referred for elctrophysiological testing	12	2	0	0
Hiromasa (12)	Case series (selection criteria not specified)	10	0	0	3
Olofsson (6)	Consecutive case series	65	7	0	0
Nguyen (11)	Case series of patients undergoing autopsy for whom cardiac tissue was available for study	12	2	3	1
Hawley (9)	Case series (selection criteria not specified)	37	2	0	0
Fragola (7)	Consecutive case series	56	1	2	0

Table 24.3B
Cardiac Arrhythmias in Myotonic Dystrophy (24-Hour Ambulatory Monitoring)

Reference	Study population	n	Number of patients with abnormalities on 12-lead ECG	Atrial fibrillation/ flutter	Supraventricular tachycardia	Ventricular tachycardia	Premature ventricular complexes
Motta (13)	Case series (selection criteria not specified)	8	BBB (n = 1) 1st degree AVB (n = 1)	1[a]	0	0	2[b]
Perloff (16)	Case series (selection criteria not specified)	25	Not reported	2[c]	1[c]	1[c]	1[c]
Hiromasa (12)	Case series (selection criteria not specified)	10	1st degree AVB in all BBB (n = 1) Hemiblock (n = 1)	3[a]	0	2[b]	2[b]
Melacini (33)	Case series (selection criteria not specified)	42	Not reported	0	0	0	3[c]

ECG, electrocardiogram; AVB, atrioventricular block; BBB, bundle branch block.
[a]One patient with cardiovascular symptoms.
[b]Two patients with cardiovascular symptoms.
[c]Presence or absence of cardiovascular symptoms not specified.

tom. With one exception *(17)*, the available studies are relatively small *(18–20)*. In the largest series to date, Laberge and colleagues reported the frequency and characteristics of EDS in 157 consecutive patients with DM1 *(17)*. Thirty-three percent of patients met criteria for EDS *(17)*. In another series of 36 patients with genetically proven MD (DM1) who responded to a mailed questionnaire, Rubinsztein and colleagues noted that EDS was present in 16 (44%) patients, with 2 of these reporting symptoms suggestive of sleep apnea *(18)*. Manni similarly noted the presence of EDS in 5 of 10 consecutive patients with MD *(19)* and van der Meche and colleagues found that 17 of 22 consecutive patients with MD described symptoms of EDS *(20)*. These small series, therefore, suggest that the prevalence of EDS among patients with MD ranges from 44% *(18)* to 77% *(20)* whereas the largest series suggests a slightly lower prevalence of approximately 33% *(17)*. The differences in estimates of the prevalence of EDS are likely due to the different criteria used to define EDS in these various studies, as well as the potential for bias (e.g., selection bias in the study that utilized a mailed questionnaire *[18]*) and random error (i.e., due to small sample size *[18–20]*). The study with the larger sample size and which recruited consecutive patients and employed a uniform definition of EDS likely provides the most accurate estimate of the prevalence of this symptom—33% *(17)*.

2.7. What Is the Cause of EDS in MD?

There has been some controversy about the cause of EDS amongst patients with MD, as several potential mechanisms have been proposed. One possibility is that respiratory muscle weakness causes hypoventilation and CO_2 retention. Others have suggested that patients with MD are more susceptible to developing obstructive sleep apnea, due in part to their generally increased body mass index and in part due to weakness of pharyngeal muscles. The third possibility is that EDS results from some central disorder of arousal that might be a primary manifestation of the disease given the systemic nature of MD. The studies that have formally addressed these possibilities are few in number, and the published studies are relatively small (Table 24.4). These data suggest that EDS in MD is accompanied by a short latency to sleep onset *(21,22)* and that it is typically not caused by underlying sleep apnea *(19–23)*. There are conflicting data regarding the question of whether sleep-onset rapid eye movement (REM) occurs in these patients *(19,21,22)*. These findings are most consistent with the hypothesis that EDS in MD reflects some central disturbance of maintaining wakefulness and that a distinction should be drawn between this phenotype and the narcolepsy phenotype in which EDS, short sleep latency, and sleep-onset REM are accompanied by sleep paralysis, cataplexy, and hyponogogic/hypopompic hallucinations. The frequency of these narcoleptic symptoms is not increased among patients with DM *(17)*. Finally, the observation that DM patients with EDS tend to report long sleep periods, nonrestorative sleep, and difficulty being alert and receptive following morning awakening as well as the absence of sudden and uncontrollable attacks of deep sleep during normal awake times *(17)* provide further evidence for the distinction between narcolepsy and the EDS seen in patients with DM.

Table 24.4
Excessive Daytime Sleepiness in Myotonic Dystrophy

Reference	n	Study population	EDS	Sleep apnea (RDI >5)	MSL (<8 min)	SOREM	Daytime CO_2 retention
Van der Meche (20)	22	Consecutive patients with MD (11) referred specifically for EDS	17	5 (all central)—only 3 complained of EDS	Not reported	Not reported	Not reported
Gibbs (21)	19	Patients with MD who were referred for evaluation of EDS	19	5 (1 central, 1 obstructive, 1 mixed, 3 UARS)	12 of 13 who underwent MSLT (including 4 with sleep apnea) 5	8 of 13 (62%)	Not reported
Manni (19)	10	Consecutive patients with MD (unselected for EDS)	5	1 (mixed)		None	Not reported
Park (22)	7	Patients with MD referred for evaluation of EDS	7	2	5 of 5 who underwent MSLT	3 of 5	Not reported
Gilmartin (23)	7	Patients with MD not selected for sleep disturbance or EDS	3	3 (1 obstructive, 2 central); only 1 complained of EDS	Not reported	Not reported	1

RDI, respiratory disturbance index; MSL, mean sleep latency; SOREM, sleep-onset rapid eye movement; CO_2, carbon dioxide; MSLT, multiple sleep latency test; UARS, upper airways resistance syndrome.

3. TREATMENT

3.1. How Should MD Patients With Cardiac Conduction Disturbances be Managed?

Although MD patients are usually asymptomatic, it is worth asking specifically about symptoms that might suggest underlying cardiovascular disease such as dyspnea on exertion, presyncope, syncope, and palpitations. Given the frequent lack of symptoms and the high prevalence of cardiac conduction disturbances in MD patients (such as atrioventricular [AV] block and intraventricular conduction delays), a standard 12-lead ECG should be obtained regularly. The available data (*see* "Prognosis") suggest that most abnormalities evolve gradually over a period of many months *(7,9)*, and so routine ECG should probably be performed on at least an annual basis. The indications for 24-hour ambulatory ECG monitoring are less clear, but could certainly be justified in patients with symptoms and/ or those with abnormalities on routine ECG. The indications for invasive electrophysiological testing and pacemaker placement are less clear. In their 1998 evidence-based practice guideline, the American College of Cardiology recommended pacemaker placement for patients with third-degree AV block and patients with His–ventricular interval >100 ms (on electrophysiological studies) *(24)*. In their revised guidelines, published 4 years later, they added to this list the recommendation for pacemaker placement for MD patients with second- or even first-degree heart block irrespective of symptoms *(25)*. Interestingly, this change in the guidelines was not based on any new published data, but this guideline was rated as *class IIb* (condition for which there is conflicting evidence and/or a divergence of opinion about the usefulness/efficacy of a procedure with the weight of evidence/opinion in favor of usefulness/efficacy).

Given the uncertainty surrounding the need for a pacemaker in subjects without symptoms or those with relatively mild forms of atrioventricular and intraventricular conduction delay, a reasonable approach would seem to involve discussion of the issues with the patient and family and, if necessary, referral to a cardiologist with an interest and expertise in myotonic heart disease.

3.2. Is There Any Effective Treatment for EDS in MD?

There are two randomized placebo-controlled trials that have examined the efficacy of modafinil for the treatment of EDS in patients with myotonic dystrophy *(26,27)* as well as a single study of selegiline *(28)*. The study of selegiline showed no benefit.

The two studies of modafinil both employed a cross-over study design, but differed in the dosage used, the duration of therapy, and choice of primary efficacy variables (Table 24.5A). In the study by MacDonald, the dose of modafinil was increased to a maximum of 200 mg twice per day for the second week of the 2-week treatment period *(26)*. In the study by Talbot, subjects received half of this dose (200 mg per day), but were treated for 4 weeks *(27)*. Both studies used the Epworth Sleepiness Scale (ESS) as a primary outcome measure, but MacDonald and colleagues chose to report the mean ESS scores at the end of the study period whereas Talbot and colleagues used the mean change in ESS score between baseline and the end of each study period. Talbot and colleagues also used a modification of the Maintenance of Wakefulness Test (MWT) as a primary outcome measure. Subjects were asked to resist sleep while lying semi-recumbent in a dark room for a maximum of 40 minutes on three occasions during the day (9:30 AM, 11:30 AM,

Table 24.5A
Modafinil for the Treatment of Excessive Daytime Sleepiness (EDS) in Myotonic Dystrophy

Reference	n	Design	Dosage	Primary efficacy variable	Outcome
MacDonald (26)	40	Cross-over design 2 × 2wk 1 wk wash-out	100 mg bid × 1 wk 200 mg bid × 1 wk	Epworth Sleepiness Scale (ESS)	Mean ESS score 9.9 (modafinil) vs 12.4 (placebo)
Talbot (27)	20	Cross-over design 2 × 4 wk 2-wk wash-out	200 mg qd × 4 wk	Change in Maintenance of Wakefulness Test (MWT) score Change is ESS score	Significant change in MWT at 1.30pm, but not other times Nonsignificant reduction in ESS score

Bid, twice per day; qd, once per day.

Table 24.5B
Quality of Randomized Controlled Trials of Modafinil for EDS in Myotonic Dystrophy

Reference	Randomization	Allocation concealment	Observer binding	Patient blinding	Explicit inclusion/ exclusion criteria	Loss to follow-up
MacDonald (26)	Adequate	Adequate	Unclear	Adequate	Adequate	n = 4 (10%)
Talbot (27)	Adequate	Unclear	Unclear	Adequate	Adequate	n = 1 (5%)

443

and 1:30 PM). The change in MWT score between baseline and the end of the treatment period was used as one of the primary outcome measures. Both studies were of high methodological quality (Table 24.5B).

MacDonald and colleagues reported a significant reduction in mean ESS among subjects treated with modafinil, although they did not report the proportion of patients who improved or who achieved an ESS score reduction of a particular magnitude *(26)*.

In the study by Talbot and colleagues, significant improvement with modafinil was seen only with the change in MWT score at the third time point (1:30 PM), but efficacy was not demonstrated using the other primary outcome measures. The authors had not specified in advance which time point in the MWT would be used, with the result that they were in fact testing four primary outcome measures—change in MWT at three time points and the change in ESS—making it a little more difficult to interpret their findings. The benefits of modafinil were also evident on the secondary outcome measures (Stanford Sleepiness Scale, Profile of Mood States and the RAND 36-item Health survey) in the study by MacDonald *(26)*, but the secondary outcome measures in the study by Talbot and colleagues (driving simulation test and SF-36 quality of life score) showed no benefit *(27)*. It is possible that the benefits of modafinil were less clear in the study by Talbot and colleagues because a lower dose of modafinil was used.

Overall, therefore, there is some evidence (albeit somewhat conflicting) for the efficacy of modafinil (200 mg twice daily) for the treatment of EDS in patients with DM.

4. PROGNOSIS

4.1. How Severe Is the Skeletal Muscle Weakness in MD and How Rapidly Does It Progress?

There are limited data from which to gauge the severity and progression of skeletal muscle weakness in MD. In one study, Johnson and colleagues performed both manual muscle testing (MMT) and quantitative strength measures in 92 patients with MD *(29)*. The average MMT score for all muscle groups combined was 4.0 (on a scale of 0 to 5, with 4 indicating the ability to overcome gravity and resistance). The neck and trunk flexors were the weakest muscle groups, with only one-half of the patients able to move the neck and trunk against gravity (MMT score >3.0). Although not used in routine clinical practice and therefore less intuitively understood, quantitative measurement of strength in a subset of 36 patients showed that isometric strength was reduced between 26% and 72% for different muscle groups *(29)*.

There are no large studies that provide longitudinal (follow-up) data regarding muscle strength in patients with MD. Some insight into the rate of progression of skeletal muscle weakness, however, can be derived from cross-sectional data that relate muscle strength to age. In a subset of 51 patients (out of a total of 91), Johnson and colleagues found a linear decline in MMT scores with advancing age, with an average of 0.36 unit decline per decade of age *(29)*. These authors did not find a decline over time in their longitudinal analysis (i.e., in those patients for whom MMT scores were available at more than one point in time), but this may have been a reflection of the small sample size studied (longitudinal analysis was available in only a subset of 34 patients) *(29)*.

In a large cross-sectional study of 295 patients with MD living in the Saguenay–Lac–Saint-Jean region in Quebec, Mathieu and colleagues also found a linear decline in muscle strength with advancing age *(30)*. They also found a correlation between the duration of disease and the severity of muscle weakness. Although variability was wide, on average distal weakness developed after approximately 9 years' disease duration, proximal weakness developed after approximately 18 years, and patients become wheelchair bound after approximately 27 years *(30)*.

These data indicate that muscle weakness in patients with MD is quite variable, but does tend to decline gradually over time. Weakness tends to begin in distal muscles and progresses to involve proximal muscles over time. Although in the early stages of disease patients retain the ability to move muscles against gravity and against resistance, the weakness does become more severe with advancing age (and duration of disease) at a rate of approximately 0.36 units per decade.

4.2. Are There Any Factors That Reliably Predict the Progression of Muscle Weakness?

In their large cross-sectional study, Mathieu and colleagues examined the effects of age at disease onset, the sex of the patient, and the sex of the affected parent and found that none of these factors were predictive of the rate of disease progression *(30)*. Although in general, there is a correlation between the severity of the MD phenotype and the degree of expansion of the underlying CTG expansion, there has been no investigation into the question of whether larger CTG expansions are associated with more rapidly progressive disease. In summary, then, there do not appear to be any factors that reliably predict the progression of muscle weakness in MD.

4.3. What Is the Natural History of Cardiac Disease in MD?

A number of studies have followed patients longitudinally to determine the natural history of cardiac disease among those with MD (Table 24.6) *(7–9)*. Consecutive series of patients were followed in two of these series *(7,8)*, and mean follow-up ranged from 4.5 to 6 years. Conduction disturbances developed in those patients with normal ECG at the outset and the conduction abnormalities present initially became more severe over time *(7–9)*. In two of these studies there was a tendency for these conduction abnormalities to gradually worsen over time *(7,9)*. The authors of the third study did not comment on the rate at which conduction abnormalities evolved *(8)*. Hawley and colleagues concluded that the single death in their study might have been predicted on the basis of serial ECG changes, as "sudden death" was preceded by progressive prolongation of the PR interval and QRS complex over a period of 18 months *(9)*. Similarly, the patient who died in another series was known to have a history of atrial fibrillation and had a four-beat run of ventricular tachycardia. He died suddenly while awaiting electrophysiological investigation *(7)*.

There are, therefore, relatively little data on which to base firm conclusions about the natural history of cardiac conduction abnormalities in MD. The available literature suggests that there is a tendency for these conduction disturbances to progress over time, with two studies indicating that these changes tend to develop gradually. Sudden death is relatively uncommon, although the risk of fatal outcome may well have been mitigated by pacemaker placement in a significant minority of patients. There are too few reports of sudden death in patients with MD to determine the true risk of this complication.

Table 24.6
Natural History of Cardiac Disease in Myotonic Dystrophy

Reference	n	Study population	Mean follow-up (range)	ECG changes	PM	Adverse outcome
Florek (8)	45	Consecutive series	55 mo (12–177)	New 1st degree AVB (n = 6) Widening of QRS (n = 11) New BBB (n = 4)	5	Sudden death in one patient with PM (pacing spikes without ventricular capture). No deaths in non-PM group.
Fragola (7)	56	Consecutive series	56 mo (2–192)	New 1st degree AVB (n = 5) New BBB (n = 7)	9	One cardiac death in the non-PM group (patient with AF and history of a 4-beat run of VT)
Hawley (9)	31	Case series	72 mo (18–110)	New 1st degree AVB (n = 10) New BBB (n = 7)	1	Sudden death in 1 patient Atrial flutter/fibrillation in 2 patients

ECG, electrocardiogram; PM, pacemaker; AVB, atrioventricular block; BBB, bundle branch block; AF, atrial fibrillation; VT, ventricular tachycardia.

Similarly, there are limited studies that describe serial ECGs in advance of sudden death, and so it is not possible to draw any reliable conclusions regarding whether this complication might reliably have been predicted based on the increasing severity of conduction disturbances over time.

4.4. Is Life Expectancy Reduced in MD?

Data from a number of studies indicate that life expectancy is reduced in patients with MD *(31,32)*. In their large study of patients with MD living in the Saguenay–Lac–Saint-Jean region in Quebec, Mathieu and colleagues followed 367 patients longitudinally over a 10-year period and reviewed death certificates to determine the frequency and cause of death. Mortality was compared with that in the general population of the same region by calculating standardized mortality ratios *(31)*. During the 10-year follow-up period, 75 patients (20%) died. The mortality rate was 7.3 times higher than expected for the age-matched population. Deaths were mostly due to respiratory disease, although cardiovascular disease and neoplasia contributed to the excess mortality *(31)*. The risk of death was greatest among those with more severe weakness and for those with a younger age of onset of disease *(31)*.

In their follow-up study of 180 patients with MD living in Southern Limburg, a geographically isolated part of the Netherlands, de Die-Smulders and colleagues estimated survival using the Kaplan-Meier method. The attained age was used as the survival time and was compared with the expected survival among the general Dutch population. Median age at death was 59 and 60 years for men and women, respectively *(32)*. Survival to age 45 was comparable between MD patients and the general population, but survival of MD patients to age 65 was markedly reduced (18%) compared with that expected from the general population (78%) *(32)*. The most frequent causes of death were respiratory (pneumonia) and cardiac (arrhythmias), each accounting for approximately 30% of deaths *(32)*.

Life expectancy, therefore, is significantly reduced among patients with MD, with respiratory and cardiac disease being the most common causes of death. Younger age of onset and more severe muscle weakness are associated with an increased risk of death.

5. SUMMARY

- Facial muscles, eyelids, and neck flexors as well as forearm flexor muscles are the most commonly affected muscles in DM1.
- The high frequency of weakness of hip flexors and the low frequency of facial weakness in DM2 help to distinguish DM2 from DM1 clinically.
- Myotonia can be demonstrated most easily both clinically and electromyographically in distal muscles of the hands.
- Cardiac symptoms are unusual in MD, occurring in 16–23% of patients.
- Atrioventricular and intraventricular conduction delays are the most common electrocardiographic abnormalities. First-degree AV block occurs in 20–30% of patients and bundle branch block in 5–15%.
- These conduction abnormalities tend to worsen gradually over a period of months to years.
- Atrial flutter and fibrillation are the most common arrhythmias. Supraventricular and ventricular tachycardia may also occur, but less commonly.

- Surface ECG should be performed at least annually, and 24-hour ambulatory ECG is appropriate for patients with symptoms and/or those with abnormalities on routine 12-lead ECG.
- Sudden cardiac death does occur in MD, but the frequency with which it occurs and whether it might be predicted by prior changes on 12-lead ECG are not clear.
- Pacemaker placement is recommended for those with third-degree AV block; although some controversy persists, the American College of Cardiology has recommended pacemaker placement even for those with first- and second-degree AV block.
- EDS is a common symptom in MD, reported by approximately 33% of patients.
- EDS is infrequently due to sleep apnea and more likely represents a form of "idiopathic" hypersomnolence that is distinct from narcolepsy by virtue of the absence of "sleep attacks," cataplexy, sleep paralysis, and hallucinations.
- There is some evidence from randomized controlled trials to support the use of modafinil (200 mg twice daily) for the treatment of EDS in MD.
- Muscle weakness is typically mild in the early stages of the disease (Medical Research Council [MRC] grade 4) and affects distal muscles before proximal muscles (at least in DM1). Muscle strength declines at a rate of approximately 0.36 units per decade and may lead to significant proximal and distal weakness with increasing age and duration of disease. Many patients become wheelchair-bound in the later stages of the disease.
- There are no factors that reliably predict which patients will develop severe weakness and become wheelchair-bound.
- Life expectancy is reduced in MD. The median age of death is approximately 60 years.
- The most common causes of death in MD are respiratory and cardiac.

REFERENCES

1. Harper PS. Myotonic Dystrophy. Major Problems in Neurology. Vol. 21. W. B. Saunders Company, London: 1989.
2. Avaria M, Patterson V. Myotonic dystrophy: relative sensitivity of symptoms, signs and abnormal investigations. Ulster Med J 1994;63:151–154.
3. Day J, Ricker K, Jacobsen J, et al. Myotonic dystrophy type 2. Molecular, diagnostic and clinical spectrum. Neurology 2003;60:657–664.
4. Streib E, Sun SF. Distribution of electrical myotonia in myotonic muscular dystrophy. Ann Neurol 1983;14:80–82.
5. Church SC. The heart in myotonia atrophica. Arch Int Med 1967;119:176–181.
6. Olofsson BO, Forsberg H, Andersson S, Bjerle P, Henriksson A, Wedin I. Electrocardiographic findings in myotonic dystrophy. Br Heart J 1988;59:47–52.
7. Fragola PV, Luzi M, Calo L, et al. Cardiac involvement in myotonic dystrophy. Am J Cardiol 1994;74:1070–1072.
8. Florek RC, Triffon DW, Mann DE, Ringel SP, Reiter MJ. Electrocardiographic abnormalities in patients with myotonic dystrophy. West J Med 1990;153:24–27.
9. Hawley RJ, Milner MR, Gottdiener JS, Cohen A. Myotonic heart disease: a clinical follow-up. Neurology 1991;41:259–262.
10. Melacini P, Villanova C, Menegazzo E, et al. Correlation between cardiac involvement and CTG trinucleotide repeat length in myotonic dystrophy. J Am Coll Cardiol 1995;25:239–245.
11. Nguyen HH, Wolfe JT, Holmes DR, Edwards WD. Pathology of the cardiac conduction system in myotonic dystrophy: a study of 12 cases. J Am Coll Cardiol 1988;11:662–671.
12. Hiromasa S, Ikeda T, Kubota K, et al. Myotonic dystrophy: ambulatory electrocardiogram, electrophyisiologic study, and echocardiographic evaluation. Am Heart J 1987;113:1482–1488.
13. Motta J, Guilleminault C, Billingham M, Barry W, Mason J. Cardiac abnormalities in myotonic dystrophy. Electrophysiologic and histopathologic studies. Am J Med 1979;67:467–473.

14. Griggs RC, Davis RJ, Anderson DC, Dove JT. Cardiac conduction in myotonic dystrophy. Am J Med 1975;59:37–42.
15. Komajda M, Frank R, Vedel J, Fontaine G, Petitot JC, Grosgogeat Y. Intracardiac conduction defects in dystrophia myotonica. Electrophysiological study of 12 cases. Br Heart J 1980;43:315–320.
16. Perloff JK, Stevenson WG, Roberts NK, Cabeen W, Weiss J. Cardiac involvement in myotonic muscular dystrophy (Steinert's disease): a prospective study of 25 patients. Am J Cardiol 1984;54:1074–1081.
17. Laberge L, Begin P, Montplaisir J, Mathieu J. Sleep complaints in patients with myotonic dystrophy. J Sleep Res 2004;13:95–100.
18. Rubinsztein J, Rubinsztein D, Goodburn S, Holland A. Apathy and hypersomnia are common features of myotonic dystrophy. J Neurol, Neurosurg Psychiatry 1998;64:510–515.
19. Manni R, Zucca C, Martinetti M, Ottolini A, Lanzi G, Tartara A. Hypersomnia in dystrophica myotonica: a neurophysiological and immunogenetic study. Acta Neurol Scand 1991;84:498–502.
20. van der Meche F, Bogaard J, van der Sluys J, Schimsheimer R, Ververs C, Busch H. Daytime sleep in myotonic dystrophy is not caused by sleep apnoea. J Neurol, Neurosurg Psychiatry 1994;57:626–628.
21. Gibbs JW, Ciafaloni E, Radtke RA. Excessive datyime somnolence and increased rapid eye movement pressure in myotonic dystrophy. Sleep 2002;25:662–665.
22. Park YD, Radtke RA. Hypersomnolence in myotonic dystrophy: demonstration of sleep onset REM sleep. J Neurol, Neurosurg Psychiatry 1995;58:512–513.
23. Gilmartin J, Cooper B, Griffiths C, et al. Breathing during sleep in patients with myotonic dystrophy and non-myotonic respiratory muscle weakness. Q J Med 1991;78:21–31.
24. Gregoratos G, Cheitlin M, Conill A, et al. ACC/AHA Guidelines for Implantation of Cardiac Pacemakers and Antiarrhythmia Devices: Executive Summary—a report of the American College of Cardiology/American Heart Association Task Force on Practice Guidelines (Committee on Pacemaker Implantation). Circulation 1998;97:1325–1335.
25. Gregoratos G, Abrams J, Epstein AE, et al. ACC/AHA/NASPE 2002 guideline update for implantation of cardiac pacemakers and antiarrhythmia devices—summary article: a report of the American College of Cardiology/American Heart Association Task Force on Practice Guidelines (ACC/AHA/NASPE Committee to Update the 1998 Pacemaker Guidelines). J Am Coll Cardiol 2002;40:1703–1719.
26. MacDonald J, Hill J, Tarnopolsky M. Modafinil reduces excessive somnolence and enhances mood in patients with myotonic dystrophy. Neurology 2002; 59:1876–1880.
27. Talbot K, Stradling J, Crosby J, Hilton-Jones D. Reduction in excess daytime sleepiness by modafinil in patients with myotonic dystrophy. Neuromuscul Disord 2003;13:357–364.
28. Antonini G, Morino S, Fiorelli M, Fiorini M, Giubilei F. Selegiline in the treatment of hypersomnolence in myotonic dystrophy: a pilot study. J Neurol Sci 2002;147:167–169.
29. Johnson ER, Abresch RT, Carter GT, et al. Profiles of neuromuscular diseases—myotonic dystrophy. Am J Phys Med Rehabil 1995;74 (5 Suppl):S104–S116.
30. Mathieu J, De Braekeleer M, Prevost C, Boily C. Myotonic dystrophy: clinical assessment of muscular disability in an isolated population with presumed homogeneous mutation. Neurology 1992;42:203–208.
31. Mathieu J, Allard P, Potvin L, Prevost C, Begin P. A 10–year study of mortality in a cohort of patients with myotonic dystrophy. Neurology 1999;52:1658–1662.
32. de Die-Smulders C, Howeler C, Thijs C, et al. Age and cause of death in adult-onset myotonic dystrophy. Brain 1998;121:1557–1563.
33. Melacini P, Buja G, Fasoli G, et al. The natural history of cardiac involvement in myotonic dystrophy: an eight year follow-up in 17 patients. Clin Cardiol 1988;11:231–238.

25 Facioscapulohumeral Muscular Dystrophy

1. INTRODUCTION

Facioscapulohumeral (FSH) muscular dystrophy is the third most common dystrophy, after myotonic dystrophy and the dystrophinopathies (Duchenne and Becker), with a prevalence of approximately 1 in 20,000. It is inherited in an autosomal-dominant fashion and has been linked to microsatellite markers on chromosome 4q35. A deletion of a variable number of repetitive elements (known as D4Z4 repeats) leads to the generation of a small EcoRI restriction fragment that is recognized by the p13E-11 probe. The precise mechanism whereby this genetic abnormality results in disease is unclear, but it is thought that the deletion alters chromosomal structure and influences the expression of more centromerically located genes. Because of its slow progression and relatively benign course, FSH is the second most common dystrophy (after myotonic dystrophy) in adults.

What are the typical clinical manifestations of FSH muscular dystrophy, and which laboratory studies are most helpful in confirming the diagnosis? Are facial and scapular weakness essential components of the clinical syndrome? How useful is genetic testing for confirming or excluding the diagnosis and how often does FSH result from a new sporadic mutation? Are steroids or β-agonists of any therapeutic value in FSH and under what circumstances should scapular fixation be considered? What is the long-term prognosis for patients with FSH, and are there any clinical or genetic factors that might predict the course of the disease? These and other questions are the focus of this chapter.

2. DIAGNOSIS

2.1 What Is the Typical Clinical Phenotype of FSH Muscular Dystrophy?

Padberg has provided one of the most comprehensive descriptions of the clinical phenotype of patients with FSH muscular dystrophy (1). He examined 190 people in 19 families to identify 107 affected individuals. The gold standard by which these subjects were determined to have the disease is not entirely clear. It is stated that all 107 were gene carriers, and although the genetic data are not provided, he explains that the study began with 19 probands and the remaining affected individuals were identified by screening the family members of these probands. Some information on the clinical phenotype is also obtained from Tyler and Strephens' study of 58 individuals from a single kindred (2) and from Lunt and Harper's study of 146 patients from 41 families (3).

From: *Neuromuscular Disease: Evidence and Analysis in Clinical Neurology*
By: M. Benatar © Humana Press Inc., Totowa, NJ

Of the 107 affected subjects studied by Padberg, 73 were symptomatic, with the most common symptom being difficulty keeping the arms sustained above the shoulder level in various tasks (indicating shoulder girdle weakness), which was present in 82% of subjects *(1)*. Shoulder girdle weakness was similarly the most common symptom in the subjects evaluated by Tyler and Stephens *(2)*. Less common symptoms were facial weakness (10%) and weakness of foot extensors (8%) *(1)*.

Because patients were examined a mean of 28 years after the onset of disease, Padberg described separately the clinical findings in the 34 asymptomatic subjects in an effort to provide a description of the early features of the disease. Among these asymptomatic subjects, facial weakness was present in 91%, occurring in isolation in 24%. Shoulder weakness was present in 76% and foot extensor weakness in 26%. Various combinations of facial, shoulder girdle and foot extensor weakness were encountered with the most common being that of facial and shoulder girdle weakness (41%) *(1)*.

Among all of the affected subjects, facial weakness was present in 94% and was asymmetric in 53% of patients *(1)*. The asymmetry might affect one side more than the other or be mixed (with some muscle groups more severely affected on one side and other muscle groups more severely affected on the other side). In an effort to get a sense of the relative involvement of different muscle groups, the Medical Research Council (MRC) strength scores for each muscle were summed across the 74 patients in whom every muscle had been examined. These summed scores were then expressed as a percentage of the total possible score to obtain an average percentage that expressed the severity of muscle weakness (with lower percentages indicating more severe muscle weakness). Muscles with lower scores were presumed to have been affected in advance of muscles with higher scores. Based on this premise, the scapular fixators, latissimus dorsi, and pectoralis major muscles (as well as facial muscles) were deemed to be affected earliest in the course of the disease (Fig. 25.1), a finding also noted by Tyler and Stephens *(2)*. Anterior compartment muscles in the lower leg (tibialis anterior, extensor muscles of the toes, and the peroneii muscles) as well as the spinatii (supraspinatus and infraspinatus), triceps, deltoid, and teres major were affected next *(1)*. Pelvic girdle weakness as well as weakness of neck flexors and extensors, wrist extensors and intrinsic hand muscles were affected only late in the course of the disease (Fig. 25.1) *(1)*. Asymmetric muscle involvement was common (64%), frequently affecting some muscles groups on one side and others on the opposite side. Asymmetry of scapular and upper limb involvement was similarly present in 65% of patients studied by Lunt and Harper *(3)*. Padberg noted variable loss of deep tendon reflexes, often not related to the severity of muscle weakness *(1)*. Contractures were rare, except for ankle contractures, which were present in 10% of patients. Scoliosis was seen in 32% *(1)*.

The overall clinical picture, therefore, is that of early involvement of facial and shoulder girdle muscles that is frequently asymmetric. Although typical, facial weakness is not invariable. With progression of the disease, weakness of anterior compartment muscles in the legs and eventually the pelvic girdle as well as neck flexors and extensors may be seen.

Facial weakness
Shoulder girdle weakness
(scapular fixators, latissimus dorsi, pectoralis major muscles)
↓
Abdominal muscles (difficulty sitting up from a lying position)
↓
Peroneal muscular weakness (tibialis anterior, toe extensors, peroneii)
↓
Further shoulder girdle (supraspinatus and infraspinatus)
Proximal arm weakness (deltoid, triceps and teres major)
↓
Pelvic girdle weakness
Neck flexors/extensors
Wrist extensors
Intrinsic hand muscles

Fig. 1. Temporal and spatial progression of weakness in facioscapulohumeral muscular dystrophy. Data from ref. *1*.

2.2. What Is the Broader Spectrum of Clinical Manifestations of FSH Muscular Dystrophy?

The advent of reliable genetic testing for FSH has made it possible to examine the broader clinical phenotype that may accompany the integral deletion of D4Z4 repeats on 4q35. The most common clinical variant appears to that of a facial-sparing scapular myopathy *(4–6)*. In their initial study of this variant, Felice and colleagues retrospectively reported their experience of patients with myopathic scapular weakness, usually associated with proximal myopathy, but excluding those with a personal or family history of facial weakness. They identified 17 such patients, 14 of whom consented to undergo genetic testing for FSH. Ten of these patients had restriction fragments consistent with the 4q35 deletion *(4)*. In eight of these patients, the initial symptom was shoulder weakness. In one patient the initial symptom was leg weakness and one described asymmetric chest weakness and atrophy *(4)*.

Other variants appear less common, given that they are the subject of isolated case reports *(5,6)*. Felice and colleagues, for example, described a 51-year-old man with a limb-girdle pattern of weakness in the absence of either facial or scapular weakness, a 78-year-old woman with progressive bilateral foot drop, and a 29-year-old man with right shoulder weakness and atrophy *(5)*. Others have described the typical FSH phenotype in association with progressive external ophthalmoplegia *(6)*.

High-frequency hearing loss *(7)* and retinal vascular abnormalities (ranging from vascular tortuosity to exudative telangiectasia) *(8)* have increasingly been recognized to be a part of the FSH phenotype. Symptomatic cardiac involvement is thought to be uncommon in FSH. In one study of 100 genetically confirmed cases of FSH, five patients were found to have conduction defects or arrhythmias in the absence of known cardio-vascular risk factors *(9)*. Four of these patients had symptoms suggestive of cardiac disease including dyspnea on exertion, episodic palpitations at night, episodic light-headedness with bradycardia, and episodic ventricular tachycardia *(9)*.

Finally, although the age of onset of FSH is typically in the first or second decade of life, an early (infantile) onset form of the disease has also been recognized *(10)*. Apart from the earlier age of onset, the clinical phenotype is no different from the typical form of the disease.

In conclusion, therefore, FSH has a fairly broad phenotype that includes a facial-sparing scapular myopathy, a limb-girdle pattern of weakness with sparing of both facial and scapular muscles, and a form characterized by unilateral shoulder weakness and atrophy. More typical FSH may be accompanied by high-frequency hearing loss and retinal vascular abnormalities as well as a chronic progressive external ophthalmoplegia. Finally, the age of onset is typically within the first two decades of life. The relative frequency of these less common presentations is not yet known.

2.3. How Often is Serum Creatine Kinase Increased Among Patients With FSH?

A number of studies have examined the frequency with which serum creatine kinase (CK) is increased. Hughes assayed serum CK in the serum of 19 patients with FSH in whom the diagnosis was based on the typical clinical phenotype in conjunction with a positive family history *(11)*. CK was increased in 77% of patients, and mean values for both men and women were increased about twofold above the upper limit of normal *(11)*. Similar findings were reported in the larger series by Lunt and Harper of 150 patients with FSH *(3)*. These investigators found increased CK in 47–63% of patients, depending on the severity of the disease. As shown in Table 25.1, it seems that CK is more often increased among affected men than among affected women ($x^2 = 11.5$, $p < 0.001$) *(3)*. Padberg reported increased CK in 64% of the 77 patients in whom it was measured *(1)*. Mean CK in affected men (106 U/L) was approximately double that in affected women (54 U/L) *(1)*. CK levels tended to decline with increasing duration of the disease.

The overall impression is that CK is elevated in the majority (but not all) of patients with FSH, that the increase tends to be mild (1–2 times normal), that CK levels may be slightly higher in men, and that CK concentration tends to fall as the diseases progresses. It is unlikely that the presence or absence of an elevation in CK will assist in the diagnosis of FSH, unless the increase is marked, in which case a diagnosis other than FSH should be considered.

2.4. How Common Are Inflammatory Changes in Muscle of Patients With FSH?

A number of investigators have reported the presence of inflammatory changes in muscle biopsy specimens from patients with FSH *(8,12–14)* and it has been tempting to speculate that there may be some correlation between the finding of inflammatory infiltrates and the presence of increased serum CK values *(13)*. Munsat and colleagues

Table 25.1
Proportion of Facioscapulohumeral Muscular Dystrophy Patients With Increased Creatine
Kinase Values

Disease severity	Male	Female	Totals
Mild	15/20 (75%)	10/27 (37%)	25/47 (47%)
Moderate	22/28 (79%)	19/37 (51%)	41/65 (63%)
Severe	12/19 (63%)	7/19 (37%)	19/38 (50%)

Data from ref. *3*.

reported the presence of inflammatory infiltrates in four families with FSH and specu-
lated that these findings may have been present because muscle biopsy was performed
relatively early in the course of disease. They suggested that FSH might progress through
an early inflammatory phase that would be missed if biopsy were only performed later
in the disease *(12)*. Other investigators have disagreed. Molnar and colleagues, for example, examined muscle biopsy specimens from 15 patients with FSH *(13)*. They found
that inflammatory infiltrates were not characteristic of any particular stage of the disease,
but noted that the presence or absence of such infiltrates was consistent among various
members of a particular family. They suggested, therefore, that the inflammatory changes
might be genetically determined *(13)*. Unfortunately, there are no large studies that
provide a reliable estimate of the frequency with which inflammatory infiltrates may be
found in patients with FSH.

2.5. How Reliable Is the Genetic Diagnosis of FSH?

In the vast majority of cases, linkage for FSH has been established to a marker on the
subtelomeric region of chromosome 4 (4q35). This chromosomal region contains a series
of 3.3kb D4Z4 tandem repeats. DNA fragments resulting from restriction digest using the
EcoRI enzyme may be identified using the p13E-11 probe. FSH is characterized by the
deletion of an integral number of these 3.3 kb D4Z4 repeats. The result is a smaller
fragment than normal amongst patients with FSH that is recognized by the p13E-11
probe. The molecular diagnosis of FSH was initially complicated by the observation that
the p13E-11 probe also identifies 3.3 kb D4Z4 repeats from a region on chromosome
10q26. Subsequent recognition that the 10q26 D4Z4 repeats, but not the 4q35 repeats,
contains a BlnI restriction site, has proven useful for the molecular diagnosis of FSH.
Double digest with EcoRI and BlnI leaves only fragments derived from 4q35. A number
of investigators have examined the diagnosed accuracy of this "double digest" molecular
diagnostic test *(15,16)*. Each of these studies relied on the clinical phenotype of FSH as
the gold standard for the diagnosis. Orrell and colleagues examined 113 subjects with
FSH and 205 controls. All 113 patients had fragment sizes ≤38 kb and all controls had
fragment sizes ≥41 kb, suggesting sensitivity and specificity each of 100% using a
fragment size of 38 kb as the cut off *(15)*. Upadhyaya and colleagues examined 130 FSH
patients and 200 controls using the same double-digest technique. Using a cut-off fragment size of 38kb their results, summarized in Table 25.2, show a sensitivity of 95.6%
and a specificity of 100% *(16)*.

Table 25.2
Sensitivity and Specificity of the Molecular Diagnosis of Facioscapulohumeral
Muscular Dystrophy

| | FSH clinical phenotype | | |
	Present	Absent	TOTAL
Fragment <38 kb	123	0	123
Fragment ≥38 kb	7	200	207
TOTAL	130	200	330

Sensitivity = true positive / (true positive + false negative) = 123 / (123+7) = 94.6%
Specificity = true negative / (true negative + false positive) = 200 / (200+0) = 100%
Data from ref. *16*.

As with any diagnostic test, it must be compared to some other gold standard. The studies of the accuracy of molecular tests for the diagnosis of FSH have relied upon the clinical phenotype as the gold standard. As discussed elsewhere in this chapter, improved molecular diagnosis has subsequently led to an appreciation of the broader clinical phenotype of FSH. The high diagnostic sensitivity and specificity of the molecular assays such as those described here, are relevant to patients who have the typical clinical phenotype. The diagnostic accuracy of these tests for those with an unusual clinical phenotype remains unknown.

2.6. What Is the Differential Diagnosis for FSH Muscular Dystrophy?

The spectrum of disorders that may manifest with a pattern of weakness similar to that encountered in FSH is somewhat limited, and the relevant literature comprises a series of case reports and small case series. It has been claimed that polymyositis may occasionally present with a pattern of weakness mimicking FSH *(17,18)*. It is, however, difficult to ascertain whether these reports genuinely describe patients with polymyositis rather than typical FSH with inflammatory infiltrates on muscle biopsy. One of these patients did show some improvement in response to corticosteroid therapy *(18)*, but the other did not show significant response *(17)*. A number of authors have drawn attention to what has been described variably as "neurogenic FSH" *(19)* or spinal muscular atrophy of the "FSH type" *(20,21)*. The distinguishing clinical feature of the patients described in these reports is the presence of fasciculations in combination with an FSH pattern of muscular weakness. The picture is further complicated by the finding of both neurogenic and myopathic motor units on electromyographic examination *(19,20)*. Finally, there is the report of a family with a mitochondrial myopathy, in which some family members presented initially with an FSH-like pattern of muscle weakness *(22)*.

The differential diagnosis, therefore, in patients who present with the typical FSH-pattern of muscle weakness is quite limited. It is not possible to determine the true frequency with which these other disorders mimic FSH, but the rarity of the case reports seems to suggest that they are all uncommon.

2.7. How Common Are Sporadic Mutations in FSH Muscular Dystrophy?

In the majority of cases, FSH is inherited as an autosomal-dominant trait. There are, however, at least two circumstances under which an individual with FSH may have unaffected parents. One possibility is that the proband represents an instance of a sporadic or *de novo* mutation. The alternative possibility is that of germline or somatic mosaicism. Germline mosaicism implies that the one of the parents harbors the genetic mutation only in gonadal tissue. Somatic mosaicism implies that the mutation is present in some tissues but, crucially, not in muscle tissue, and so does not manifest the phenotype of FSH. So long as the mutation is present in the germline, it will be possible for the offspring to be affected.

In a study of patients with FSH in Brazil, the authors identified 34 families, including 19 multigenerational families and 15 probands, who were the first affected individuals in their families. In seven of these families, both parents were tested and neither was found to harbor the small EcoRI fragment that was present in the affected individual *(23)*. In four further families, the parents were deceased or not available for testing, but the likelihood of a spontaneous mutation seems high given that each of the probands had 6–10 unaffected siblings all over the age of 20 *(23)*. Based on these data, the rate of spontaneous mutations would be estimated to be approximately 30%.

3. TREATMENT

3.1. Is There a Role for Steroids in the Treatment of FSH Muscular Dystrophy?

A number of early case reports suggested that some patients with FSH might benefit from treatment with corticosteroids. This hypothesis was formally tested in a small prospective study in which eight patients with FSH were treated with prednisone 1.5 mg/kg/day for 12 weeks. Patients were selected for participation in the study irrespective of whether inflammatory changes were present on muscle biopsy. Manual muscle testing (MMT) and maximal voluntary isometric contraction testing (MVICT) were performed at baseline and following the treatment period. The change in average MMT score from baseline to 12 weeks was used as the primary measure of efficacy. Eighteen muscles were scored using the MRC scale from 0 to 5, with each grade assigned a numeric value. Scores for each muscle were then averaged to produce a final score. Secondary outcome measures included the change in MVICT scores between baseline and 12-week follow-up and changes in body muscle mass. No changes were observed for any of these outcome measures. The authors had estimated that a sample size of eight patients would yield a power of 80% to detect a change in average MMT score of 0.22 units. Although this study showed no benefit of high-dose oral steroids over a period of 12 weeks, the duration of treatment and follow-up was insufficient to determine whether such treatment might affect the natural history of the disease. Given the authors' previous observation that MMT scores decline by 0.05 units over a period of 6 months, any study designed to detect a slowing of the rate of progression of the disease would need to extend over a prolonged period.

In conclusion, therefore, despite the few case reports suggesting a beneficial effect, the available data do not support the use of steroids for patients with FSH. Whether steroids might retard the progression of disease, however, remains unanswered.

3.2. Is There a Role for β-agonists in the Treatment of FSH Muscular Dystrophy?

A possible role for β_2-agonists in the treatment of muscular dystrophy has been proposed based on their known anabolic effects. Based on the promising results of a small open-label study of albuterol, the FSH-DY study group undertook a larger randomized, placebo-controlled trial to more formally evaluate the efficacy of sustained-release albuteraol, administered daily over the course of a year, in improving muscle strength in patients with FSH *(24)*. Patients were recruited based on clinical phenotype, as reliable genetic testing was not available at the time the trial was begun. Block randomization led to 30 patients being assigned to the placebo group, 30 patients being assigned to the low-dose albuterol group (8 mg twice daily), and 30 subjects being assigned to the high-dose group (16 mg twice per day). Randomization resulted in differences between the three groups in terms of gender distribution, grip strength, and lean body mass at baseline. Treatment was continued for 52 weeks. The primary outcome measure was the change in maximum voluntary isometric contraction testing (MVICT) between baseline and 52 weeks. Other outcome measures included the results of MMT, grip strength, and lean body mass. Eighty-four patients completed the study, with four drop-outs in the high-dose group and one in each of the other two groups. Data were analyzed on an intention-to-treat basis. There were no significant differences in the primary outcome measure, and of the secondary outcome measures, a mild beneficial effect was seen in terms of grip strength and lean body mass *(24)*.

This was a well designed study that was adequately powered to detect a beneficial effect of albuterol. The significance of the finding of improved grip strength and lean body mass is unclear. However, the absence of an effect on muscle strength or functional status argues that albuterol offers no real benefit to patients with FSH.

3.3. Is There Any Evidence for the Efficacy of Scapular Fixation Surgery in the Treatment of FSH Muscular Dystrophy?

The prominent and selective weakness of the muscles responsible for scapular fixation in FSH impairs functional shoulder abduction despite relatively preserved strength in the muscles responsible for shoulder abduction, at least in the early stages of the disease. This provides the rationale for surgical fixation of the scapula to the chest wall, with the intention of improving the range and strength of shoulder abduction, which in turn should lead to improved independence with daily activities such as combing hair, brushing teeth, and reaching for objects above the head. Broadly speaking, there are two procedures that have been used to fix the scapula to the thorax—scapuloplexy and scapulodesis. Scapuloplexy employs slings to surgically anchor the scapular to the chest wall whereas scapulodesis involves scapular fixation using screws, wires, and plates with or without a bone graft. There are no randomized controlled trials that have examined the efficacy of these surgical techniques. The nonrandomized literature has recently been presented in a systematic review from the Cochrane collaboration *(25)*. The authors of this review conclude that although operative intervention offers significant benefits, these must be balanced against the potential complications and postoperative rehabilitative demands.

4. PROGNOSIS

4.1. What Is the Long-Term Prognosis for Patients With FSH Muscular Dystrophy?

Although there are limited studies that inform the long-term prognosis in FSH, the degree of disability that evolves over time seems to be quite variable. In their study of 54 familial cases of FSH, Lunt and Harper classified patients into one of three categories, with mild disability defined as no proximal muscle with MRC grade strength less than 4, moderate disability defined as one or more proximal muscles with MRC grade 4 or weaker, and severe disability defined as pelvic girdle weakness less than or equal to MRC grade 2 or the requirement for a wheelchair *(3)*. The data are summarized in Table 25.3. Overall, 50% of patients will remain mildly affected, 35% develop moderate disability, and only 15% require the use of a wheelchair. The data in Table 25.3 also illustrate that the prognosis for disability is strongly influenced by age *(see* Subheading 4.2.). In considering the prognosis for patients with familial FSH, it is also relevant to note that the penetrance of the disease varies according to age, being <5% at 0–4 years, 21% at 5–9 years, 58% at 10–14 years, 86% at 15–19 years, and 95% over the age of 20 *(3)*. The implications of these data are that if disease has not become manifest by age 20, then it is extremely unlikely that it will develop later in life, and that if it does begin after the age of 20, that disability is likely to remain mild.

4.2. Are There Any Clinical Parameters That Predict Long-Term Disability?

There are a number of clinical parameters that have been studied to determine whether they are predictive of the severity of the disease and the development of long-term disability. These include the age of onset of the disease, whether the gene mutation is inherited or arises from a spontaneous mutation, the presence of affected family members in previous generations, the size of the DNA fragment hybridized by the p13E-11 probe, and the serum CK level.

4.2.1. AGE OF ONSET

Studies of the correlation between the age of onset and the severity of the disease may be confounded by a number of factors. Chief among these is the question of how age of onset is determined. This is a particularly difficult issue in a disease such as FSH, in which facial weakness may have been present for many years prior to clinical presentation for medical evaluation because of the development of muscle weakness affecting the shoulder girdle or proximal arm. For adults, most studies have relied on the age at which the patient first noticed any evidence of muscle weakness. For children, the age at which the parents first notice signs of muscle weakness is typically chosen as the age of onset. For family members of symptomatic probands who were found to have weakness on clinical examination (despite the absence of symptoms), the date of case ascertainment may be taken as the age of onset. Such a strategy, however, does pose certain problems, as family members of affected probands may be more likely to be diagnosed at a younger age once the affected proband has sought medical consultation. Notwith-

Table 25.3
Disability in Facioscapulohumeral Muscular Dystrophy

Age category	n	Age of onset	Severity (% in each grade)		
			Mild	Moderate	Severe
<20 yr	8	52	100	0	0
20–40 yr	25	28	48	36	16
>40 yr	21	14	33	48	19
All ages	54	–	50	35	15

See text for definitions of what constitutes mild, moderate, and severe disease.
Data from ref. 3.

Table 25.4
Correlation Between Age of Onset and the Severity of the Disease

Disease severity	Sample size	Mean age of onset (range)	Mean age at evaluation
Mild	13	52 (37–70)	57
Moderate	30	28 (10–71)	55
Severe	26	14 (5–21)	52

Data from ref. 3.

standing these methodological issues, the available data suggest that increasing disease severity correlates with younger age of onset (3). In one study of 69 affected individuals, there was an inverse correlation between increasing age of onset and increasing disease severity (Table 25.4) (3).

4.2.2. SERUM CK LEVEL

In their large series of 41 families with FSH, Lunt and Harper reported the results of serum CK in 150 affected subjects and tried to determine whether there was any correlation between the presence and degree of serum CK elevation on the one hand, and the severity of disease on the other. In general, there was a tendency for higher CKs to be detected in affected men, and the authors postulated that this might related to a greater tendency towards physical exercise. There was, however, no correlation between serum CK level and the severity of the disease. Serum CK, therefore, cannot be used to comment on current or expected disease severity and disability.

4.2.3. INHERITANCE PATTERN

For the most part, FSH is transmitted in an autosomal-dominant fashion. Cases related to new mutations are defined on the basis of an affected individual whose parents are both unaffected (with the caveat that they have both undergone careful evaluation for asymptomatic disease). Some authors have suggested that the disease tends to be more severe in new (sporadic) cases than in familial cases (3,23,26). The mean age of onset among 25 new mutation cases was reported to be 6.9 years; and by the time of clinical evaluation (mean age of 20) 92% had significant weakness in the legs and 28% required the use of a wheelchair *(26)*. Among the 28 probands of familial cases, these authors reported a mean age of onset of 14 years *(3)*. Significant proximal lower limb weakness was reported in 39% of those less than 20 years of age, 46% of those aged 20–40 years, and 68% of those over the age of 40. Only 8 of 54 subjects (15%) required a wheelchair *(3)*. One concern that might be raised with regard to these data is that there may be a bias toward identification of milder familial cases given the presence of a family history whereas *de novo* cases only come to clinical attention when relatively severe. This bias is probably not relevant to these data, however, because the comparison is made between *de novo* cases and familial probands. There would appear, therefore, to be little or no ascertainment bias, and the data suggest that sporadic mutations tend to be associated with a more severe clinical phenotype.

4.2.4. ANTICIPATION

The term "anticipation" has been used primarily to describe the earlier age of onset of an inherited disease with successive generations. The term may also be used to describe the phenomenon of increasing disease severity with successive generations. A number of studies have suggested that anticipation occurs in FSH *(23,27)*. In a study of 34 Brazilian families, the authors found that the onset of the disease occurred at a significantly younger age among affected offspring (mean age 15 years) compared with their parents (mean age 32 years). With the recognition that there might be ascertainment bias due to the inclusion of probands who might be expected to have more severe disease, the analysis was repeated with the probands excluded. The difference remained significant, with the age of onset amongst the parents and offspring being 34 and 15 years, respectively *(23)*. Tawil and colleagues used quantitative muscle testing to ascertain the severity of disease in 23 affected parent–offspring pairs. They found that the offspring were more severely affected than their parents in 15/23 pairs, but noted that parents were more severely affected in 7/23 pairs *(27)*. These data would seem to suggest that there is a tendency for symptoms to begin at an earlier age in successive generations. It may be that the increasing disease severity with passing generations simply reflects the earlier age of onset, but this conclusion cannot be reached with any degree of certainty based on the available data.

4.3. Are There Any Genetic Parameters That Predict Long-Term Disability?

It will be recalled that the molecular pathogenesis of FSH involves the deletion of an integral number of 3.3 kb tandem repeats in the subtelomeric region of chromosome 4. It has been suggested that disease severity may be greatest among those with the largest deletion, and hence the smallest DNA fragments, detected by probe p13E-11 *(26)*. In a large study of 124 affected individuals from 16 families and including 34 *de novo* cases, the authors found a correlation between the presence of a smaller fragment and an earlier age of onset (Table 25.5). Based on these data, it might argued that a dichotomization could be made between fragments smaller or larger than 18 kb, with the age of onset significantly younger among those with fragments less than 18 kb in size. At any rate, the data do suggest that there is a correlation between smaller fragment size and earlier age of onset. In the same paper, Lunt and colleagues showed that there was a linear relationship between fragment size and the age at which a wheelchair was required, that age being less than 30 years for fragments smaller than 18 kb *(26)*.

Table 25.5
Correlation Between Age of Onset and DNA Fragment Size

Fragment size	Mean of median onset age	Number of subjects
15–18 kb	6.5 yr	8
19–22 kb	17 yr	29
23–26 kb	18.9 yr	78
27–30 kb	19 yr	9

Data from ref. 26.

5. SUMMARY

- FSH is typically inherited in an autosomal-dominant fashion, although approximately 30% of cases are sproradic.
- Shoulder girdle weakness is the most common clinical symptom in FSH.
- The typical clinical phenotype of FSH includes early involvement of facial and shoulder girdle muscles (often asymmetrically). Peroneal muscular weakness develops later and is followed by proximal arm, pelvic girdle, neck flexion/extenstion, and distal upper limb muscle weakness.
- The most common variant of FSH is a facial-sparing scapular myopathy.
- Serum CK is frequently elevated one- to twofold in FSH, more commonly in men.
- Polymyositis and spinal muscular atrophy may also produce scapuloperoneal patterns of weakness and may thus mimic FSH clinically.
- Muscle biopsy may show inflammatory infiltrates, but these are of little (if any) clinical significance.
- Molecular diagnosis of FSH using a double digest with EcoRI and BlnI and a fragment length of 38 kb as cutoff between normal and abnormal, provides a sensitivity of >95% and a specificity of 100%.
- There is no evidence that steroids improve strength in FSH. Their role in slowing progression of disease has not been evaluated.
- There is evidence from a single randomized controlled trial that β_2-agonists do not improve clinical outcome in FSH.
- There are no randomized controlled data to support the use of scapular fixation procedures.
- Penetrance of the FSH phenotype varies with age, but is >95% by age 20.
- Approximately 50% of FSH patients will develop mild disability, 35% will be moderated disabled, and only 15% will require the use of a wheelchair.
- Younger age of onset, the presence of a *de novo* (sporadic) mutation (rather than an inherited mutation), and a larger deletion of D4Z4 repeats on 4q35 are all associated with a more severe clinical phenotype.

REFERENCES

1. Padberg G. Facioscapulohumeral disease (Thesis). Inercontinental Graphics, Leiden: 1982.
2. Tyler FH, Stephens F. Studies in disorders of muscle II. Clinical manifestations and inheritance of facioscapulohumeral dystrophy in a large family. Ann Int Med 1950;32:640–660.

3. Lunt P, Harper P. Genetic counselling in facioscapulohumeral muscular dystrophy. J Med Genet 1991;28:655–664.
4. Felice KJ, North WA, Moore SA, Mathews KD. FSH dystrophy 4q35 deletion in patients presenting with facial-sparing scapular myopathy. Neurology 2000;54:1927–1931.
5. Felice KJ, Moore SA. Unusual clinical presentations in patients harboring the facioscapulohumeral dystrophy 4q35 deletion. Muscle Nerve 2001;24:352–356.
6. Krasnianski M, Eger K, Neudecker S, Jakubiczka S, Zierz S. Atypical phenotypes in patients with facioscapulohumeral muscular dystrophy 4q35 deletion. Arch Neurol 2003;60:1421–1425.
7. Brouwer O, Padberg G, Ruys C, Brand R, de Laat J, Grote JJ. Hearing loss in facioscapulohumeral muscular dystrophy. Neurology 1991;41:1878–1881.
8. Wulff JD, Lin JT, Kepes JJ. Inflammatory facioscapulohumeral muscular dystrophy and Coats syndrome. Ann Neurol 1982;12:398–401.
9. Laforet P, de Toma C, Eymard B, et al. Cardiac involvement in genetically confirmed facioscapulohumeral muscular dystrophy. Neurology 1998;51:1454–1456.
10. Brouwer OF, Padberg GW, Bakker E, Wijmenga C, Frants RR. Early onset facioscapulohumeral muscular dystrophy. Muscle Nerve 1995;2:S67–S72.
11. Hughes B. Creatine phosphokinase in facioscapulohumeral muscular dystrophy. Br Med J 1971;3:464–465.
12. Munsat TL, Piper D, Cancilla P, Mednick J. Inflammatory myopathy with facioscapulohumeral distribution. Neurology 1972;22:335–347.
13. Molnar M, Dioszeghy P, Mechler F. Inflammatory changes in facioscapulohumeral muscular dystrophy. Eur Arch Psychiatry Clin Neurosci 1991;241:105–108.
14. Bacq M, Telerman-Toppet N, Coers C. Familial myopathies with restricted distribution, facial weakness and inflammatory changes in affected muscles. J Neurol 1985;231:295–300.
15. Orrell R, Tawil R, Forrester J, Kissel J, Mendell J, Figlewicz D. Definitive molecular diagnosis of facioscapulohumeral dystraophy. Neurology 1999;52:1822–1826.
16. Upadhyaya M, Maynard J, Rogers M, et al. Improved molecular diagnosis of facioscapulohumeral muscular dystrophy (FSHD): validation of the differential double digestion for FSHD. J Med Genet 1997;34:476–479.
17. Rothstein TL, Carlson CB, Sumi SM. Polymyositis with facioscapulohumeral distribution. Arch Neurol 1971;25:313–319.
18. Bates D, Stevens J, Hudgson P. "Polymyositis" with involvement of facial and distal musculature. One form of the facioscapulohumeral syndrome. J Neurol Sci 1973;19:105–108.
19. Furukawa T. Neurogenic FSH muscular atrophy. Muscle Nerve 1995;2:S96–S97.
20. Furukawa T, Toyokura Y. Chronic spinal muscular atrophy of facioscapulohumeral type. J Med Genet 1976;13:285–289.
21. Siddique T, Roper H, Pericak-Vance M, et al. Linkage analysis in the spinal muscular atrophy type of facioscapulohumeral disease. J Med Genet 1989;26:487–489.
22. Hudgson P, Bradley W, Jenkison M. Familial "mitochondrial" myopathy. A myopathy associated with disordered oxidative metabolism in muscle fibers. 1. Clinical, electrophysiological and pathological findings. J Neurol Sci 1972;16:343–370.
23. Zatz M, Marie SK, Passos-Bueno MR, et al. High proportion of new mutations and possible anticipation in Brazilian facioscapulohumeral muscular dystrophy families. Am J Med Genet 1995;56:99–105.
24. Kissel J, McDermott M, Mendell J, et al. Randomized, double-blind, placebo-controlled trial of albuteral in facioscapulohumeral dystrophy. Neurology 2001;57:1434–1440.
25. Mummery C, Copeland S, Rose M. Scapular fixation in muscular dystrophy. Cochrane Database Syst Rev 2003;3:CD003278..
26. Lunt PW, Jardine PE, Koch MC, et al. Correlation between fragment size at D4F104S1 and age at onset or at wheelchair use, with a possible generational effect, accounts for much phenotypic variation in 4q35-facioscapulohumeral muscular dystrophy (FSHD). Hum Mol Genet 1995;4:951–958.
27. Tawil R, Forrester J, Griggs RC, et al. Evidence for anticipation and association of deletion size with severity in facioscapulohumeral muscular dystrophy. The FSH-DY Group. Ann Neurol 1996;39:744–748.

INDEX

AU: Are entries or page nos. missing from under "lactate dehydrogenase deficiency"?